Date Due

NOV 1 4 2003		
FEB 1 7 2005		
Mar 14 2005		
3-1-06		
NOV 2 6		
FEB 1 1 2017		

DISCARDED

BRODART, CO.   Cat. No. 23-233-003   Printed in U.S.A.

D1560510

DISEASES OF THE SPINE
AND SPINAL CORD

CONTEMPORARY NEUROLOGY SERIES

DISEASES OF THE SPINE AND SPINAL CORD

Thomas N. Byrne, M.D.

Clinical Professor of Neurology and Internal Medicine
Yale University School of Medicine
Assistant Chief, Department of Neurology
Yale-New Haven Hospital
New Haven, CT

Edward C. Benzel, M.D.

Director of Spinal Disorders
Department of Neurosurgery
Cleveland Clinic Foundation
Cleveland, OH

Stephen G. Waxman, M.D., Ph.D.

Professor and Chairman, Department of Neurology
Yale University School of Medicine
Neurologist-in-Chief
Yale-New Haven Hospital
Director, PVA/EPVA Neuroscience Research Center
and Rehabilitation Research Center
VA Medical Center
West Haven, CT
Visiting Professor
Institute of Neurology
University College London

OXFORD
UNIVERSITY PRESS
2000

OXFORD
UNIVERSITY PRESS

Oxford   New York
Athens Auckland Bangkok Bogotá Buenos Aires Calcutta
Cape Town Chennai Dar es Salaam Delhi Florence Hong Kong Istanbul
Karachi Kuala Lumpur Madrid Melbourne Mexico City Mumbai
Nairobi Paris São Paulo Singapore Taipei Tokyo Toronto Warsaw

and associated companies in
Berlin Ibadan

Copyright ©2000 by Oxford University Press, Inc.

Published by Oxford University Press, Inc.
198 Madison Avenue, New York, New York 10016

Oxford is a registered trademark of Oxford University Press

Library of Congress Cataloging-in-Publication Data
Byrne, Thomas N.
Diseases of the spine and spinal cord /
Thomas N. Byrne, Edward Benzel, Stephen G. Waxman.
p. cm. — (Contemporary neurology series ; 58)
Includes bibliographical references and index.
ISBN 0-19-512968-7 (cloth : alk. paper)
1. Spine—Diseases.   2. Spinal cord—Diseases.
I. Benzel, Edward C.   II. Waxman, Stephen G.
III. Title.   IV. Series.
[DNLM: 1. Spinal Diseases.   2. Spinal Cord Diseases.   W1 C0769N   v.58 2000 /
WE 725 B995d 2000]   RC400.B97   2000   616.793—dc21
DNLM/DLC   for Library of Congress   99-26448

The science of medicine is a rapidly changing field. As new research and clinical experience broaden our knowledge, changes in treatment and drug therapy do occur. The author and the publisher of this work have checked with sources believed to be reliable in their efforts to provide information that is accurate and complete, and in accordance with the standards accepted at the time of publication. However, in light of the possibility of human error or changes in the practice of medicine, neither the author, nor the publisher, nor any other party who has been involved in the preparation or publication of this work warrants that the information contained herein is in every respect accurate or complete. Readers are encouraged to confirm the information contained herein with other reliable sources, and are strongly advised to check the product information sheet provided by the pharmaceutical company for each drug they plan to administer.

9 8 7 6 5 4 3 2 1
Printed in the United States of America
on acid-free paper

PREFACE

This book is an outgrowth of *Spinal Cord Compression,* written by two of us for the Contemporary Neurology Series one decade ago. Since its publication, there have been dramatic advances in both the imaging as well as the treatment of many spine and spinal cord diseases. Accordingly, in this new book we have expanded the scope to include a neurosurgical perspective and a more in-depth discussion of the management of spine and spinal cord diseases.

In the preface of *Spinal Cord Compression,* we noted that the book had its origin when, on rounds, one of us was presented with an all-too-common scenario: a 50 year-old man with known prostatic cancer presented to the Emergency Room in a paraplegic condition. Tragically, the patient had been seen in another clinic 2 weeks previously, complaining of back pain and leg weakness. The outcome in this case may have been preventable by earlier diagnosis and treatment.

Spinal cord compression from neoplastic or nonneoplastic disease is a common clinical problem. As in the case cited above, if undiagnosed and untreated it frequently progresses to permanent paraparesis and sphincter disturbances. Many times, spinal cord compression is treatable. This book offers house officers and practicing clinicians an optimal approach for evaluating and managing patients with spine and spinal cord diseases.

Since the publication of *Spinal Cord Compression,* magnetic resonance imaging (MRI) and computerized tomography (CT) have replaced myelography as the preferred definitive imaging techniques of the spine and spinal cord. MRI provides images of the spine and neural structures in multiple planes showing neural compression to great advantage. For intramedullary diseases, such as multiple sclerosis and acute transverse myelitis, MRI may demonstrate the lesion and help to determine prognosis in some patients. Furthermore, the use of contrast enhancement may help distinguish active from remote lesions in patients with multiple sclerosis. Contrast enhancement may also help to characterize intradural-extramedullary lesions such as leptomeningeal metastases and arachnoiditis, or to distinguish recurrent disc herniation from postoperative scar.

Rapid technological advances in imaging the spine are welcome, but we believe that they cannot replace clinical judgment. For example, because most individuals over 50 years of age harbor radiographic evidence of spondylosis, the clinician must often decide whether such a finding is incidental or responsible for a patient's neurological symptoms and signs. In cases where findings are not recognized as only incidental, a patient may undergo unnecessary surgery for "abnormalities," when the actual cause of a clinical syndrome remains undiagnosed and untreated. We believe that an understanding of pathophysiology is an essential prerequisite to clinical judgment.

In writing this volume, we have first reviewed the relevant anatomy and clinical pathophysiology of the spine and spinal cord. Because pain is the most common presenting complaint of patients with spine disease, we have devoted a chapter to pain and its evaluation. Subsequent chapters examine degenerative diseases of the spine, such as spondylosis and disc disease, and neoplastic forms of spinal cord compression. Noncompressive forms of myelopathy such as inflammatory diseases, both noninfectious and infectious, and vascular diseases of the spine are presented. The final chapters review evaluation and management principles of traumatic spine injury.

The three authors bring different backgrounds to this book. Following a fellowship in neuro-oncology at Memorial Sloan-Kettering Cancer Center, Dr. Byrne has been engaged in clinical aspects of neurology and neuro-oncology at Yale. Dr. Benzel completed his neurosurgical and spine fellowship at Medical College of Wisconsin and is currently the Director of Spinal Disorders in the Department of Neurosurgery at the Cleveland Clinic Foundation. Dr. Waxman has spent the past 2 decades at Stanford and Yale, combining a university-based practice with research focusing on molecular aspects of neurological disease. In bringing together perspectives gained from each of our professional experiences, we have attempted to present a single, coherent approach to the evaluation and management of spine and spinal cord diseases.

Many colleagues have helped us in the writing of this volume and we are indebted to them. We wish to thank Dr. Sid Gilman, who read the entire manuscript and provided superb advice and encouragement. We are indebted to Dr. Richard Becker who contributed previously unpublished imaging material. We also thank Dr. Timothy Vollmer for his thoughtful advice regarding treatment of multiple sclerosis. We are grateful to Lauren Enck, Nancy Wolitzer, and the staff at Oxford University Press, for their diligence, patience, and editorial support during the development of this book.

Finally we thank Susan Hockfield, Elizabeth Byrne, Mary Benzel, Morgan Culverhouse, Jason Culverhouse, Brian Benzel, Matthew Benzel, Merle Waxman, Matthew Waxman, and David Waxman. They know why we thank them.

September 1999

T.N.B.
E.C.B.
S.G.W.

CONTENTS

DISEASES OF THE SPINE
AND SPINAL CORD

Chapter 1

ANATOMY AND BIOMECHANICS OF THE SPINE AND SPINAL CORD

The spine is a segmented structure consisting of a precisely aligned column of vertebrae and their intervertebral articulations. Its primary functions are (1) to provide support for the trunk and head; (2) to provide a protective covering for the spinal cord; and yet, (3) to permit enough flexibility to allow movement. In humans, these functions are achieved through an architecture based on a column of articulated vertebrae that affords both structural support and mobility.

The spinal cord is also segmented, both functionally and anatomically. Sherrington first recognized that the nervous system is hierarchically organized. He suggested that the spinal cord is the first level of organization, where the most primitive motor reflexes are mediated through the spinal nerve roots.[1] Disturbed function of these spinal roots often indicates disease processes affecting the spine and spinal cord. For example, patients with spinal mass lesions frequently present with radicular pain at the level of the injured nerve root and with radicular motor, sensory, and reflex disturbances. As spinal cord compression ensues, ascending and descending tracts are injured, resulting in neurologic disturbances caudal to the level of the lesion. Although the localization and differentiation of these diseases are frequently vexing problems that require imaging and laboratory studies for confirmation, the physician is guided by the patient's clinical history and physical examination.

VERTEBRAL COLUMN ANATOMY: AN OVERVIEW

The vertebral column (Fig. 1–1) normally consists of 7 cervical, 12 thoracic, and 5 lumbar individual vertebrae; the sacrum, which is usually formed by the fusion of 5 vertebrae; and the coccyx. Variations in the number and distribution of the cervical, thoracic, and lumbar presacral vertebrae have been found in approximately 10% of skeletons.[2] Most of these variations are radiographically confusing but clinically insignificant.

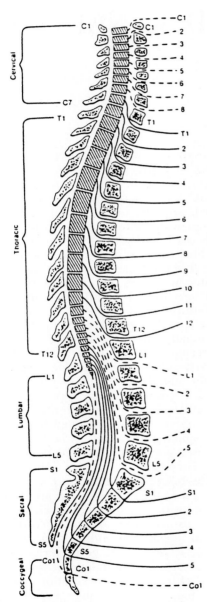

Figure 1–1. The anatomical relationships between the spinal cord segments, vertebral bodies, and intervertebral foraminae. Note the disparity between spinal segmental level and localization of corresponding vertebrae. (From DeJong, RN,[130] p. 61, with permission.)

Ventral Segment and the Intervertebral Disc

The functional spinal unit consists of two vertebral bodies separated by an intervertebral disc (Fig. 1–2). The intervertebral disc, which unites the adjacent vertebral bodies to complete the functional ventral segment, is attached to the apposing vertebral end plates.

The combined height of the intervertebral discs normally contributes approximately 25% to the height of the spine above the sacrum. There is a difference in the vertical shape of the intervertebral discs in the cervical region compared with that in the lumbar region. In the lumbar region, the vertical height of the intervertebral discs is slightly greater ventrally than dorsally, contributing to lumbar lordosis. In the cervical region, this difference is even greater: The vertical height of the intervertebral disc ventrally measures approximately two times that dorsally.[3] This greater height in the ventral region substantially contributes to the lordotic curve of the cervical spine.

The intervertebral disc is composed of a central nucleus pulposus encircled by the annulus fibrosus (Fig. 1–3). Fibers of the annulus fibrosus insert into the cartilaginous end plates of the vertebral bodies and the bony rim of the vertebral body. The hyaline cartilaginous end plates form the rostral and caudal borders of the nucleus pulposus, and the encircling annulus fibrosus forms the lateral border. The annulus consists of a series of concentric rings of fibroelastic fibers that course obliquely between the vertebral bodies (at about 30° with respect to each other). The obliquity of each successive ring is different from that of the adjacent rings, providing for a

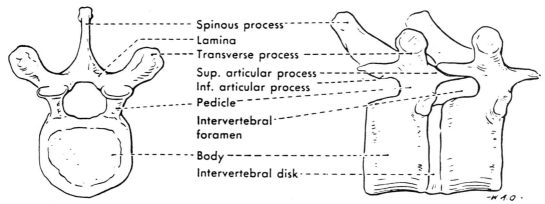

Figure 1–2. Anatomy of a typical vertebra. (From Hollinshead, WH,[2] p. 304, with permission.)

strong and elastic annulus that unites the vertebral bodies and confines the nucleus pulposus.

In addition to its weight-bearing ability, the ventral segment of the spine provides shock absorption. This is accomplished through the nucleus pulposus, which is placed slightly dorsal to the center of the intervertebral disc space in the lumbar spine. The nucleus pulposus, a mucopolysaccharide gel, is composed of 70% to 88% water in the young healthy adult and is deformable but not compressible.[2] The incompressible nucleus pulposus,

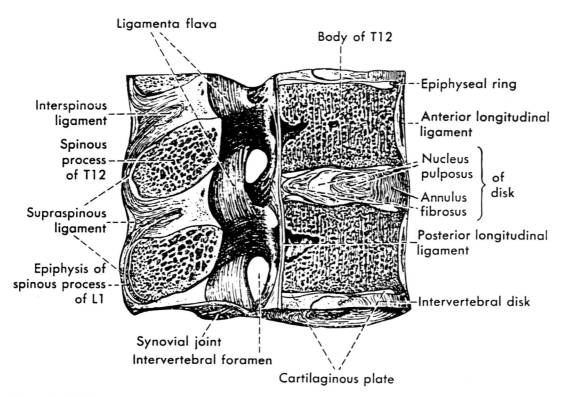

Figure 1–3. Sagittal section through two vertebral levels demonstrating the location of ligaments. (From Hollinshead, WH,[2] p. 315, with permission.)

surrounded by the elastic annulus fibrosus, permits the intervertebral disc to change its shape and thereby permits intervertebral movement. For example, when the spine is flexed, the nucleus pulposus moves from ventral to dorsal. The intervertebral discs do not limit the direction of movement.

The mechanical stresses experienced by the lumbar intervertebral discs have practical importance. Using a needle connected to a pressure transducer, Nachemson measured the lumbar intradiscal pressures of healthy and degenerated discs in individuals during the assumption of different postures.[4] The intradiscal pressure increased as the individual moved from the supine, to standing, to sitting position. Furthermore, the pressure rose when the trunk was flexed in the standing or sitting position (Fig. 1–4). The weight-bearing, shock-absorbing capacity and mobility of the ventral segment of the spine depends on the deformable, but incompressible, nature of the nucleus pulposus.

As the water content of the nucleus pulposus declines with age, individual discs lose height. This contributes to the development of osteophytes (spondylosis) of the vertebral bodies, particularly at sites of greatest mobility. The decline in water content of intervertebral discs can be appreciated in vivo with magnetic resonance imaging (MRI), a technique very sensitive to water content.[5] On T_2-weighted MRI images, the normal hydrated disc is white and the desiccated, degenerated disc is black ("black disc").

Dorsal Segment

The dorsal spine segment protects the spinal cord and establishes the direction and extent of spine movement. The dorsal segment consists of pedicles, lamina, transverse processes, spinous processes, and articulating facets (see Fig. 1–2). The pedicles and lamina form the lateral and dorsal walls of the spinal canal.

Each dorsal segment contains a superior and inferior articular facet and a pars interarticularis. At the intervertebral level, each inferior articular facet articulates with the superior articular facet of its caudal neighbor. Unlike the intervertebral disc joint, facet joints are true synovial joints, consisting of cartilage-covered apposing articular facets enclosed in a synovial capsule. The plane of the apposing articular facets determines the direction of movement of the spine. Whereas the intervertebral disc permits limited movement in all directions, the

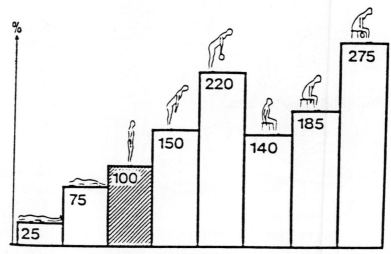

Figure 1–4. The relative change in pressure in the third lumbar disc during different postures. (From Nachemson, AL,[4] p. 61, with permission.)

facet joints limit direction to that governed by the orientation of the plane of the apposing facets.

Like other synovial joints, the facet joints may be the seat of inflammation. Each synovial joint is innervated by branches of the posterior division of two spinal nerves.[6] Since the facet joints are adjacent to the exiting spinal nerve roots at the intervertebral foramen, inflammation or spur formation may cause compression of the nerve root and radicular pain.

COMPONENT-SPECIFIC ANATOMY AND BIOMECHANICS

The Vertebral Body

Both the width and depth of the vertebral bodies (see p. 1–13) increase from the rostral to the caudal segments of the spine.[7–11] The vertebral body height also increases in a similar manner, with the exception of a slight reversal of this relationship at the C6 and lower lumbar levels.[7–11] In the cervical spine, the uncinate process projects from the rostral–dorsal–lateral aspect of each vertebral body (C3–7) (Fig. 1–5). This forms part of the uncovertebral joint, which allows an articulation of this process with the vertebral body above.

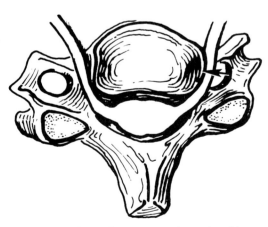

Figure 1–5. The uncinate process (arrow) and its relationship to the rostral–dorsal–lateral aspect of the vertebral body and exiting nerve root (From Benzel, EC,[7] with permission.)

The uncovertebral joint is, in fact, essentially a dorsolateral extension of the intervertebral disc. It participates in complex neck movements[7,12]

The increase in vertebral body size from rostral to caudal correlates with the strength of the vertebral body (resistance to failure). Spine fractures are less frequent in the lower lumbar spine compared to other regions. This is, at least in part, related to the increased size of the individual vertebra. This is corroborated by laboratory studies (Fig. 1–6).[11,13–16]

The Facet Joints

The facet joints bear a portion of axial loads. They do so more actively when the spine is in an extended posture. They are apophyseal joints; each has a loose capsule and a synovial lining. The orientation of the facet joints changes from rostral to caudal, significantly affecting spinal movement.[7,11,17,18] In the cervical spine, the facet joints are essentially oriented in the coronal plane, which does not particularly restrict most movements.[7,11]

In the lumbar region, however, the facet joints are oriented sagitally.[11,19,20] Their ability to resist flexion or subluxation in this region is minimal, whereas their ability to resist rotation is substantial (see Fig. 1–7).

The facet joints absorb a greater fraction of axial load bearing if the spine is oriented in extension (see below). This varies with the type and orientation of the load.[21]

The Lamina, Spinal Canal, and Contents

The lamina provides dorsal protection for the dural sac and a foundation for the spinous processes, thus allowing for the solid attachment of muscles and ligaments. They move the spine by forces applied via the spinous processes.

In the normal spine, the spinal canal dimension, and hence the extramedullary

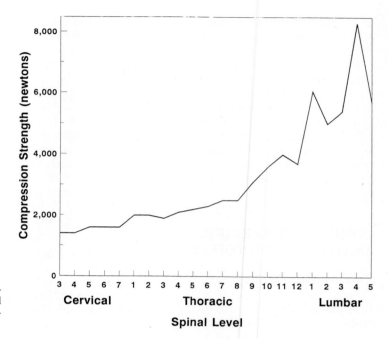

Figure 1–6. Vertebral compression strength versus spinal level (From Benzel, EC,[7] with permission.)

space, is generous. It is most generous in the upper cervical region, and least in the upper thoracic region. In the lumbar region, both the epidural and intradural spaces are generally capacious (Fig. 1–8),[7–10] but the safety margin may be small in patients with a relative spinal stenosis. The lumbar spinal canal depth does not change significantly, but the width increases from upper to lower lumbar regions (Fig. 1–8). This region contains the cauda equina, which is relatively

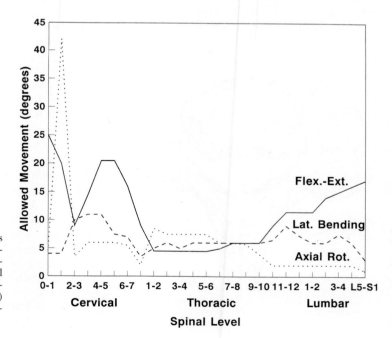

Figure 1–7. Segmental motions allowed at the various spinal levels. (Combined flexion and extension, solid line; unilateral lateral bending dashed line; unilateral axial rotation, dotted line) (From Benzel, EC,[7] with permission.)

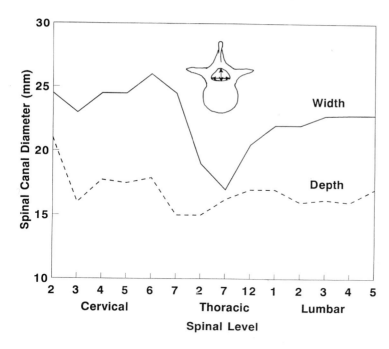

Figure 1–8. Spinal canal diameter versus spinal level. The average width (solid line) and average depth (dashed line) of the canal are depicted separately. (From Benzel, EC,[7] with permission.)

resistant to neurological insults (compared with the spinal cord proper). This is so because of the "peripheral nerve nature" (e.g., the presence of collagen) in the cauda equina. Therefore, post-traumatic lumbar neural element injury is less common than that associated with comparable spinal column deformation elsewhere. The shape of the spinal canal itself changes from rostral to caudal. The triangle-like "balloon" configuration of most of the subaxial spine assumes a shape more like "Napoleon's hat" toward the lumbosacral junction.[19]

The Pedicle

The pedicles of the cervical spine are shorter and proportionally of greater diameter than other regions of the spine; i.e., they have a relatively small length/width ratio. The transverse pedicle width gradually decreases from the cervical to the midthoracic region. It then increases progressively in the lumbar spines.[7,9,22,23] The pedicle height (sagittal pedicle width) gradually increases (with the exception of C2) from the cervical to the thoracolum-

bar junction region. It then decreases progressively in the lumbar spine.[7,9,22,23]

The transverse pedicle angle decreases from the cervical spine to the thoracolumbar region. It then increases progressively in the lumbar spine.[7,9,22,23]

The pedicles of the thoracic spine are smaller than their lumbar counterparts. From a surgical perspective, this is compounded by the variable orientation of the pedicles.[7,9,22–24] In the upper lumbar and thoracic spine, the sagittal pedicle angle is relatively steep. The relationship of the thoracic pedicle to the transverse process changes as the thoracic spine is descended.[24]

The Intervertebral Disc

The ability of intervertebral discs to resist axial loads is great, but it decreases with age.[20] The vertebral end plates incompletely resist herniation of the disc into the vertebral body (Schmorl's nodule— "prolapse of a nucleus pulposus into an adjoining verterbra" [*Dorland's*, 28th edition]).

The annulus fibrosus consists of several layers of radiating fibers that are oriented

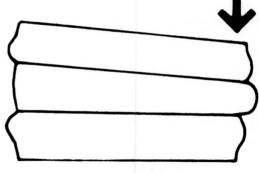

Figure 1–9. An eccentric force application (arrow) results in annulus fibrosus bulging on the side of the greatest force application—i.e., the concave side of the bend (A). (From Benzel, EC,[7] with permission.) An anterior-posterior radiograph of the spine showing osteophytes (arrows) on the concave side of a scoliotic curve (B).

A

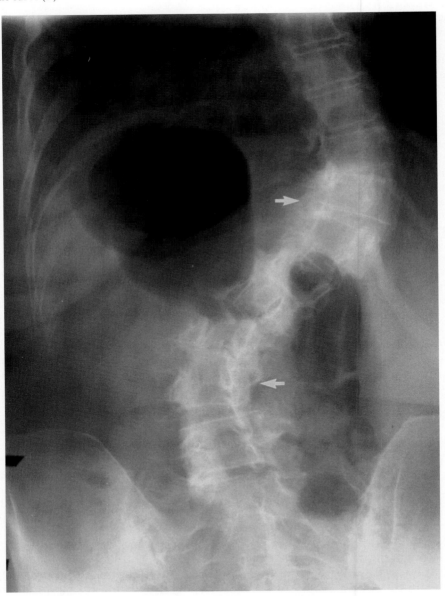

B

10

at an angle of about 30° to each other. They are attached to the cartilaginous end plates (inner fibers) and the cortical bone on the walls of the vertebral body (Sharpey's fibers). These components usually allow some, but not excessive, deformation.

Disc bulging occurs on the concave side of a curve or the side toward which the spine bends (Fig. 1–9). This correlates with osteophyte formation; i.e., osteophytes form predominantly on the concave side of spinal curvatures (Fig. 1–9).

When compression forces are applied to one side of the disc, the annulus fibrosus is distorted and bulges, and osteophytes are formed. Disc herniation, on the other hand, is caused by the migration of the nucleus pulposus from its normal location toward the side of the disc away from where the compression is applied. Thus bulging of the annulus (toward the concavity of a spinal bend) is in the opposite direction from nucleus pulposus migration (Fig. 1–10). Flexion, therefore, causes the annulus fibrosus to bulge in a ventral direction, while the nucleus pulposus migrates dorsally. Significant strains thus are placed on the annulus fibrosus during the application of physiological loads.[25]

The Transverse Process

The transverse processes provide sites for attachment of paraspinous muscles.

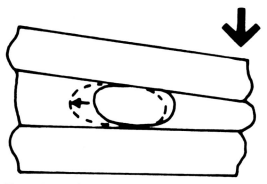

Figure 1–10. The nucleus pulposus moves in the opposite direction of an eccentrically applied force (arrow). Dashed lines indicate the positions of the nucleus pulposus during force application (From Benzel, EC,[7] with permission.)

Therefore, they function as a site of attachment for the application of leverage that causes lateral bending. Transverse processes are easily fractured because of their small diameter. Their susceptibility to fracture is greatest in the lumbar region.

They originate at the junction of the pedicle and the lamina. In the mid to low thoracic region, the processes are moderately robust and project in a lateral and slightly rostral direction. In the lower thoracic region, they are smaller.

In the lumbar region, they are situated more ventrally than at thoracic levels. They also become more substantial as one descends the spine. They can, therefore, be utilized more effectively as sites for bone fusion. Their utility as a site for bony fusion, however, is adversely affected by their relatively poor vascularity and an often less-than-optimal robustness.

The upper six cervical vertebrae usually transmit the vertebral artery through their respective foramina transversarium, which is in continuum with the cervical transverse process. The foramina transversarium is in close proximity to the uncovertebral joint. Therefore, it is subject to encroachment by osteophyte formation.

The Spinous Processes

The spinous processes project dorsally and caudally from the dorsal arch (laminae) of each vertebral segment. The C3–6 spinous processes are usually bifid. In the cervical spine, they become longer as the spine is descended. In the cervical and upper to midthoracic spine, they are oriented in a more caudal direction than in the thoracolumbar and lumbar regions. During surgical procedures, this caudal orientation often dictates the resection of the overhanging spinous process (and interspinous ligament) in order to gain access to the interlaminar space.

The Ligaments

A variety of spinal ligaments provide support (via tension) for the spine.

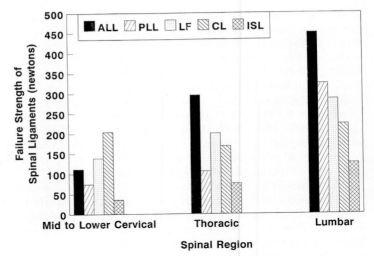

Figure 1–11. Failure strength of spinal ligaments versus spinal region. (ALL = anterior longitudinal ligament; PLL = posterior longitudinal ligament; LF = ligamentum flavum; CL = capsular ligament; ISL = interspinous ligament) (From Benzel, EC,[7] with permission.)

These include the interspinous ligament, the ligamentum flavum, the anterior and posterior longitudinal ligaments, and the capsular ligaments. Their ability to resist deformation and failure varies (Fig. 1–11).[7,11,20,26–34]

The effectiveness of a ligament depends on its morphology and the length of its effective moment arm.[7] One should think of a moment arm as a lever. The moment arm through which a ligament functions is extremely important in determining the efficacy of a ligament, just as a long crowbar (which has a longer moment arm, or lever) is more effective than a short crowbar (Fig. 1–12). This is as important as the strength of the ligament. The length of the moment arm (lever arm) is the perpendicular distance between the applied force and the instantaneous axis of rotation (IAR), the point about which each segment of the spine rotates. The IAR is usually located in the midvertebral body region. A very strong ligament that functions through a relatively short moment arm may contribute less to stability than a weaker ligament that has a mechanical advantage because it functions through a longer moment arm.

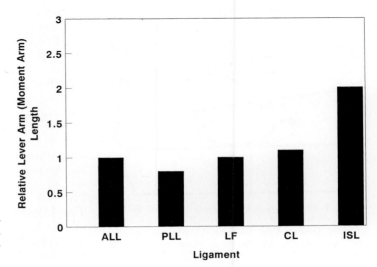

Figure 1–12. The relative lever arm (moment arm) length for ligaments (see Fig. 1–13). (From Benzel, EC,[7] with permission.)

For example, although the *interspinous ligament* is not strong (see Fig. 1–11), its attachment to a bone with a relatively long moment arm (spinous process) allows for the application of a significant bending moment (flexion resistance force) to the spine. In this case, the moment arm is defined as the perpendicular distance from the point of attachment of the ligament (spinous process; site of applied force) to the IAR of the affected vertebral body (Fig. 1–13). The interspinous ligament may be absent at the L5–S1 level and deficient at the L4–L5 level.

The *ligamentum flavum* is a strong ligament that functions through a short moment arm (see Figs. 1–11 and 1–13). It is a discontinuous ligament that attaches the ventral-caudal border of the rostral laminae to the rostral border of the caudal laminae. It extends from C2 to S1 and is deficient in midline. It has the highest percentage of elastic fibers of any human tissue. It is also, except in extreme extension, under tension at all times. This minimizes the chance of ligament buckling and spinal canal encroachment during extension.

The *anterior longitudinal ligament* is a relatively strong ligament that is firmly attached to the margins of the vertebrae (and not so firmly attached to the annulus fibrosus) at each segmental level of the spine. Its position, which is ventral to the IAR, minimizes extension (see Fig. 1–13). Rostrally, it attaches to the ventral basiocciput. Caudally, it attaches to the sacrum.

The *posterior longitudinal ligament* is not as strong as the anterior longitudinal ligament. Its location (dorsal to the IAR) and its short moment arm result in only a mediocre ability to resist flexion (see Figs. 1–11 through 1–13). As opposed to the anterior longitudinal ligament, the posterior longitudinal ligament is predominantly attached to the annulus fibrosus, which is firmly attached to the vertebrae. Its relatively narrow width, in part, permits dorsolateral (paramedian) disc herniation.

The *capsular ligaments* are relatively strong. They, therefore, play a significant role with regard to spinal stability, particularly in the cervical spine. They have a short effective moment arm (Fig. 1–12), but their relative strength, compared to the stresses placed upon them, is significant.

The concept of the neutral zone, as outlined by Panjabi[35] and recently emphasized by Dickman et al.,[36] is essential to the understanding of both the importance and limitations of spinal ligaments in conferring spinal stability. The neutral zone is that component of the physiologic range of motion that is associated with significant flexibility and minimal stiffness at low loads.[7] The neutral zone combined with the elastic zone compose the physiologic range of motion (Fig. 1–14). Stretching a ligament can increase the neutral zone by increasing ligament laxity. Similarly, it is increased in cases of ligamentous injury. In the latter situation, the ligament is pathologically lengthened, and as a result the flexibility of the spine is pathologically increased. When a ligament is stretched during a "warm-up" exercise, the range of motion is increased by virtue of the increase of the neutral zone. This facilitates joint mobility. Under unloaded conditions, the spine is lax (i.e., it is within the neutral zone). The assumption of the upright pos-

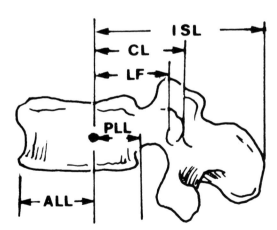

Figure 1–13. The ligaments and their effective moment arms. Note that this length depends on the location of the instantaneous axis of rotation (IAR). An "average" location is used in this illustration. (Dot = IAR; ALL = anterior longitudinal ligament; PLL = posterior longitudinal ligament; LF = ligamentum flavum; CL = capsular ligament; ISL = interspinous ligament.) (From Benzel, EC,[7] with permission)

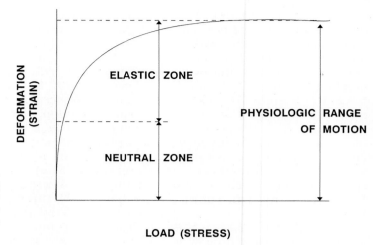

Figure 1–14. A typical load deformation curve depicting the neutral and elastic zones (deformation, or strain, versus load, or stress) (From Benzel, EC,[7] with permission.)

ture, however, is not possible if the spine remains lax (floppy). Continuous muscular tension functions as a compensatory mechanism by limiting intervertebral movement, thus decreasing the size of the neutral zone by applying tension to lax ligaments, and increasing stability.

The Muscles

The muscles move the torso by either directly or indirectly imparting forces to the spine. The morphology[14] and geometry[37] of these muscles have been studied extensively. The erector spinae muscles cause spinal extension and lateral bending. The psoas muscle contributes to flexion. The rectus abdominous muscle causes spinal flexion, despite its lack of direct spinal attachments. It is a strong torso flexor because of its long moment arm (from the ventral abdominal wall to the spine).[37]

The rib cage plays a major role in the maintenance of spinal stability. The maintenance of the bony shell is vital to stability. This stabilizing effect is greatest in extension and least in flexion. It is augmented by the rib attachments to an intact sternum.[38]

Bone

The vertebral body is the component of the spine that bears the majority of ap-

plied loads. Vertebral body dimensions are proportional to load-bearing capacity.

The cortical–cancellous bone ratio of a vertebral body affects its weight-bearing potential. This ratio increases with age. It is also greater in the pedicles than in the vertebral bodies and in small pedicles (thoracic and upper lumbar) than in larger pedicles (sacrum). Bone density (proportional to the cortical/cancellous ratio) correlates with screw pullout resistance. Therefore, pedicles resist screw pullout better than vertebral bodies, and smaller pedicles are more resistant than larger ones.[7] A 50% decrease in the mass of osseus tissue results in a 25% reduction of the tissue's original strength.[11]

Epidural Space

The epidural space is located between the periosteum of the vertebrae and the dura mater. It therefore surrounds the spinal cord and cauda equina. It contains fat, connective tissue, and a venous plexus. The fat can be visualized by computed tomography (CT) scanning, which can be helpful in determining whether lesions within the spinal canal are intradural or epidural.

The epidural venous plexus is extensive and communicates with the dural venous sinuses within the cranium. According to Field and Brierley,[39] there are no

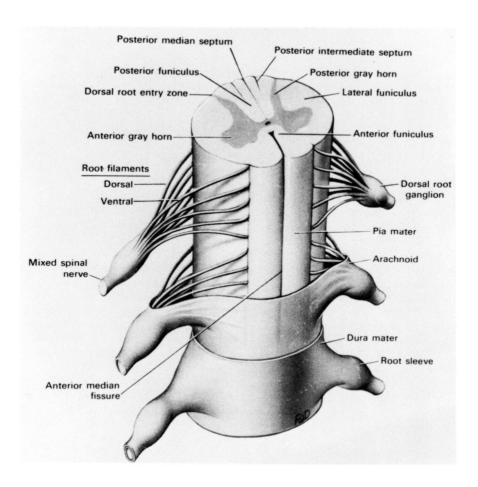

Figure 1–15. The gross anatomy of the spinal cord, gray matter, white matter, and nerve roots. (From Carpenter, MB,[40] p. 215, with permission.)

lymph nodes in the epidural space. The regional lymph nodes of the spinal subarachnoid space are the prevertebral nodes.

Meninges

The meninges consist of dura mater, arachnoid, and pia mater (Fig. 1–15). The dura mater extends from the foramen magnum, where it is continuous with the cranial dura, to the level of the second sacral vertebra, where it fuses with the sacral periosteum. The dura follows each nerve root to fuse with the epineurium and with the periosteum in the intervertebral foramen. Between the dura mater and the arachnoid is a potential space, the subdural space.

The arachnoid is a membrane that is continuous with the intracranial arachnoid. It extends caudally with the dura mater to the second sacral vertebra. The term arachnoid arose because of the similarity between its numerous delicate trabeculae that course between the outer arachnoid membrane and the pia mater and the trabeculated pattern of a spider's web. These trabeculae course through the subarachnoid space, which contains the cerebrospinal fluid. The cross-sectional area of subarachnoid space is smallest in the thoracic spine and greatest in the lumbar region below the conus me dullaris where the cauda equina is located.

The pia mater is adherent to the spinal cord and follows penetrating blood vessels into the cord. Below the conus medullaris, the pia mater continues caudally as the filum terminale to attach to the dura mater at the level of second sacral vertebra. At the second sacral level, the filum merges with the dura to form the coccygeal ligament. The dentate ligaments arise from the pia along the lateral aspect of the spinal cord (via the lateral band) and pass through the arachnoid to attach to the dura mater. The ligaments begin just above the first cervical root and are found between successive roots to approximately the first lumbar root. These ligaments suspend the spinal cord within the spinal canal via their attachment to the dura mater laterally.

SPINAL CORD

Gross Anatomy

The spinal cord begins at the level of the foramen magnum, which demarcates the caudal level of the medulla. Although early in fetal life the spinal cord occupies the entire length of the spinal canal, the growth of the vertebral column exceeds that of the spinal cord so that by the ninth month of gestation, the spinal cord usually terminates at the level of the L3 vertebra. In the adult, the conus medullaris (conical termination of the spinal cord) ends between the T12 and L3 vertebrae; the lower end of the L1 level is the most common site of termination. The conus medullaris is anchored to the sacrum via the filum terminale.

The cervical and lumbar enlargements reflect the greater number of nerve cell bodies and synapses in the gray matter, which gives rise to the brachial and lumbosacral plexi. They provide innervation to the upper and lower extremities. The anterior–posterior (A–P) and lateral di-

mensions of the spinal cord at the cervical enlargement are 9 and 13 mm; in the midthoracic region, the dimensions are 8 and 10 mm; and at the lumbar enlargement, they are 8–9 and 12 mm.[40]

There are 31 paired nerve roots: 8 cervical, 12 thoracic, 5 lumbar, 5 sacral, and 1 rudimentary coccygeal. Each nerve root is composed of ventral and dorsal filaments that carry motor and sensory axons, respectively, except for the first cervical and coccygeal nerves, which usually lack a sensory filament. In the cervical spine, the numbered nerve roots exit *above* the similarly numbered vertebral bodies. The nerve root between C7 and T1 is numbered C8. This explains why there are 8 cervical roots and yet only 7 cervical vertebrae. In the remainder of the spine, the numbered nerve roots exit below the appropriately numbered vertebral body (Fig. 1–1). Each spinal nerve root passes through its corresponding intervertebral foramen, occupying up to 50% of the cross-sectional area of the foramen.[41]

Below the conus medullaris is the cauda equina (horse's tail). The nerve roots are arranged such that the lower sacral segments are located most medially, and the exiting upper lumbar segments are oriented most laterally (Fig. 1–16).[7,42]

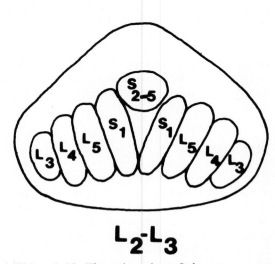

Figure 1–16. The orientation of the nerve roots within the dural sac at the L2–3 level.

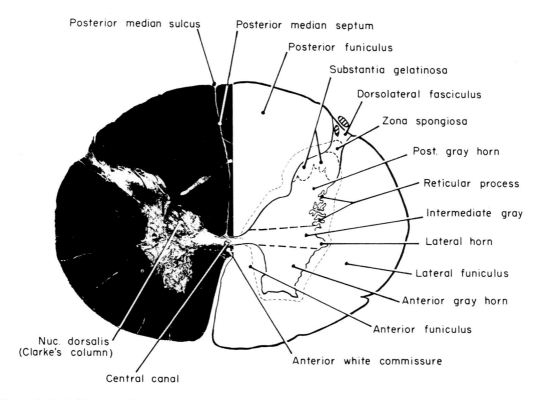

Figure 1–17. Axial section through the lower thoracic spinal cord. The left side is stained with Weigert's myelin stain and the right shows a schematic drawing of the tracts and gray matter subdivisions. The dotted area surrounding the gray matter contains short ascending and descending fibers of the fasciculus propius system. (From Carpenter, MB,[40] p. 219, with permission.)

The spinal cord gray matter is a butterfly-shaped structure surrounded by white matter, which contains the axons of ascending and descending tracts (Fig. 1–17). The central canal is a vestigial lumen lined by ependymal cells. The white matter tracts of the spinal cord are divided into the posterior, lateral, and anterior funiculi.

Gray Matter

The gray matter may be subdivided into an anterior horn, posterior horn, and intermediate zone (see Fig. 1–17). The somatic efferent neurons are located within the anterior horn and give rise to the axons that traverse the ventral roots. These neurons may be divided into the larger (alpha) and smaller (gamma) mo-

tor neurons. The former innervate extrafusal muscle fibers, and the latter innervate small intrafusal fibers of the muscle spindles. The alpha motor neurons are important in mediating individual muscle movements. The gamma efferent system is important in setting the gain of the spindles and maintaining normal or abnormal muscle tone (e.g., spasticity or rigidity) through supraspinal influences.

The visceral efferent fibers of the autonomic nervous system exit the spine with the somatic motor neurons in the ventral root. Within the spinal cord, the perikarya of the preganglionic sympathetic neurons are primarily located in the intermediolateral nucleus from the level of C8 through L3, with axons exiting in ventral roots T1–L3. These axons terminate in the peripheral sympathetic ganglia. The parasympathetic neurons in the spinal cord are located at the S2, S3, and S4 levels in the lateral region of the gray matter. Preganglionic axons exit the spine through the ventral roots at these same levels to synapse in the peripheral ganglia located at or near the pelvic viscera, i.e., the bladder, colon, rectum, and genitalia.

The posterior horn of the spinal gray matter receives afferent input from axons in the dorsal root; the cell bodies for these axons lie in the dorsal root ganglia. The dorsal root ganglia are located in the intervertebral foramina, along the dorsal roots. The dorsal root has two divisions. The lateral division contains small-diameter fibers mediating sensation for pain and temperature. The medial division contains large-diameter fibers mediating other sensory modalities such as proprioception. The axons carrying different sensory modalities terminate and synapse in different locations within the posterior horn or pass through it to enter ascending tracts (e.g., posterior columns). Afferent fibers mediating the stretch reflex pass through the posterior horn to synapse on motor neurons and interneurons in the anterior horn. In the thoracic and upper lumbar region, the intermediate zone also contains the nucleus dorsalis, which receives input from the muscle spindles and joint receptors. This information is relayed ipsilaterally in the spinal white matter in the posterior spinocerebellar tract and may explain why patients with spinal cord compression can, though rarely, present with gait ataxia.[43]

Muscle Stretch Reflex

The muscle stretch, or myotatic, reflex is tested as a part of all neurological examinations. In its simplest form, the stretch reflex is a monosynaptic reflex in which a sensory afferent neuron synapses directly onto a motor efferent neuron in the anterior horn of the gray matter. The sensory afferent (group 1a) is stimulated when the muscle spindle that it innervates is stretched, as occurs with percussion of a deep tendon. This 1a afferent makes direct excitatory monosynaptic connections with the alpha motor neurons of the same muscle and synergistic muscles, which are activated and cause muscle contraction (see Chapter 2).

The monosynaptic reflex depends on the temporal, as well as the spatial, summation of impulses impinging on the motor neuron. Temporal summation requires the temporal synchrony of incoming impulses. Disease processes that interfere with this synchrony, such as those which result in the demyelination of peripheral nerve or spinal roots, result in the loss of deep tendon reflexes.[44] In peripheral neuropathies, there can be a temporal dispersion of impulses (due to unequal involvement of the axons within a nerve) even prior to the slowing of nerve conduction below the lower limit of normal. This probably accounts for the early loss of deep tendon reflexes.[45] The loss of synchrony is greatest for those impulses that must be conducted over the largest distances, accounting for the early loss of distal reflexes such as ankle jerks.[46]

Integrated into this monosynaptic reflex are other interneurons and connections that can modulate its responsiveness. For example, the 1a afferents also synapse with interneurons that inhibit the alpha motor neurons of antagonistic muscles. Furthermore, the threshold of the muscle spindles depends upon the degree of contraction of the intrafusal muscle fibers at the poles of the muscle spindle. The intrafusal muscle fibers are under the control of the gamma efferent motor neurons. The result is that descending supraspinal pathways are responsible for modulating muscle tone and the stretch reflex through the gamma motor system.

Finally, the muscle tendon contains another sensory fiber, the Golgi tendon organ. This receptor measures the tension of the entire muscle. When excess muscle contraction occurs, it inhibits the alpha motor neurons via an inhibitory interneuron in the spinal gray matter.

White Matter

The white matter of the spinal cord surrounds the gray matter and includes well-defined myelinated tracts that are somatotopically organized. The white matter of the spinal cord is divided into three major regions: the posterior, lateral, and anterior funiculi. The funiculi, which contain ascending and descending axons, are sometimes referred to as columns.

Close to the gray matter there are propriospinal tracts in the white matter, in which intraspinal axons run in a rostral–caudal direction and integrate information between segments into reflex patterns. These axons provide both crossed and uncrossed pathways linking neurons in one part of the spinal cord with those in others. They thus provide a basis for coordinated reflex activity, cyclic patterns of activity, and pattern generation within the spinal cord.[47,48]

Ascending Pathways

POSTERIOR COLUMNS

The posterior columns, each of which consists of the medially located fasciculus gracilis and the laterally located fasciculus cuneatus, contain the centrally directed axons of a large proportion of the myelinated sensory fibers within the dorsal roots. The axons within the posterior columns are somatotopically organized so that the fibers from the more caudal regions of the body are located medial (fasciculus gracilis) to those representing the more rostral areas (fasciculus cuneatus) (Figs. 1–18 and 1–19). The cell bodies of these first-order sensory neurons are located in the dorsal root ganglia. The axons of these neurons, which ascend uncrossed in the posterior columns, synapse with second-order neurons in the gracile and cuneate nu-

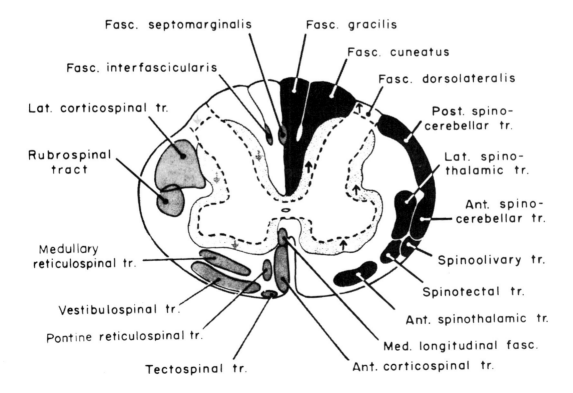

Figure 1–18. The relationships of the ascending tracts (on the right) and the descending tracts (on the left). (From Carpenter, MD,[40] p. 270, with permission.)

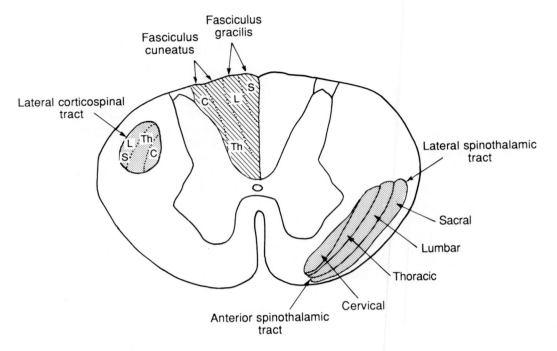

Figure 1–19. The lamination of the corticospinal tract, spinothalamic tract, and posterior columns.

clei in the medulla. Axons from these nuclei transmit sensory information rostrally via a pathway that decussates and ascends as the medial lemniscus and synapses in the ventral posterolateral (VPL) nucleus of the thalamus. Neurons in the VPL nucleus send their axons to the cortex.

The posterior columns have classically been thought to conduct impulses concerned with position and movement of the extremities. Since these fibers mediate the discrimination of spatial and temporal cutaneous stimuli, their function is usually clinically tested by vibration, position, and two-point discrimination. However, there is a dispute over whether the posterior columns solely mediate these sensibilities.[49–52]

LATERAL SPINOTHALAMIC TRACT

Cutaneous pain and temperature sensation are mediated by the lateral spino thalamic tract, which ascends in the lateral funiculus. Evidence suggests that at least some of the fibers in the lateral

spinothalamic tract transmit information related to bowel and bladder fullness and pain from the lower urinary tract (lower ureter, urethra, and bladder), mediating the desire to micturate.[53] Nonmyelinated or thinly myelinated axons mediating pain and temperature sensation enter the spinal cord at the posterior horn and synapse, either at the level of entry into the cord or after ascending or descending for one or two segments, with second-order neurons in the deep layers of the posterior horn. The axons of the second-order neurons decussate in gray matter just ventral to the spinal canal to form the spinothalamic tract. Within the brain, the lateral spinothalamic tract axons synapse in the VPL nucleus and the posterior intralaminar nuclei of the thalamus.[54–56]

The spinothalamic tracts are somatotopically organized such that the sacral dermatomes run most laterally and the cervical dermatomes are ultimately represented most medially in the upper cervical spine (Fig. 1–20). Unilateral complete lesions of the lateral spinothalamic tract

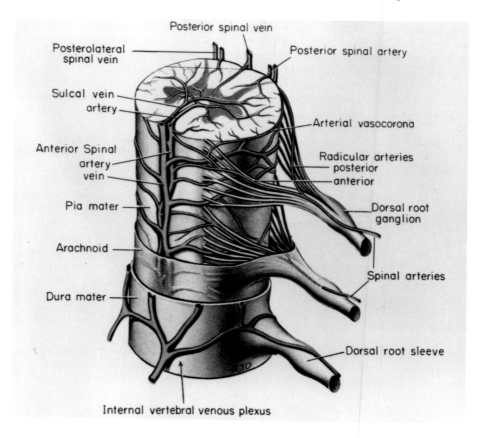

Figure 1–20. The arterial and venous anatomy of the spinal cord. (From Carpenter, MB,[40] p. 603, with permission.)

produce a contralateral loss of somatic pain and temperature sensibility that often (as a result of the pattern of decussation of the fibers) extends one to two segments below the level of the lesion. In some cases after the lateral spinothalamic tract is transected, there is some return of sensibility to pain, possibly reflecting the presence of a small uncrossed spinothalamic pathway.[40]

Descending Pathways

CORTICOSPINAL TRACT

The descending pathways are divided into the corticospinal tract (generally corresponding to the pyramidal tract) and non-pyramidal pathways. The corticospinal neurons are located in the cerebral cortex and their axons descend to terminate within the spinal cord, directly on lower motor neurons, or on other interposed neurons within the gray matter.

Phylogenetically speaking, the corticospinal tracts first appeared in mammals. The great majority of fibers in the corticospinal tract arise from pyramidal neurons (mostly the large Betz cells in cortical layer IV) in the precentral gyrus, and to a lesser extent, from the premotor area and the parietal lobe (especially the somatosensory cortex). Many of these axons project directly to alpha motor neurons innervating the distal extremities,[57,58] which subserve discrete appendicular movements.

The corticospinal tract of each side is composed of approximately 1 million fibers, most of them myelinated. After passing into the medullary pyramids, 75%

to 90% of the corticospinal fibers decussate to form the lateral corticospinal tract, which is in the dorsal portion of the lateral funiculus (Fig. 1–20). Fibers within the lateral corticospinal tract exhibit a distinct lamination which has important clinical implications. Fibers controlling lumbar- and sacral-innervated musculature run in the dorsolateral aspect tracts, and fibers controlling cervical-innervated musculature are located ventromedially, closer to the central gray. As a result of this lamination, in the central cervical cord syndrome, one often finds impairment of the upper extremities with relative sparing of the legs.

Usually, 10% to 25% of the corticospinal fibers do not decussate but rather descend in the spinal cord ipsilateral to the cerebral hemisphere of origin. Most of these fibers descend in the anterior corticospinal tract within the anterior funiculus of the spinal cord white matter. These fibers, after descending, either cross the midline in the anterior white commissure to terminate in the centromedial portion of the contralateral anterior horn or, less commonly, terminate in the same area of the ipsilateral anterior horn[59,60] to synapse with neurons innervating neck and trunk musculature.

There is also evidence for the existence of some recrossed fibers in the lateral corticospinal tract. Evidence from postmortem examinations of patients who had undergone spinal cordotomies for relief of intractable pain suggests that recovery of motility of the leg after damage to the ipsilateral corticospinal tracts is due to activity in descending fibers in the contralateral lateral corticospinal tract.[61] According to this view, most corticospinal fibers innervate motor neurons contralateral to the cerebral hemisphere from which they originate, but a small proportion descend from the cerebral cortex into the contralateral lateral corticospinal tract and subsequently recross to activate ipsilateral leg motor neurons controlling proximal musculature, possibly via interneuronal chains within the spinal gray matter. These proximal muscles, while not mediating fine or discrete motor ac-

tivity, appear sufficient for some aspects of stance and, in some patients, gait. This recrossing of a small number of fibers from the lateral corticospinal tract could provide a neuroanatomic basis for the recovery of motility observed after spinal cord hemisections in experimental animals,[62,63] and after damage to the cerebral peduncle in humans. In comparison to discrete activity of distal limb muscles, this recovery involves gross postural movements, suggesting that the more medially located motor neuron pools may receive bilateral innervation from the cerebral cortex.

The hallmark of corticospinal function is the movement of individual muscle groups to perform skilled movements of the distal extremities. This clinical observation is reflected in the pattern of distribution of corticospinal fibers. Weil and Lassek[64] estimated that 55% of corticospinal fibers project to the cervical region, 20% to the thoracic spine, and 25% to the lumbosacral area. The disproportionately large number of fibers projecting to the upper extremity and to a lesser extent the lower extremity, compared with the thoracic spinal cord, is due to the large contribution of fibers mediating discriminative movements of the distal extremity. In testing corticospinal function in patients with spinal cord disease, therefore, there is usually a loss of individual toe or finger movement long before there is loss of proximal muscle strength and control.

Corticospinal tract dysfunction results in release phenomena, such as the Babinski response (a withdrawal response). The Babinski sign is observed more often with the loss of skilled movements of the foot than with hyperreflexia. Gijn[65] has described the Babinski sign as due to a disturbance of direct pyramidal tract projections to distal motor neuron.

Spasticity is generally considered a sign of corticospinal disturbance, however experiments in monkeys[66] and observations in humans[67] have shown that sectioning of the corticospinal tracts at the level of the medullary pyramids or cerebral peduncles results in decreased muscle tone

and reduced or normal reflexes. Gilman and colleagues demonstrated in the monkey that medullary pyramidotomy caused (1) hypotonia, (2) loss of contactual orienting responses such as grasping, and (3) defective use of fine toe and hand movements.[67a] These authors concluded that hypotonia is due to decreased tonic fusimotor innervation of muscle spindles, resulting in a depression of the afferent responses to passive extension of muscle spindles.[67b] Spasticity, therefore, appears to result from disturbance of pathways to the spinal cord that have been termed parapyramidal.[68] Nevertheless, because pure lesions of the corticospinal tract occur only rarely in clinical practice,[69] in practical terms, spasticity suggests corticospinal damage.

NONPYRAMIDAL TRACTS

Nonpyramidal pathways are phylogenetically older than the pyramidal pathways. These pathways originate in the brain stem and project to spinal gray matter. The major nonpyramidal pathways located in the anterior funiculus of the spinal cord are the reticulospinal tracts, the vestibulospinal tract, and the tectospinal tract (Fig. 1–18). These pathways project to spinal gray matter, innervating axial musculature and control muscle tone, reflex activity, posture, and balance.

AUTONOMIC PATHWAYS

Descending pathways for autonomic control of breathing, blood pressure, sweating, and urinary bladder control are located primarily in the ventrolateral quadrant of white matter in the spinal cord. Segmental innervation of the diaphragm most commonly occurs at levels C3–5. Sympathetic fibers arising in the upper lumbar segments, parasympathetic fibers from S2–4, and somatic efferents originating at S2–4 innervate the urinary bladder. The anal sphincter and genitalia share pathways similar to those of the urinary bladder.

Vascular Anatomy

The detailed studies of Adamkiewicz in the late 19th century form the basis of our understanding of the vascular anatomy of the human spinal cord. These findings have been extended by recent injection studies.[70-72] The arterial supply to the spinal cord is provided by the unpaired anterior spinal artery and the paired posterior spinal arteries (Fig. 1–20). Rostrally, the anterior spinal artery is most commonly formed in the region of the foramen magnum or upper cervical spine from branches of the vertebral arteries. Although radicular arteries accompany each spinal nerve root, only a few (usually fewer than 10) serve as tributaries to the anterior spinal artery.[73]

Different anterior radicular arteries vary considerably in the degree to which they contribute to perfusion of the anterior spinal artery, especially in the cervical and thoracic regions.[73] Despite this variability, the artery of Adamkiewicz has come to be recognized as the largest and most constant in the region. It is an unpaired vessel and is located on the left side in two-thirds of all cases. It often accompanies the spinal root of L1 or L2 but may accompany any root from T7 to L3.[74,75] The artery of Adamkiewicz is the major source of blood flow to the anterior spinal artery region for 50% of the spinal cord in 50% of individuals.[75a]

The anterior spinal artery gives rise to a number of sulcal branches that enter the anterior median fissure and then divide into left and right branches to perfuse the gray matter and central white matter (see Fig. 1–20).[73] The sulcal branches are least numerous in the thoracic region; this arrangement may contribute to the already tenuous blood supply to this region. In addition to the vascular supply arising from the sulcal branches, the arterial vasocorona surrounding the spinal cord supplies another source of blood flow. Through the two arterial systems, the anterior spinal artery perfuses the anterior and lateral horns, the base of the posterior horn and the central gray matter, and the anterior

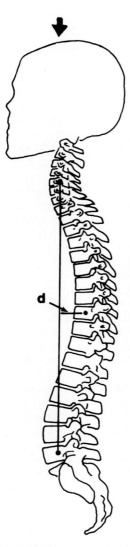

Figure 1–21. A kyphotic posture (as is normally present in the thoracic region) has a large natural moment arm (d); and, thus, the magnitude of the bending moment resulting from an axial load (arrow) is significant. (From Benzel, EC,[7] with permission.)

terruption of blood flow to the spinal cord, therefore, often is clinically manifest in this region, resulting in an anterior spinal artery syndrome in the thoracic region near the level of T4.[76,77] This syndrome is characterized by paraplegia and a middle-to-upper thoracic pin and temperature sensory level, with preservation of posterior column function due to perfusion by the posterior spinal arteries. Spinal cord ischemia has been considered to be a rare phenomenon in the past but is increasingly reported.[78] Some causes of spinal cord infarction include cardiac arrest, aortic dissection, aortic surgery, coarctation operation, and intra-aortic balloon pump counterpulsation.[78–84]

The posterior spinal arteries are paired structures often forming a network of

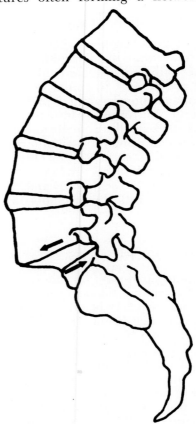

Figure 1–22. Axially oriented translational deformation, resulting in a dislocation. This occurs when two parallel, but noncoincident, apposed force vectors (arrows) are applied. (From Benzel, EC,[7] with permission)

and lateral funiculi. The remaining portion of the posterior horn and the posterior funiculi are perfused by the posterior spinal arteries.

The cervical and lumbar regions are the locations of the most copious blood flow from radicular arteries, making the anterior spinal artery supply of the thoracic spinal cord a watershed region. In-blood vessels in which none is dominant. Rostrally, the posterior spinal arteries arise from the vertebral or the posterior inferior cerebellar arteries.[77] Caudally, they are fed by the radicular arteries. In the cervical region the blood flow is caudally directed, but in the thoracic and lumbar spine, blood flows rostrally.[70] The posterior spinal arteries perfuse the posterior columns and lateral aspects of the posterior horns.

In general, the draining venous system follows a similar pattern to that of the arterial system, although there are more individual variations. An anterior spinal vein is fed by sulcal veins and accompanies the anterior spinal artery. A single prominent median posterior draining vein is usually found near the posterior median septum. Radicular veins drain the anterior and posterior median veins. As is the case with radicular arteries, some of these veins are more prominent than others; in the lumbar region the most prominent vein is the vena radicularis magna.[72]

A network of veins termed the internal vertebral venous plexus or Batson's plexus courses in the epidural space. Batson's plexus forms a collateral valveless route for venous return from intra-abdominal and intrathoracic organs to the heart. Venous effluent from these organs enters the valveless system when intrathoracic and intra-abdominal pressure is increased, such as occurs during straining, coughing, and sneezing. Neoplasms and infections in the viscera of these locations may thus metastasize to the spine through this collateral circulation.

CONFIGURATION OF THE SPINE

The normal (nonpathologic) cervical and lumbar spine assumes a lordotic posture. A kyphosis, as is commonly present in the thoracic and thoracolumbar regions, predisposes the spine to exaggerated stresses (via an imposed long moment arm). This long moment arm

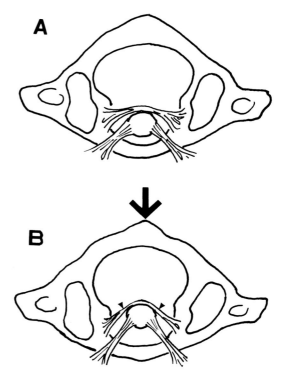

Figure 1–23. The mechanism of injury of a rupture of the transverse ligament of the atlas. (A) C1 vertebral ring (atlas) with transverse ligament dorsal to the dens. (B) A dorsally directed force (arrow), applied to the head, causes a dorsally directed force vector applied to C1. The transverse ligament of the atlas (arrowheads) stretches (B) if this dorsally directed force vector (arrow) is applied to the ring of C1. (From Benzel, EC,[7] with permission.)

(lever arm) creates an excessive bending moment (bending moment = applied force × movement arm length) (Fig. 1–21). Therefore, the intrinsic configuration of the spine contributes substantially to the type of spinal column injury incurred (via an effect of applied forces through existing moment arms). For example, at the thoracolumbar junction, the lower terminus of the thoracic kyphosis (with an accompanying absence of the protective support of the rib cage and the absence of the more massive lower lumbar vertebral body support) fosters vertebral column injury. The intrinsic bending moment allowed by the kyphosis, and the abrupt change in mechanics result in focally increased amounts of strain and in an increased incidence of compression fractures in this region (see below).[7,85]

At the lumbosacral junction, the angle of the sacrum in relation to the L5 vertebral body (the lumbosacral joint angle) may substantially affect pathological processes related to both traumatic and degenerative processes.[7] This joint is exposed to significant axial stresses. There-fore, it must resist substantial translational forces. A translational force results in a tendency toward subluxation or dislocation perpendicular to the long axis of the spine. Subluxation is caused by two parallel but noncoincident apposed force vectors. The axial and translational stresses applied to the lumbosacral junction are depicted in Figure 1–22. The greater the lumbosacral joint angle the greater are the

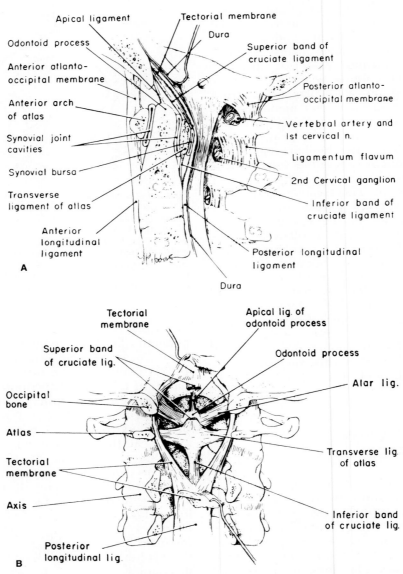

Figure 1–24. The anatomical relationships of the atlantoaxial complex are illustrated. (A) Midsagittal section. (B) Coronal section. (From Makela, A-L, et al.,[131] p. 489, with permission.)

applied translational forces. The ability of the spine to resist these translational forces is diminished by the common vertical (sagittal) lumbosacral facet joint orientation, as well as the tensile characteristics of the supporting ligaments. Patients with an exaggerated lumbar lordosis are particularly prone to the sequelae of these stresses, such as degenerative joint disease and spondylolisthesis.[7]

BIOMECHANICS OF THE SPINAL COLUMN AND SPINAL COLUMN FAILURE

Regional Characteristics and Variations From a Biomechanical Perspective

THE ROSTRAL CERVICAL SPINE AND CRANIOCERVICAL JUNCTION

The rostral cervical spine deserves attention because of its unique morphology. C1 has no centrum. The presence of the dens (of C2) between its two lateral masses makes this spinal level unique among all other levels of the spine. The dens articulates with the dorsal aspect of the ventral aspect of the ring of C1 and with the transverse ligament of the atlas. These attachments occur via separate synovial joints.

The lateral masses of C1 join with the occipital condyles and C2 by means of kidney-shaped articulations. These articulations are both rounded. This results in a joint in which the facets glide rather easily past each other. The superior facet of C1 faces a rostral and medial direction, while the inferior facet faces a caudal and medial direction. This unique relationship assumes a wedge-like configuration that results in a lateral transmission of force vectors resulting from axial loads which may cause a C1 burst (Jefferson) fracture.

The transverse ligament of the atlas attaches to the tubercles located on the medial aspect of the ring of C1. This anatomical arrangement, along with the confines created by the ventral aspect of the ring of C1, provides for the containment of the

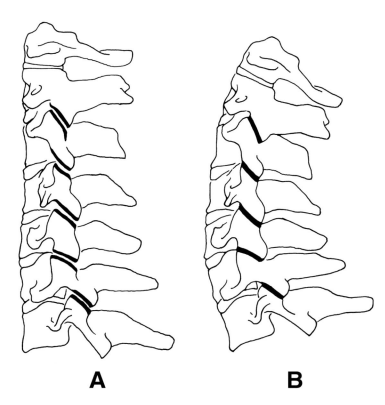

A **B**

Figure 1–25. (A) In a neutral spinal orientation, the facet joints of the cervical spine are unloaded during moderate axial loading. (B) In a lordotic orientation (relative extension), however, they are loaded. (From Benzel, EC,[7] with permission.)

Table 1–1. **Average Movements Allowed in the Craniocervical Region**[*]

Joint	Motion	Range of Motion (Degrees)
Occiput–C1	Combined flexion/extension	25
	Lateral bending (unilateral)	5
	Axial rotation (unilateral)	5
C1–2	Combined flexion/extension	20
	Lateral bending (unilateral)	5
	Axial rotation (unilateral)	40

*From Benzel EC,[7] p. 13, with permission.

intruding dens of C2 (Fig. 1–23). The short (and strong) transverse process of C2 provides a site of attachment for the rotators of the upper cervical spine. Also, the ventral aspect of the ring of C1 is composed of strong, dense cortical bone. In fact, a circumferentially intact ring of C1 is not necessary for the attainment of stability if the ventral portion of the ring is intact. C2 has many of the attributes of the subaxial cervical vertebrae, but it also has a rostral extension, the dens. The pars interarticularis (not to be confused with the pedicle) is substantial and projects from the lamina toward the vertebral body in a rostral and ventral direction (to attach to the lateral mass). The occipital nerve passes dorsal to the atlanto-axial joint.

C2 is connected directly to the occiput by the alar and apical ligaments and the tectorial membrane (Fig. 1–24). C1 functions, as an intermediate "fulcrum" or "spacer" that regulates movement between the occiput and C2.[86] The atlanto-occipital joint permits flexion, extension, and a minimal degree of lateral bending. Rotation is significantly restricted. The atlanto-axial joint allows moderate lateral bending, coupled with rotation.[87] Most of the rotation allowed in the cervical spine, which occurs about the dens, is permitted at the level of this joint. The amount of movement at each segmental level of the craniocervical region is depicted in Table 1–1.[7,11,12,18]

Surgery on the upper cervical spine is complicated by the difficulties associated with calvarial fixation for spinal implants and by the unique anatomy of the upper cervical vertebrae, as well as by the substantial spinal movement allowed in this

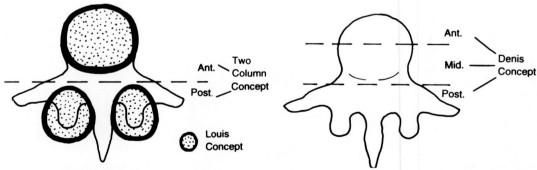

Figure 1–26. The "column" concepts of spinal instability. The concept described by Louis (left) assigns significance to the vertebral body and the facet joint complexes (lateral masses) on either side of the dorsal spine. The two-column construct (left) relies on anatomically defined structures; i.e., the vertebral body (anterior column) and posterior elements (posterior column). Louis's three-column concept (left) similarly relies on anatomically defined structures. Denis's three-column concept (right) assigns significance to the region of the neutral axis and the integrity of the dorsal vertebral body wall (the middle column). (From Benzel, EC,[7] with permission.)

region. The sum of the movements from the occiput to C2 is greater than in any other region of the spine.

THE MIDDLE AND LOWER CERVICAL SPINE

The vertebrae of the mid and lower cervical spine are relatively uniform and have a similar morphology. They are unique in their contribution to the attainment of the cervical lordosis. This, perhaps, aids in spinal cord injury prevention by distributing axially applied loads symmetrically so that a significant bending moment is not applied. Because the addition of a flexion component to an axial load greatly increases the probability of vertebral body failure and the retropulsion of bone and disc fragments into the spinal canal, the lordotic posture also tends to protect against catastrophic injury.

The orientation of the facet joints in the coronal plane does not significantly limit spinal movement in any direction except extension and ventral translation. With the cervical spine in an extension posture, the spine's ability to resist axial loading is greatest because the applied load is shared between the ventral vertebral bodies and discs, and the dorsal facet joint complexes (Fig. 1–25).

THE THORACIC SPINE

The thoracic spinal cord is shielded from injury by the paraspinal muscle masses and by the thoracic cage. The small diameter of the rostral thoracic spinal canal, however, complicates the issue. The former attributes protect the neural elements, while the latter facilitates neural injury. This perhaps explains the increased incidence of catastrophic neurological injuries associated with spine fractures in this region. The paraspinous muscles and rib cage relatively protect the spine from failure, thus causing a relative all-or-nothing neural injury phenomenon. Significant kinetic energy is required to fracture the upper thoracic spine, but if such a fracture occurs, the narrow spinal canal leaves little room to

spare for neural element protection.[7,85] The natural kyphotic posture of the thoracic spine, with its associated predisposition to spine fracture, complicates all of these factors.

THE THORACOLUMBAR JUNCTION

The thoracolumbar junction is located at a point of spinal configuration and bony morphology transition that makes it vulnerable to excessive force application. At this junctional region of the spine, the rib cage no longer provides support, and the kyphotic curvature of the spine predisposes the spine to fracture. In addition, the vertebral bodies of the thoracolumbar junction are not as massive as those of the mid to low lumbar region and thus do not share the latter's increased ability to resist deformity. Therefore, an increased incidence of fractures occurs at this junction.[7,85] The transverse processes of the lower thoracic region are usually rudimentary.

THE UPPER AND MIDDLE LUMBAR SPINE

The upper and mid lumbar spine vertebral bodies are larger and more massive than those at more rostral spinal levels. This, combined with the lordotic curvature of the lumbar spine, makes the lumbar spine relatively resistant to excessive force application, as incurred via trauma. Furthermore, the transition of the spinal cord into the cauda equina (which is more tolerant to trauma than the spinal cord) makes catastrophic neural element injury less likely.[85]

THE LOW LUMBAR SPINE AND LUMBOSACRAL JUNCTION

The caudal terminus of the spinal column is associated with significant logistic therapeutic dilemmas. A frequently observed inability to obtain substantial points of sacral fixation during spinal surgical procedures creates a multitude of surgical problems. Furthermore, the relatively steep orientation of the lumbosacral joint exposes the lumbosacral junction to a proclivity to translational deformation (see Fig. 1–22).

Spinal Stability and Instability

A variety of schemata have been employed theoretically and clinically to assist in the determination of spinal stability. They can be broken down into (1) bony column models,[88] (2) functional column models,[89] and (3) combination models.[90,91,92] These are illustrated in Figure 1–26.

White and Panjabi[11] define clinical stability of the spine as "the ability of the spine under physiologic loads to limit patterns of displacement so as not to damage or irritate the spinal cord or nerve roots and, in addition, to prevent incapacitating deformity or pain due to structural changes." Spinal stability is not absolute. It should be measured in increments, regarding its absolute presence or absence. Depending upon the circumstance, the spine is expected to provide varying degrees of support (stability). Therefore, spinal stability should be defined differently under these varying circumstances.[7]

The converse of stability is, obviously, instability. The former evades definition, whereas the latter is somewhat more easily assessed and quantitated; point systems have been described in quantitating instability.[11] Instability should, perhaps, be generally defined, with significant consideration given to the type of instability and the existing circumstances. In general, instability is defined as the inability to limit excessive or abnormal spinal displacement.[7]

The two fundamental categories of moderate instability are acute and chronic. Acute instability may be subdivided into overt (gross instability) and limited (moderate) instability. Chronic instability can similarly be subdivided into glacial instability (gradual slippage, such as with isthmic spondylolisthesis) and the instability associated with dysfunctional segmental motion (e.g., that instability associated with a significantly unstable disc).

Overt instability is associated with a circumferential disruption of the spine. This results not only in the loss of spinal integrity but also in the creation of a nidus for pain. The spine cannot safely support the torso during the assumption of the upright posture.[7]

Limited instability is similar to overt instability, with the exception that the instability is of a lesser magnitude and is not associated with a significant risk of further acute spinal failure during the assumption of the upright posture.

Glacial instability is associated with a gradual movement of one segment upon another (i.e., progressive subluxation such as with isthmic spondylolisthesis). However, overt instability that results in a significant chance of acute instability with the assumption of the upright posture is not present. This type of instability is akin to a glacier in that gradual movement occurs independent of external forces.

The instability associated with dysfunctional segmental motion may result from inadequately treated overt or limited instability. It also can be associated with glacial instability. However, it is most commonly associated with degenerative spine disease. It is related to pathological degeneration of a motion segment and is manifested by (1) excessive segmental motion, (2) a fixed subluxation (recognizing that motion may be difficult to elicit due to guarding), or (3) excessive segmental degenerative changes (a manifestation of previous or ongoing dysfunctional motion).

THE MECHANISMS AND BIOMECHANICS OF NEURAL ELEMENT INJURY

External influences can cause a cell to become dysfunctional or die via several mechanisms: (1) cell disruption, (2) cell distortion, or (3) metabolic derangements.[7,93] The physical disruption of a cell membrane usually results in the cell's death. Both cell distortion and metabolic derangements

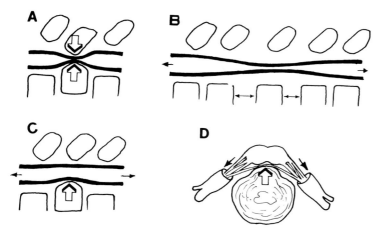

Figure 1–27. The four mechanisms of neural element distortion-related injury. (A) Neural element compression; (B) simple distraction, resulting in spinal cord stretching and narrowing; (C) tethering over an extrinsic mass in the sagittal plane ("sagittal bowstring" effect); and (D) tethering of neural elements over an extrinsic mass in the coronal plane ("coronal bowstring" effect; axial depiction). Solid arrows depict "distractive" forces; hollow arrows depict forces applied directly to the dural sac. (From Benzel, EC,[7] with permission.)

can cause either temporary dysfunction or the death of the cell. Cell disruption can be the result of an initial injury such as the impact (*primary injury*), or the exaggeration of cell distortion caused by CNS tissue shift, such as those related to edema or hematoma formation (e.g., herniation). This is termed *ongoing primary injury.* Loss of cell membrane integrity (resulting in cell death) can also be caused by metabolic derangements, such as extracellular osmotic shifts and autodestructive processes that follow the primary injury. The latter is termed *secondary injury.* Thus, cell distortion (alteration of course or shape) and metabolic derangements can lead to cell disruption (loss of cell wall integrity).[7,93]

The mechanisms responsible for secondary cell injury in the central nervous system differ in gray and white matter. Injury to gray matter, with resultant loss of neuronal cell bodies and synapses in the surrounding neuropil, produces *segmental* deficits (e.g., the loss of motor axons at the C6 level with resultant weakness and atrophy in the biceps, brachioradialis, etc.). Secondary injury of cellular elements within the gray matter depends, in large part, on excitotoxic mechanisms that reflect the inappropriate release of excitatory amino acid neurotransmitters, which trigger abnormal ion fluxes (including abnormal calcium influx) into nerve cells and glial cells.

Secondary injury to white matter, in contrast, impairs the transmission of in-

formation, up and down the spinal cord within *ascending* and *descending* spinal cord tracts. Thus injury to white matter produces symptomatic deficits that are not confined to the level of the lesion but account for clinical dysfunction at many spinal levels below the lesion. Damage to white matter accounts for the brunt of symptomatic deficit following various insults to the spinal cord. Since synapses are not present within white matter, excitotoxic mechanisms do not play a major role in producing secondary cell death. Recent studies have demonstrated that, despite the lack of excitotoxic injury mechanisms within the white matter, secondary cell death does occur, and is calcium-mediated.[94,95] The underlying molecular cascade involves activation of a particular class of sodium channels, which collapses the transmembrane gradient for sodium ions, thereby driving the Na/Ca-exchanger (a specialized antiporter molecule that exchanges sodium ions for calcium ions) to operate in a "reverse" mode, exporting sodium from the cell interior and importing injurious amounts of calcium into axons.[96,97]

This mechanism has been most rigorously demonstrated in CNS white matter following anoxic insult, but it is also likely to participate in secondary injury of spinal cord axons following trauma and in spinal cord compression.[98,99]

There is evidence that even in mechanical injuries to the spinal cord (e.g., trau-

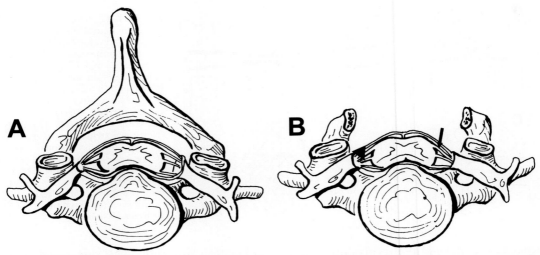

Figure 1–28. Coronal plane tethering ("coronal bowstring" effect). The nerve roots (arrow) or, more commonly, the dentrate ligaments (arrowhead) may tether the spinal cord in the coronal plane (A). Laminectomy may not relieve the distortion (B). (From Benzel, EC,[7] with permission.)

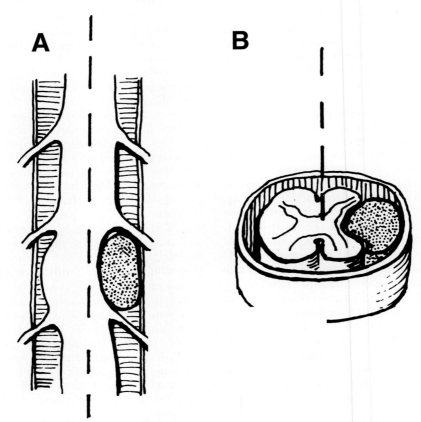

Figure 1–29. A laterally impinging mass may be missed by sagittal imaging through the dotted line of this coronal image (A). Therefore, axial images are critical (B).

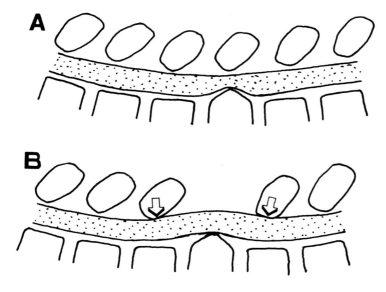

Figure 1–30. Kinking of the spinal cord may occur after laminectomy if an inadequate length of the spinal canal is decompressed A = Prelaminectomy, B = Post laminectomy (From Benzel, EC,[7] with permission.)

matic spinal cord injury and spinal cord compression) ischemia can supervene, thus reducing adenosine triphosphate (ATP) levels so that secondary cell injury occurs.[100] Spinal cord axons are not the only target for traumatic injury. There is substantial evidence for the presence of a subpopulation of axons that maintains continuity through traumatic and compressive injuries, but fails to conduct as a result of demyelination.[101–103] Recently, apoptosis (or programmed cell death), of oligodendrocytes within the spinal cord has been demonstrated following trauma.[104–106]

There is also evidence that inflammatory mechanisms, triggered by trauma, may contribute to the death of myelin-forming oligodendrocytes in the spinal cord. Irrespective of the underlying mechanism, the existence of axons that run without interruption through injured segments of the spinal cord with impaired conduction as a result of demyelination may be important for the development of new therapeutic strategies. Restoration of function in these demyelinated axons may lead to functional improvement in some patients who appear, on clinical grounds, to be harboring "complete" spinal cord lesions.

The removal of a mass lesion by surgical means can relieve distortion of the cell and may also improve nervous tissue perfusion, which can relieve metabolic derangements. The evidence available at this time indicates that the secondary response to injury can be diminished by rapid administration of high doses of methylprednisolone.[107] A complex cascade of cellular and biomechanical events contributes to neurological impairment,[93,108–112] and pharmacologic interventions at any of a number of steps in this injurious cascade may provide useful therapeutic strategies in the future.

Biomechanics of Neural Injury

From a practical clinical perspective, four mechanisms of persistent neural element distortion-related injury exist: (1) extrinsic neural element compression, (2) simple distraction, (3) tethering of the the of the neural elements over extrinsic masses in the sagittal plane ("sagittal bowstring effect"), and (4) tethering of the neural elements over extrinsic masses in the coronal plane ("coronal bowstring effect") (Fig. 1–27).[7] Each must be considered and accounted for during the management decision-making process.

EXTRINSIC NEURAL ELEMENT COMPRESSION

Spinal cord compression is arguably the most important cause of neurological dysfunction associated with degenerative disease (annular constriction)[113] and trauma (unidirectional compression or ventrodorsal "squeeze") (Fig. 1–27A). The annular constriction associated with degenerative disease is a result of compression by a ventral osteophyte, dorsolateral facet, or dorsal hypertrophied ligamentum flavum. In the case of trauma, the compression is most commonly caused by a ventral mass lesion. The distortion of neural elements, combined with their exposure to repetitive movement (chronic spinal cord irritation), can result in persistence of distortion and in repeated insults.[7,114–120]

SIMPLE DISTRACTION

The distraction of neural elements may cause electrophysiological and metabolic dysfunction or cell death. Distraction results in two fundamental potentially harmful occurrences: neuronal distortion and impediment of the blood supply.[7]

Cusick et al.[121,122] and Brieg[123,124] have made significant observations regarding spinal cord distraction. Distraction alone requires the application of significant force in order to cause neural dysfunction. However, a variety of injury mechanisms combine to exaggerate the neural injury. For example, the distraction of the spinal cord over an impinging mass (tethering, depicted in Fig. 1–27C and D) requires much less distractive force to cause an equivalent neuronal impairment compared to simple distraction (depicted in Fig. 1–27B).[7]

"SAGITTAL BOWSTRING" EFFECT

An underestimated cause of neurological dysfunction is related to the tethering of the spinal cord over extrinsic structures. In the sagittal plane, this may be related to either ventral or dorsal structures.[7] However, extrinsic masses located ventral to the spinal cord are most often implicated. A patient with a focal kyphotic deformity and an associated neurological deficit often has spinal cord tethering in the sagittal plane ("sagittal bowstring effect") as a factor that contributes to the neurological deficit.[7,125] Spinal cord tethering in the sagittal plane may be implicated in some patients who are neurologically worse following dorsal decompression procedures. Thus, a kyphosis associated with cervical spondylosis may cause neural injury in part by tethering of the spinal cord over a ventral mass via the sagittal bowstring effect. In such cases, dorsal decompression (e.g., via laminectomy) may worsen the deformation. Morgan et al. documented this clinically in patients with posttraumatic ventral mass lesions.[126] He observed that many patients undergoing a dorsal decompression procedure for posttraumatic ventral spinal cord compression worsened neurologically.

"CORONAL BOWSTRING" EFFECT

The spinal cord also can be tethered in the coronal plane (see Fig. 1–27D).[125] This "coronal bowstring" effect is caused by the tethering of the spinal cord ventrally by lateral extensions of the spinal cord; i.e., by nerve roots or the dentate ligaments (Fig. 1–28).[7] If a coronal bowstringing is present, a laminectomy may fail to relieve spinal cord distortion (Fig. 1–28B).[125] A ventral decompression operation, or a dorsal operation combined with an untethering procedure, is thus required to adequately relieve the spinal cord distortion. This may be achieved by employing a ventral decompression of the spinal cord or by sectioning the dentate ligament.[125] Kahn detailed the anatomical and biomechanical factors involved with the latter.[113]

Laterally placed masses such as a neurofibroma can cause bow-stringing as well. In this case, the bow-stringing can occur in both the sagittal (via the dentate ligaments) and the coronal planes (Fig. 1–29).

Multiple angled imaging is critical (Fig. 1–29).

Iatrogenic Neural Element Injury

INAPPROPRIATE WIDTH OF DECOMPRESSION

The width of spinal decompression is critical. For example, a laminectomy that is not wide enough to adequately decompress the spinal canal may result in persistent neurological dysfunction. Conversely, a laminectomy that is too wide or that is performed in conjunction with a wide foraminotomy may result in spinal instability, or even neurological deficit.[127] Nevertheless, a laminectomy should be extended laterally to the lateral extent of the dural sac. This should not significantly injure the integrity of the facet joints.[128]

INAPPROPRIATE LENGTH OF DECOMPRESSION

A laminectomy can be too long or too short. If it is too long, spinal instability or deformity may occur.[7,129] On the other hand, a laminectomy that is not extended far enough rostral and caudal may result in a neurological worsening, due to a dorsal kinking (distortion) of the spinal cord. (Fig. 1–30).[7]

SUMMARY

The most clinically relevant aspects of vertebral column and spinal cord anatomy are reviewed in Chapter 1. Back and neck pain affect the majority of individuals at some time in our lives. Such pain is often due to spondylosis and intervertebral disc disease, which invariably occur to a greater or lesser extent in older individuals in the lower cervical and lumbar spine. The reasons for this finding can be understood in terms of the anatomy and biomechanics of the vertebral column.

Spinal cord anatomy including the white matter tracts, gray matter, and roots are described in clinically-oriented terms. The anatomical basis of the muscle stretch reflex is presented as well as the descending tract influence on the is reflex such as the pyramidal pathways. Furthermore, an overview of the mechanisms and biomechanics of spinal cord and nerve root injury due to mass lesions, distraction, "sagittal bowstring," and "coronal bowstring" effect are described. The anatomical basis of spinal cord function and dysfunction which is presented in Chapter 1 serves as a prelude to the physiological basis which is presented in Chapter 2.

REFERENCES

1. Sherrington CS. *The Integrative Action of the Nervous System*. New Haven: Yale University Press; 1923.
2. Hollinshead WH. *Textbook of Anatomy*. New York: Hoeber: Harper & Row; 1967.
3. Cailliet R. *Neck and Arm Pain*. Philadelphia: F.A. Davis; 1981.
4. Nachemson A. In vivo discometry in lumbar discs with irregular nucleograms. *Acta Orthop Scand* 1965;36:418–34.
5. Modic MT, Masaryk T, Paushter D. Magnetic resonance imaging of the spine. *Radiol Clin North Am* 1986;24:229–45.
6. Bogduk N. The innervation of the lumbar spine. *Spine* 1983;8:286–93.
7. Benzel EC. Biomechanics of Spine Stabilization: Principles and Clinical Practice. New York: McGraw-Hill; 1995, p. 278.
8. Berry JL, Moran JM, Berg WS, Steffee AD. A morphometric study of human lumbar and selected thoracic vertebrae. *Spine* 1987;12:362–6.
9. Panjabi MM, Duranceau J, Goel V, Oxland T, Takata K. Cervical human vertebrae: quantitative three-dimensional anatomy of the middle and lower regions. *Spine* 1991;16:861–9.
10. Panjabi MM, Takata K, Goel V, Federico D, Oxland T, Duranceau J, Krag M. Thoracic human vertebrae: quantitative three-dimensional anatomy. *Spine* 1991;16:888–901.
11. White AA, Panjabi MM. Clinical Biomechanics of the Spine. 2nd Edition. Philadelphia, PA: JB Lippincott; 1990.
12. Penning L, Wilmink JT. Rotation of the cervical spine: a CT study in normal subjects. *Spine* 1987;12:732–8.
13. Bell GH, Dunbar O, Beck JS, Gibb A. Variation in strength of vertebrae with age and their relation to osteoporosis. *Calcif Tissue Res* 1967;1:75.
14. Macintosh JE, Nikolai B. The morphology of the lumbar erector spinae. *Spine* 1987;12:658–68.

15. Perry O. Fracture of the vertebral end-plate in the lumbar spine. *Acta Orthop Scand* 1957;25 (Suppl).

16. Perry O. Resistance and compression of the lumbar vertebrae. In Encyclopedia of Medical Radiology. New York: Springer-Verlag; 1974.

17. Lin HS, Liu YK, Adams KH. Mechanical response of the lumbar intervertebral joint under physiological (complex) loading. *JBJS* 1978; 60A:41–55.

18. Panjabi M, Dvorak J, Duranceau J, Yamamoto I, Gerber M, Rauschning W, Bueff HU. Three-dimensional movements of the upper cervical spine. *Spine* 1988;13:726–30.

19. Van Schaik JPJ, Verbiest H, Van Schaik FDJ. The orientation of laminae and facet joints in the lower lumbar spine. *Spine* 1985;10: 59–63.

20. White AA, Panjabi MM. The basic kinematics of the human spine: a review of past and current knowledge. *Spine* 1978;3:12–20.

21. Shirazi-Adl A. Finite element evaluation of contact loads on facets of an L2–L3 lumbar segment in complex loads. *Spine* 1991;16: 533–41.

22. Krag MH, Weaver DL, Beynnon BD. Morphometry of the thoracic and lumbar spine related to transpedicular screw placement for surgical spinal fixation. *Spine* 1988;13:27–32.

23. Zindrick MR, Wiltse LL, Doornik A, et al. Analysis of the morphometric characteristics of the thoracic and lumbar pedicles. *Spine* 1987; 12:160–6.

24. McCormack BM, Benzel EC, Adams MS, Baldwin NG, Rupp FW, Maher DJ. Anatomy of the thoracic pedicle. *Neurosurgery* 1995; 37:303–8.

25. Broberg KB. On the mechanical behavior of intervertebral discs. *Spine* 1983;8:151–165

26. Chazal J, Tanguy A, Bourges M, et al. Biomechanical properties of spinal ligaments and a histological study of the supraspinal ligament in traction. *J Biomech* 1985;18:167.

27. Dvorak J, Schneider E, Saldinger P, Rahn B. Biomechanics of the craniocervical region: the alar and transverse ligaments. *J Orthop Res* 1988;6:452.

28. Goel VK, Njus GO. Stress-strain characteristic of spinal ligaments, 32nd *Trans Orthop Res Soc* New Orleans, 1986.

29. Myklebust JB, Pintar F, Yoganandan N, Cusick JF, Maiman D, Myers TJ, Sances A. Tensile strength of spinal ligaments. *Spine* 1988;13:526.

30. Nachemson A, Evans J. Some mechanical properties of the third lumbar inter-laminar ligament (ligamentum flavum). *J Biomech* 1968;1: 211.

31. Panjabi MM, Hausfeld JN, White AA. A biomechanical study of the ligamentous stability of the thoracic spine in man. *Acta Orthop Scan* 1981;52: 315–26.

32. Panjabi MM, Jorneus L, Greenstein G. Lumbar spine libaments: an in vitro biomechanical study. Tenth meeting of the international society for the study of the lumbar spine, Montreal, 1984.

33. Posner I, White AA III, Edwards WT, et al. A biomechanical analysis of the clinical stability of the lumbar and lumbosacral spine. *Spine* 1982; 7:374–89.

34. Tkaczuk H. Tensile properties of human lumbar longitudinal ligaments. *Acta Orthop Scand* 1968;115 (Suppl).

35. Panjabi MM. The stabilizing system of the spine. Part II: neutral zone and instability hypothesis. *J Spinal Disord* 1992;5:390–7.

36. Dickman CA, Greene KA, Sonntag VK. Injuries involving the transverse atlantal ligament: classification and treatment guidelines based upon experience with 39 injuries. *Neurosurgery* 1996; 38:44–50.

37. Tracy MF, Gibson MJ, Szypryt PE, Rutherford A, Corlett EN. The geometry of the muscles of the lumbar spine determined by magnetic resonance imaging. *Spine* 1989;14: 186–93.

38. Andriacchi TP, Schultz AB, Belytschko TB, Galante JO. A model for studies of mechanical interactions between the human spine and rib cage. *J Biomech* 1974;7:497.

39. Field EJ, Brierley JB. The lymphatic connexions of the subarachnoid space: an experimental study of the dispersion of particulate matter in the cerebrospinal fluid, with special reference to the pathogenesis of poliomyelitis. *Br Med J* 1948;1:1167–71.

40. Carpenter MB. *Human Neuroanatomy, 7th Edition.* Baltimore: William and Wilkins; 1976.

41. Sunderland S. Anatomical perivertebral influences on the intervertebral foramen. *The Research Status of Manipulative Therapy. NINCDS Monograph 15.* Washington, DC: US Dept Health, Educ, Welfare; 1975:129–40.

42. Wall EJ, Cohen MS, Massie JB, et al. Cauda equina anatomy 1: Intrathecal nerve root organization. *Spine* 1990;15:1244–7.

43. Karp SJ, Ho RTK. Gait ataxia as a presenting symptom of malignant epidural spinal cord compression. *Postgrad Med J* 1986;62:745–7.

44. Waxman SG. Pathophysiology of nerve conduction: relation to diabetic neuropathy. *Ann Int Med* 1981;92(Part 2):297–301.

45. Gilliatt RW, Willison RG. Peripheral nerve conduction in diabetic neuropathy. *J Neurol Neurosurg Psychiat* 1962;25:11–18.

46. Waxman SG, Brill M, Geschwind N, et al. Probability of conduction deficit as related to fiber length in random-distribution models of peripheral neuropathies. *J Neurol Sci* 1976;29: 39–53.

47. Coghill GE. *Anatomy and the Problem of Behavior.* London: Oxford University Press; 1929.

48. Grillner S. Locomotion in vertebrates: central mechanisms and reflex interaction. *Physiol Rev* 1975;55:247–304.

49. Cook AW, Browder EJ. Function of the posterior column. *Trans Am Neurol Assoc* 1964;89: 193–4.

50. Gilman S, Denny-Brown D. Disorders of movement and behavior following dorsal column lesions. *Brain* 1966;89:397–418.

51. Netsky M. Syringomyelia: a clinicopathologic study. *AMA Arch Neurol Psychiatr* 1953;70: 741–77.
52. Wall P. The sensory and motor role of impulses traveling in the dorsal columns towards the cerebral cortex. *Brain* 1970;93: 505–24.
53. Nathan PW, Smith MC. The centripetal pathway from the bladder and urethra within the spinal cord. *J Neurol Neurosurg Psychiat* 1951;14: 262–80.
54. Mehler WR, Feferman ME, Nauta WJ. Ascending axon degeneration following anterolateral cordotomy. An experimental study in the monkey. *Brain* 1960;83:718–50.
55. Bowsher D. Termination of the central pain pathway: the conscious appreciation of pain. *Brain* 1957;80:606–22.
56. Bowsher D. The termination of secondary somatosensory neurons within the thalamus of Macaca mulatta: an experimental degeneration study. *J Comp Neurol* 1961;177:213–27.
57. Kuypers HGJM. Central cortical projections to motor and somato-sensory cell groups. *Brain* 1960;83:161–84.
58. Liu CN, Chambers WW. An experimental study of the corticospinal system in the monkey (Macaca mulatta). The spinal pathways and preterminal distribution of degenerating fibers following discrete lesions of the pre- and postcentral gyri and bulbar pyramid. *J Comp Neurol* 1964;123:257–84.
59. Nathan PW, Smith MC. Long descending tracts in man: review of present knowledge. *Brain* 1955;78:248–303.
60. Schoen JHR. Comparative aspects of the descending fibre systems in the spinal cord. *Progr Brain Res* 1964;11:203–22.
61. Nathan PW, Smith M. Effects of two unilateral cordotomies on motility of the lower limb. *Brain* 1973;96:471–94.
62. Jane JA, Evans JP, Fisher LE. An investigation concerning the restitution of motor function following injury to the spinal cord. *J Neurosurg* 1964;21:167–71.
63. Lassek AM, Anderson P. Motor function after spaced contralateral hemisections in the spinal cord. *Neurology* 1961;11:362–5.
64. Weil A, Lassek A. Quantitative distribution of pyramidal tract in man. *Arch Neurol Psychiat* 1929;22:495–510.
65. Gijn J. The Babinski response and the pyramidal syndrome. *J Neurol Neurosurg Psychiat* 1978; 41:865–73.
66. Bucy PC, Ladpli R, Ehrlich A. Destruction of the pyramidal tract in the monkey: the effects of bilateral destruction of the cerebral peduncles. *J Neurosurg* 1966;25:1–20.
67. Bucy PC, Keplinger JE, Siqueira EB. Destruction of the pyramidal tract in man. *J Neurosurg* 1964;21:385–98.
67a. Gilman S, Marco, LA. Effects of medullary pyramidotomy in the monkey. I. Clinical and electromyographic abnormalities. *Brain* 1971;94: 495–514.
67b. Gilman S, Marco LA, Ebel HC. Effects of medullary pyramidotomy in the monkey. II. Abnormalities of spindle afferent responses. *Brain* 1971;94:515–30.
68. Lance JW. The control of muscle tone, reflexes and movement: Robert Wartenberg Lecture. *Neurology* 1980;30:1303–13.
69. Burke D. Spasticity as an adaptation to pyramidal tract injury. In Waxman SG, editor. *Functional Recovery in Neurological Disease*. New York: Raven Press; 1988.
70. Bolton B. Blood supply of the human spinal cord. *J Neurol Neurosurg Psychiatry* 1939;2: 137–48.
71. Herren TY, Alexander I. Sulcal and intrinsic blood vessels of human spinal cord. *Arch Neurol Psych* 1939;41:678–87.
72. Stoltman HF, Blackwood W. The role of ligamenta flava in the pathogenesis of myelopathy in cervical spondylosis. *Brain* 1964; 87:45–50.
73. Gillilan LA. The arterial supply of the human spinal cord. *J Comp Neurol* 1958;110:75–103.
74. Craige EH. Vascular Supply of the Spinal Cord. *The Spinal Cord: Basic Aspects and Surgical Considerations*. Springfield: Charles C. Thomas; 1961; pp 217–43.
75. Champlin AM, Rael J, Benzel EC, Kesterson L, King JN, Orrison WW, Mirfakhraee M. Preoperative spinal angiography for lateral extra cavitary approach to thoracic and lumbar spine. *AJNR Am J Neuroradiol* 1994;15:73–4.
75a. Haymaker W. *Bing's Local Diagnosis in Neurological Disease, 15th Edition*. St. Louis: C.V. Mosby; 1969.
76. Domisse GF. The blood supply of the spinal cord. A critical vascular zone in spinal surgery. *J Bone Joint Surg* 1974;56-B:225–35.
77. Henson RA, Parsons M. Ischaemic lesions of the spinal cord: an illustrated review. *Q J Med* 1967;36:205–22.
78. Buchan AM, Barnett HJM. Infarction of the spinal cord. In Barnett HJM, Mohr JP, Stein BM, Yatsu FM, editors. *Stroke: Pathophysiology, Diagnosis and Management*. New York: Churchill Livingstone; 1986; pp. 707–19.
79. Albert ML, Greer WER, Kantrowitz W. Paraplegia secondary to hypotension and cardiac arrest in a patient who has had previous thoracic surgery. *Neurology* 1969;19:915–8.
80. Blackwood W. Discussion on the vascular disease of the spinal cord. *Proc R Soc Med* 1958;51: 543–7.
81. Gilles FH, Nag D. Vulnerability of human spinal cord in transient cardiac arrest. *Neurology* 1971;21:833–9.
82. Hogan EL, Romanul FCA. Spinal cord infarction occurring during insertion of aortic graft. *Neurology* 1966;16:67–74.
83. Hughes JT, MacIntyre AG. Spinal cord infarction occurring during thoracolumbar sympathectomy. *J Neurol Neurosurg Psychiatry* 1963;26: 418–21.
84. Silver JR, Buxton PH. Spinal stroke. *Brain* 1974;97:539–50.
85. Benzel EC, Larson SJ. Functional recovery after decompressive operation for thoracic and lumbar spine fractures. *Neurosurgery* 1986;19: 772–7.

86. Jofe MH, White AA, Panjabi MM. Clinically relevant kinematics of the cervical spine. In The Cervical Spine Research Society: The Cervical Spine, 2nd Edition. Philadelphia: J. B. Lippincott; 1989.

87. Shapiro R, Youngberg AS, Rothman SLG. The differential diagnosis of traumatic lesions of the occipito-atlanto-axial segment. *Radiol Clin North Am* 1973;11:505.

88. Louis R. Spinal stability as defined by the three-column spine concept. *Anat Clin* 1985;7:33–42.

89. Denis F. The three-column spine and its significance in the classification of acute thoracolumbar spine injuries. *Spine* 1983;8:817–31.

90. Bailey RW. Fractures and dislocations of the cervical spine: orthopedic and neurosurgical aspects. *Postgrad Med* 1964;35:588–99.

91. Holdsworth FW. Fractures, dislocations and fracture dislocation sof the spine. *J Bone Joint Surg* 1963;45B:6–20.

92. Kelly RP, Whitesides TE. Treatment of lumbodorsal fracture-dislocation. *Ann Surg* 1968;167(5):705–17.

93. Benzel EC, Wild GC. Biochemical mechanisms of neural injury. In Barrow D, editor. Perspectives in Neurological Surgery. 1991;2(2):95–126.

94. Ransom BR, Waxman SG, Davis PK. Anoxic injury of CNS white matter: protective effect of ketamine. *Neurology* 1990;40:1399–1404.

95. Waxman SG, Ransom BR, Stys PK. Non-synaptic mechanisms of calcium-mediated injury in CNS white matter. *Trends Neurosci* 1991;14:461–8.

96. Stys PK, Waxman SG, Ransom BR. Ionic mechanisms of anoxic injury in mammalian CNS white matter: Role of Na^+ channels and Na^+-Ca^{2+} exchanger. *J Neurosci* 1992;12:430–9.

97. LoPachin RM, Jr., Stys PK. Elemental composition and water content of rat optic nerve myelinated axons and glial cells: effects of *in vitro* anoxia and reoxygenation. *J Neurosci* 1995;15:6735–46.

98. Agrawal SK, Fehlings MG. Mechanisms of secondary injury to spinal cord axons *in vitro*: role of Na^+-Na^+-K^+-ATPase, the Na^+-H^+ exchanger, and the Na^+-Ca^{2+} exchanger. *J Neurosci* 1996;16:545–52.

99. Imaizumi T, Kocsis JD, Waxman SG. Anoxic injury in the rat spinal cord: pharmacological evidence for multiple steps in Ca^{2+}-dependent injury of the dorsal columns. *J Neurotrauma* 1997;14:293–312.

100. Young W, DeCrescito V, Tomasula JJ. Effect of sympathectomy on spinal blood flow autoregulation and posttraumatic ischemia. *J Neurosurg* 1982;56:706–10.

101. Blight AR. Cellular morphology of chronic spinal cord injury in the cat: analysis of myelinated axons by line-sampling. *Neuroscience* 1983;10:521–43.

102. Blight AR. Delayed demyelination and macrophage invasion: a candidate for secondary cell damage in spinal cord injury. *Central Nervous System Trauma* 1985;2:299–306.

103. Waxman SG. Demyelination in spinal cord injury and multiple sclerosis: what can we do to enhance functional recovery? *J Neurotrauma* 1992;9:S15–S117.

104. Crowe MJ, Bresnahan JC, Shuman SL, Masters JN, Beattie MS. Apoptosis and delayed degeneration after spinal cord injury in rats and monkeys. *Nature Med* 1997;3:73–6.

105. Beattie MS, Shuman SL, Bresnahan JC. Apoptosis and spinal cord injury. *Neuroscientist* 1998;4:163–71.

106. Liu XZ, Xu XM, Hu R, Du C, Zhang SX, McDonald JW, Dong HX, Wu YJ, Fan GS, Jacquin MF, Hsu CY, Choi DW. Neuronal and glial apoptosis after traumatic spinal cord injury. *J Neurosci* 1997;17:5395–406.

107. National Acute Spinal Cord Injury Study Group. A randomized controlled trial of methylprednisolone or naloxone in the treatment of acute spinal cord injury. *N Engl J Med* 1990;332:1405–11.

108. Benoist G, Kausz M, Rethelyi M, Pasztor E. Sensitivity of the short-range spinal interneurons of the cat to experimental spinal cord trauma. *J Neurosurg* 1979;51:834–40.

109. Dohrmann GJ, Panjabi MM, Banks D. Biomechanics of experimental spinal cord trauma. *J Neurosurg* 1978;48:993–1001.

110. Hung T-K, Lin H, Bunegin L, Albin MS. Mechanical and neurological response of cat spinal cord under static loading. *Surg Neurol* 1982;17:213–7.

111. Tunturi AR. Elasticity of the spinal cord dura in the dog. *J Neurosurg* 1977;47:391–6.

112. Tunturi AR. Elasticity of the spinal cord, pia, and denticulate ligament in the dog. *J Neurosurg* 1978;48:975–9.

113. Shapiro K, Shulman K, Marmarou A, Poll W. Tissue pressure gradients in spinal cord injury. *Surg Neurol* 1977;7:275–9.

114. Kahn EA. The role of the dentate ligaments in spinal cord compression and the syndrome of lateral sclerosis. *J Neurosurg* 1947;4:191–9.

115. Nurick S. The pathogenesis of the spinal cord disorder associated with cervical spondylosis. *Brain* 1972;95:87–100.

116. Payne EE, Spillane JD. The cervical spine. An anatomico-pathological study of 70 specimens (using a special technique) with particular reference to the problem of cervical spondylosis. *Brain* 1957;80:571–96.

117. Reid JD. Effects of flexion-extension movements of the head and spine upon the spinal cord and nerve roots. *J Neurol Neurosurg Psychiatry* 1960;23:214–21.

118. Stoops WL, King RB. Neural complications of cervical spondylosis: their response to laminectomy and foraminotomy. *J Neurosurg* 1962;19:986–9.

119. Taylor AR. The mechanism of injury to the spinal cord in the neck without damage to the vertebral column. *JBJS* 1951;33-B:543–7.

120. Wilkinson HA, LeMay ML, Ferris EJ. Clinical-radiographic correlations in cervical spondylosis. *J Neurosurg* 1969;30:213–8.

121. Convery FR, Minteer MA, Smith RW, Emerson SM. Fracture-dislocation of the dorsal-lumbar spine. Acute operative stabilization by Harrington instrumentation. *Spine* 1978;3:160–6.
122. Cusick JF, Ackmann JJ, Larson SJ. Mechanical and physiological effects of dentatotomy. *J Neurosurg* 1977;46:767–75.
123. Breig A. Adverse mechanical tension in the central nervous system. An analysis of cause and effect: relief by functional neurosurgery. Stockholm: Almqvist and Wiksell; 1978, pp. 264.
124. Breig A. Biomechanics of the Central Nervous System. Chicago: Year Book Medical, 1960, p. 183.
125. Benzel EC, Lancon J, Kesterson L, Hadden T. Cervical laminectomy and dentate ligament section for cervical spondylotic myelopathy. *J Spinal Disord* 1991;4:286–95.

126. Morgan TH, Wharton GW, Austin GN. The results of laminectomy in patients with incomplete spinal cord injuries. *Paraplegia* 1971;9: 14–23.
127. Saunders RL. On the pathogenesis of the radiculopathy complicating multilevel corpectomy. *Neurosurgery* 1995;37:408–12.
128. Raynor RB, Pugh J, Shapiro I. Cervical facetectomy and its effect on spine strength. *J Neurosurg* 1985;63:278–82.
129. Benzel EC. Cervical spondylotic myelopathy: posterior surgical approaches. In Cooper PR, editor. Degenerative Disease of the Cervical Spine. Park Ridge, Illinois: American Association of Neurlogical Surgeons: 1992; pp. 91–104.
130. De Jong RN. *The Neurologie Examination*, ed. 4, Hagerstown: Harper and Row, 1979.
131. Makela A-L, Lang H, Sillanpas M. *Handbook of Clinical Neurology*, Volume 38. Amsterdam: Noah Holland; 1979.

Chapter 2

CLINICAL PATHOPHYSIOLOGY OF SPINAL SIGNS AND SYMPTOMS

The first task of the physician examining a patient with suspected spinal cord disease is to establish the presence or absence of such disease and, if present, then the location(s) of the lesion(s). The lesion's anatomical coordinates are its (1) "level" in the rostrocaudal axis, and (2) the extent of the lesion in the transverse plane of the spinal cord. These coordinates are determined by clinically testing specific functions of the myotomes and dermatomes served by both nerve roots and tracts that may be involved. A third coordinate is the time-course of evolution of spinal cord dysfunction; this is often important in predicting the etiology and the physiological response of the cord to compression, and in determining prognosis. For example, a patient with a long-standing lesion, such as a benign meningioma, may manifest few signs, whereas a patient with a malignancy of comparable size that is rapidly enlarging may be paraplegic. The purpose of this chapter is to provide an understanding of the clinical pathophysiology of the spinal cord and to demonstrate the methods of history-taking and physical ex-

40

amination that are helpful in assessing the patient with suspected spinal cord disease.

SEGMENTAL INNERVATION

The spinal cord is divided into 31 segments; one spinal nerve root represents each segmental level. A segment is defined as the entire region innervated by a single nerve root. Segments are further generally characterized by dermatomes, myotomes, and angiotomes.[1] (Not every segment has all three tomes.) A dermatome is the cutaneous area innervated by the sensory nerves of a single nerve root. A myotome refers to the skeletal musculature innervated by the motor nerves of one spinal root. An angiotome refers to the blood vessels innervated via the autonomic efferents in a spinal nerve. Autonomic efferents also have other autonomic functions, such as sudomotor and pilomotor activity. As discussed below, the distribution of segmental autonomic innervation differs significantly from that of dermatomal innervation.

Traversing the ventral roots of spinal nerves along with motor axons are unmyelinated axons that are probably sensory.[2] At levels from C7 to L2 and S2 to S4, autonomic fibers also traverse the ventral root. The dorsal roots convey myelinated and unmyelinated sensory fibers.

Ventral Root Dysfunction

A disturbance of ventral root function usually results in characteristic motor disturbances distinct from those arising from corticospinal tract disease or from plexus or peripheral nerve dysfunction. Although there may be a variety of signs and symptoms, in most cases the presenting chief complaint is weakness. The localization of this complaint to the ventral root is determined by the pattern of weakness and associated physical findings.

Those aspects of physical examination that are most helpful are the assessment of muscle strength, bulk, and tone. The discussion below briefly reviews these physical signs and then focuses on features of

the examination important in differentiating ventral root disturbance from other causes of weakness.

MUSCLE STRENGTH

Muscle strength may be determined by individual muscle testing or by functional assessment. Three methods of muscle strength testing are described here.

Individual muscle strength is commonly graded according to the British Medical Research Council[3] classification as shown in Table 2–1. This classification is helpful but it is insufficiently sensitive to accurately describe the many grades of weakness commonly observed. It is often necessary to assign a plus (+) or minus sign (−) to these grades. For example, a supine patient who can maintain an extended leg at the knee with the thigh supported off the bed, but who is unable to elevate the leg independently, would be assigned a grade of 3 for quadriceps strength. If the individual can elevate the leg against gravity but can't resist any further force, a grade 3+ might be assigned. We have found this modification to be helpful in following the clinical evolution of patients as well as in comparing patients.

Another potentially useful scale of strength is the modified scheme of Vignos and Archibald[4] shown in Table 2–2. Like the Karnofsky index,[5] it is a measure of overall performance that may be particularly valuable in evaluating patients with spinal cord disease because it is sensitive to disturbances in ambulation.

Table 2–1. **British Medical Research Council Scale of Muscle Strength**[3]

0:	No muscular contraction
1:	A flicker of contraction, either seen or palpated, but insufficient to move joint
2:	Muscular contraction sufficient to move joint horizontally but not against the force of gravity
3:	Muscular contraction sufficient to maintain a position against the force of gravity
4:	Muscular contraction sufficient to resist the force of gravity plus additional force
5:	Normal motor power

Table 2–2. **Scale of Muscle Strength**[*]

Grade 0:	Preclinical. All activities normal
Grade 1:	Walks normally. Unable to freely run
Grade 2:	Detectable defect in posture or gait. Climbs stairs without using bannister
Grade 3:	Climbs stairs only with bannister
Grade 4:	Walks without assistance. Unable to climb stairs
Grade 5:	Walks without assistance. Unable to rise from a chair
Grade 6:	Walks only with calipers or other aids
Grade 7:	Unable to walk. Sits erect in a chair. Able to roll a wheelchair and eat and drink normally
Grade 8:	Sits unsupported in a chair. Unable to roll a wheelchair or unable to drink from a glass unassisted
Grade 9:	Unable to sit erect without support or unable to eat or drink without assistance
Grade 10:	Confined to bed. Requires help for all activities

[*]From Walton, J,[7] p. 452, with permission.

Finally, a recently reported assessment of motor strength of the lower extremities measures the time required for an individual to rise from a standard chair ten times.[6] Although this may not be helpful in patients suffering from pain or marked weakness, it is often useful in following patients longitudinally and is particularly helpful in measuring proximal muscle strength, which is often diminished by corticosteroids or chronic disease.

MUSCLE BULK

Causes of muscular atrophy include disuse, endocrinological disturbance, malnutrition, and loss of innervation (neurogenic atrophy) such as in cases of radiculopathy. In cases of monoradiculopathy, atrophy is not prominent since most muscles receive innervation from multiple nerve roots. In cases of chronic radiculopathy (such as cervical spondylosis), atrophy may precede weakness, whereas weakness may precede atrophy in cases of acute radiculopathy (such as acute disc herniation).

Neurogenic atrophy may be associated with fasciculations, which represent the spontaneous contraction of a group of muscle fibers innervated by a single motor neuron. Fasciculations are not sufficiently strong to move a joint but can usually be seen as a rippling movement just beneath the skin. They may be difficult to see if the period of observation is brief or if the lighting is poor. It is generally best to observe the muscle obliquely rather than perpendicularly to take advantage of the shadows created by the rippling movements. Fatigue, cold, medications, and metabolic derangements often cause similar movements.

In cases of compressive root lesions, fasciculations may occur in the myotomal distribution of the compressed root. Fasciculations are also commonly observed in patients with anterior horn cell disease; however these fasciculations are different in that they don't occur repetitively in the same fasciculus during minimal contraction, and are present during complete rest.[7] Spontaneous benign fasciculations occasionally are observed in healthy individuals. Typically, they occur only after contraction of the muscle and are not associated with weakness or atrophy.[7]

MUSCLE TONE

Muscle tone, the resistance that a muscle presents to passive limb movement, is often a very valuable sign in distinguishing the site of a lesion causing weakness. When measuring muscle tone, it is imperative that the muscles be relaxed, and it is often helpful to distract the patient's attention.

Spasticity and rigidity refer to common forms of increased muscle tone due to central nervous system disease. In spasticity, the increased tone is due to an exaggeration of the stretch reflex. If the muscle is slowly stretched, increased tone may not be found. However, if the muscle is stretched more rapidly, increasing amounts of resistance are found. Spasticity has been referred to as "rate-sensitive" for this reason. When due to cortical disease, spasticity preferentially involves the flexors in the upper extremities and extensors in the lower extremities.

Rigidity refers to increased muscle tone that is not rate-sensitive—that is, not dependent on the rate of movement. Unlike spasticity, it is found equally in both extensors and flexors. Rigidity is commonly seen in patients with Parkinson's disease.

Spasticity usually results from dysfunction of the descending tracts, including the corticospinal tract.[8–11] Spinal shock is one very important condition in which interruption of descending motor tracts results in flaccid weakness.

SPINAL SHOCK

When patients present with weakness associated with reduced muscle tone or flaccidity, the examiner is usually directed to diseases of the peripheral nerves or multiple nerve roots (although other causes such as cerebellar lesions are known). If the lesion is in the thoracic spine, it may give the appearance of a cauda equina syndrome or peripheral neuropathy. A critically important diagnostic error may be made in evaluating patients in which all spinal reflexes caudal to an acute transection are lost. The clinical manifestation of spinal shock is flaccid paralysis with loss of deep tendon reflexes below the level of the lesion. When this occurs in the cervical spine, it may resemble the clinical picture of an acute polyneuropathy or polyradiculopathy, such as Guillain-Barré syndrome. These errors will delay the correct diagnosis of spinal shock and appropriate intervention, which in many cases may require surgical decompression of the cord. The clinical differentiation of spinal shock from peripheral nerve or root disease can usually be made on the basis of a sensory level, which is only present in patients with spinal cord transection. Severe bowel dysfunction and bladder dysfunction early in such a course also suggest cord involvement rather than peripheral nerve disease.

DIFFERENTIATION FROM OTHER CAUSES OF WEAKNESS

The pattern of weakness, and associated neurological findings, is of considerable localizing value. Individual nerve roots generally project to several different muscles, and individual skeletal muscles usually receive their innervation from multiple roots. An important clinical corollary is that muscle paresis is common after injury to a single nerve root but frank paralysis is unusual. Also, corticospinal and peripheral nerve dysfunction often present with paralysis of several muscles or muscle groups.

Atrophy, often severe, develops in peripheral nerve lesions as well. Atrophy is generally less prominent in isolated root lesions because multiple nerve roots innervate single muscles, and there is usually reinnervation of chronically denervated muscle fibers from adjacent roots. In some cases of radiculopathy, denervation may only be seen with electrodiagnostic studies. The most sensitive clinical finding in diagnosing root lesions, however, is a depressed deep tendon reflex of the muscle that receives much of its innervation from the injured root.

"SEGMENT-POINTER" MUSCLES

Although most muscles are innervated from multiple roots, in many cases a single muscle suffers the greatest dysfunction from a monoradiculopathy. Schliack has termed such muscles segment-pointer muscles.[1] Table 2–3 lists a group of muscles that may point the examiner to a specific nerve root. Because some individuals have prefixed and some have postfixed innervation, this listing, although very helpful as a screening examination, should not be considered infallible. A more detailed review is found in the Appendix.

PAIN

Pain is not often considered to be a manifestation of ventral root dysfunction. However, recent clinical reports suggest that irritation of the ventral root may result in

Table 2–3. **Segment-Pointer Muscles***

Root	Muscle	Primary Function
C3	Diaphragm	Respiration
C4	Diaphragm	Respiration
C5	Deltoid	Arm abduction
C5	Biceps	Forearm flexion
C6	Brachioradialis	Forearm flexion
C7	Triceps	Forearm extension
L3	Quadriceps femoris	Knee extension
L4	Quadriceps femoris	Knee extension
L4	Tibialis anterior	Foot dorsiflexion
L5	Extensor hallucis longus	Great toe dorsiflexion
S1	Gastrocnemius	Plantar flexion

*Adapted from Schliack, H,[1] p. 172.

pain that is distinct in character from the pain experienced from dorsal root irritation.[12,13] According to the theory advanced by Sir Charles Bell,[14] the ventral roots are responsible for conveying impulses controlling muscular contraction, and the dorsal roots conduct those for sensation. Magendie[15] provided the most extensive experimental support for this doctrine, which has come to be called the law of Bell and Magendie. However, pain can be induced in experimental animals through the stimulation of the ventral root. Some sensory afferents are present in the ventral roots and enter the spinal cord.[16,17]

In a series of patients undergoing operation for cervical ventral root compression, mechanical stimulation of the ventral roots evoked deep and diffuse pain, whereas stimulation of the dorsal root caused a rapid electric-like shock sensation.[18] The pain arising from the ventral roots was termed myalgic and that from the dorsal root, neuralgic. Ventral roots that had been pathologically compressed were more susceptible to eliciting pain than those which had not been pathologically compressed prior to stimulation. Furthermore, if the dorsal roots were anesthetized, the pain was not experienced.

These experimental findings in animals and humans may explain some of the myalgic-type pain that some patients report. For example, several publications have cited the cervical spine as the source for pain that may be difficult to differentiate from angina pectoris.[12,13,19,20] Because the lower cervical myotomes extend to the chest wall (see Chapter 3), and the pain arising from ventral root irritation may be similar to that arising from coronary ischemia, the designation of cervical angina has been applied.[13,21] There is little doubt that pain, perhaps of a myalgic character, may result from compression of the ventral roots elsewhere. In such cases, other signs of nerve root dysfunction such as motor, sensory, and reflex loss are often present.[12]

AUTONOMIC FIBERS

Preganglionic autonomic projections within the ventral root contain fibers that project to ganglia outside the spine. Lesions of individual roots may not disturb sweating or vasomotor control, but more extensive lesions may cause such abnormalities as hypohydrosis and hyperhydrosis. Sympathetic innervation nerves exit the spine from C8 to L2. Therefore lesions in this region may have distant effects. For example, the trigeminal region and C2 to C4 receive sympathetic innervation from C8 to T3. For this reason, a patient with a lesion in the paravertebral region of the upper thoracic spine, such as a superior sulcus tumor, may present with Horner's syndrome.[22] Table 2–4 lists the dermatomal distribution of sympathetic (sudomotor) efferents.

The parasympathetic efferents in the spine exit from the sacral roots 2–4 to innervate the pelvic viscera, genitalia, and bladder. Within the spinal cord, the nerve cell bodies for these efferents are located within the conus medullaris. Disease processes involving the conus or cauda equina may therefore present with disturbances of these functions.

Dorsal Root Dysfunction

The dorsal roots convey sensory information to the spinal cord, and disturbance of

Table 2–4. Cutaneous Distribution of Sympathetic Efferents (Sudomotor Fibers)*

Ventral Spinal Root	Corresponding Dermatomal Areas Receiving Sweat Gland Innervation
C8	C2–C4
T1–T3	Trigeminal area and C2–C4
T4	C5–C6
T5–T7	C5–T9
T8	T5–T11
T9	T6–L1
T10	T7–L5
T11	T9–S5
T12	T10–S5
L1	T11–S5
L2	T12–S5

*From Schliack, H,[1] p. 164, with permission.

their function is most commonly manifested by pain and, to a lesser extent, by sensory impairment. It is now well established that, following damage to sensory axons within peripheral nerves, there are changes in the cell bodies of dorsal root ganglion neurons that include the down-regulation of certain sodium channel genes and include the activation of other, previously silent, sodium channel genes.[23,24] As a result, inappropriate combinations of sodium channels are produced, poising nociceptive dorsal root ganglion neurons to generate inappropriate bursts of impulses that produce pain and paraesthesia.[25-27] In addition, following damage to nociceptive axons within the dorsal roots, there can be sprouting of non-nociceptive (A) afferents onto pain-signaling neurons within the superficial laminae of the dorsal horns so that ordinary tactile stimuli activate central pain pathways.[28] Pain may be local, it may be in a radicular or nonradicular distribution, and/or secondary to muscle spasm.

Back symptoms are often caused by mechanical disease of the spine, such as the common problem of spondylosis. Low back pain is the second most common cause for absenteeism in industrial settings.[29] It is usually self-limited and often responds to bed rest,[30] however, it may be the first symptom of a much more serious underlying disease. For example, as will be seen in Chapter 5, back pain and/or radicular pain is reported in approximately 95% of such patients at the time of diagnosis of cord compression.[31,32] Pain may also be a sign of serious visceral disease manifested in the spine or elsewhere. In some cases, this pain may be confused with benign regional pain, resulting in a delay in diagnosis. Clinical clues discussed below and in Chapter 3 suggest those cases where pain is more likely to be due to a serious pathology.

PAIN

Local Pain

Local or regional back or neck pain is secondary to irritation or damage of innervated structures of the spine. The periosteum, ligaments, dura, and apophyseal joints are innervated structures. However, the central regions of the vertebral body and nucleus pulposus are not innervated and cannot, therefore, be a source of pain. For this reason, the central region of a vertebral body may be replaced by tumor and yet the patient does not complain of pain. If the tumor invades the periosteum, however, pain will be reported.

Local pain is appreciated in the region of the spine and is deep, aching, and exacerbated by activity that places an increased load on diseased structures. Patients suffering from pain due to epidural tumor generally report that their pain is made worse by a supine position,[33,34] whereas those suffering from spondylosis and musculoligamentous strain generally favor bed rest. The reason for pain exacerbation in the reclining position in patients with epidural tumor is uncertain, although Rodriguez and Dinapoli[35a] suggest that a recumbent position is associated with lengthening of the spine, which presumably would cause increased traction of compressed nerve roots and spinal cord.

Palpation of the involved structures may exacerbate the local pain regardless of the cause. Surprisingly, however, percussion tenderness may not always be elicited in patients with metastatic disease. In one study[36] of 43 patients with spine metastases demonstrated by computed tomography (CT), only 20 (46%) had spinal percussion tenderness. Furthermore, of 20 patients whose tumor extended into the epidural space, only 13 (65%) had spinal percussion tenderness. The absence of percussion tenderness should not reassure the examiner that metastatic disease is unlikely.

In addition to irritation of local innervated structures, muscle spasm often causes local pain. Such pain is usually diffuse and aching, and spasm is often found on examination. Myofascial pain syndromes[37,38] may cause both local and referred pain.

Projected Pain

Projected pain arises from one anatomical site but is projected or referred to a site some distance from the site of pathology. Projected pain arising from irritation of dorsal nerve roots is of a radicular type, whereas that due to irritation of other spinal structures is usually of a nonradicular type. Although these forms of pain are not always easy to differentiate, it is important to distinguish between them because radicular pain has strong localizing value but nonradicular pain does not. Radicular pain will be used to describe pain arising from nerve root irritation with projection in that root distribution. Nonradicular referred pain (called simply referred pain in the interest of brevity) will be discussed separately.

Referred Pain

Referred pain arising from disease of the spine has been studied by several investigators.[39-41] After injecting hypertonic saline in the region of the interspinous ligament, Kellgren concluded that pain arising from pathology of this region was referred in a segmental distribution. This study was criticized by Sinclair and associates,[41] who concluded that the pattern of

segmental pain referral was, in fact, due to nerve root irritation.

In one study,[40] the pattern of pain referral was examined in normal volunteers after injection of 6% saline into the apophyseal joints of L1–2 and L4–5. The pain exhibited was cramping and aching in quality. As shown in Figure 2–1, there was overlap in the regions of pain referral

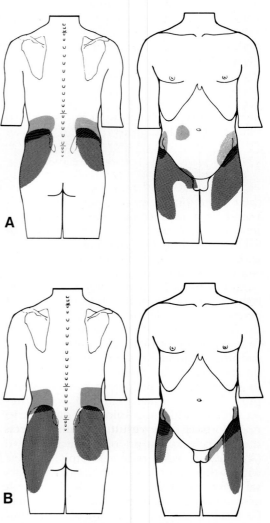

Figure 2–1. Patterns of referred pain. The distribution of pain referral from L1–2 (diagonal lines) and L4–5 (crosshatching) are superimposed following intracapsular (A) and pericapsular (B) injections. Overlap of the patterns is shown in the region of the iliac crest and groin. (From McCall, IW, et al.,[40] p. 18, with permission.)

from upper and lower lumbar injections, with most of the pain being referred to the flanks, buttocks, groin, and thighs. It is of clinical interest that referred pain did not project below the knee despite the fact that the L4–5 level was stimulated. McCall concluded that unlike radicular pain, referred pain does not follow segmental dermatomes and is not helpful in localization.

Although there may be paresthesias in the cutaneous area of pain referral as well as tenderness to deep palpation of the muscles, there are no neurologic abnormalities found in cases with referred pain of nonradicular origin. (This situation is unlike radicular pain, where disturbance of the nerve root may often be present in the form of sensory loss, hyporeflexia, and/or ventral root dysfunction.) Referred pain is generally aggravated and relieved by the same maneuvers that alter local pain.

Referred pain arising from disease of visceral structures may mimic referred pain from the spine. The autonomic nervous system provides both efferent and afferent innervation of the viscera. Up to 10% of all dorsal root afferents are visceral in origin.[42] Visceral pain may thus be referred in segmental distributions. The skin in these areas of referral may be hypersensitive. Head's zones and muscles may be tender in the region of pain referral.[43] Table 2–5 lists patterns of pain referral from common causes of visceral disease, which often create diagnostic problems.

Radicular Pain

Radicular pain arises from irritation of the dorsal roots. The resulting pain projects to the region of segmental innervation of the respective nerve. As noted above, unlike other forms of referred pain, radicular pain has great specificity for localizing disease causing irritation of a nerve root. Since it is diagnostically so valuable, it is important to recognize and accurately diagnose the level of radicular involvement. Table 2–6 lists the common sites to which pain of radicular origin is projected.

Radicular pain is often sharp and stabbing, and it can be associated with a

Table 2–5. **Patterns of Visceral Pain Referral**[*]

Visceral Source of Pain	Roots	Pain Referred to
Heart	T1–5	Chest and arm
Stomach	T5–9	Region of xiphoid
Duodenum	T6–10	Xiphoid to umbilicus
Pancreas	T7–9	Upper abdomen or back
Gallbladder	T6–10	Right upper abdomen
Appendix	T11–12	Right lower quadrant
Kidney, glans	T9–L2	Costovertebral angle, penis
Prostate region	S2–4	Glans penis, lumbar

*Adapted from Haymaker, W,[67] p. 67.

chronic ache that radiates from the spine to the distribution of the involved nerve root. Maneuvers that stretch or further compress the nerve root, such as coughing, sneezing, straight leg raising and neck flexion, generally aggravate the pain. The patient may avoid certain activities and postures that place further stretch on the nerve. For example, in the case of sciatica, the patient may prefer to maintain the leg in a flexed posture at the hip and knee and to plantar flex the foot. Such a posture results in a rather characteristic gait in these patients. Cutaneous paresthesias and tenderness of tissues in the region of pain projection, as in referred pain, are common. However, in cases of radicular pain there may also be sensory disturbances and, at times, reflex and motor abnormalities corresponding to the injured nerve root. Motor disturbances are described in the section on ventral root disorders.

CASE ILLUSTRATION

A 62-year-old man with lymphoma was referred for evaluation of pain in the right buttock, which radiated down the lateral aspect of the thigh to the region of the patella. The pain

Table 2–6. **Differential Diagnosis of Lesions on Nerve Roots***

				Roots		
	C5	C6	C7	C8	D1	
Sensory supply	Lateral border upper arm	Lateral forearm including thumb	Over triceps, mid-forearm and middle finger	Medial forearm to include little finger	Axilla down to the olecranon	
Sensory loss	As above	As above	Middle fingers	As above	As above	
Area of pain	As above and medial scapula border	As above esp. thumb and index finger	As above and medial scapula border	As above	Deep aching in shoulder and axilla to olecranon	
Reflex arc	Biceps jerk	Supinator jerk	Triceps jerk	Finger jerk	None	
Motor deficit	Deltoid Supraspinatus Infraspinatus Rhomboids	Biceps Brachioradialis Brachialis (Pronators and supinators of forearm)	Latissimus dorsi Pectoralis major Triceps Wrist extensors Wrist flexors	Finger flexors Finger extensors Flexor carpi ulnaris (thenar muscles in some patients)	*All* small hand muscles (in some thenar muscles via C8)	
Some causative lesions	Brachial neuritis Cervical spondylosis Upper plexus avulsion	Cervical spondylosis Acute disc lesions	Acute disc lesions Cervical spondylosis	Rare in disc lesions or spondylosis	Cervical rib Outlet syndromes Pancoast tumour Metastatic carcinoma in deep cervical nodes	

Roots

	L2	L3	L4	L5	S1
Sensory supply	Across upper thigh	Across lower thigh	Across knee to medial malleolus	Side of leg to dorsum and sole of foot	Behind lateral malleolus to lateral foot
Sensory loss	Often none	Often none	Medial leg	Dorsum of foot	Behind lateral malleolus
Area of pain	Across thigh	Across thigh	Down to medial malleolus	Back of thigh, lateral calf—dorsum of foot	Back of thigh, back of calf lateral foot
Reflex arc	None	Adductor reflex	Knee jerk	None	Ankle jerk
Motor deficit	Hip flexion	Knee extension Adduction of thigh	Inversion of the foot	Dorsiflexion of toes and foot (latter L4 also)	Plantar flexion and eversion of foot
Some causative leisions		Neurofibroma Meningioma Neoplastic disease Disc lesions very rare (except L4 <5 percent *all*)			Disc lesions Metastatic malignancy Neurofibromas Meningioma

*From Patten, J,[37] p. 195 and 211, with permission.

was provoked by neck flexion and occasionally was present in the recumbent position. Neurological examination was remarkable for an equivocal reduction of the right patellar reflex and positive reverse straight leg raising that provoked the leg pain. Plain films of the spine were unrevealing but a CT scan with intravenous contrast enhancement demonstrated a small mass lesion in the region of the L3–4 foramen compressing the L3 nerve root. This was considered to be lymphoma and radiation therapy was commenced. Following radiation therapy, the pain resolved entirely and the knee reflex returned to normal.

Comment. This case illustrates the sensitivity and specificity of radicular pain in localizing an epidural neoplasm. The pain, which was primarily present on neck flexion, convinced the examiner that the lesion was most probably in the spinal axis and not in the pelvis, hip, or elsewhere. The workup, therefore, was immediately directed to the spine despite the fact that there were only equivocal reflex findings.

SENSORY DISTURBANCES

Just as referred pain from the spine or from visceral sources may mimic radicular pain, so may irritation of peripheral nerves cause diagnostic confusion. For example, carpal tunnel syndrome may commonly cause pseudoradicular symptoms in the proximal arm. Similarly, the piriformis muscle in the pelvis may compress the sciatic nerve, causing sciatica that may be difficult to differentiate from radicular syndromes. In cases of nerve root injury and peripheral nerve injury, pain may be associated with sensory loss, unlike other forms of referred pain in which true sensory loss is not found. Careful attention to the sensory exam may help distinguish between these various causes of radicular and nonradicular projected pain and pain arising from peripheral nerve injury.

Although there can be sensory loss in both radicular pain and pain secondary to peripheral nerve injury, the type and pattern of sensory loss are different in the two situations. A knowledge of dermatomal and peripheral nerve cutaneous innervation is, of course, helpful in distin-

guishing the two causes. It is important to recognize that since there is considerable overlap in dermatomal areas of tactile sensation, loss of touch does not generally occur as a result of monoradiculopathy. However, since the dermatomal representation of pain sensation has less overlap, monoradiculopathies result in a greater area of pinprick analgesia than of tactile anesthesia. Alternatively, in the case of a peripheral nerve lesion, one will often find an area of tactile anesthesia due to lack of overlap of peripheral nerve cutaneous distribution. However, individual variations in cutaneous innervation occur frequently.

Dermatomes

A knowledge of the dermatomal map is crucial for recognizing and localizing radicular syndromes. As in many other areas of neurophysiology, Sherrington laid the groundwork for our current anatomical knowledge of dermatomes.[44] Using the method of residual sensibility, he mapped the dermatomes in primates by sectioning the adjacent dorsal roots above and below a single dorsal root. The remaining area of sensibility was considered to be the dermatome of the intact dorsal root. Modern knowledge of dermatomal maps in humans dates back to Foerster's work,[45] which utilized this strategy in monkeys. Foerster demonstrated that there is significant overlap in dermatomal representations in humans.

More recent physiological studies in monkeys have demonstrated even greater variability in the dermatomal maps than previous studies had suggested.[46] Recent studies suggest that the axons of each dorsal root innervate the cutaneous region of up to five adjacent dermatomes.[47] This would mean that each area of skin may be innervated by several adjacent dorsal root ganglia. Thus, our current definition of a dermatome may need to be reformulated.[48]

Although these newer findings are expected to lead to changes in our concepts and definitions of dermatomes, Figure 2–2 illustrates a currently recognized dermatomal map that has considerable clinical value. A few points deserve emphasis:

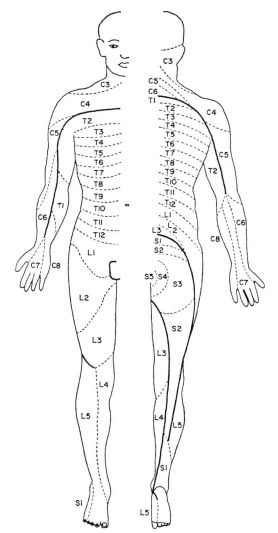

Figure 2–2. A dermatomal map. (From Sinclair, D,[183] p. 41, with permission.)

1. There is no C1 dermatome.
2. On the trunk, the C4 and T2 dermatomes are contiguous.
3. The thumb, middle finger, and fifth digits are innervated by C6, C7, and C8, respectively.
4. The nipple is at the level of T4.
5. The umbilicus is at the T10 level.
6. In the posterior axial line of the leg (medial thigh), the lumbar and sacral dermatomes are contiguous.

Finally, there are variations in dermatomal maps between individuals that may make clinical conclusions based upon sensory testing alone problematic.

Deep Tendon Reflexes

In addition to motor and sensory disturbances, deep tendon reflex abnormalities can be of precise localizing value in spine disease. As demonstrated in Figure 2–3, the stretch, or myotatic reflex, is a monosynaptic reflex that requires both ventral and dorsal roots to function normally. When deep tendon reflexes are focally hypoactive, they can be sensitive indicators of specific root disturbance. When they are hyperactive below a specific level (or acutely hypoactive or absent in spinal shock), they may indicate a myelopathy at some more rostral level.

The combination of hypoactive reflexes at a segmental level and hyperactive reflexes caudal to this level is commonly found in patients with cervical spine disease. For example, although a variety of diseases may be responsible, cervical spondylosis in the lower cervical spine may result in the combination of hyporeflexia of the brachioradialis due to impingement on C5 and C6 roots and hyperreflexia below this level secondary to an associated myelopathy. When the brachioradialis reflex is stimulated in this case, one paradoxically finds contraction of the finger flexors (rather than flexion) and supination of the hand.[35] Such a response is called inversion of the radial reflex. Table 2–6 identifies nerve roots and their associated deep tendon reflexes.

The superficial reflexes also require intact spinal roots as well as intact descending tracts from the brain through the spinal cord. The most commonly tested superficial reflexes are shown in Table 2–7. Diminution or absence of the abdominal, cremasteric, or anal reflexes may occur due to lesions interrupting the nerve roots subserving such reflexes or as a consequence of lesions of pyramidal and/or other descending tracts. When there is a reduction in these superficial reflexes and an increase in deep tendon reflexes, the lesion is generally found in the descending tracts within the brain or spinal cord. A pathological plantar response, the

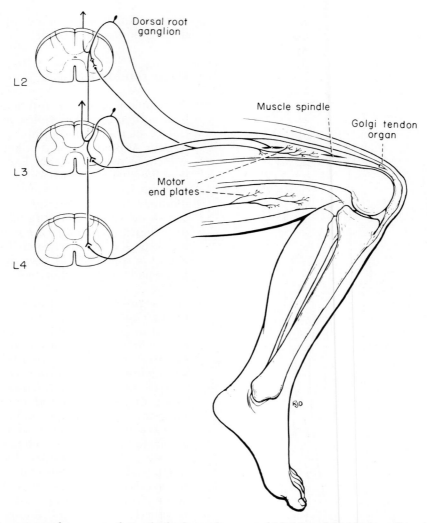

Figure 2–3. The motor and sensory pathways in the femoral nerve and L2, L3, and L4 which mediate the patellar myotatic reflex. The muscle spindles, which respond to a brisk stretching of the muscle as occurs with tapping the patella, are shown entering the L3 spinal segment. These afferent nerves synapse with anterior horn cells at the same levels to complete the reflex arc. Excessive stretching stimulates the Golgi tendon organs which are shown entering the L2 spinal segment and which inhibit the extrafusal muscle fibers via an interneuron. A pathway for reciprocol inhibition of the antagonistic muscle, the hamstring, is also shown. (From Carpenter, MB,[180] p. 236, with permission.)

Table 2–7. **Commonly Tested Superficial Reflexes and Corresponding Spinal Roots**

Abdominal, T7–T12
Cremasteric, L1–L2
Anal, S2–S4
Plantar, S1–S2

Babinski sign, indicates corticospinal tract dysfunction and is discussed below.

Nerve Root versus Peripheral Nerve Lesion

As indicated above, monoradiculopathies rarely cause frank paralysis of a single muscle or muscle group, whereas such paralysis is quite common in cases of peripheral nerve damage. A knowledge of innervation of muscle groups is important in making the distinction (Table 2–8; see Table 2–6).

The sensory examination may be helpful in distinguishing peripheral nerve lesions from radiculopathies. Knowledge of the peripheral nerve sensory distributions and of dermatomal anatomy is important. In addition, as already discussed, cutaneous tactile loss is more frequent in peripheral nerve lesions than in monoradiculopathies; in radiculopathies, loss of tactile sensation is unusual due to overlap of dermatomes.[1]

Finally, whereas peripheral nerve injuries frequently are associated with autonomic complaints, monoradiculopathies ordinarily are not. This distinction is due to the fact that the sympathetic ganglia are located peripheral to the spine and receive their preganglionic input from several segmental levels. The postganglionic efferents then join the peripheral nerves, so injuries to peripheral nerves generally are associated with loss of sweating.[1]

LOCALIZATION AND CHARACTERIZATION OF THE SEGMENTAL LEVEL OF SPINAL CORD DYSFUNCTION

Motor Disturbances

Following pain, the most common symptom of patients suffering from neoplastic spinal cord compression is weakness.[31] Weakness, particularly of the legs, must always be viewed as a possible early manifestation of spinal cord disease. The pattern of weakness as well as the associated reflex findings and muscle tone can direct the physician to the anatomical localization and may suggest the etiology as well. In spinal cord disease, weakness is classified as either due to lower motor neuron or corticospinal tract dysfunction.

As mentioned above, the findings of lower motor neuron dysfunction are weakness associated with atrophy, hypotonia, fasciculations, and depressed reflexes of a single extremity (myotome). Upper motor neuron disease often manifests with spasticity, hyperreflexia, and Babinski sign (note the exception of spinal shock), as well as weakness involving more than a single extremity. In the case of cervical spine disease, one may find a combination of lower motor neuron disturbance involving the upper extremity and upper motor neuron findings in one or both lower extremities.

Perhaps the most important clue in suggesting a spinal origin to weakness is the pattern of weakness. In individuals with hemiparesis involving the face, arm, and leg, there is usually no confusion that the site of localization is in the brain. Similarly in patients with definite paraparesis or quadriparesis, the examiner is usually directed to the spinal cord. The occurrence of monoparesis creates the most diagnostic confusion. In diagnosing spinal cord tumors at an eary stage, the patient may present with unilateral leg weakness, and examination may not reveal findings in the contralateral leg or the arms. In such cases, the physician may erroneously attribute the disorder to an anterior cerebral artery stroke, especially if the patient indicates that it was acute in onset. In our experience, anterior cerebral artery strokes are a relatively uncommon cause of unilateral leg weakness in comparison with the frequency of cases due to spinal pathology.

Lesions of the craniocervical junction and cervical spine often present with a pattern of unilateral arm weakness before progressing to ipsilateral leg weakness and finally contralateral involvement.[49,50] Although weakness involving an ipsilateral arm and leg with sparing of the face suggests a high cervical lesion, cerebral disturbances or pyramidal infarction[51] may account for this localization. Finally, not all cases of apparent lower extremity weakness are due to spinal cord disease. Many patients treated with corticosteroids or who have generalized cachexia appear to present with leg weakness because their chief complaint is often gait difficulty.

Table 2–8. **Differential Diagnosis of Lesions of Peripheral Nerves***

Nerves	Axillary	Musculocutaneous	Radial	Median	Ulnar
Sensory supply	Over deltoid	Lateral forearm to wrist	Lateral dorsal forearm and back of thumb and index finger	Lateral palm and lateral fingers	Medial palm and 5th and medial half ring finger
Sensory loss	Small area over deltoid	Lateral forearm	Dorsum of thumb and index (if any)	As above	As above but often none at all
Area of pain	Across shoulder tip	Lateral forearm	Dorsum of thumb and index	Thumb, index and middle finger. Often spreads up forearm	Ulnar supplied fingers and palm distal to wrist. Pain occasionally along course of nerve
Reflex arc	Nil	Biceps jerk	Triceps jerk and supinator jerk	Finger jerks (flexor digitorum sublimis)	Nil
Motor deficit	Deltoid (teres minor cannot be evaluated)	Biceps Brachialis (coracobrachialis weakness not detectable)	Triceps Wrist extensors Finger extensors Brachioradialis Supinator of forearm	Wrist flexors Long finger flexors (thumb, index and middle finger) Pronators of forearm. Abductor pollicis brevis	All small hand muscles excluding abductor pollicis brevis. Flexor carpi ulnaris. Long flexors of ring and little finger
Some causative lesions	Fractured neck of humerus, Dislocated shoulder Deep I.M. injections	Very rarely damaged	Crutch palsy. Saturday night palsy. Fractured humerus. In supinator muscle	Carpal tunnel syndrome Direct trauma to wrist	Elbow: trauma, bed rest, fractured olecranon. Wrist: local trauma, ganglion of wrist joint

Nerves	Obturator	Femoral	Sciatic Nerve	
			Peroneal Division	**Tibial Division**
Sensory supply	Medial surface of thigh	Anteromedial surface of thigh and leg to medial malleolus	Anterior leg, dorsum of ankle and foot	Posterior leg, sole and lateral border of foot
Sensory loss	Often none	Usually anatomical	Often just dorsum of foot	Sole of foot
Area of pain	Medial thigh	Anterior thigh and medial leg	Often painless	Often painless
Reflex arc	Adductor reflex	Knee jerk	None	Ankle jerk
Motor deficit	Adduction of thigh	Extension of knee	Dorsiflexion, inversion and eversion of the foot (+ lateral hamstrings)	Plantar flexion and inversion of foot (+ medial hamstrings)
Some causative lesions	Pelvic neoplasm Pregnancy	Diabetes Femoral hernia Femoral artery aneurysm Posterior abdominal neoplasm Psoas abscess	Pressure palsy at fibula neck Hip fracture/dislocation Penetrating trauma to buttock Misplaced injection	Very rarely injured even in buttock Peroneal division more sensitive to damage

*From Patten, J.,[37] p. 195 and 211, with permission.

CASE ILLUSTRATION

A 75-year-old man with a several-year history of lymphoma was referred for progressive gait difficulty over a two-month period. The patient had a history of bone marrow involvement with lymphoma and had received multiple courses of chemotherapy. His most recent course of chemotherapy was completed three months earlier and had included vinca alkaloids and corticosteroids. His extent of disease evaluation just prior to neurological referral had included no evidence of lymphoma on physical examination and a negative chest–abdominal CT scan, negative bone marrow, and negative cerebrospinal fluid (CSF) cytology, although the CSF protein was mildly elevated at 75 mg per dl. The patient denied any pain but complained of leg weakness out of proportion to weakness elsewhere.

His neurological examination revealed a normal mental status and cranial nerves, and the motor examination resulted in a grade 6 score (Vignos Archibald scale[4]) with only apparent mild to moderate weakness of the upper extremities. The patient had no deep tendon reflexes (due to vinca alkaloids) and had only minimal sensory loss distally in the upper and lower extremities. Sphincters were intact. There was no evidence of spinal tenderness or Lhermitte's sign, and straight leg raising provoked no pain. Total spine films were unrevealing. The patient died within a few days of referral.

Autopsy demonstrated a pulmonary embolus as the proximate cause of death. There was no evidence of brain or spinal involvement by lymphoma. There was no evidence of motor neuronopathy on histological examination of the spinal cord.[49] Muscle histological examination revealed no sign of polymyositis. The patient had a massive amount of lymphoma in the mesentery and retroperitoneal space that was not evident in imaging studies three weeks before death.

Comment. This case illustrates apparent paraparesis due to advanced malignancy without spinal cord involvement. The absence of back or radicular pain made a diagnosis of cord compression less likely but, of course, did not exclude it. The pathophysiological basis for such cases of severe gait difficulty is not usually satisfactorily explained, although the cases are often attributed to a paraneoplastic syndrome without further pathological or physiological definition. The important lesson is that without definitive imaging of the spine one could not be confident that the cause of weakness was not cord compression from lymphoma.

Superficial Reflexes

Superficial reflexes, which occur in response to stimulation of the skin or mucous membranes, are often abnormal in patients suffering from spinal cord or cauda equina disease. The most commonly tested superficial reflexes in the patient suspected to have spine disease are the superficial abdominal, anal, cremasteric, and Babinski reflexes. The superficial abdominal reflexes are tested by stimulating the abdominal wall with a blunt or sharp object unilaterally and observing for contraction of the ipsilateral abdominal muscles. The normal response is contraction of the underlying abdominal muscles resulting in deviation of the umbilicus or linea alba to the ipsilateral side. Each of the four quadrants of the abdominal wall is stimulated independently. The upper abdominal, or supraumbilical, reflex is innervated by nerve roots T7–9. The umbilical reflex is innervated by nerve roots T9–11 and the lower abdominal, or infraumbilical, is innervated by the lower thoracic and upper lumbar roots.

As with deep tendon reflexes, if there is injury or compression of the spinal roots subserving the reflex, then there may be selective diminution of that specific abdominal reflex. There is a pathway that facilitates the superficial abdominal reflexes. This pathway ascends the spinal cord to the brain, where it synapses with neurons, giving rise to descending fibers that course within or adjacent to the pyramidal tracts. If this cerebral loop is interrupted, then the superficial abdominal reflex is diminished or abolished. If the lesion is above the decussation of the pyramidal tract, then the absent abdominal reflexes will be contralateral to the lesion. If the lesion is within the spinal cord, then the reflex loss will be ipsilateral to the pathology. Such damage to the pyramidal pathways may give rise to dissociation of reflexes, that is, absent superficial abdominal reflexes with exaggerated deep tendon reflexes.

Superficial abdominal reflexes may, however, be absent for a number of reasons other than neurological disease. Complicating factors can include deep sleep, anesthesia, coma, obesity, multiparous females, the acute abdomen, postsurgical abdominal incisions, childhood, advanced age, and others. It is important to recognize that the reflex may fatigue easily after a few stimuli. When there is unilateral loss of the reflex in the absence of a local cause (such as abdominal incision), neurological etiologies are usually responsible.

The superficial abdominal reflexes are often lost in cases of intrinsic cord disease such as demyelination, as well as in cases of cord compression from extramedullary disease. Although considered a sign of pyramidal tract disease, they are not involved in most cases of amyotrophic lateral sclerosis, suggesting that the pathways subserving the superficial abdominal reflex are not dependent on the upper motor neuron pathways.

The cremasteric reflex is elicited by stimulating the skin of the upper, inner thigh from proximal to distal and observing for ipsilateral elevation of the testicle as a result of contraction of the cremasteric muscle. The nerve roots innervating the reflex are L1 and L2 via the ilioinguinal and genitofemoral nerves. The cremasteric reflex may be absent in the elderly man or when a varicocele, epididymitis, or other urological diseases are present. As above, one may find a loss of the cremasteric reflex in association with exaggeration of the deep tendon reflexes. This finding also suggests disturbance in the ascending or descending tracts of spine or brain.

The cutaneous anal reflex is the contraction of the external anal sphincter upon stimulation of the perianal tissues. This reflex is innervated by nerve roots S2–4 via the inferior hemorrhoidal nerve.[5] The cutaneous anal reflex is to be distinguished from the internal anal sphincter reflex, which is elicited by introduction of a finger into the anus.

BABINSKI SIGN

The Babinski response, or upgoing toe, is recognized as a very useful sign of corticospinal tract disease. Plantar stimulation is, therefore, tested in patients with leg weakness in an attempt to differentiate upper motor neuron causes from other etiologies. Landau, Gijn, and others have studied the pathophysiological basis of the plantar response extensively.[52–54]

There are many pitfalls in the method of testing. If the stimulus is applied to the medial or tender palm of the sole, then a flexor response may falsely be elicited.[37] Alternatively, if the flexor creases of the toes are stimulated directly, then an extensor response with no diagnostic value can generally be expected. The examiner should stimulate the lateral aspect of the foot from the heel towards the toes and then move the stimulating object across the ball of the foot in order to avoid false-positive or false-negative results.

The Babinski sign may be found in otherwise asymptomatic patients with no neurological complaints. For example, a Babinski sign was reported in approximately 4% of a series of 2500 nonneurological hospitalized patients.[55] In addition, a Babinski reflex developed in over 7% of normal individuals after a 14-mile march.[56]

Sensory Disturbances

The sensory examination is generally recognized as the most difficult part of the neurological examination for two reasons: First, it is often difficult to know whether the slight alterations in sensation that the patient reports are clinically significant. The second, and perhaps more important, reason is that subjective sensory complaints generally precede objective sensory signs and therefore may be the first sign of serious underlying neurological disease. One corollary is that in the absence of sensory complaints, the sensory examination is usually normal. Thus in the patient with no sensory complaints, a survey of sensory function by testing position and vibration sense in the toes and fingers and pin sensation of the face, trunk, and extremities is usually sufficient. If abnormalities are found or there is evidence of spinal root or peripheral nerve dysfunction, then a more detailed examination is, of course, required.

Some techniques are helpful in performing the sensory exam: (1) test pinprick from the area of reduced sensation to the normal area; (2) test pinprick sensation over the entire limb, from distal to proximal, in the patient who does not report decreased sensation; (3) watch the patient's facial expression (i.e., look for a wince) when testing pinprick sensation, especially in the encephalopathic or demented patient; (4) ask the patient to use his or her own index finger to outline the area of subjectively reduced sensation.

As already discussed, radicular sensory complaints may be the first manifestation of spinal root pathology. Dysfunction of the posterior columns or lateral spinothalamic pathways also may first present with characteristic symptoms. Tingling paresthesias that may be vibratory in nature are sometimes reported below the level of a posterior column lesion.[37] Subjective reports of the skin being too tight or an extremity or trunk being wrapped in bandages also may be due to posterior column disturbances.[37]

Spinothalamic tract disturbance is often first manifested, especially in chronic cases such as intramedullary lesions, by poorly characterized and localized pain. We have seen one patient with an intramedullary neoplasm involving the lateral spinothalamic tracts who complained of burning, searing pain of the arms and trunk. Convinced that she had visceral disease, she underwent bone scans, mammography, electrocardiograms (ECGs), and other imaging studies until it was clear that her pain was spinal in origin. Many complaints of patients with intramedullary lesions are not associated with any abnormal signs early in their course, so the complaints may be inappropriately dismissed after what is considered a negative workup of the suspected organ. Since the descriptions of the sensation often seem atypical, they may incorrectly be ignored by the physician when the physical examination is normal.

When signs of sensory disturbance are present, the cause of sensory symptoms is more readily recognized. Pain sensation, usually measured by pinprick and temperature, is conveyed via the lateral spinothalamic tract. As noted in Chapter 1, these pathways are somatotopically organized so that the sacral fibers are most peripheral and the cervical fibers are most central. Since a laterally placed extramedullary lesion will compress the peripheral fibers before the more centrally located fibers, a lesion in the rostral spine may give rise to an apparently ascending myelopathy. The pin and temperature sensory disturbance is, of course, contralateral to the involved spinothalamic tract.[15]

Position and vibration sensations, transmitted through the posterior columns, are generally easily evaluated. Ataxia due to spinal lesions is not as readily recognized. A bizarre ataxic gait may result from disturbances of posterior columns or possibly the spinocerebellar tracts[57] and may be particularly evident in combined systems disease. Light touch is conveyed by both lateral columns and posterior columns and usually is not impaired as early in spinal cord disease as the more specific modalities.

CHARACTERISTIC SENSORY DISTURBANCE PATTERNS

Immediately after complete transverse lesions of the spinal cord, a sensory level with loss of all sensation caudal to the lesion is found (Fig. 2–4A). In time, however, the area of analgesia extends higher than the area of complete anesthesia,[58] owing to the wider distribution of tactile sensibility than pain sensibility of nerve roots.

Several incomplete lesions of the spinal cord result in characteristic sensory signs. A hemisection of the spinal cord results in the so-called Brown-Séquard syndrome, in which there is loss of pain and temperature sense contralateral to the lesion and loss of position and vibration senses and paralysis ipsilateral to the lesion (Fig. 2–4B).

An early intramedullary lesion of the cord may give rise to a dissociated sensory loss in which the decussating fibers at the

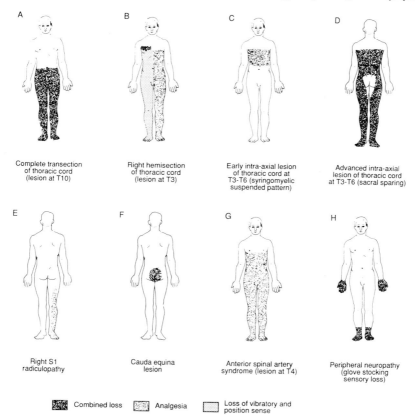

Figure 2–4. Characteristic sensory disturbances found in various spinal cord lesions in comparison to peripheral neuropathy.

level of the lesion mediating sensation of pin and temperature are lost or decreased, whereas the position and vibratory sensibilities remain unimpaired (Fig. 2–4C). In the cervical spine, such a clinical presentation may be caused by a syrinx, or by a neoplasm or central contusion of the cord. Central cord lesions may also result in a suspended sensory level (Fig. 2–4D). In such cases, sacral sensation is preserved until late in the course because these fibers are most peripheral in the lateral spinothalamic tracts and tend to be involved later. Similarly, a lateral brain-stem lesion may rarely give rise to a rostral sensory level over the contralateral trunk or a suspended sensory level with the lower border over the trunk.[59]

FALSE LOCALIZING SIGNS

Infrequently, a centrally placed anterior epidural lesion, such as a central cervical

disc herniation, may result in a sensory level several segments below the level of the spinal cord compression. Simmon described five cases of radiographically proven painless, central cervical disc herniations between C3 and C6 with the clinical examination demonstrating thoracic levels of hypalgesia between T5 and T7 (Table 2–9[60]). Some patients had other signs of myelopathy, such as spasticity, leg weakness, and hyperreflexia. The progressive neurological complaints of numbness and, when present, weakness, resolved with surgical excision of the offending disc material. The pathophysiology of this discrepancy could not be confidently explained, nor could the authors attribute the discrepancy in the level of cord compression from the sensory level on the basis of the lamination of the tracts, since each mass was anterior, not lateral. These findings, and similar falsely localizing sensory levels with laterally placed ex-

Table 2–9. **Examples of Painless Cervical Myelopathy with Sensory Levels***

Case	Sensory Level	Level of Cord Compression
1	T5–T12 bilaterally	C3–C4
2	T5 bilaterally	C5–C6
3	T7 left	C5–C6
4	T6 right	C3–C4
5	T6 right	C5–C6

*From Simmon, Z, et al.,[60] p. 871, with permission.

tramedullary lesions, underscore the importance of recognizing that a rostral lesion may give rise to a sensory level far below the site of compression. In practical terms, therefore, one may need to image the entire spine rostral to the sensory level in order to exclude a higher lesion with certainty.

Autonomic Disturbances

Disturbances of spinal cord and caudal equina function are often manifested as symptoms and signs of bladder, bowel, and sexual dysfunction and, less commonly, as respiratory compromise. The anatomy and pathophysiology of these pathways are discussed in this section.

Although the diaphragm, intercostal muscles, and abdominal muscles all are used for normal respiration, individuals may ventilate adequately with only the diaphragm intact. This massive muscle is usually innervated by nerve roots C3–5 (though it may be prefixed, innervated by nerve roots C2–4, or postfixed, innervated by nerve roots C4–6). With complete transection of the cord between the cervicomedullary junction and C3, respiration cannot be maintained. In partial transections involving bilateral anterolateral quadrants, a condition referred to as Ondine's curse occurs.[61–63] Since the pathways for voluntary control of respirations in the lateral quadrant of the spinal cord are intact but the pathways for automatic control in the anterior quadrant are lost,

the patient must remain awake in order to avoid apnea, which occurs upon falling asleep.[64] Foramen magnum tumors, atlanto-axial dislocation,[65] and congenital disturbances of the craniocervical junction are frequent causes of upper cervical spine compression.

The urinary bladder is innervated by (1) sympathetic nerves beginning in the intermediolateral cell column at the lumbar level (primarily L1 and L2 with some contribution from L3 and L4), (2) parasympathetic nerves exiting at S2–4, and (3) the somatic efferent nerves to the skeletal muscles of the external urethral sphincter, exiting at S2–4 to form the pudendal nerves. In complete transverse lesions of the cord, an immediate flaccid bladder ensues. In unilateral lesions, as demonstrated by anterolateral cordotomy,[66] voluntary control of micturition is not lost. Thus it is unusual to have sphincter function disturbed early in spinal cord compression when there is only unilateral or equivocal bilateral lower extremity weakness or sensory disturbance. The most common exception to this rule is when the conus medullaris or sacral nerve roots alone are compressed.

In infancy and early development, bladder contraction occurs as a reflex mediated largely via S2–4. Voluntary bladder control involves the development of inhibition of the bladder evacuation reflex. Micturition is initiated by voluntary modulation of this inhibition and requires the integrity of descending axons. The majority of these fibers run in the lateral columns near the equatorial plane, lateral to the central canal and just anterior to the corticospinal tract.[66] The descending micturition pathways are just posterolateral to the descending pathways for automatic breathing in the cervical spine and just medial to the ascending spinothalamic pathways.[66] When the cord is injured above the spinal segment S1, descending inhibition is lost and the sacral (S2–4) reflex arc for bladder emptying reverts to a reflexic mode of functioning. As a result, after an initial period of spinal shock, which is often accompanied by urinary retention and overflow incontinence, a reflex (neurogenic) bladder develops. If the disturbance of upper motor neuron function evolves slowly, then the reflex bladder may develop without a preceding period of spinal shock and flaccid bladder.

The reflex or spastic bladder is characterized by overactivity of both the detrusor muscle and the external sphincter, causing incontinence of urine or precipitant micturition. In addition, the bladder capacity is diminished due to the detrusor contraction. The sensation of bladder distention may be lost if ascending tracts are also involved. The anal reflex is often intact in cases of reflex bladder. On cystometrogram testing, the detrusor muscle demonstrates excessive contraction to small increments of fluid volume.

In contrast to the reflex bladder, when spinal damage occurs in the region of the conus medullaris or the cauda equina, a decentralized or autonomous flaccid bladder ensues. Voluntary control over bladder function is impaired or abolished. Detrusor tone is lost and the bladder distends so that overflow incontinence occurs. Bladder sensation is impaired. Control over the anal sphincter and the anal reflex are usually lost. A region of saddle anesthesia may be present. The cystometrogram usually demonstrates diminished or absent contractions of the detrusor muscle.

The anatomical pathways subserving bowel function are similar to those controlling the urinary bladder. Spinal shock is generally associated with ileus and a neurogenic megacolon may develop. The anal reflex is usually lost. In slowly evolving lesions above the sacral level, voluntary control of the sphincter ani may be lost, but the anal reflex remains intact unless complete cord transection occurs, in which case it may be absent. In disturbances of the conus medullaris and cauda equina (nerve roots S3–5), fecal incontinence and a flaccid anal sphincter with loss of the anal reflex may be a presenting manifestation. Saddle anesthesia is often seen in such cases. Partial impairment may be present in any of these syndromes before frank paralysis and a flaccid sphincter ensue.

Disturbances of sexual function are common in spinal cord disease, especially in men. The descending pathways from the neocortex, limbic system, and hypo-

thalamus course adjacent to the corticospinal tracts in the lateral funiculi. Penile erection occurs through the sacral parasympathetics (S3 and S4), the pudendal nerves, and nervi erigentes, and by inhibition of the sympathetic vasoconstrictor center located in the intermediolateral cell column at L1–2 and then through the superior hypogastric plexus.[67] Vascular channels in the penis dilate in response to parasympathetic innervation and tumescence occurs. Ejaculation is performed via the reflex arc beginning with the afferent limb arising in the genital epithelium and passing centrally via the dorsal nerve of the penis and pudendal nerve to the S3 and S4 dorsal roots. These afferent impulses synapse with two centers: a sympathetic center from T6 to L3 and a parasympathetic center at S3–4, which together form the efferent limb of the reflex arc. The perineal branch of the pudendal nerve is an important peripheral efferent pathway.[67]

CHARACTERIZATION AND QUANTITATION OF SPINAL CORD DYSFUNCTION: SPECIAL CONSIDERATIONS FOR TRAUMA PATIENTS

Tator has developed a list of "safe assumptions" to make when initially evaluating a trauma victim in order to avoid missing "occult" injuries.[68] One should assume that all multiple trauma victims have spinal cord injury (SCI) until proven otherwise, particularly in the cerebrally impaired patient (via head injury, intoxication, etc.) (Table 2–10). He also provides "spinal clues" that can be obtained from detailed testing and observation. These include an assessment of vital signs, strength, sensation, and reflexes in all four limbs (Table 2–11). Palpation of the entire dorsal surface of the neck and back overlying the spine is mandatory. Regarding vital signs, the observation of hypotension is particularly important. This, obviously may indicate hemorrhagic shock, but it also may indicate the presence of a cervical or upper thoracic SCI. Hypotension, bradycardia, and warm extremities

Table 2–10. "Safe Assumptions"—To Aid in the Diagnosis of SCI*

1. Every patient with a head injury and every unconscious patient has an SCI
2. Every patient with multiple trauma has an SCI
3. Every motor-vehicle accident victim has an SCI
4. Every victim of a sports or recreational accident has an SCI
5. Every severely injured worker has an SCI
6. Every victim of a fall at home has an SCI
7. Every SCI has an unstable spinal column and any movement of the spinal column after trauma will cause further damage to the spinal cord

*SCI = spinal cord injury.

together indicate an underlying SCI.[68] Although these concerns are particularly related to trauma, their application to other potential causes of myelopathy is relevant.

Table 2–11. "Spinal Clues"—To Aid in the Diagnosis of SCI (especially useful in patients who are uncooperative or have impaired consciousness)

1. Hypotension and bradycardia occur in spinal shock
2. Paradoxical respiration
3. Low body temperature and high skin temperature
4. Priapism
5. Bilateral paralysis of arms and legs, especially flaccid
6. Bilateral paralysis of either arms only or arms more than legs, especially flaccid
7. Bilateral paralysis of legs, especially flaccid
8. Lack of response to painful stimuli
9. Detection of an anatomic level in response to painful stimuli
10. Painful stimulation produces only head movement or facial grimacing
11. Sweating level
12. Horner's syndrome
13. Brown-Séquard syndrome

Clinical Examination

Appropriate evaluation of the spinally impaired patient must begin with a reliable method of assessment. This method must have significant interobserver reliability, be of utility with respect to serial examinations, and allow results to be compared with those from other patients. The precursor of the schemes that have been designed to assess the extent of functional disability related to spinal cord dysfunction is the Frankel scale (Table 2–12).[69] This method lacks specificity with regard to the definition of extent of neurological dysfunction. To address this problem, the American Spinal Injury Association (ASIA) and the International Medical Society of Paraplegia (IMSOP) have published a modified scale as the International Standards for Neurologic and Functional Classification of Spinal Cord Injury (Table 2–13 and Fig. 2–5).[70]

Benzel and Larson revised the Frankel scale by expanding it to seven from five grades. This was accomplished by expanding grades C and D into two grades each,

Table 2–12. Frankel Classification of Neurological Deficit After Spinal Cord

	INJURY
Frankel Grade	Description
A	Complete: no motor or sensory function below level of lesion
B	Sensory only: complete motor paralysis below level of lesion with some preservation of sensory function; includes sacral sparing
C	Motor useless: some motor power present below level of lesion, but it is of no practical use
D	Motor useful: useful motor power below level of lesion; these patients can move lower limbs and many can walk, with or without aids
E	Recovery: free of neurological symptoms, i.e., no weakness, sensory loss, or sphincter disturbance; abnormal reflexes may be present

Table 2–13. SCI Based on the International Standards for Neurologic and Functional Classification by ASIA and IMSOP

ASIA/IMSOP Impairment Scale*

Grade A	Complete	No motor or sensory function is preserved in the sacral segments S4–5
Grade B	Incomplete	Sensory but not motor function is preserved below the neurologic level and extends through the sacral segments S4–5
Grade C	Incomplete	Motor function is preserved below the neurologic level, and the majority of key muscles below the neurologic level have a muscle grade less than 3
Grade D	Incomplete	Motor function is preserved below the neurologic level, and the majority of key muscles below the neurologic level have a muscle grade 3 or greater
Grade E	Normal	Motor and sensory function are normal

*ASIA = American Spinal Injury Association; IMSOP = International Medical Society of Paraplegia; SCI = spinal cord injury.

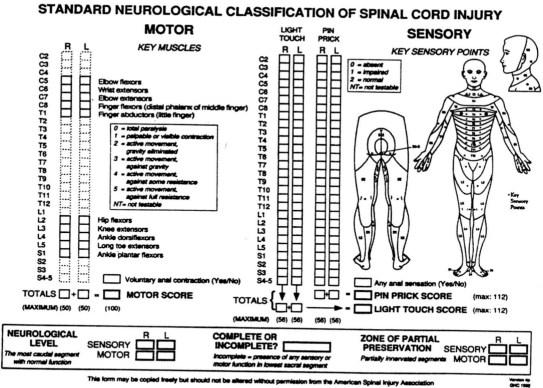

Figure 2–5. Neurologic classification of SCI (ASIA/IMSOP). This diagram contains the principal information about motor, sensory, and sphincter function necessary for accurate classification and scoring of acute SCI. The ten key muscles to be tested for the motor examination are shown on the left along with the Medical Research Council grading system, and the 28 dermatomes to be tested on each side for the sensory examination are shown on the right. The system for recording the neurologic level(s), the completeness of the injury, and the zone of partial preservation (in complete injuries) is shown at the bottom. (From ASIA,[70] with permission.)

thus increasing the ability to separate functional grades and to more clearly define the extent of dysfunction.[71] This scheme, however, did not allow the precise quantitation of function in the patient confined to bed. Therefore, a modification of this scheme was devised, and it is currently being employed by the GM1 Ganglioside trial (Table 2–14).

It is emphasized that lesions that result in an incomplete myelopathy are associated with a far better prognosis than are lesions that are associated with a complete myelopathy. Therefore, their careful differentiation is obligatory. Tator emphasizes that the clinician must test touch and pinprick sensation in the lowest sacral dermatomes, i.e., at the mucocutaneous junction perianally. Furthermore, voluntary motor contraction of the external anal sphincter must be assessed by digital rectal examination.[68]

THE SEGMENTAL LEVEL OF SPINAL CORD INJURY

The ASIA/IMSOP classification scheme mentioned above provides a method of determining the segmental level of injury (neurological level), defined by Tator as "the most caudal segment of the spinal cord with normal sensory and motor function on both sides of the body."[68] This definition is necessary because symmetry of injury is often not present, and differences must be determined by motor and sensory examination. The assessment involves 28 right and 28 left dermatomes and 10 myotomes by the evaluation of 10 "key" muscle groups (Fig. 2–5).

Table 2–14. **Neurological Grading System of Thoracic and Lumbar Spine Injuries With Regard to Myelopathic Function**[*]

Grade I	Complete Functional Neural Transection
	No motor or sensory function below the level of injury
Grade II	Motor Complete
	No voluntary motor function below the level of injury with preservation of some sensation
Grade III	Motor Incomplete-Nonfunctional
	Minimal nonfunctional voluntary motor function below the level of injury
Grade IV	Motor Incomplete-Functional (Nonambulatory)
	Some functional motor control present below the level of injury that is significantly useful (for use with transfers, etc.) but not sufficient for independent walking
Grade V	Motor Incomplete-Functional (Limited Ambulation)
	Motor function allows walking with assistance or unassisted, but significant problems secondary to lack of endurance or fear of falling limit patient mobility
Grade VI	Motor Incomplete-Functional (Unlimited Ambulation)
	Ambulatory without assistance and without significant limitations other than one or more of the following:
	1. Difficulties with micturition
	2. Loss of nerve root function that significantly impedes ease of ambulation
	3. Slightly discoordinated gait
Grade VII	Normal
	Neurologically intact with the exception of minimal deficits that cause no functional difficulties

[*]Because of the occasional limitation related to spinal instability, "ambulatory" is defined as the motor and sensory function consistent with the ability to walk.

THE SEGMENTAL LEVEL OF SPINAL COLUMN INJURY

The vertebral level of injury is defined as the level with the greatest spinal column integrity disruption, as defined by imaging studies.

COMMON SPINAL CORD SYNDROMES

Spinal Shock

The term "spinal shock" has been used in a variety of circumstances, some of which are inappropriate. It has at least two commonly utilized general definitions. These are (1) hypotension associated with SCI and (2) the transient (several days to several months) loss of intrinsic spinal cord reflex activity. Spinal shock occurs, according to this second definition, when a patient demonstrates manifestations of lower motor neuron dysfunction for days to months after the onset of myelopathy; however, ultimately upper motor neuron dysfunction (with the associated spinal reflex activity) develops. This latter definition is employed here.

A complete transverse section of the spinal cord results in the loss of motor and sensory function below the level of that lesion. If the lesion is slow to develop, as may occur with a benign tumor or cervical spondylosis, or is incomplete, spinal reflexes such as hyperactive deep tendon reflexes and Babinski signs generally are present. If the lesion develops acutely, spinal shock ensues and there is loss of all spinal reflex activity below the level of the lesion. Spinal shock is characterized by flaccid, areflexic paralysis of skeletal and smooth muscles. There is a complete loss of autonomic functions below the level of the lesion, resulting in a loss of urinary bladder tone and paralytic ileus. Sweating and piloerection are also diminished or absent below the lesion. Since vasomotor tone is lost, dependent lower extremities may become edematous and temperature regulation may be a major problem. Genital reflexes are lost. Sensation below the level of the lesion is completely absent.

Sherrington performed initial transections of the spinal cord on animals.[72] He then waited for the animal to recover spinal reflex activity before sectioning the cord again, this time below the initial level of the injury. Following the second transection, he found that no spinal shock ensued, which showed that it was the acute loss of facilitatory supraspinal influences rather than trauma itself that was responsible for spinal shock. The specific pathways responsible for providing this facilitatory influence on spinal neurons are as yet unknown. Sherrington's studies showed that the duration of spinal shock is longer in primates than in more primitive mammals. In humans, the duration is quite variable. In the majority of cases, spinal reflex activity begins to return after one to six weeks. In one series, spinal shock was reported to be permanent in five out of 29 patients.

EVOLUTION OF SPINAL SHOCK

A period of spinal shock typically evolves into a stage of heightened reflex activity.[73] Thus the Babinski response, which usually involves only dorsiflexion of the great toe and fanning of the remaining toes, may develop into a triple flexion response involving the hip, knee, and foot after only minimal tactile stimulation. Simple withdrawal reflexes may develop into flexor spasms.

When these reflexes occur together in response to various stimuli, such as touch or a distended or infected bladder, the resulting flexor spasms, hyperhydrosis, and piloerection form the mass reflex. In addition to a reduction in the threshold of stimulation that will evoke a spinal reflex, there is an enlargement of the reflexogenic zone to a level just caudal to the transection of the cord. The deep tendon reflexes below the lesion also become hyperactive.

The mechanism of this heightened reflex response after spinal shock is not understood. One hypothesis is that hyperreflexia is secondary to sprouting of afferent neurons below the level of transection.[74] It is thought that after degeneration of the descending supraspinal tracts, spinal motor neurons and interneurons are left with many postsynaptic vacancies, which presumably are innervated by sprouting of intact afferent neurons. Based on this hypothesis, the heightened reflex activity is not, therefore, an exaggeration of a normal reflex but rather a new, abnormal reflex.

In the evolution of spinal shock, thermoregulatory sweating is impaired below the lesion but it may be exaggerated, resulting in hyperhydrosis, above the lesion. In fact, autonomic disturbances above the level of the lesion are common. Bradycardia, hypertension resulting in headache, and flushing of the skin are often seen in patients, and are thought to be due to a release of norepinephrine from disinhibited sympathetic neurons caudal to the lesion and due to a release of epinephrine from the adrenal medulla.

Riddoch's studies[73] during World War I led to the belief that, following spinal shock, complete transverse lesions of the spinal cord ultimately developed into paraplegia-in-flexion, while incomplete lesions developed into paraplegia-in-extension. Thus, one could determine the extent of the transection on such a clinical basis. Although this view was supported by some experimental work,[75] Sherrington[58,72] had earlier shown in experimental animals that following complete transections of the cord a preponderance of extensor tone was sometimes found, and Kuhn[76] demonstrated that 18 of 22 patients with complete cord transection eventually developed extensor reflexes after they had fully developed flexor reflexes.

The experience of World War II demonstrated that, with the avoidance of decubiti and urinary tract infections (which provoke flexor spasms) and with other forms of improved medical care, paraplegia-in-extension often ultimately evolves after complete transection of the cord.[77,78] Guttmann[58,79] found other factors important in determining the ultimate posture, such as the posture of individuals in the early period following cord transection. He found that if the lower extremities of patients were maintained in an adducted and flexed position (as with a pillow beneath the knees), paraplegia-in-flexion would more commonly develop. Alternatively, if the legs were maintained in an abducted and extended position, then paraplegia-in-extension was more common. The extensor posture is also favored if the patient is maintained in a prone position. These observations and the changes in medical care for spinal-cord-injured patients that derived from those observations have had an important impact on the outcome of patients with spinal cord injuries.

The level of the lesion also is important in determining the ultimate posture of the legs. Higher lesions, such as at the level of the cervical spine, are much more likely to result in paraplegia-in-flexion than more caudal lesions. Intermittent extensor posturing is much more likely in patients with incomplete cord transections than in those with complete transverse lesions.[80]

Spinal Cord Injury Syndromes

Spinal cord distortion or disruption results in neurological deficit that may result in a variety of spinal cord injury syndromes. An understanding of their characteristic features is mandatory for the clinician to appropriately diagnose and manage this patient population.

COMPLETE MYELOPATHY

In the purest sense, complete myelopathy is associated with no evidence of long tract neural transmission across the injury site. This can be difficult to document clinically, and in some cases, efficacy of putative intervention has been erroneously reported in patients with an incomplete myelopathy, in which some degree of recovery of neurological function might have been expected.

Complete myelopathy is a functional description. It has classically been considered to be an indication of a spinal cord transection. Although researchers are searching for cures for spinal cord transection and are making rapid progress, it is conceded by most investigators that spinal cord transection remains, at this time, a neurologically irreversible process.

However, in some cases of clinically complete myelopathy a population of axons survives and runs through the lesion but fails to conduct impulses as a result of demyelination and in these cases some recovery may occur.[81]

Careful and serial motor and sensory (including saddle sensation, lower sacral, perianal sensation) examinations are mandatory. Appropriate consideration should be given to the inaccuracies of the examination that can occur in the cerebrally impaired or intoxicated patient. Their examination may inappropriately reflect a disproportionately decreased level of neurological function.

The definition of complete myelopathy is further confused by the inclusion of patients with some sensory preservation, when they are indeed not "complete."[82] If one "rigorously" employs the schemes for neurological assessment depicted in this chapter, there should be no confusion.

ANTERIOR SPINAL CORD ARTERY AND ANTERIOR SPINAL CORD INJURY SYNDROMES

Although first described in 1904[83] as syphilitic paraplegia with dissociated sensibility, spinal cord infarction had been considered a clinical rarity. In a series of over 3700 postmortem examinations at a London hospital between 1909 and 1958, no cases of arterial infarction of the spinal cord were found.[84] More recently, however, it has been recognized much more frequently. This is partly a result of an increased number of invasive procedures such as vascular[85,86] and thoraco-abdominal surgery[87] and partly due to improved survival after cardiac arrest and hypotension.[88–91]

The anterior horns and anterolateral tracts are involved in the anterior spinal artery syndrome (Figs. 2–6 and 2–7). Initially spinal shock is expected. Subse-

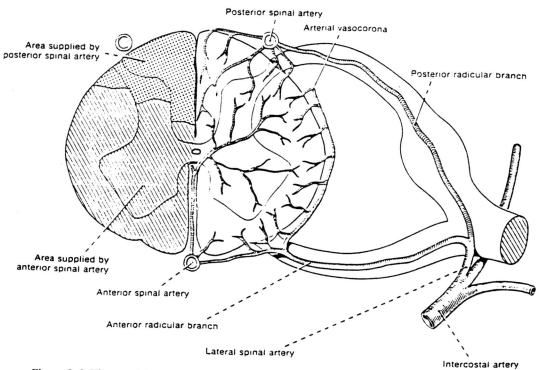

Figure 2–6. The arterial supply of the spinal cord. (From DeJong, RN,[35] p. 580, with permission.)

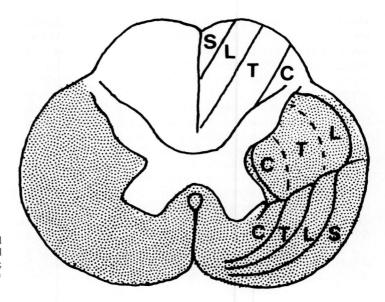

Figure 2–7. The tracts involved (shaded area) in anterior spinal artery infarction. (C = cervical; T = thoracic; L = lumbar; S = sacral.)

quently, motor examination shows lower motor neuron weakness in the region of ischemia and corticospinal deficits below the level of the infarction. Autonomic pathways are also involved, so there is loss of bowel, bladder, and sexual function. The sensory disturbance is dissociated in that posterior column function is intact but the spinothalamic tracts are disrupted.

Anterior spinal artery syndrome is differentiated from acute central cord syndrome[92] by the sacral sensory sparing that tends to occur in the latter. Moreover, the intact posterior column function seen in the anterior spinal artery syndrome differentiates it from the syndrome of acute complete transverse myelopathy.[93]

Commonly, a ventral injury to the spinal cord is caused by the retropulsion of a disc and/or bone fragments into its substance. This insult can result in dysfunction of the ventral spinal cord tracts, predominantly the spinothalamic (pain and temperature) and corticospinal (motor) tracts, with preservation of the posterior columns (joint position sense and gross touch). The preservation of at least some sensory function drastically alters the overall prognosis.[71,94]

BROWN-SÉQUARD SPINAL CORD INJURY SYNDROME

A unilateral lesion or hemisection of the spinal cord produces Brown-Séquard syndrome.[15] In reality, such pure unilateral lesions are rare (except in pure stab injuries), and most clinical cases are described as a modified Brown-Séquard syndrome.

The clinical presentation of pure Brown-Séquard syndrome is that of ipsilateral weakness and a loss of position and vibration below the lesion, with contralateral loss of pain and temperature (Fig. 2–4B). The loss of pain and temperature is usually manifest a few segments below the level of the lesion because the decussating fibers enter the spinothalamic tract a few segments rostral to the level of entry of the nerve root. At the level of the insult, there may be a small ipsilateral area of anesthesia, analgesia, and lower motor neuron weakness because the segmental afferent and efferent pathways are disrupted. Both axial and sagittal imaging techniques may be particularly useful for evaluating patients with this syndrome.

There are many known causes of the pure syndrome; trauma is probably the most common.[67,95] Radiation necrosis has also been reported as a cause.[96] Patients with spinal metastases rarely present with Brown-Séquard syndrome. In one large series of patients with spinal metastases,[97] of 106 patients with signs of myelopathy, only two had a pure Brown-Séquard syndrome. An additional eight had greater weakness ipsilateral to the lesion and more marked pain and temperature loss contralateral to the lesion, but no dorsal column signs. This group would be considered to have a "modified Brown-Séquard syndrome."

CENTRAL SPINAL CORD SYNDROME

A sudden annular constriction of the spinal cord will often lead to an injury of the central portion of the spinal cord. A stenotic spinal canal, combined with traumatic insult, appears to be necessary for its traumatic inducement. Other causes, such as primary spinal cord tumors and syringomyelia, are also common. Regardless of the etiology, the central portion of the spinal cord is injured, thus providing an anatomical explanation for the neurological picture.[98-103]

Because of the somatotopic distribution of function in spinal cord long tracts in the axial plane, a central injury to the cervical spinal cord results in a characteristic clinical picture, i.e., a loss of motor and sensory function in the upper extremities that is out of proportion to that lost in the lower extremities (Fig. 2–8).

The central cord syndrome is due to an intra-axial lesion disturbing the normal structures of the central or paracentral region of the spinal cord. Such disturbances may be acute, usually due to hemorrhage or contusion following trauma,[92] or chronic, due to tumor or syringomyelia. Although a demyelinating process may occasionally cause a similar syndrome, it is usually not confused with the more typical causes. The clinical presentations of these disorders share some common features. Contusions following trauma and syringomyelia frequently occur in the cervical spine and cervicothoracic junction. Spontaneous hematomyelia generally presents with the acute onset of severe back or neck pain, followed by paralysis. It can occur at any level of the cord and may be due to an arteriovenous malformation or coagulopathy.

When the cervical spine or cervicothoracic junction is the site of a central cord syndrome, the upper extremities show weakness of a lower motor neuron type. Characteristically, there is loss of sensation in the upper extremities of a dissociated type—i.e., loss of pin and temperature with preservation of position and vibration—because the decussating fibers destined for the spinothalamic tracts are interrupted while those projecting within

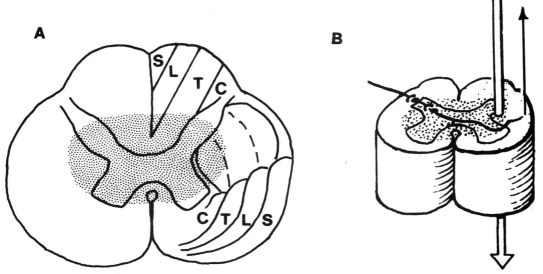

Figure 2–8. Somatotopic organization of the cervical spinal cord revealing the anatomic explanation for central cord syndromes causing sacral sparing. Shaded area represents region of dysfunction (A), axial view. (B) Longitudinal view. Arrows denote ascending and descending tracts.

the posterior columns are spared. As a result of the laminated structure of the spinothalamic tract, sensation from the more caudal regions is preserved, and sacral sparing of pin and temperature sensation is the rule (see Fig. 2–4D).

In slowly developing lesions, the lower extremities ultimately exhibit signs of weakness of an upper motor neuron type. In acute lesions, there is usually initial spinal shock. Bowel, bladder, and sexual function are generally impaired immediately in acute lesions and later in chronic lesions. In cases involving the cervical and cervicothoracic spine, there may also be Horner's syndrome unilaterally or bilaterally.

ANTERIOR HORN SYNDROME

Prior to development of the polio vaccine, the acute anterior horn syndrome was commonly encountered due to invasion of the spinal cord by poliomyelitis virus. Rarely, other enteroviruses may cause the acute syndrome. The chronic anterior horn syndrome in the adult population is commonly seen in conjunction with degenerative diseases such as amyotrophic lateral sclerosis and in post-polio syndrome. Paraneoplastic conditions may also present as an anterior horn syndrome, such as the subacute motor neuronopathy that has been reported as a remote effect of lymphoma.[49] Finally, there are several forms of inherited spinal muscular atrophy that may present as an anterior horn syndrome.

These patients present clinically with lower motor neuron weakness that may be asymmetric, especially in the acquired forms. The muscles become areflexic and flaccid. Fasciculations may occur. Sensory and autonomic disturbances are not generally seen. A similar clinical syndrome may, of course, be due to intramedullary lesions such as syringomyelia or tumors, but this must be differentiated from ventral root disturbances such as those due to spondylosis.

ANTERIOR HORN AND PYRAMIDAL TRACT SYNDROME

Disturbances of the anterior horns and pyramidal tracts with sparing of the sen-

sory functions and autonomic nervous system are seen in motor neuron disease. Clinically, one typically finds a combination of lower motor neuron weakness patients with its attendant atrophy and fasciculations (and fibrillations on EMG) and upper motor weakness with spasticity, hyperreflexia, and Babinski signs. Either the lower motor neuron or upper motor neuron disturbance may predominate for months or years. Ultimately, as the lower motor neuron disease progresses, there is increasingly severe atrophy and evolution from hyperreflexia to hyporeflexia.

COMBINED POSTERIOR AND LATERAL COLUMN DISEASE

The patients who lose posterior column and lateral column (pyramidal) function clinically present with a spastic ataxic gait. Although Friedreich's ataxia may cause such a syndrome, the classic cause is subacute combined degeneration[104] associated with pernicious anemia. When symptoms such as paranoia and megaloblastic madness accompany a gait that appears nonorganic or hysterical, the patient often is referred for psychiatric evaluation.

CASE ILLUSTRATION

A 52-year-old woman presented with a three-month history of distal extremity paresthesias and weakness manifested by difficulty walking. Her internist found her depressed and suspicious. Her gait was unsteady and she had depressed reflexes. She was uncooperative for the remainder of the examination. She believed that she had injured both knees but could not relate any specific injury. When her knee roentgenograms were reported as negative, she refused a further workup and was lost to follow-up. Several months later she was seen by a psychiatrist who recognized the need for neurological assessment. On mental status examination, the patient manifested agitation and suspiciousness. Her gait was both ataxic and spastic; each step was associated with choreoathetoid arm movements as though she was walking a tightrope. She could not tandem walk, had poor foot position sense, and a positive Romberg. Her deep tendon reflexes were diminished, but her lower extremity muscle tone was increased. Babinski signs were present, and vibration sensation was impaired in both legs.

A CBC (complete blood count) showed a mild anemia and an MCV (mean corpuscular volume) of 110 (82–92, normal range). A serum vitamin B_{12} level was 13 μgs per ml (200–800, normal range). A diagnosis of subacute combined degeneration of the spinal cord was made. The Schilling test was positive and confirmed the clinical impression. Intramuscular injections of vitamin B_{12} were begun. The patient's neurological status did not significantly change after one month, although she had a hematological response. She remained insistent that her problem was due either to a knee disturbance or to a lumbar spine problem because she had had a long history of back pain. She sought the care of other physicians unfamiliar with her medical history and underwent knee arthroscopy and a lumbar myelogram. When these studies were reported normal, she returned for her vitamin B_{12} injections. Her gait and mental status improved but she continued to have mild gait ataxia and depression and required psychiatric counseling and physical therapy.

Comment. This case illustrates the predominance of neuropsychiatric as well as sensorimotor findings in patients with subacute combined degeneration.[105] The patient's persistent delusion that she had back and knee disease, despite evidence to the contrary, was a manifestation of suspiciousness and paranoia secondary to the vitamin B_{12} deficiency. This delayed her workup and treatment. Subacute combined degeneration is a treatable disorder that can be diagnosed noninvasively. It should be considered in all patients with signs of posterior column and pyramidal tract dysfunction.

CHARACTERISTIC CLINICAL FEATURES OF LESIONS AT DIFFERENT LEVELS

Spinal tumors at different levels often present with characteristic symptoms and signs referable to the segmental levels involved. In cases of extramedullary tumors, disturbances at the segmental level usually herald the presentation of the neoplasm. Intramedullary tumors frequently do not present with segmental disturbances but rather with tract dysfunction.[106]

Foramen Magnum

Lesions of the foramen magnum, which include tumors, syringomyelia, multiple sclerosis, Arnold-Chiari malformation, atlanto-axial dislocation, and other bony abnormalities of the craniocervical junction, present one of the most challenging diagnostic problems for the clinician because the symptoms are often vague or may be distant from the foramen magnum. For example, although patients with Arnold-Chiari malformation type 1 (without meningocele) often present with progressive cerebellar dysfunction, increased intracranial pressure, or lower cranial nerve dysfunction, they may also present with a syndrome of syringomyelia.

Since many foramen magnum lesions, such as benign tumors, neurofibromas or meningiomas, or atlanto-axial dislocation, are surgically treatable, there is a high premium on early diagnosis and treatment.[65] Congenital bony abnormalities in the region of the foramen magnum may be entirely asymptomatic, but when found, they often lead to difficult clinical decision making.[107,108]

FORAMEN MAGNUM TUMORS

When the foramen magnum lesion is a tumor (Fig. 2–9), occipital or neck pain, often increased by neck movement, is the most common initial manifestation.[109] The pain may also radiate into the shoulders or the ipsilateral arm. In the latter situation, the pain may be difficult to differentiate from that secondary to cervical spondylosis. In many such cases the latter diagnosis may be suspected clinically, only to be confirmed by plain films of the cervical spine. As documented elsewhere,[110] cervical spondylosis as diagnosed on plain radiographs is found in 50% of individuals over 50 years of age and 75% of those over 65 years old, many of whom are asymptomatic. This high prevalence of spondylosis in the general population may result in delay in diagnosing a rare condition such

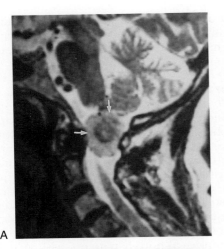

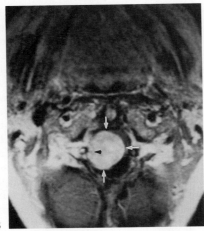

Figure 2–9. An MRI scan of a meningioma at the cranio-cervical junction. (A) Sagittal view. (B) Axial view. In the sagittal view, the tumor is seen occupying the entire anteroposterior extent of the spinal canal. In the axial view, the spinal cord (black arrowhead) is severely compressed by the tumor (white arrows). (Courtesy of Dr. Richard Becker.)

as a foramen magnum tumor, which constitutes only approximately 1% of intracranial and intraspinal tumors.[111] In other cases of foramen magnum tumors, the pain may also radiate into the lower back.[111]

The neurological signs associated with foramen magnum tumors may also be perplexing. Cranial nerve symptoms and signs are variable; nystagmus, impaired sensation over the face (due to involvement of the descending tract of cranial nerve V), and dysarthria, dysphonia, and dysphagia are present in some patients.[109]

Motor system involvement characteristically presents itself as spastic weakness. The corticospinal tracts are compressed by the extramedullary intradural neurofibroma or meningioma, so weakness typically begins in the ipsilateral arm, followed in order by weakness of the ipsilateral leg, the contralateral leg, and contralateral arm.[109]

It has been long recognized, however, that foramen magnum tumors may cause signs of lower motor neuron weakness, atrophy, and depressed reflexes in the arms and hands.[109] The mechanism of this lower motor neuron disturbance well below the level of the tumor has never been fully elucidated, but it may be secondary to circulatory disturbances affecting the distribution of the anterior spinal artery. It is important to recognize that atrophy of the hand muscles may arise from tumors above C4, since the findings could be mistaken for a syrinx, motor neuron disease, or pathology at the level of the lower cervical spine.[109]

Sensory disturbances consisting of pain and numbness are early manifestations of foramen magnum tumors. Remarkably, the paresthesias are often reported along the ulnar aspect of the forearm and hand, despite the fact that the lesion is several segments above the C8–T1 dermatomes. In one series,[109] early findings were pain and paresthesias affecting the same upper extremity first involved by spastic weakness. The mechanism whereby the upper motor neuron weakness and sensory loss occur in the same upper extremity has not been explained but is thought to be secondary to a disturbance of an intramedullary pathway.[109]

The sensory disturbances found in these patients are often of the dissociated type, so patients suffer from loss of pin and temperature, but have preserved tactile sensation. A suspended sensory loss also has been reported in some cases. This pattern often leads to the mistaken clinical impression that the patient has an intramedullary lesion such as a syrinx. Lhermitte's sign is frequently reported and some patients exhibit loss of vibration sensibility over the clavicle or acromion process.[109] In the past, myelography was the imaging modality of choice. Scanning by CT has been helpful in defining lesions of this region, especially if bone such as the skull base is being imaged. With the advent of MRI, this area may be now readily and noninvasively visualized.[112,113]

ATLANTO-AXIAL DISLOCATION

Atlanto-axial dislocation is another important craniocervical abnormality that may result in spinal cord compression. It may be caused by incompetence of either the odontoid process or of the transverse atlantal ligament. When posterior atlanto-axial subluxation is due to congenital and developmental causes, there also may be a variety of anomalies of the spine and craniocervical junction. Some of the disorders associated with atlanto-axial instability and dislocation include craniocervical junction anomalies, basilar impression, neurofibromatosis, congenital scoliosis, and others.[114]

Metastatic cancer to the dens is becoming a more frequently recognized cause of atlanto-axial dislocation, especially in patients harboring malignancy.[115] Rheumatoid involvement of the transatlantal ligament is another acquired cause and is seen in patients with rheumatoid arthritis.[116]

With atlanto-axial subluxation, the spinal cord may be compressed. Compression is reported to occur regularly when the sagittal diameter of the spinal canal at this level is 14 mm or less and may occur at 15–17 mm.[65] This measurement is considerably greater than that at which compression occurs in the lower cervical spine (10–13 mm).[117] As the sagittal diameter of the spinal cord varies by only 1 mm from C1 to C7, this difference probably is due to the sagittal diameter of the transverse atlantal ligament (4–5 mm), which is interposed between the odontoid process and spinal cord.

The mechanism of neural injury in many cases of atlanto-axial subluxation is reported to be compression of the medullocervical junction by the odontoid process.[118] The clinical presentation of atlanto-axial instability and subluxation may be perplexing. Symptoms are often intermittent and may include weakness of an upper motor neuron type or muscle wasting of the upper extremities, ataxia, dizziness, lower cranial nerve symptoms, and pain. Priapism is seen in some patients. Patients are often considered to have demyelinating disease or motor neuron disease before the correct diagnosis is made. Patients with atlanto-axial instability, especially if not recognized, are at risk for deterioration when undergoing general anesthesia.[114] A great many articles have been devoted to atlanto-axial instability and subluxation.[65,107,114,118,119]

CASE ILLUSTRATION

A 16-year-old mildly retarded young man was brought to the emergency room after suddenly falling to the ground, while at a dance. He did not lose consciousness but was unable to move. The emergency room physician noted a sustained penile erection but could find no other abnormalities on examination. The emergency room staff asked the neurological consultant to rule out a hysterical pseudoseizure.

Examination revealed an alert young man with dulled mental capacities. When questioned, he stated he had lost control of his arms and legs after hyperextending his neck while dancing. The weakness resolved over several hours. Examination revealed no cranial nerve abnormalities. Motor examination was normal except for decreased muscle tone in all extremities. Sensory examination revealed inconsistent results, but a spinal level could not be appreciated. Deep tendon reflexes were moderately brisk bilaterally and plantar responses were mute. Abdominal reflexes were absent. There was a sustained penile erection.

Because of the suspicion of an atlanto-axial dislocation, the patient's neck was immobilized. Cervical spine X-rays showed nonfusion of the dens, which was minimally displaced at the time of the examination.

Comment. This case illustrates several points. First, in atlanto-axial dislocation, neurological dysfunction can be transient, presumably reflecting the variable anatomy of the unstable atlanto-axial junction. Thus, in the patient with a history of transient tetraparesis, pathology of this crucial region must be sought. The absence of signs of spinal cord compression on examination does not rule out atlanto-axial pathology. Second, this case illustrates the importance of priapism as a localizing sign in disorders of the high cervical spine. This sign was well known to professional hangmen, who in the past were paid by the families of convicted criminals to hang their victims privately so as to avoid the embarrassment of the penile erection reflex in response to the hangman's fracture at C1–2.

Upper Cervical Spine

Neoplasms involving the upper cervical spine have similar clinical characteristics to those arising at the foramen magnum. Pain in the neck, occipital region, or shoulder is a very common presenting complaint. The first cervical root does not have a sensory dermatomal distribution, but the second cervical root innervates the posterior aspect of the scalp, explaining the pattern of radicular pain to this location. If the tumor is at the third or fourth cervical level, radicular pain may be projected to the neck or top of the shoulder. When pain occurs, it is usually provoked by neck movements, resulting in marked limitation of spontaneous head turning and nodding. This may be apparent on casual inspection.

Furthermore, since the descending tract of the trigeminal nerve may be irritated, sensory disturbances and funicular pain in the face may occur. Sensory disturbances in the face are rare presenting manifestations of spinal tumors; when they are the initial complaint of such a patient, they are much more likely to be secondary to an intramedullary rather than an extramedullary tumor. For example, Elsberg[50] described a patient harboring a high cervical intramedullary tumor who had an early symptom of numbness and shooting pain on the side of the face. In the absence of numbness, one might consider a diagnosis of tic douloureux in such a patient.

Usually following the initial complaint of pain, upper extremity weakness becomes apparent on the same side. The weakness may be of an upper or lower motor neuron type. Some patients, therefore, may have spasticity and hyperreflexia, whereas others may have atrophy and hyporeflexia of a portion or of the entire upper extremity including the hand.[50] The cause of lower motor neuron findings in patients with foramen magnum and upper cervical lesions several segments above the disturbed segmental levels is unknown. It has been attributed to circulatory disturbances, although this has not been proven. When upper motor neuron findings develop in the ipsilateral leg, a spinal hemiplegia is present. Weakness may progress to the contralateral lower extremity and then to the contralateral upper extremity. The weakness in both lower extremities may be of the upper motor neuron type, and that of the upper extremities may be either of the lower motor neuron variety or a combination of both upper and lower motor neuron. If attention is limited to the lower cervical spine using CT scanning or other imaging procedures, an upper cervical mass lesion may be missed.

Frequently, sensory disturbances do occur. Sensory loss may appear initially in the same upper extremity as the weakness, and it may be quite variable in distribution and type. Cases have been reported[106] that present with upper extremity astereognosis interpreted as suggesting a parietal lesion. Lhermitte's sign also often occurs.

Cranial nerve symptoms and signs are infrequent in upper cervical spine disease.[50] Reference to involvement of the descending trigeminal tract has already been made. In addition, atrophy and weakness involving the trapezius and sternocleidomastoid may occur owing to the spinal component to the 11th cranial nerve. Nystagmus may be present. Other cranial neuropathies such as facial and tongue weakness have also rarely been reported. Unequal pupils may occur secondary to a central Horner's syndrome if the descending pathways are injured en route to the neurons involved in ciliospinal reflexes situated at the intermediolateral horn at C8, T1, and T2. Horner's syndrome may be incomplete, in which case loss of sweat and vasodilatation due to vasoconstrictor paralysis, and enophthalmos may not uniformly be present.

Weakness or paralysis of the diaphragm may occur at lesions at or above the C4 level. Complete transverse lesions at the C4 level may not be associated with paralysis of the diaphragm if the innervation of the phrenic nerve at the C3 level is adequate.[58] The weakness may of course be unilateral or bilateral. Emphasizing that diaphragmatic paralysis is the most life threatening of complications of lesions of the spine. Degenerative disease of the cervical spine may present with similar but characteristic findings.

Lower Cervical and Upper Thoracic Spine

Extramedullary neoplasms and nonneoplastic lesions at the levels of C5–T1 frequently cause radicular symptoms at the affected level in the shoulder or upper extremity in the form of pain and later reflex, motor, and sensory disturbances. With lesions at the C4–6 level, pain and sensory disturbances are frequently reported along the radial aspect of the arm, forearm, and thumb. Pain is also frequent with intramedullary growths at these levels but the localization is usually more diffuse and less typically radicular in nature.

Pain and sensory symptoms at the C7–T1 levels frequently are localized to the ulnar aspect of the arm, forearm, and hand. As demonstrated in the dermatomal map, the C7 dermatome usually includes the middle finger and the T1 and T2 dermatomes are located at the ulnar border of the hand and forearm. Tumors at the T1 and T2 levels often cause pain to radiate into the elbow and hand along with sensory complaints along the ulnar border of the hand. Such complaints are often attributed to an ulnar neuropathy at the elbow or to orthopedic problems. As at other locations, intramedullary growths usually give rise to more diffuse symptoms that are often bilateral, while extramedullary neoplasms frequently present with exquisite localizing symptoms.

Weakness usually follows pain in extramedullary tumors, with a preponderance of weakness often present at the affected

segmental level. As might be expected based on the myotomal map of the upper extremity, intramedullary and extramedullary lesions at C4–6 tend to involve the muscles in the shoulder and upper arm. As with foramen magnum and upper cervical spine tumors, atrophy and weakness of the hand are also seen occasionally with lesions at C4–6, possibly due to vascular factors affecting the lower cervical segments. Such a pattern of weakness and atrophy may lead the examiner to consider a lesion at the C7–T2 level instead, for tumors at these levels typically cause muscle symptoms and signs in the forearm and hand.

The pattern of extremity weakness may be a guide in distinguishing intramedullary from extramedullary disorders. Although there are exceptions, extramedullary lesions tend to affect the ipsilateral upper and lower extremity before involving the contralateral side. In contrast, intramedullary lesions may involve both upper extremities before the lower extremities or show bilateral arm and leg involvement from the onset.[50]

The deep tendon reflexes are very helpful in localizing the segmental level of involvement in the cervical spine. Disease at the C5–6 levels often is associated with depressed biceps (C5) and/or brachioradialis reflex (C6) (see Table 2–6). One may encounter cases of a depressed biceps reflex associated with a hyperactive brachioradialis reflex if there is a compressive myelopathy at the C5 level. Although not specific for cervical spondylosis, a depressed brachioradialis (C6) reflex with hyperactive finger flexors (C8–T1) is often seen in individuals who have a C6 radiculopathy with myelopathy; neoplasms or other diseases at the C6 level may cause a similar clinical presentation. When the lesion is at the C7 level, the triceps reflex may be affected.

With lesions at C8 and T1, the finger flexor response, the Hoffmann sign, may be impaired. The Hoffmann sign is evoked by dorsiflexing the patient's wrist and then flicking the distal phalanx of the middle finger with the examiner's thumb.[35] The patient's middle finger is thus flexed and suddenly extended. When the Hoffmann sign is present, this maneuver is followed by sudden flexion of the patient's thumb and other fingers. When present bilaterally, it usually indicates hyperactive deep tendon reflexes. Although there may be disease of the pyramidal pathways, healthy individuals may have bilateral Hoffmann signs in conditions such as anxiety, hyperthyroidism, and use of CNS-stimulating drugs. When unilaterally present, it usually signifies disease of the nervous system, and the examiner must distinguish between disease of the pyramidal tract and disease of the peripheral nervous system, such as of the C8-T1 nerve roots or the lower brachial plexus (e.g., Pancoast tumor). For example, a Pancoast tumor may present with loss of a Hoffmann reflex and with hyperreflexia below the cervical cord due to cord compression. The associated physical findings and history are usually helpful.

Although Horner's syndrome may develop with a neoplasm at any level of the cervical spine, it is most commonly seen as an early manifestation of tumors near the intermediolateral cell column at the C7–T2 segmental levels.[67] In addition, the close anatomical relationship with the sympathetic ganglion near the T1 level makes Horner's syndrome an early hallmark of epidural tumors in this region. For example, among cancer patients with brachial plexus lesions, the presence of Horner's syndrome is a risk factor for the extension of paravertebral tumor into the epidural space.[121]

Thoracic Levels

As with lesions at other levels of the cord, pain is the most frequent presenting manifestation.(Fig. 2–10) The pain may be local, radicular, or both. The thoracic dermatomal landmarks that guide the examiner to the level of involvement are the nipple (T4), the umbilicus (T10), and the inguinal ligament (L1). Pain or sensory alterations in a radicular distribution are localized to a specific dermatome using these levels as points of reference. Pain in the upper thoracic level may be mis-

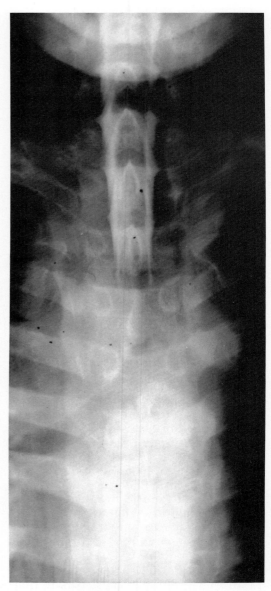

Figure 2–10. Myelogram following C1–2 puncture demonstrates an epidural block from lymphoma at the T3 level.

taken for pleural disease, whereas in the right upper abdominal quadrant, attacks of radicular pain may be considered symptoms of cholelithiasis. Other abdominal or thoracic viscera might be suspected as the source of pain at other levels. Radicular pain may also be bilateral, creating a girdle sensation.

When the lesion is in the lower thoracic spine, the segmental level of involvement sometimes may be determined by the presence of Beevor's sign. Since tensing the abdominal musculature (as in elevating the head off the bed in the supine position) requires the supraumbilical and infraumbilical muscles, a lesion at or adjacent to the level of T10 may be associated with upward movement of the umbilicus with such a maneuver.

The relatively small vertebral canal and the vascular watershed area of the spinal cord in the thoracic region make the thoracic spinal cord extremely vulnerable to injury from compression.[122] Consequently, the temporal course of symptoms of cord compression is often shorter in this region than elsewhere.[106,122] Pain often evolves rapidly into weakness, sensory loss, and reflex abnormalities caudal to the lesion. Sphincter disturbances ultimately develop.

Lesions in the region of the thoracolumbar junction may present with clinical manifestations of a myelopathy, conus medullaris syndrome, or cauda equina syndrome.

Conus Medullaris and Cauda Equina

Lesions of the cauda equina and conus medullaris cause similar symptoms and signs including local, referred, and radicular pain; sphincter disturbances; loss of buttock and leg sensation; and leg weakness. It may be relatively easy to establish the level of a single radiculopathy, but it is much more difficult to assign the cause and localization when there are several lumbosacral levels involved. In such situations, the examiner must consider the possibility of a lower spinal cord lesion or a cauda equina syndrome. There has been a long effort to differentiate conus medullaris lesions from those of the cauda equina,[30,123] but some authors conclude that it usually is not possible to discriminate between neoplasms arising from the lower spinal cord and those arising from the cauda equina[124,125] because in most cases, both anatomical regions are involved. This section describes features traditionally considered valuable in differentiating these lesions.

Table 2–15. **Differentiation of Conus/Epiconus From Cauda Equina Lesions**[*]

	Conus Medullaris/ Epiconus	**Cauda Equina**
Spontaneous pain	Unusual and not severe; bilateral and symmetric in perineum or thighs	Often very prominent and severe, asymmetric, radicular
Motor findings	Not severe, symmetric Fibrillary twitches are rare	May be severe, asymmetric, fibrillary twitches of paralyzed muscles are common
Sensory findings	Saddle distribution, bilateral, symmetric, dissociated sensory loss (impaired pin and temperature sensibility with sparing of tactile sensibility)	Saddle distribution, may be asymmetric, no dissociation of sensory loss
Reflex changes	Epiconus: Only Achilles absent Conus: Achilles and patellar present	Patellar and Achilles may be absent
Sphincter disturbance	Early and marked (both urinary and fecal incontinence)	Late and less severe
Male sexual function	Impaired early	Impairment less severe
Onset	Sudden and bilateral	Gradual and unilateral

*Adapted from DeJong, RN[35] and Haymaker, W.[67]

The conus medullaris consists of levels S3–Coc1 and the epiconus, as well as levels L4–S2.[67] Disturbances of epiconus function involve weakness, sensory loss, and reflex loss in the lower extremities subserved by L4–S1 roots, along with sphincter disturbances. Patients, therefore, experience difficulty with external rotation and extension of the thigh at the hip, flexion of the knee, and weakness of all muscles below the knee. Although rare in its pure form, patients with conus medullaris syndrome present with sphincter disturbances, saddle anesthesia (S3–5), impotence, and absence of lower extremity abnormalities. Pure conus medullaris syndrome is usually due to an intramedullary lesion such as a tumor, cyst, or infarct or trauma.[67,126] Injury disturbs spinal cord and cauda equina function. Therefore low lumbar and sacral (spinal cord; conus medullaris) function is lost, while more proximally exiting (cauda equina) roots are also impaired.. Table 2–15 attempts to identify the clinical features that may help in differentiating conus and epiconus lesions from cauda equina lesions.

DISTINGUISHING INTRAMEDULLARY FROM EXTRAMEDULLARY TUMORS

Neoplasms of the spine may be classified on the basis of location (Fig. 2–11 and Table 2–16). Intramedullary tumors consist of neoplasms arising from neuroectodermal tissues such as ependymoma, astrocytoma, or glioblastoma. Extramedullary–intradural growths are usually histologically benign meningiomas and nerve sheath tumors, although metastatic neoplasms to the leptomeninges also occur. Epidural tumors are usually metastatic deposits to the vertebral column with extension into the spinal canal and secondary cord/cauda compression, or, less frequently, epidural tumors may be primary tumors of the skeletal tissues such as multiple myeloma, or osteogenic sarcoma.

The relative frequency of epidural, extramedullary–intradural, and intramedullary tumors is difficult to ascertain. This

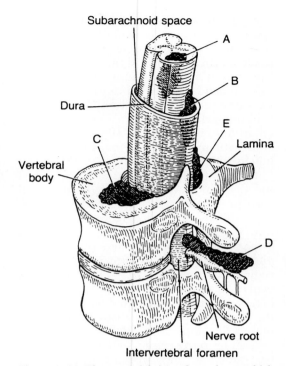

Figure 2–11. The potential sites of neoplasms which may cause myelopathy. The neoplasm may arise in or metastasize to the spinal cord (intramedullary)(A). The neoplasm may be extramedullary but intradural (B). Epidural tumors may begin in the vertebral column (C), in the paravertebral space (D), or, rarely, in the epidural space itself (E). (From Byrne, TN,[182] with permission.)

problem arises because the patients discussed in the neurosurgical literature much more commonly suffer from primary spinal tumors than from metastatic lesions; the converse is true in oncologic series. Since the majority of metastatic spinal neoplasms occur in the epidural space, whereas primary spinal tumors are more frequently intradural lesions, some estimate of the relative frequency of these locations for neoplastic growth may be determined by histological type. Based on population studies, metastatic cancer to the spine is much more common than primary spinal tumors. For example, Alter[127] has reported that primary spinal tumors occur at an annual incidence rate of 0.9–2.5 per 100,000 individuals. For a population of 250 million in the United States, this would mean a maximum annual incidence of 6250 individuals. The

Table 2–16. Classification of Spinal Neoplasms According to Location with Some Examples of Histological Types

Intramedullary Neoplasms
  Ependymoma
  Astrocytoma
  Glioblastoma
  Vascular neoplasm
  Metastasis
Extramedullary–Intradural Neoplasms
  Meningioma
  Nerve sheath tumor
  Vascular neoplasm
  Metastasis
Epidural Neoplasms
  Metastasis
  Multiple myeloma
  Osteogenic sarcoma (osteoma)
  Chondrosarcoma (chondroma)
  Lipomas
  Teratoma

annual mortality rate for cancer in 1980 was 184 per 100,000 individuals in the United States (data from Center for Environmental Health, Centers for Disease Control [CDC]). Approximately 5% of patients dying from cancer develop spinal cord compression,[128] so the annual incidence of metastatic spinal cord compression is approximately 9 per 100,000. For a population of 250 million, this corresponds to an annual incidence of 22,500 in the United States. Therefore, it appears, based on available epidemiological data, that metastatic spinal tumors are 3 to 4 times more common than primary spinal tumors. This calculation is very similar to other reports of relative frequency.[129]

Distinguishing among intramedullary, extramedullary–intradural, and epidural tumors of the spinal cord may be a vexing clinical problem that ultimately requires radiographic confirmation. The explanation for this clinical experience has been provided by a clinicopathological study of extramedullary spinal neoplasms[130] which demonstrated that extramedullary tumors can cause ischemia and demyelination in the posterior and lateral column with relative sparing of the anterior columns regardless of the location of the extramedul-

lary tumor. Both coup and contrecoup injuries occurred in the spinal cord. The areas of infarction and demyelination were often deep and did not follow a specific pattern. In some instances the pathological findings were more marked ipsilateral to the tumor; in other cases, they were primarily contralateral. Therefore, definite clinical patterns of evolution would not be expected. Nevertheless, at times clinical presentations may be helpful in evaluating patients (Table 2–17).

Pain

Pain is a common initial symptom of all types of spinal tumors. Although the pain is usually progressive, it has been reported to remit transiently in some cases.[50] Guidetti and Fortuna state, "It is pointless to try to predict the type of growth from the presence or absence of pain,"[122] but there are some characteristics of pain that may be helpful in the evaluation.

As already mentioned, approximately 90% of patients with metastatic epidural tumors complain of vertebral or radicular pain at the time of diagnosis.[131] In cases of extramedullary–intradural tumors, radicular pain is often a prominent complaint and may be present for months or years prior to diagnosis.[132,133] With neurofibromas, the pain is usually unilateral, whereas it may be bilateral in meningiomas.

Typical radicular pain is much less common in cases of intramedullary tumor.[134] Individuals with intramedullary tumors rarely present with root symptoms or signs alone.[106] The projected pain is usually burning, biting, and pinching.[50,135] Funicular pain is much more common than radicular pain in these patients and it is often bilateral.[136] It is typically poorly localized, diffuse, and burning, and often involves large areas of the body. Funicular pain may be triggered by tactile stimulation or movement of the spine.

Funicular pain is rare in cases of epidural tumors; it was found in only 3% of Torma's series.[137] However, in Guidetti's series,[122] funicular pain was the initial symptom in 22% of his patients and

Table 2–17. Characteristics That Can Help in Differentiation Between Extramedullary and Intramedullary Tumors of the Spinal Cord*

	Extramedullary Tumors	Intramedullary Tumors
Spontaneous pain	Radicular or regional (local) in type and distribution; an early and important symptom	Funicular; burning in type; poorly localized
Sensory changes	Contralateral loss of pain and temperature; ipsilateral loss of proprioception; (Brown-Séquard type)	Dissociation of sensation; spotty changes
Changes in pain and temperature sensations in saddle area	More marked than at level of lesion. Sensory level may be located *below* site of lesion	Less marked than at level of lesion. Sensory loss can be suspended
Lower motor neuron involvement	Segmental	Can be marked and widespread with atrophy and fasciculations
Upper motor neuron paresis and hyperreflexia	Prominent	Can be late and less prominent
Trophic changes	Usually not marked	Can be marked
Spinal subarachnoid block and changes in spinal fluid	Early and marked	Late and less marked

*Adapted from DeJong, RN.[35]

appeared later in 45%. Lhermitte's sign, a commonly encountered neurologic complaint, is thought to be due to demyelinated ascending tracts of the spinal cord that discharge spontaneously when mechanically stimulated.[138] Although Lhermitte[139] recognized its common occurrence in patients with multiple sclerosis,[140] it is now recognized to occur in a variety of clinical settings involving spinal cord disease, including cervical spondylosis and disc herniation,[141] head injuries,[142] following radiation injury,[143,144] and in subacute combined degeneration.[145,146] Furthermore, cisplatin has been reported to cause Lhermitte's sign. Lhermitte's sign has been reported in patients with both extramedullary and intramedullary tumors and is not, therefore, helpful in distinguishing between them.[122]

Motor Disorders

Motor disorders are second only to pain as the most common presenting manifestation of spinal cord tumors, perhaps be-cause the pyramidal pathways may be more sensitive to the compressive and ischemic effects of neoplasms than the sensory pathways.[122] The rate of evolution of weakness is not helpful in distinguishing between intramedullary and extramedullary tumors. Slow progressive weakness is frequently seen in both types of neoplasms. Similarly, rapid deterioration in motor function has been reported in cases of intramedullary tumors, extramedullary–intradural tumors, and extradural tumors.[31,122] Hemorrhage into the tumor has been found in some cases of intramedullary tumors, such as glioblastoma.[122,147] Vasogenic edema and circulatory disturbances have been reported to occur experimentally in epidural tumors[148,149] and probably also play a role in intramedullary and extramedullary–intradural tumors. Although progressive weakness is the rule in all spinal neoplasms, transient remissions may occur,[122] reflecting secondary mechanical and vascular factors.

Weakness has been found in 13%–60% of cases of intramedullary tumors at the time of diagnosis.[122] Weakness due to intramedullary tumors may characteristically spread in the limbs from a proximal to a distal location.[50,136] This pattern is due to the lamination of the corticospinal tract. Intramedullary lesions in the cervical spine, such as gliomas or syringomyelia, may cause unilateral or bilateral arm paresis with sparing of the lower extremity strength early in their course[136] (suspended area of weakness). Except for foramen magnum tumors, extramedullary cervical neoplasms infrequently give a clinical picture of bilateral arm weakness with preservation of leg strength. As discussed earlier, neoplasms of the foramen magnum often present with unilateral arm weakness before progressing to leg weakness.[122,150,151]

Unlike the case in intramedullary tumors, in cases of extramedullary–intradural tumors of the cervical spine such as neurofibromas and meningiomas, lower extremity strength is usually impaired to a comparable degree to that in the arms.[152,153] In addition, the weakness at the level of the neoplasm may be radicular as well. In epidural tumors, signs of weakness are frequently seen at the time of diagnosis; the prevalence is approximately 85% in one series.[31] Other series of epidural metastases have reported a lower incidence of weakness,[154] but only pain is a more frequent complaint in patients with metastatic spinal cord compression.[30,155]

Sensory Disturbances

Sensory disturbances may begin with subjective complaints of paresthesias. For unknown reasons, paresthesias are unusual presenting manifestations in most patients with spinal tumors. Frequencies of less than 10% have been reported in cases of epidural tumors, nerve sheath tumors, and intramedullary tumors.[122,132,137] In cases of meningiomas, though, the complaint of paresthesia appears to be common, with frequencies of 23%–37% reported.[122,137,152]

On examination, isolated sensory loss in the absence of other complaints and signs is a rare presenting manifestation of either intramedullary or extramedullary spinal

tumors. The cutaneous pattern and evolution of sensory loss may be helpful in distinguishing between these tumors. Dissociated sensory loss—preservation of posterior column function with loss of spinothalamic functions—is considered characteristic of intramedullary lesions; however, extramedullary tumors also have been reported to cause this pattern.[50,122] Extramedullary neoplasms may present with an ascending sensory level and intramedullary growths may cause a suspended sensory level most prominent at the level of the tumor.[156] This difference is due to the lamination of the spinothalamic tracts. Because the fibers conducting the caudal dermatomes are most posterolateral and those mediating rostral regions are more anteromedial, extramedullary compressive lesions tend to injure the fibers representing the caudal locations initially. Conversely, intramedullary growths tend to involve the more medial fibers initially and later invade the more laterally placed pathways. Thus, intramedullary tumors may appear to cause a descending sensory loss.

The evolution of sensory loss does not necessarily follow the classical patterns. For example, an eccentric intramedullary growth may give rise to an ascending sensory level rather than a suspended sensory loss. Exceptions to the ascending sensory levels are frequently found with epidural growths. Benign extramedullary tumors in the region of the foramen magnum frequently cause position sense loss more marked in the upper extremity than in the lower extremity ipsilateral to the tumor.[151,157] These examples of variability are probably explained on the basis of the tracts affected by ipsilateral and contralateral injuries. In a clinicopathological study of extramedullary spinal tumors, McAlhany and Netsky[130] found that regions of spinal ischemia and demyelination cannot be predicted on the basis of the location of the tumor in relationship to the cord.

Autonomic Disorders

Sphincter disturbances are considered unusual early manifestations of extramedullary and intramedullary tumors unless the conus or cauda equina is the site of involvement.[122,137,158] In one large series of intramedullary tumors,[147] only 3% of patients presented with sphincter disturbances as their first symptom. Of 130 patients with epidural tumor reported by Gilbert and associates,[31] none had sphincter disturbances as an initial complaint. However, sphincter disturbances were present in 57% of these cases by the time patients were seen in neurological consultation. Most authors report that sphincter disturbance occurs after motor and sensory disturbances are already manifest[136,147] unless the lesion is in the region of the conus or cauda equina.[122] Thus with either intramedullary or extramedullary mass lesions of the conus or mass lesions compressing the cauda equina, sphincter disturbances may be the initial manifestation.[125,158]

Other autonomic disorders generally do not help distinguish between intramedullary and extramedullary disorders, as they are found in both instances. For example, Horner's syndrome has been found in both types of growths.[122] The superior sulcus tumor as described by Pancoast is a common cause of Horner's syndrome.[22] Both primary tumors of the lung and metastases to this region commonly cause a combination of lower brachial plexopathy and Horner's syndrome.[121,159,160] In this setting, the tumor can extend into the epidural space by invading through the intervertebral foramina; thus, the radionuclide bone scan and plain films can be unremarkable.[121] Disturbances of sweating, cyanosis, and edema have been reported in both intramedullary and extramedullary tumors and do not appear to be helpful in discriminating between them.[122]

AUTONOMIC DYSREFLEXIA

Autonomic dystreflexia is a paroxysmal syndrome. It is a manifestation of an exaggerated and, to some degree, uncontrolled sympathetic nervous system response to noxious stimuli. These stimuli include, but by no means are limited to, bladder distension and infection, urethral instrumentation, defecation and rectal distention, or cutaneous stimulation and cutaneous sores or infections. Patients with lesions in the cervical and upper thoracic spine (T6 or above) may lack cerebral (supraspinal) inhibitory control of the thoracolumbar sympathetic outflow. Sympathetic overactivity of a reverberating nature may ensue. This can result in hyperhydrosis, increased cardiac output, and an increase in peripheral vascular resistance with hypertension and headache. Reflex bradycardia as well as other vagal manifestations may result (due to uninhibited vagal tone). Dangerous levels of rapid onset and persistent hypertension can occur. Intracranial hemorrhage may result, even in young patients.

The management of autonomic dysreflexia should focus on the elimination of the inciting stimulus and the management of hypertension. Prophylactic calcium channel blockers may be administered to patients susceptible to autonomic dysreflexia during high-risk situations, such as childbirth or awake surgical procedures. Patients who do not have plausible explanation for an episode of autonomic dysreflexia should undergo a urological workup.[161]

Temporal Course

Intramedullary tumors cannot be differentiated from extramedullary benign growths such as meningiomas and nerve sheath tumors, or from malignant epidural tumors, on the basis of the time course of symptoms and signs. While there are differences in the average period of time in which the clinical spinal syndrome evolves, frequent individual exceptions preclude definite conclusions. For example, while most malignant epidural tumors have a time course measured over days, and may range to weeks or months, intramedullary growths as well as meningiomas and nerve sheath tumors may have a similar acute or subacute presentation. Occasionally, they may evolve over many years.

Spinal tumors of any location may present with a remitting/relapsing course often mistaken for multiple sclerosis. Schliack and Stille[106] cite a neurinoma in a young man that caused a progressive paraparesis with sphincter involvement over a few months and subsequently resolved to a complete remission lasting four years, at which time the symptoms recurred rapidly to a near-complete transection of the cord. The same authors cite several other cases of meningiomas and intramedullary tumors that presented with relapsing and remitting courses over several years. When a relapsing and remitting clinical syndrome involves one location of the nervous system, one should consider a structural etiology as responsible. Although the side of the clinical involvement may vary during subsequent attacks owing to the close anatomical relationship of the tracts, when the same segmental level is repeatedly involved, a mass lesion needs to be considered.

UNUSUAL CLINICAL FEATURES OF SPINAL TUMORS

Raised Intracranial Pressure and Dementia

Rarely, spinal tumors present with symptoms and signs of intracranial disease.[55,162–168] For example, headache and papilledema secondary to raised intracranial pressure has rarely been reported as a presenting complaint. As of 1984, Michowiz and associates[169] found 53 cases of papilledema in association with spinal lesions. In each case, the papilledema resolved upon surgical removal of the spinal lesion.

The majority of reported spinal tumors causing increased intracranial pressure papilledema have been ependymomas–ependymoblastomas.[122,170] However, extramedullary tumors have also been found to cause papilledema.[122,168,171] Most spinal tumors causing increased intracranial pressure have been in the lower spinal canal: Half of the cases reviewed by Schliack and Stille[106] occurred in the lumbar area.

Among the patients with elevated intracranial pressure secondary to spinal

neoplasms, approximately 50% have associated ventriculomegaly.[163,172,173] Recently, Feldman and colleagues[163] reported a case of hydrocephalic dementia secondary to a benign lumbar schwannoma. Removal of the schwannoma resulted in a rapid resolution of the hydrocephalus and dementia. These authors reviewed five other cases[174–176] in which a caudal intradural tumor was associated with increased intracranial pressure, ventriculomegaly, and dementia. While over 50% of cases of papilledema due to spinal tumors are due to ependymomas–ependymoblastomas,[169] the spinal tumors in these six cases of dementia were two cases of neurofibroma, three of schwannoma, and one of oligodendroglioma.

The pathophysiological mechanism of elevated intracranial pressure secondary to spinal tumors has not been adequately explained. Although elevated CSF protein content has been suggested as a cause of impaired CSF resorption,[177] experimentally induced elevated CSF protein in monkeys did not cause papilledema.[178] Another explanation is that CSF normally absorbed in the lumbar subarachnoid region cannot be absorbed in such cases, resulting in increased intracranial pressure.[106] Intracranial basilar arachnoiditis may be the cause in some cases.[162]

Cranial Nerve Disturbances and Nystagmus

Surprisingly, lesions of the high cervical spine seldom give rise to lower cranial nerve symptoms and signs.[50] In one report of foramen magnum lesions,[109] disturbances of cranial nerves V (sensory loss), XI, and XII; vertigo; and nystagmus were only occasionally seen. After reviewing their own experience and that of others,[179] the authors commented on the relative rarity of these complaints in patients with foramen magnum tumors. They concluded that when cranial nerve symptoms did occur, they were overshadowed by the symptoms of spinal cord compression unless the lesion was located primarily in the posterior fossa.

Sensory disturbances involving the trigeminal distribution may occur in high cervical lesions, including both intramedullary and extramedullary tumors, since the descending trigeminal tract extends as far as the upper cervical spine.[180] Although high cervical intramedullary tumors may cause sensory loss in the distribution of the trigeminal nerve alone before long tract signs develop, extramedullary spinal growths produce long tract signs before trigeminal sensory loss is found.[106]

Nystagmus has been reported in several cases of both intramedullary and extramedullary cervical spine tumors.[50,106,109] The mechanism may be due to involvement of the medial longitudinal fasciculus in the cervical spine, extension of the tumor into the posterior fossa, distant vascular effects in the medulla, or other reasons.[106]

Cranial nerve symptoms and signs and elevated intracranial pressure also may occur in patients with spinal tumors when the tumor has spread to the intracranial space. This may occur due to a second primary tumor intracranially, as is often seen in neurofibromatosis. Intracranial metastases may occur from primary spinal tumors or may develop independently in cases where the spinal tumor is itself a metastasis. Finally, cerebral and brain-stem symptoms and signs may, of course, be due to an independent, unrelated disease.

Subarachnoid Hemorrhage

Spontaneous spinal subarachnoid hemorrhage is responsible for less than 1% of all cases of subarachnoid hemorrhage.[181] Unlike intracranial causes, in which aneurysm is the most important etiology, spinal aneurysms are rare.[181] Spinal arteriovenous malformations are the most common cause of spinal subarachnoid hemorrhage. Rarely, spinal tumors may be responsible. According to one review,[122] the neoplasm is usually found in the lower spinal cord or cauda equina. The most common histological tumor type appears to be ependymoma. Other intramedullary tumors may also be responsible, and

meningiomas and neurinomas have been reported to cause spinal subarachnoid hemorrhage. The same review[122] fails to cite any cases caused by epidural spinal tumors, and we are unaware of any such cases.

SUMMARY

Spinal cord dysfunction whether it be due to compression, inflammation, trauma, ischemia, or other cause presents with clinical patterns that can be understood, in most cases, based on a knowledge of the anatomy and physiology of the spinal cord. This chapter has reviewed those clinical presentations that are most commonly encountered. The clinical presentations were generally separated on the basis of (1) the anatomical level of spinal cord and/or root involvement and (2) the spinal tracts involved (transverse plane).

The spinal cord is divided into 31 segments from the first cervical through first coccygeal levels. Segmental (or root) dysfunction is determined on the basis of motor, sensory, and/or reflex loss. Some muscles have been described as "segment-pointer" muscles, such as the triceps that is innervated by C7 or the extensor hallucis longus that is innervated by L5. The distribution of pain referral, sensory disturbance, or reflex loss is also helpful in localizing the level of segmental dysfunction.

Localization of spinal cord disease in the transverse plane is determined on the basis of white matter tract involvement (e.g., a "sensory level" may distinguish a spinal cord lesion from peripheral neuropathy). Furthermore, the secondary examination in an intramedullary cord lesions may spare the buttocks because the ascending sponothalamic tracts are laminated with the sacral dermatomes most peripherally represented. This pattern of "sacral sparing" has been associated with syringomyelia but may occur with other etiologies such as intramedullary cord tumors or cord injury following trauma. Alternatively, a Brown-Sequard syndrome is defined as a hemisection of the cord with upper motor neuron (weakness) and posterior column (position and vibratory sensation) dysfunction ipsilateral to the lesion and contralateral loss of spinothalamic tract (pin and temperature sensation) below the lesion.

There are several characteristic clinical syndromes that can be recognized. For example, cervical spondylotic myelopathy commonly presents with loss of segmental function at the C5, C6, and C7 level and myelopathic findings below the lesion. In such a case where there is a C6 radiculopathy and myelopathy below this level, tapping the brachioradialis reflex (C6) may cause the finger flexors to contract but no brachioradialis response because of the hyperreflexia below the C6 level. Furthermore, the clinical presentation of "sciatica" with L5 or S1 radiculopathy can usually be recognized based on the history and clinical examination. Finally, special consideration was given to etiologies such as trauma and distinguishing intramedullary from extramedullary lesions that cause spinal cord and cauda equina dysfunction.

REFERENCES

1. Schliack H. Segmental innervation and the clinical aspects of spinal nerve root syndromes. In Vinken PJ, Bruyn GW, editors. *Handbook of Clinical Neurology, Volume 2*. Amsterdam: North-Holland 1969; pp. 157–77.
2. Coggeshall RE, Applebaum ML, Fazen M, et al. Unmyelinated axons in human ventral roots, a possible explanation for the failure of dorsal root rhizotomy to relieve pain. *Brain* 1975;98: 157–66.
3. MRC. *Aids to the Investigation of Peripheral Nerve Injuries*. London: Her Majesty's Royal Stationery Office; 1953.
4. Vignos PJ, Archibald KC. Maintenance of ambulation in childhood muscular dystrophy. *J Chronic Dis* 1960;12:273–90.
5. Karnofsky DA, Burchenal JH. The clinical evaluation of chemotherapeutic agents in cancer. In McCleod CM, editor. *Evaluation of Chemotherapeutic Agents*. New York: Columbia University Press; 1949; pp. 191–205.
6. Csuka M, McCarty DJ. Simple method for measurement of lower extremity muscle strength. *Am J Med* 1978;78:77–81.
7. Walton J. Clinical examination of the neuromuscular system. In Walton J, editor *Disorders of Voluntary Muscle*. Edinburgh: Churchill Livingstone; 1981; pp. 448–80.
8. Bucy PC, Keplinger JE, Siqueira EB. Destruction of the pyramidal tract in man. *J Neurosurg* 1964;21:385–98.
9. Bucy PC, Ladpli R, Ehrlich A. Destruction of the pyramidal tract in the monkey: the effects of bilateral destruction of the cerebral peduncles. *J Neurosurg* 1966;25:1–20.
10. Burke D. Spasticity as an adaptation to pyramidal tract injury. In Waxman SG, editor. *Functional Recovery in Neurological Disease*. New York: Raven Press; 1988.
11. Tower SS. Pyramidal lesion in the monkey. *Brain* 1940;63:36–90.
12. Booth RE, Rothman RH. Cervical angina. *Spine* 1976;1:28–32.
13. Brodsky A. Cervical angina: a correlative study with emphasis on the use of coronary arteriography. *Spine* 1985;10:699–709.
14. Brown-Sequard CE. Truth of Sir Charles Bell's theory as regards the existence of two distinct sets of nervous conductors: the sensitive and the motor. In Brown-Sequard CE, editor. *Physiology and Pathology of the Central Nervous System*. Philadelphia: Collins, Printer; 1860; pp. 1–12.
15. Brown-Sequard CE. *Physiology and Pathology of the Central Nervous System*. Philadelphia: Collins, Printer; 1860.
16. Maynard CW, Leonard RB, Coulter JD, et al. Central connections of ventral root afferents as demonstrated by the HRP method. *J Comp Neurol* 1977;172:601–8.
17. Yamamoto T, Takahashi K, Satomi H, et al. Origins of primary afferent fibers in the spinal ventral roots in the cat as demonstrated by the horseradish peroxidase method. *Brain Res* 1977;126:350–4.
18. Frykholm R, Norlen G, Skoglund CR. On pain sensations produced by stimulation of ventral roots in man. *Acta Physiol Scand* 1953;29:455–69.
19. Nachlas I. Pseudo-angina pectoris originating in the cervical spine. *JAMA* 1934;103:323.
20. Phillips J. The importance of examination of the spine in the presence of intrathoracic or abdominal pain. *Proc Int Postgrad MA North Am* 1927;3:70.
21. Roofe PG. Innervation of annulus fibrosus and posterior longitudinal ligament. *Arch Neurol Psych* 1940;44:100–3.
22. Pancoast HK. Superior pulmonary sulcus tumor: tumor characterized by pain, Horner's syndrome, destruction of bone and atrophy of hand muscles. *JAMA* 1932;99:1391–6.
23. Waxman S, Kocsis J, Black J. Type III sodium channel mRNA is expressed in embryonic but not adult spinal sensory neurons, and is re-expressed following axotomy. *J Neurophysiol* 1994; 72:466–71.
24. Dib-Hajj S, Black J, Felts P, Waxman S. Down-regulation of transcripts for Na channel alpha-SNS in spinal sensory neurons following axotomy. *Proc Natl Acad Sci* 1996;93:14950–4.
25. Rizzo M, Kocsis J, Waxman S. Selective loss of slow and enhancement of fast Na⁺ currents in cutaneous afferent DRG neurons following axotomy. *Neurobiol Dis* 1995;2:87–97.

26. Rizzo M, Kocsis J, Waxman S. Mechanisms of paraesthesiae, dysaesthesiae and hyperesthesiae: role of Na channel heterogeneity. *Eur Neurol* 1996;36:3–12.

27. Cummins T, Waxman S. Down-regulation of tetrodotoxin-resistant sodium currents and up-regulation of a rapidly repriming tetrodotoxin-sensitive sodium current in small spinal sensory neurons following nerve injury. *J Neurosci* 1997; 17:3504–14.

28. Woolf C, Shortland P, Coggeshall R. Peripheral nerve injury triggers central sprouting of myelinated afferents. *Nature* 1992;355:75–7.

29. Rowe ML. Low back pain in industry: a position paper. *J Occup Med* 1969;11:161–9.

30. Deyo RA, Diehl AK, Rosenthal M. How many days of bed rest for acute low back pain? A randomized clinical trial. *N Engl J Med* 1986;315: 1064–70.

31. Gilbert RW, Kim JH, Posner JB. Epidural spinal cord compression from metastatic tumor: diagnosis and treatment. *Ann Neurol* 1978;3:40–51.

32. Portenoy R, Lipton RB, Foley KM. Back pain in the cancer patient: an algorithm for the evaluation and management. *Neurology* 1987; 37:134–7.

33. Nicholas JJ, Christy WC. Spinal pain made worse by recumbency: a clue to spinal cord tumors. *Arch Phys Med Rehabil* 1986;67:598–600.

34. Rasmussen TB, Kernohan JW, Adson AW. Pathologic classification, with surgical consideration, of intraspinal tumors. *Ann Surg* 1940; 111:513–30.

35. DeJong RN. *The Neurologic Examination, 4th Edition.* Hagerstown: Harper & Row; 1979.

35a. Rodriguez M, Dinapoli RP. Spinal cord compression. With special reference to metastatic epidural tumors. Mayo Clin Proc 1980;55: 442–8.

36. O'Rourke T, George CB, Redmond J, et al. Spinal computed tomography and computed tomographic metrizamide myelography in the early diagnosis of metastatic disease. *J Clin Oncol* 1986;4:576–83.

37. Patten J. *Neurological Differential Diagnosis.* New York: Springer-Verlag; 1977.

38. Simons DG, Travell JG. Myofascial pain syndromes. In Wall PD, Melzack R, editors. *Textbook of Pain.* Edinburgh: Churchill Livingstone; 1984; pp. 263–76.

39. Kellgren JH. On the distribution of pain arising from deep somatic structures with charts of segmental pain areas. *Clin Sci* 1939;4:35–46.

40. McCall IW, Park WM, O'Brien JP. Induced pain referral from posterior lumbar elements in normal subjects. *Spine* 1979;4:441–6.

41. Sinclair DC, Feindel WH, Falconer MA. The intervertebral ligaments as a source of segmental pain. *J Bone Joint Surg* 1948;30-B:515–21.

42. Fitzgerald M. The course and termination of primary afferent fibers. In Wall PD, Melzack R, editors. *Textbook of Pain.* Edinburgh: Churchill Livingstone; 1984; p. 40.

43. Head H. On disturbances of sensation with special reference to visceral disease. *Brain* 1893;16: 1–132.

44. Sherrington CS. Experiments in the examination of the peripheral distribution of the fibers of the posterior roots of some spinal nerves Part II. *Philos Trans B* 1898;190:45–186.

45. Foerster O. The dermatomes in man. *Brain* 1933;56:1.

46. Dykes Rw, Terzis JK. Spinal nerve distribution in the upper limb: the organization of the dermatome and afferent myotome. *Philos Trans R Soc Lond Biol* 1981;293:509–54.

47. Denny-Brown D, Kirk EJ, Yanigasawa N. The tract of Lissauer in relation to sensory transmission in the dorsal horn of spinal cord in the macaque monkey. *J Comp Neurol* 1973;151: 175–200.

48. Willis WD, Coggeshall RE. Peripheral nerves, sensory receptors, and spinal cord. In Willis WD, Coggeshall RE, editors. *Sensory Mechanisms of the Spinal Cord.* New York: Plenum Press; 1978; pp. 9–52.

49. Schold SC, Cho E-S, Somasundaram M, Posner JB. Subacute motor neuronopathy: a remote effect of lymphoma. *Ann Neurol* 1979;5:271–87.

50. Elsberg CA. *Surgical Diseases of the Spinal Cord, Membranes and Nerve Root* New York: Hoeber; 1941.

51. Ropper AH, Fisher CM, Kleinman GM. Pyramidal infarction in the medulla: a cause of pure motor hemiplegia sparing the face. *Neurology* 1979;29:91–5.

52. Gijn J. The Babinski response and the pyramidal syndrome. *J Neurol Neurosurg Psychiat* 1978; 41:865–73.

53. Landau WM, Clare MH. The plantar reflex in man, with special reference to some conditions where the extensor response is unexpectedly absent. *Brain* 1959;82:321–55.

54. Nathan PW, Smith MC. The Babinski response: a review and new observations. *Brain* 1955;18: 250–9.

55. Savitsky N, Madonick MJ. Statistical control studies in neurology: Babinski sign. *Arch Neurol Psych* 1943;49:272–6.

56. Yakovlev P, Farrell MJ. Influence of locomotion on the plantar reflex in normal and in physically and mentally inferior persons: theoretic and practical implications. *Arch Neurol Psych* 1941;46:322–30.

57. Karp SJ, Ho RTK. Gait ataxia as a presenting symptom of malignant epidural spinal cord compression. *Postgrad Med J* 1986;62:745–7.

58. Guttman L. Clinical symptomatology of spinal cord lesions. In Vinken PJ, Bruyn GW, editors. *Handbook of Clinical Neurology, Volume 2.* Amsterdam: North-Holland; 1969; pp. 178–216.

59. Matsumoto S, Okuda B, Imai T, Kameyama M. A sensory level on the trunk in lower lateral brainstem lesions. *Neurology* 1988;38:1515–9.

60. Simmons Z, Biller J, Beck DW, et al. Painless compressive cervical myelopathy with false localizing sensory findings. *Spine* 1986;11:869–72.

61. Brooker AE, Barter AW. Cervical spondylosis. Clinical study with comparative radiology. *Brain* 1965;88:925–36.

62. Good DC, Couch JR, Wacasar L. "Numb, clumsy hands" and high cervical spondylosis. *Surg Neurol* 1984;22:285–91.

63. Plum F. Neurological integration of behavioural and metaboloic control of breathing. In Porter R, editor. *Breathing: Hering-Breuer Centenary Symposium.* London: Churchill; 1970; pp. 159–75.

64. Berger L, Mitchell RA, Servinghaus JW. Regulation of respiration (3 part series). *N Engl J Med* 1977;297:92–7;138–43;194–201.

65. Greenberg AD. Atlanto-axial dislocations. *Brain* 1968;91:655–84.

66. Nathan P, Smith M. The centrifugal pathways for micturition within the spinal cord. *J Neurol Neurosurg Psychiatry* 1958;21:177.

67. Haymaker W. *Bing's Local Diagnosis in Neurological Disease, 15th Edition.* St. Louis: C.V. Mosby; 1969.

68. Tator C. Clinical manifestations of acute spinal cord injury. In Benzel E, editor. *Contemporary Management of Spinal Cord Injury.* Park Ridge, Illinois: American Association of Neurological Surgeons; 1995; pp. 238–46.

69. Frankel H, Hancock D, Hyslop G, others. The value of postural reduction in the management of closed injuries of the spine with paraplegia and tetraplegia, part 1. *Paraplegia* 1969;7:179–92.

70. ASIA. *American Spinal Injury Association, International Medical Society of Paraplegia: International Standards for Neurological and Functional Classification of Spinal Cord Injury (Revised, 1992).* Chicago, IL: ASIA/IMSOP; 1992.

71. Benzel E, Larson S. Functional recovery after decompressive operation for thoracic and lumbar spine fractures. *Neurosurgery* 1986;19:772–8.

72. Sherrington CS. *The Integrative Action of the Nervous System.* New Haven: Yale University Press; 1923.

73. Riddoch G. The reflex functions of the completely divided spinal cord in man, compared with those associated with the less severe lesions. *Brain* 1917;40:264.

74. Chambers WW, Liu CN, McCouch GP. Anatomical and physiological correlates of plasticity in the central nervous system. *Brain Behav Evol* 1973;8:5–26.

75. Fulton JE, Liddell EGT, Rioch DM. The influence of the vestibular nuclei upon posture and the knee jerk. *Brain* 1930;53:327–43.

76. Kuhn RA. Functional capacity of the isolated human spinal cord. *Brain* 1950;73:1–51.

77. Elkins CW, Wegner WR. Newer concepts in the treatment of the paralyzed patient due to wartime injuries of the spine. Neurosurgical complications. *Ann Surg 1946;123:516–22.*

78. Guttman L. Rehabilitation after injury to the spinal cord and cauda equina. *Br J Phys Med 1946;9:130.*

79. Guttman L. Studies on reflex activity of the isolated spinal cord in spinal man. *J Nerv Ment Dis* 1946;116:957–72.

80. Adams RD, Victor M. Diseases of The spinal cord. In Adams RD, Victor M, editors. *Principles of Neurology.* New York: McGraw-Hill; 1985: 665–98.

81. Waxman S. Demyelinating diseases—new pathological insights, new therapeutic targets. *N Engl J Med* 1998;338:323–5.

82. Benzel E. *Biomechanics of Spine Stabilization: Principles and Clinical Practice.* New York: McGraw-Hill; 1995.

83. Preobrajensky PA. Syphilitic paraplegias with dissociated disturbances of sensibility. *J Neuropat Psikhiat* 1904;4:594.

84. Blackwood W. Discussion on the vascular disease of the spinal cord. *Proc R Soc Med* 1958; 51:543–7.

85. Djindjian R. Angiography in angiomas of the spinal cord. In Pia HW, Djindjian R, editors. *Spinal Angiomas: Advances in Diagnosis and Therapy.* New York: Springer-Verlag; 1978; p. 98.

86. Hogan EL, Romanul FCA. Spinal cord infarction occurring during insertion of aortic graft. *Neurology* 1966;16:67–74.

87. Hughes JT, MacIntyre AG. Spinal cord infarction occurring during thoracolumbar sympathectomy. *J Neurol Neurosurg Psychiatry* 1963;26:418–21.

88. Albert ML, Greer WER, Kantrowitz W. Paraplegia secondary to hypotension and cardiac arrest in a patient who has had previous thoracic surgery. *Neurology* 1969;19:915–8.

89. Gilles FH. Hypotensive brain stem necrosis. *Arch Pathol* 1969;88:32.

90. Gilles FH, Nag D. Vulnerability of human spinal cord in transient cardiac arrest. *Neurology* 1971;21:833–9.

91. Silver JR, Buxton PH. Spinal stroke. *Brain* 1974;97:539–50.

92. Schneider RC, Cherry G, Pantek H. The syndrome of acute central cervical spinal cord injury with special reference to mechanisms involved in hyperextension injuries of the cervical spine. *J Neurosurg* 1954;11:546–77.

93. Ropper AH, Poskanzer DC. The prognosis of acute and subacute transverse myelopathy based on early signs and symptoms. *Ann Neurol* 1978;4:51–9.

94. Benzel E, Larson S. Functional recovery after decompressive spine fractures. *Neurosurgery* 1987;20:742–6.

95. John JRS, Rand CW. Stab wounds of the spinal cord. *Bull Los Angeles Neurol Soc* 1953;18:1–24.

96. Dynes JB, Smedal MI. Radiation myelitis. *AJR Am J Roentgenol* 1960;83:78–87.

97. Stark RJ, Henson RA, Evans SJW. Spinal metastases: a retrospective survey from a general hospital. *Brain* 1982;105:189–213.

98. Kahn E. The role of dentate ligaments in spinal cord compression and the syndrome of lateral sclerosis. *J Neurosurg* 1947;4:191–9.

99. Payne E, Spillane J. The cervical spine. An anatomico-pathological study of seventy specimens (using a special technique) with particular reference to the problem of cervical spondylosis. *Brain* 1957;80:571–96.

100. Reid J. Effects of flexion-extension movements of the head and spine upon the spinal cord and

nerve roots. *J Neurol Neurosurg Psychiatry* 1960; 23:214–21.

101. Stoops W, King R. Neural complications of cervical spondylosis: their response to laminectomy and foraminotomy. *J Neurosurg* 1962;19: 986–9.

102. Taylor A. The mechanism of injury to the spinal cord in the neck without damage to the vertebral column. *J Bone J Surg* 1951;33-B:543–7.

103. Wilkinson H, Lemay M, Ferris E. Clinical-radiographic correlations in cervical spondylosis. *J Neurosurg* 1969;30:213–8.

104. Russell JSR, Batten FE, Collier J. Subacute combined degeneration of the spinal cord. *Brain* 1900;23:39–110.

105. Lindenbaum J, Healton EB, Savage DG, et al. Neuropsychiatric disorders caused by cobalamin deficiency in the absence of anemia or macrocytosis. *N Engl J Med* 1988;318:1720–8.

106. Schliack H, Stille D. Clinical symptomatology of intraspinal tumors. In Vinken PJ, Bruyn GW, editors. *Handbook of Clinical Neurology Volume 19*. Amsterdam: North-Holland; 1975; pp. 23–49.

107. McRae DL. Bony abnormalities in the region of the foramen magnum: Correlation of the anatomic and neurologic findings. *Acta Radiol* 1953;40:335–54.

108. McRae DL. The significance of abnormalities of the cervical spine. *Am J Radiol* 1960;84:3–25.

109. Symonds C, Meadows SP. Compression of the spinal cord in the neighborhood of the foramen magnum. *Brain* 1937;60:52–84.

110. Foley KM, Sundaresan N. Management of cancer pain. In DeVita VT, Hellman S, Rosenberg SA, editors. *Cancer Principles and Practice of Oncology*. Philadelphia: J.B. Lippincott; 1985; pp. 1940–61.

111. Adams RD, Victor M. Pain in the back, neck, and extremities. In Adams RD, Victor M, editors. *Principles of Neurology*. New York: McGraw-Hill; 1985; pp. 149–72.

112. Bosley TM, Cohen DA, Schatz NJ, et al. Comparison of metrizamide computed tomography and magnetic resonance imaging in the evaluation of lesions at the cervicomedullary junction. *Neurology* 1985;35:485–92.

113. McAfee PC, Bohlman HH, Han JS, et al. Comparison of nuclear magnetic resonance imaging and computed tomography in the diagnosis of upper cervical spinal cord compression. *Spine* 1986;11:295–304.

114. Hensinger RN, Ewen GDM. Congenital anomalies of the spine. In Rothman RH, Simeone FA, editors. *The Spine* Philadelphia: W.B. Saunders; 1982; pp. 188–315.

115. Hastings DE, Macnab I, Lawson V. Neoplasms of the atlas and axis. *Can J Surg* 1968;11:290–6.

116. Lipson S. Cervical myelopathy and posterior atlanto-axial subluxation in patients with rheumatoid arthritis. *J Bone Joint Surg* 1985;67-A:593–7.

117. Wolfe BS, Kilnani M, Malis L. The sagittal diameter of the bony cervical spinal canal and its significance in cervical spondylosis. *J Mt Sinai Hosp* 1965;23:283–92.

118. Bharucha EP, Dastur HM. Craniovertebral anomalies (a report on 40 cases). *Brain* 1964;87: 469–80.

119. Spillane JD, Pallis C, Jones AM. Developmental abnormalities in the region of the foramen magnum. *Brain* 1957;80:11–48.

120. Adams RD, Victor M. Nonviral infections of the nervous system. In Adams RD, Victor M, editors. *Principles of Neurology*. New York: McGraw-Hill; 1985; pp. 510–44.

121. Kori SH, Foley KM, Posner JB. Brachial plexus lesions in patients with cancer: 100 cases. *Neurology* 1981;31:45–50.

122. Guidetti B, Fortuna A. Differential diagnosis of intramedullary and extramedullary tumors. In Vinken PJ, Bruyn GW, editors. *Handbook of Clinical Neurology, Volume 19*. Amsterdam: North-Holland; 1975; pp. 51–75.

123. Warrington WB. A case of tumor of the cauda eqina removed by operation with remarks on the diagnosis and nature of lesions in that situation. *Lancet* 1905;83(2):749–53.

124. Levitt P, Ransohoff J, Spielholz N. The differential diagnosis of tumors of the conus medullaris and cauda equina. In Vinken PJ, Bruyn GW, editors. *Handbook of Clinical Neurology, Volume 19*. Amsterdam: North-Holland; 1975; pp. 77–90.

125. Norstrom CW, Kernohan JW, Love JG. One hundred primary caudal tumors. *JAMA* 1961;178:1071–7.

126. Nassar SI, Correll JW, Housepian EM. Intramedullary cystic lesions of the conus medullaris. *J Neurol Neurosurg Psychiatry* 1968; 31:106–9.

127. Alter M. Statistical aspects of spinal cord tumors. In Vinken PJ, Bruyn GW, editors. *Handbook of Clinical Neurology, Volume 19*. Amsterdam: North-Holland; 1975; pp. 1–22.

128. Barron KD, Hirano A, Araki S, et al. Experiences with metastatic neoplasms involving the spinal cord. *Neurology* 1959;9:91–106.

129. Paillas J-E, Alliez B, Pellet W. Primary and secondary tumours of the spine. In Vinken PJ, Bruyn GW, editors. *Handbook of Clinical Neurology, Volume 20*. Amsterdam: North-Holland; 1976; pp. 19–54.

130. McAlhany HJ, Netsky MG. Compression of the spinal cord by extramedullary neoplasms: a clinical and pathological study. *J Neuropathol Exp Neurol* 1955;14:276–87.

131. Posner JB. Back pain and epidural spinal cord compression. *Med Clin North Am* 1987;71:185–204.

132. Broager B. Spinal neurinoma. *Acta Psychiatr Scand Suppl* 1953;85:1–241.

133. Iraci G, Peserico L, Salar G. Intraspinal neurinomas and meningiomas. A clinical survey of 172 cases. *Int J Surg* 1971;56:289–303.

134. Guidetti B, Fortuna A, Moscatelli G, et al. I Tumori intramidollari. Relazione al al XVI Congr Soc Ital di Neurochir Genova, Nov 1964. *Lav Neuropsychiat* 1964;35:1–409.

135. Cairns H, Riddoch G. Observations on the treatment of ependymal gliomas of the spinal cord. *Brain* 1931;54:117–46.

136. Shenkin HA, Alpers BJ. Clinical and pathological features of gliomas of the spinal cord. *Arch Neurol Psychiat* 1944;52:87–105.

137. Torma T. Malignant tumors of the spine and the spinal extradural space. *Acta Chir Scand Suppl* 1957;225:1–176.

138. Smith KJ, McDonald WI. Spontaneous and evoked electrical discharges from a central demyelinating lesion. *J Neurol Sci* 1982;55:39–47.

139. Lhermitte J, Bollak NM. Les douleurs a type de decharge electrique consecutives a la flexion cephalique dans la sclerose en plaque. *Rev Neurol (Paris)* 1924;31:36–52.

140. Khanchandani R, Howe JG. Lhermitte's sign in multiple sclerosis: a clinical survey and review of the literature. *J Neurol Neurosurg Psychiatry* 1982;45:308–12.

141. Dejong RN. Sensation. In Vinken PJ, Bruyn GW, editors. *Handbook of Clinical Neurology, Volume 1*. Amsterdam: North-Holland; 1969; pp. 80–113.

142. Chan RC, Steinboh P. Delayed onset of Lhermitte's sign following head and/or neck injuries. *J Neurosurg* 1984;60:609–12.

143. Jones A. Transient radiation myelopathy (with reference to Lhermitte's sign of electrical paresthesia). *Br J Radiol* 1964;37:727–44.

144. Word JA, Kalokhe UP, Aron BS, Elson HR. Transient radiation myelopathy (Lhermitte's sign) in patients with Hodgkin's disease treated by mantle radiation. *Int J Radiat Oncol Biol Phys* 1980;6:1731–3.

145. Sandyk R, Brennan MJW. Lhermitte's sign as a presenting symptom of subacute degeneration of the cord. *Ann Neurol* 1983;13:215–6.

146. Benninger TR, Patterson VH. Lhermitte's sign as a presenting symptom of B12 deficiency. *Ulster Med J* 1984;53:162–3.

147. Coman DR, DeLong RP. The role of the vertebral venous system in the metastasis of cancer to the spinal column. *Cancer* 1951;4:610–8.

148. Nachemson A. In vivo discometry in lumbar discs with irregular nucleograms. *Acta Orthop Scand* 1965;36:418–34.

149. Ushio Y, Posner R, Posner JB, others. Experimental spinal cord compression by epidural neoplasms. *Neurology* 1977;27:422–9.

150. Love JG, Thelen EP, Dodge HW. Tumors of the foramen magnum. *J Int Coll Surg* 1954;22:1–17.

151. Stein B, Leeds NE, Taveras J, et al. Meningiomas of the foramen magnum. *J Neurosurg* 1963;20:740–51.

152. Davis RA, Washburn PL. Spinal cord meningiomas. *Brain* 1970;90:359–94.

153. Gautier-Smith PC. Clinical aspects of spinal neurofibromas. *Brain* 1970;90:359–94.

154. Longeval E, Holdebrand J, Vollont GH. Early diagnosis of metastases in the epidural space. *Acta Neurochir* 1975;31:177–84.

155. Glasauer FE. Thoracic and lumbar intraspinal tumors associated with increased intracranial pressure. *J Neurol Neurosurg Psychiatry* 1964;27:451–8.

156. Tilney F, Elsberg CA. Sensory disturbances in tumors of the cervical spinal cord: arrangement of fibers in the sensory pathways. *Arch Neurol Psychiat* 1926;15:444–54.

157. Dodge HW, Love JG, Gottlieb CM. Benign tumors at the foramen magnum. *J Neurosurg* 1956;13:603–17.

158. Rewcastle NB, Berry K. Neoplasms of the lower spinal canal. *Neurology* 1964;14:608–15.

159. Cascino TL, Kori S, Krol G, Foley KM. CT of the brachial plexus in patients with cancer. *Neurology* 1983;33:1553–7.

160. Lederman RJ, Wilbourn AJ. Brachial plexopathy: recurrent cancer or radiation? *Neurology* 1984;34:1331–5.

161. Herchorn S, Ordorica R. Urologic management. In Benzel E, Tator C, editors. *Contemporary Management of Spinal Cord Injury*. Park Ridge, IL: AANS; 1995.

162. Arseni C, Maretsis M. Tumors of the lower spinal cord associated with increased intracranial pressure and papilledema. *J Neurosurg* 1967;27:105–10.

163. Feldman E, Bromfield E, Navia B, Pasternak GW, Posner JB. Hydrocephalic dementia and spinal cord tumor: a report of a case and review of the literature. *Arch Neurol* 1986;43:714–8.

164. Iob I, Androli GC, Rigobello L, others. An unusual onset of a spinal cord tumor: subarachnoid bleeding and papilledema. *Neurochirurgia* 1980;23:112–6.

165. Love JG, Wagner HP, Woltman HW. Tumors of the spinal cord associated with choking of the optic disks. *Arch Neurol* 1951;66:171–7.

166. Luzecky M, Siegel BA, Coxe WS, et al. Papilledema and communicating hydrocephalus: association with a lumbar neurofibroma. *Arch Neurol* 1974;30:487–9.

167. Maurice-Williams RS, Lucey JJ. Raised intracranial pressure due to spinal tumors: three rare cases with a probable common mechanism. *Br J Surg* 1975;62:92–5.

168. Mittal MM, Gupta NC, Sharma ML. Spinal epidural meningioma associated with increased intracranial pressure. *Neurology* 1970;20:818–20.

169. Michowiz SD, Rappaport HZ, Shaked I, Yellin A, Sahar A. Thoracic disc herniation associated with papilledema: case report. *J Neurosurg* 1984;61:1132–4.

170. Raynor RB. Papilledema associated with tumors of the spinal cord. *Neurology* 1969;19:700–4.

171. Schijman E, Zuccaro G, Monges JA. Spinal tumors and hydrocephalus. *Childs Brain* 1981;8:401–5.

172. Gibberd FB, Ngan H, Swann GF. Hydrocephalus, subarachnoid hemorrhage and ependymomas of the cauda equina. *Clin Radiol* 1972;23:422–6.

173. Harris P. Chronic progressive communicating hydrocephalus due to protein transudates from brain and spinal tumors. *Dev Med Child Neurol* 1962;4:270–8.

174. Bamford CR, Labadie EL. Reversal of dementia in normotensive hydrocephalus after removal of cauda equina tumor. *J Neurosurg* 1976;45:104–7.

175. Neil-Dwyer G. Tentorial block of cerebrospinal fluid associated with a lumbar neurofibroma. *J Neurosurg* 1973;38:767–70.
176. Ridsdale L, Moseley I. Thoracolumbar intraspinal tumors presenting features of raised intracranial pressure. *J Neurol Neurosurg Psychiatry* 1978;41:737–45.
177. Gardner WJ, Spitler DK, Whitten C. Increased intracranial pressure caused by increased protein content in the cerebrospinal fluid. An explanation of papilledema in certain cases of small intracranial and intraspinal tumors and in Guillain-Barre syndrome. *N Engl J Med* 1954; 250:932–6.
178. Hayreh SS. Pathogenesis of edema of the optic disc (papilledema). A preliminary report. *Br J Ophthalmol* 1964;48:522–43.
179. Elsberg CA. *Tumors of the Spinal Cord and Membranes*. New York: Paul A. Hoeber; 1925.
180. Carpenter MB. *Human Neuroanatomy, 7th Edition*. Baltimore: William and Wilkins; 1976.
181. Buchan AM, Barnett JM. Vascular malformations and hemorrhage of the spinal cord. In Barnett HJM, Mohr JP, Stein BM, Yatsu FM, editors. *Stroke: Pathophysiology, Diagnosis and Management*. New York: Churchill Livingstone; 1986; pp. 721–30.
182. Byrne TN. Spinal cord compression from epidural metastases. *N Engl J Med* 1992;327: 614–9.
183. Sinclair D. *The Physiology and Pathophysiology of the Skin*. A. Jarrett (Editor) Vol 2. London: Academic Press, 1973; p. 349.

Chapter 3

PAIN OF SPINAL ORIGIN

Back pain, neck pain, and referred pain to the trunk and extremities are common and often represent diagnostically challenging problems for the physician. In the United States, low back pain is second only to colds as the most common reason for patients' visits to physicians[1] and is reported to occur at some time in the lives of approximately 65% to 80% of individuals.[2-5] Back pain is reported to be the most expensive chronic illness among persons 30–60 years of age in our society.[4] The number of individuals reportedly disabled by low back pain grew at a rate 14 times that of the United States population growth between 1971 and 1981.[6]

Despite its major importance, in many cases the precise etiology and pathogenesis of this pain syndrome are uncertain.[7,8] While some authors report disc disease as a leading cause,[4] others cite musculoligamentous strain and degenerative osteoarthritis as the major culprits.[9-11] Fortunately, in the majority of such instances of regional back pain (i.e., those not caused by systemic illness), the pain is self-limited and the individual is able to return to normal activities in a few weeks with only rest and analgesics.[12,13]

Among the great number of individuals complaining of back and/or neck pain, with or without pain referral elsewhere, there are a few in whom it will be a manifestation of serious underlying disease. Metastatic cancer to the spine is an example of such a disease.[14] For example, in a series of 1975 outpatients with a chief complaint of back pain, 13 (0.66%) proved to have underlying cancer.[15] Findings significantly associated with cancer were:

1. Age > 50 years
2. Duration of pain greater than one month
3. Prior history of cancer or other systemic signs of underlying disease (e.g., weight loss, hematuria)
4. Lack of improvement with conservative therapy
5. Anemia
6. An elevated erythrocyte sedimentation rate

Among patients with a history of malignancy, back pain secondary to metastases frequently occurs at some time during the course of the disease. Vertebral metastases develop in nearly one-third of patients dying from cancer, and[16] in approximately 5% of dying cancer patients, vertebral metastases progress to cause epidural spinal cord compression.[17] In approximately 90% of this latter group, pain localized to the spine or referred elsewhere is the presenting manifestation of spinal cord compression.[18] It is important to detect spinal cord compression from malignancy when pain is the only symptom and the patient is ambulatory, because the prognosis for neurological function is far better than in patients who have signs of myelopathy at the time of diagnosis.

In addition to back pain arising from pathology of the spine, pain may be referred to the back from other organs. For example, back pain may be the first symptom of life-threatening intra-abdominal or intrathoracic diseases, such as dissecting aortic aneurysm, neoplasm, pleural disease, and infection.

Given the broad range of causes of back pain, radiological studies of the spine are often ordered in the expectation that they will identify the correct etiology. However, as discussed later in this chapter, radiological studies such as plain radiographs, CT scanning, or magnetic resonance imaging (MRI) performed in the evaluation of back pain may reveal clinically irrelevant information. A large number of asymptomatic individuals harbor radiological evidence of osteoarthritis and even herniated lumbar discs.[19–21] In order to be considered clinically significant, radiological findings must be correlated with the patient's clinical history and physical examination. If this is not done properly, the correct diagnosis may be delayed or, worse, laminectomy and diskectomy may be performed on a patient with an asymptomatic herniated disc who has serious disease elsewhere that is responsible for the pain.

Recognized in these terms, the diagnostic challenge of back pain, and its frequently associated referred pain, is daunting. This chapter summarizes the clinical features that are most helpful in achieving an accurate assessment of back, neck, referred, and radicular pain.

THE ANATOMICAL BASIS OF BACK AND NECK PAIN

Knowledge of the innervation of the vertebral column and its associated supporting structures is essential to understanding pain of spinal origin. Many of the pain-sensitive structures of the ventral segment of the spine are innervated by the sinuvertebral nerve,[22] whereas the facet joints of the dorsal segment are innervated by the dorsal ramus of the spinal nerve[23] (Fig. 3–1).

The sinuvertebral nerve, occasionally termed the recurrent meningeal nerve, originates as a branch of the spinal nerve just distal to the dorsal root ganglion. This branch exits the root of the spinal nerve as it passes through the intervertebral foramen. As this recurrent branch reflects back toward the intervertebral foramen, it is joined by an autonomic branch from a nearby gray ramus communicans.[24] These two branches usually fuse to form the sinuvertebral nerve, which reenters the spinal canal through the rostral aspect of the intervertebral foramen. Upon reentry into the spinal canal, the sinuvertebral nerve divides into multiple branches that innervate the periosteum of the vertebral body, posterior longitudinal ligament, the dorsal aspect of annulus fibrosus, the ventral aspect of dura mater, and blood vessels.[22,25,26]

The segmental distribution of the sinuvertebral nerves is controversial. Early studies[27] suggested that the sinuvertebral nerve courses only caudally and innervates the posterior longitudinal ligament for one or two segments below the level of entry into the vertebral canal. However, more recent investigations have failed to confirm this[28] and report that the branches of the sinuvertebral nerve course in a rostral direction for one segment and a caudal direction for two segments.[22,29,30] This results in considerable overlap of innervation between adjacent segments and may account for the fact that the section-

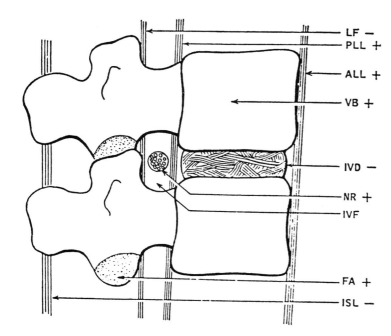

Figure 3–1. The pain-sensitive tissues of the functional unit of the spine. The tissues labeled + are pain-sensitive, containing sensory nerve endings capable of causing pain when irritated. Tissues labeled −are devoid of sensory innervation. (LF = ligamentum flavum; PLL = posterior longitudinal ligament; ALL = anterior longitudinal ligament; VB = vertebral body; IVD = annulus fibrosus of intervertebral disc; IVF = intervertebral foramen containing nerve root [NR]; FA = facet articular cartilage; ISL = interspinous ligament.) (From Cailliet, R,[37] p. 26, with permission.)

ing of a single nerve root does not result in the loss of pain from a herniated disc.

The dura mater is innervated only on its ventral surface by the sinuvertebral nerve.[29] The dorsal region of the dura mater is sparsely innervated. This may explain why puncture of the dura mater with a spinal needle is painless, although the patient may feel a pop as the needle passes through.

The nucleus pulposus and the inner layers of the annulus fibrosus are not innervated and are not, therefore, considered pain-sensitive. There has been debate over the extent of innervation of the peripheral region of the annulus fibrosus. Although early studies[27] did not identify nerve fibers, recent investigators,[31] have suggested the existence of innervation. Many of these nerve fibers have free nerve endings, which may mediate pain sensibility. Others, on the surface of the annulus, have encapsulated endings that may conduct position sensibility.[31] Despite this network of innervation of the annulus fibrosus,[32,33] there remains controversy as to whether the annulus is pain-sensitive.[34,35]

Experimental studies have demonstrated that if the intradiscal pressure is increased by injection of saline, normal subjects ex-

perience no pain. If the annulus fibrosus is degenerated (fragmented), however, pain may be experienced.[36] These experiments have been extended by anesthetizing the posterior longitudinal ligament in subjects with a degenerated disc.[37] In this situation, the same procedure does not result in pain. This led to the conclusion that the posterior longitudinal ligament is the site responsible for mediating much of the pain arising from herniated discs. According to this hypothesis, pain results from the stimulation of free nerve endings when a herniated disc dissects the posterior longitudinal ligament away from the annulus fibrosus and the vertebral body.

The ventral and lateral aspects of each annulus fibrosus and the anterior longitudinal ligament are not innervated by the sinuvertebral nerve. These structures are innervated by branches of the ventral ramus of the spinal nerves and by autonomic branches of the gray rami communicans or of the sympathetic trunk.

The synovial (facet) joints of the dorsal segment of the spine are innervated by branches of the dorsal ramus of the spinal nerve.[23] As with the ventral segments, there is considerable overlap in innervation by adjacent spinal roots. Each facet joint in the lumbar spine is innervated by three segmental levels.[38] Like synovial joints elsewhere, the facet joints may become inflamed, so conceivably they could become a source of pain. In addition to unmyelinated fibers with free nerve endings that probably mediate pain, there are myelinated fibers with complex encapsulated nerve endings that appear to mediate tension and position sensation within the facet.[34,39] These terminations are probably important in controlling posture and movement.[23]

Innervation of the ligamentum flavum and the interspinous ligament has been reported by some authors[23] but denied by others.[40] The source of innervation of the ligamentum flavum is uncertain but is thought to be the posterior ramus.[22] In the cervical spine, the supraspinous ligament expands between the spinous processes of C2 and C7 to form the nuchal ligament. Recent investigations have shown that the nuchal ligament is innervated. Proprioceptive impulses might be conducted through some of these nerve endings,[41] which could be a mechanism of controlling head and neck position and movement.

In addition to spinal pain-sensitive structures, a common source of pain is spasm of the paravertebral muscles. This pain may be local and be associated with physical findings of spasm. It also may be referred, as in cases of myofascial pain syndromes.

CLASSIFICATION OF PAIN OF SPINAL ORIGIN

Several characteristic forms of pain arise from disease of the vertebral column and its associated supporting structures, as well as from diseases of the spinal cord and the nerve roots. Pain can be classified as local, referred, radicular, funicular, or secondary to muscle spasm (myofascial pain syndromes) (Table 3–1). Each of these forms of pain has a unique pathophysiology and clinical significance. Furthermore, distinguishing the form of pain is often very helpful in determining its etiology.

Local Pain

Local back or neck pain is usually characterized by a deep, boring, and aching quality. Often this pain results from degenerative joint disease and musculoskeletal strain that is exacerbated by mechanical stresses on the weight-bearing spine. Therefore, activities that increase the load on the spine or are related to skeletal movement often exacerbate the pain, and bed rest usually alleviates it. When the pattern of pain deviates from this, etiologies of pain other than the common musculoskeletal causes should be considered. For example, back pain referred from visceral structures may share the qualities of deep, boring, aching pain, and yet this type of pain is less likely to be exacerbated by musculoskeletal movements. A gastrointestinal source of pain is likely to be temporally related to dietary and bowel habits rather than to musculoskeletal movements.

As previously discussed, local back or neck pain typically arises from irritation of the innervated portions of the vertebral column and its supporting structures. Since only innervated tissues are pain-sensitive, the cancellous region of the vertebral bodies may be invaded by tumor (as often shown by CT or MR scan) in the absence of pain. When a neoplasm invades the innervated cortical region of bone and the periosteum, however, local pain is experienced. Most cases of malignant epidural spinal cord compression originate from metastases to the vertebrae. In order for neural compression to occur, the metastasis must first invade the cortex of bone and periosteum, causing local pain as the earliest symptom in the vast majority of cases. Similarly, patients with osteoporosis experience pain when the cortex of bone is fractured and the innervated bone and periosteum are irritated.

Since degenerative joint disease (e.g., cervical and lumbar spondylosis) and herniated discs are so frequent, one of the most common clinical problems in the patient with known cancer is that of distinguishing the local pain caused by such benign disorders from local pain caused by spine metastases. Some clinical features

Table 3–1. **Classification of Pain**

1. LOCAL

- Characteristics: deep, boring, and aching
- Tenderness may be present
- If exacerbated by lying down, strongly consider tumor

2. REFERRED

- Characteristics: aching and diffuse
- Pain arising from irritation of lumbar spine referred to flank, pelvis, groin, and lower extremities but not generally below the knee
- The location of this pain is not truly segmental and does not, therefore, have localizing value
- Areas of pain referral may be tender
- Referred pain is aggravated and relieved in tandem with local pain

3. RADICULAR

- Characteristics: sharp, stabbing pain superimposed on chronic ache in the distribution of nerve root
- Commonly radiates to the distal portion of the extremity when due to cervical spondylosis at C5–7 or lumbar spondylosis at L4–S1; below knee if from L4–S1
- Has excellent localizing value
- Tenderness and sensory disturbance along the root distribution are common
- Exacerbated by stretching or further compression of root (e.g., straight leg raising, reversed straight leg raising, Valsalva maneuvers, hyperextension of spine, neck flexion)

4. FUNICULAR

- Characteristics: diffuse, poorly localized, burning sensation or abrupt stabbing pain
- Not radicular in distribution but rather involves unilateral or bilateral limbs, trunk, or entire body
- Triggered by movements of spine or incidental cutaneous sensation

5. PAIN SECONDARY TO MUSCLE SPASM

- Usually associated with local pain
- Physical findings of spasm present
- Myofascial pain syndromes (see text)

help to differentiate between these etiologies. As shown, pain due to disc disease is usually provoked by activity and alleviated by bed rest, but when the cause of local back pain is spinal tumor, the pain may be exacerbated by the recumbent position rather than relieved by it. This clinical phenomenon was recognized in an early study of intraspinal tumors: The pain "awakens the patient . . . after he has re-tired. It often becomes so severe as to compel him to walk the floor or to sleep in a sitting position."[43]

Patients with degenerative joint disease often give a history of chronic pain exacerbated and alleviated by familiar maneuvers. For example, most forms of spondylosis occur in the lower cervical and lower lumbar regions, resulting in local pain in these areas together with radicular pain radiating to distal regions of the extremities. In contrast, the thoracic spine is an infrequent location for spondylosis and disc disease but is a frequent region of spine metastases. Therefore, one should be especially wary of attributing symptoms and signs to spondylosis or degenerative disc disease in the thoracic spine.

Another important clinical clue is the chronicity and familiarity of the complaint. When patients with cancer develop a new and different form of pain, metastasis must be considered a likely cause. For example, among cancer patients, Foley[44] found that direct tumor invasion was responsible for 78% of pain problems in an inpatient population and 62% in an outpatient group. Although some complained of referred and radicular pain, many experienced local pain due to bone or viscus invasion. Thus, in the cancer patient, a new pain syndrome in the back, neck, or elsewhere is frequently due to direct tumor invasion and the workup should be so directed.

CASE ILLUSTRATION

A 30-year-old former drug abuser with a history of colon cancer treated by abdominoperineal resection presented with progressive buttock and pelvic pain. The pain did not radiate elsewhere and the Valsalva maneuver did not exacerbate it. Physical examination demonstrated no evidence for recurrent cancer, and the neurological examination was normal with no mechanical signs of spine disease. Laboratory studies were remarkable for a rising carcinoembryonic antigen (CEA), and CT scan of the abdomen and pelvis demonstrated irregularity of the posterior pelvic wall and probable postoperative scarring; however, no definite tumor was visualized. As no definite cause for the pain could be established, no specific therapy was rendered.

The patient returned three weeks later with severe pain in the same location that had developed into burning pain exacerbated by sitting. Physical examination demonstrated an enlarged liver and tenderness of the sciatic notch on the left. A repeat CEA was higher than the earlier assays. A repeat CT scan of the abdomen and pelvis demonstrated metastatic cancer in the liver and an enlarging pelvic mass in the region that had earlier been considered to be scar formation. The patient underwent radiation therapy and chemotherapy but the pain persisted unabated until he died of metastatic disease.

Comment. This case illustrates the importance of close and continued follow-up of patients with pain and known malignancy. Patients with malignancy who develop a new pain syndrome should be evaluated for recurrence of disease; if the workup proves negative and the symptoms persist, the evaluation should be repeated.

Referred Pain

Pain that arises from the spine may be projected elsewhere in a radicular or nonradicular pattern. Although both are forms of referred pain, "referred pain" in this chapter is used to denote nonradicular projected pain arising from the spine or other tissue. Myofascial pain syndromes are an example pain that may be difficult to differentiate from pain referred from the spine. As discussed in Chapter 2, these types of pain can be distinguished because radicular pain has localizing value, and referred pain usually does not. Interpreting referred pain as radicular may be misleading. Also, referred and radicular pain can coexist.[45] In one series of 1293 patients seen in a low back pain clinic over a 12-year period, referred pain was nearly twice as common as radicular pain; in some cases the two forms of pain coexisted.[45]

As reported in Chapter 2, when referred pain from the spine was studied experimentally by injecting hypertonic saline into facet joints of L1–2 and L4–5,[28] cramping, aching referred pain radiated into the flank, groin, buttocks, and thigh. Despite two noncontiguous levels of saline injection, the areas of pain referral overlapped significantly, and the pain did not radiate below the knee in either case. Although there may be paresthesias and tenderness in an area of pain referral, no objective neurological abnormalities were found. Maneuvers that exacerbate and alleviate local pain generally have the same effect on the associated referred pain.

In a study designed to identify the characteristics of back and leg pain arising from facet disease, local anesthetic was injected into the most tender facet joint in a group of patients with acute low back pain with or without associated leg pain.[46] If pain was relieved by this injection, patients were termed responders and the pain was considered to be secondary to facet disease. Responders had pain that often was exacerbated by sitting, and by flexion and extension of the lumbar spine, and sometimes was relieved by walking. Pain in the back and lower leg rarely responded to facet injection, whereas back pain associated with thigh pain often did respond. This result confirms the report[46] that spinal referred pain infrequently radiates below the knee. Although straight-leg raising often caused back pain in responders, by and large it did not cause referred leg pain. Straight-leg raising typically exacerbates radicular pain arising from the lower lumbar spine.

Somewhat different results were obtained by others in a similar series of investigations. Mooney and Robertson[47] studied the effect of saline and anesthetic injections of the lower lumbar facet joints in two groups of subjects, one without a history of back pain and sciatica and another with such symptoms. They injected facet joints at the L3–4, L4–5, or L5–S1 level with hypertonic saline and recorded the pattern of pain. The distribution of referred pain was similar for the L4–5 and L5–S1 levels and was located in the low back, greater trochanter, and posterior thigh and calf. The pain from the L3–4 facet injection usually produced pain in a more lateral distribution (Fig. 3–2). The pattern of pain referral was often that of sciatica. These authors then injected a local anesthetic into the facet joint and found that the referred pain resolved. Furthermore, in a group of patients suffering from the facet syndrome, this anesthetic injection normalized their previous positive straight-leg-raising test; in three

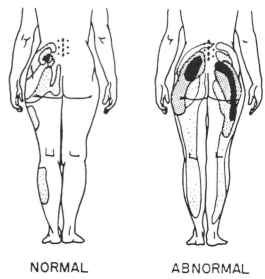

NORMAL   **ABNORMAL**

Figure 3–2. Pain referral patterns following lumbar injection in normal and symptomatic (abnormal) subjects. The investigators concluded that the pattern of pain referral from irritation of lumbar facet joints is similar to that seen in sciatica. (From Mooney, V and Robertson, J,[47] p. 152, with permission.)

patients, a depressed deep tendon reflex returned to normal. The authors speculated that the painful stimuli arising from the facet joint might inhibit the anterior horn cells innervating the reflex.

In summary, referred pain is usually poorly localized, deep, and ill-defined with respect to the distribution of a sclerotome. When arising from the low back, it can radiate into the buttock, thigh, and occasionally the calf in the same distribution as L5 or S1 radicular pain. Unlike radicular pain, however, the foot is usually not involved. Subjective motor weakness may occur, but objective weakness or atrophy is rare. Sensory loss is atypical. Deep tendon reflex abnormalities have been rarely reported. Tension signs, such as straight-leg raising, may cause an increase in low back pain or reveal tight hamstrings.[45] Referred pain into the lower extremity is often due to lumbar spondylosis; referred pain into the neck and upper extremity is frequently seen in cervical spondylosis (see Chapter 4).

Radicular Pain

DERMATOMAL PAIN

Radicular pain, which arises from irritation of the dorsal roots, is projected in the dermatomal distribution of the specific root involved. Unlike referred pain, it can have exquisite localizing value. Radicular pain is frequently sharp, stabbing, shooting, and superimposed on a chronic ache. The pain is generally aggravated by activities that increase compression of the nerve or that further stretch the root, such as coughing, sneezing, straining, straight-leg raising, external rotation and extension of the arm,[48] and hyperextension of the spine.

Since radicular pain usually radiates in the distribution of the injured nerve root, accurate localization of the site of pathology depends upon knowledge of the dermatomal map. (Exceptions to this radicular pain pattern may be due to ventral root injury, discussed below.) Unlike the case in patients with referred pain, neurological abnormalities referable to the root involved may also be found, in patients with dermatomal pain, including reflex loss, sensory disturbance, and/or motor abnormalities (discussed in Chapter 2). One of the most common causes of radicular pain is spondylosis and disc disease. Since cervical and lumbar spondylosis and disc disease typically involve nerve roots C6, C7 and L5, S1, respectively, radicular pain often is referred to the dermatomal distribution of roots in distal parts of the extremities.

MYOTOMAL PAIN

Another form of radicular pain is thought to arise from ventral spinal root irritation.[49] This pain has been described as deep, aching, diffuse, and dull in character and thus may be difficult to differentiate from visceral pain. It typically is referred to the myotome of the ventral root involved.

An example of this form of pain is anginoid pain arising from the cervical spine. Compression of the lower cervical spinal roots has been recognized as causing precordial pain that can simulate angina.[50,51]

In a large series reported from a cardiovascular referral center,[50] many patients had been carried with a diagnosis of cardiac ischemia for several years before the cervical spine was discovered as the source of pain and the condition was corrected by surgery. "Cervical angina" may be very difficult to differentiate from pain due to coronary artery insufficiency. At times, the two can coexist.

Pain in patients with cervical angina may arise from compression of the ventral nerve roots of C6, C7, and C8 because these roots innervate the chest wall muscles[50] (Fig. 3–3). This pain is, therefore, referred to the myotome rather than the dermatome of the involved nerve root. Pain of similar character may be projected to other sites (such as the leg) when ventral nerve roots at other levels are irritated. The fact that cervical spondylosis usually involves the dorsal roots and dorsal root ganglia more severely than the ventral roots[50] might explain the much greater frequency of dermatomal radicu-

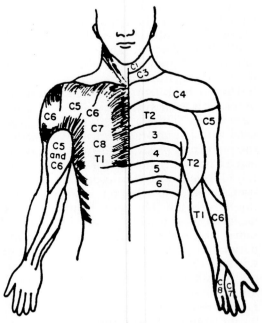

Figure 3–3. The distribution of (left) ventral (myotomal) and right dorsal (dermatomal) cervical root innervation. (From Booth, RE and Rothman, RH,[50] with permission.)

lar pain to the upper extremity from the dorsal root, as compared to the myotomal pattern of radicular pain in cervical spondylosis.

Myotomal pain referral may, of course, be due to causes other than spondylosis, such as malignancy or infection. The character of the myotomal type of pain may also be similar to referred pain from the spine. As in the case of dermatomal radicular pain, one often will find neurological signs of root dysfunction such as reflex, motor, or sensory disturbance[50] in the setting of ventral root pain.

Funicular Pain

In its complete form, funicular pain is characterized by a poorly localized, diffuse, burning pain syndrome with superimposed sharp, jabbing sensations.[52] It may be present in one or more extremities or the trunk, in a unilateral or bilateral distribution. It appears to arise from irritation or compression of the spinothalamic tracts or posterior columns and has been induced experimentally.[52,53] It is often provoked by incidental cutaneous stimulation or by movements of the spine such as neck flexion, straight leg raising, and the Valsalva maneuver—movements that cause mechanical deformation of the involved ascending tracts.

When caused by neoplasms, funicular pain appears to result more often from intramedullary than extramedullary tumors. Funicular pain was found in more than 50% of a series of patients with intramedullary tumors,[54] but in less than 5% of cases with extramedullary tumors.[55]

Another form of funicular sensation is electric-like paresthesias that radiate down the back and into the legs on neck flexion, known as Lhermitte's sign.[56] This symptom probably reflects the increased mechanosensitivity of damaged axons.[57] Similar sensations can be produced experimentally in man by stimulating the posterior funiculus.[52] Lhermitte's sign occurs in patients with demyelinating disease but may also be due to spinal cord compression from cervical spondylosis[58] or neo-

plasms of the cervical or thoracic spine as well as other causes.[59–63]

Pain Due to Muscle Spasm and Strain

A muscle strain or sprain results in a painful, tender muscle. The onset is usually acute. However, occasionally, the time of onset may be obscure. This type of pain may, indeed, be a component of the myofascial pain syndrome. It is usually associated with tender, sore paraspinous muscles.

Muscle spasm is a common response to irritation of nerves and other tissues. As mentioned earlier, injured axons are sensitive to mechanical stimulation. Paravertebral muscle spasm, which is seen in patients with spinal disorders and is reflexive in nature, guards against further mechanical irritation of the damaged tissues. When chronic, such spasm often results in a pain syndrome of its own.

The pain that arises from such spasm is of two types: The first is the well-recognized form of local pain that is cramping and aching in nature. Physical examination usually reveals evidence of muscle spasm. The second type of pain, termed myofascial pain syndrome, is both local and referred in nature.[11,64,65] Myofascial pain syndromes may not be recognized as easily as pain from local spasm because the referred pain is usually the chief complaint and is often not associated with spasm, or other abnormal findings at the site of referred pain.

Referred myofascial pain is caused by the stimulation of *trigger points*, which have been described as "self-sustaining hyperirritable foci located in skeletal muscle or its associated fascia."[11] Although the location of the projected pain does not follow a root or peripheral nerve distribution, there are several distinctive myofascial pain syndromes that may be differentiated based upon the location of the trigger point or its associated pain.

Other physical findings in patients with myofascial pain syndromes include a decreased range of motion and decreased apparent strength of the involved muscle group. Shortened tight bands of muscle fibers may give the muscle a ropey or nodular texture. Although the trigger point is typically not the site of reported pain, it is often the site of marked soft-tissue tenderness. Muscle strain and structural abnormalities such as unequal leg lengths are conditions that may initiate or perpetuate myofascial pain syndromes.

Because myofascial pain syndromes cause referred pain and are associated with subjective weakness,[11,45] they fall within the differential diagnosis of diseases of the spine or peripheral nervous system. As there are no specific laboratory tests to confirm myofacial pain syndromes the diagnosis is a clinical one. Extreme care and close follow-up should be exercised, however, because the early pain of spinal cord neoplasm or other serious pathology is often initially attributed to muscle strain.

The quadratus lumborum is the most common muscle to cause low-back myofascial pain.[11] When the trigger points of this muscle are stimulated, pain is referred downward toward the iliac crest, buttocks, and greater trochanter, and occasionally to the lower abdomen and groin. As in other cases of referred pain, the region of referred pain may be tender, resulting in the incorrect clinical impression that the pain is due to local pathology at the site of pain referral.

The gluteal muscles may also be a source of pain in the buttock and posterolateral thigh and calf, and this may be difficult to differentiate from nerve root compression or sciatica. The distinction can be made by identifying the tender spot or trigger point on the muscle and reproducing the patient's chief complaint by applying pressure on that spot.

Chronic Pain

Chronic pain is used here as a "catchall" for pain that is persistent (greater than three months in duration) and usually axial (midline) in nature. It is multifactorial but can be broken down into several components: (1) psychogenic, (2) functional, and (3) mechanical.

Psychogenic pain is usually related to depression. Back pain is a common complaint of depressed patients. Endogenous unipolar depression, which is often associated with back pain, is by definition unipolar (no manic phase). It is also associated with weight loss or weight gain, and with multiple unrelated somatic complaints (among them, neck and back pain).[42]

Etiologies of functional back pain complaints, or back pain complaint amplification, include secondary gain and malingering. These are manifestations of entities that are not structurally founded and that are not treatable by surgery. Nonoperative management schemes are most certainly appropriate in this subgroup of patients.

Mechanical back pain is pain that is associated with a dysfunctional motion segment. In this case, the dysfunctional motion segment (e.g., a degenerated disc, hypermobile motion segment) is a pain generator. The pain associated with this dysfunctional motion segment is deep and agonizing. It is not primarily associated with muscle tenderness (unless muscle spasm is an associated epiphenomenon) and is worsened by activity (loading) and lessened by rest (unloading).

Mechanical back pain, neural or dural impingement, and acute spinal instability are the only back pain types that may respond to surgical stabilization. Of these, mechanical back pain is clearly the most controversial; treatment paradigms vary considerably from physician to physician and region to region.[42]

Piriform Syndrome

Since a portion of the sciatic nerve often passes through or is extremely close to the piriform muscle,[68] the nerve may become compressed and irritated when the muscle is in spasm. The result is referred pain in a truly sciatic distribution and is called the piriform syndrome.[66] The etiology of the piriform syndrome is uncertain in most cases.[37,67]

Sciatica may also be secondary to the piriform syndrome. The pain may be poorly localized but often involves the hip, buttock, and groin and radiates down the posterolateral leg in a sciatic distribution.[67] In one large series, women were more frequently affected than men by a ratio of six to one, and they often complained of dyspareunia.[67]

The physical examination reveals normal mobility of the lumbar spine.[37] Straight-leg raising may be restricted, especially when the leg is simultaneously internally rotated, as this places the piriform muscle under tension.[37] Because the piriform muscle is an abductor and external rotator of the thigh, pain and weakness may be elicited when forced abduction and external rotation of the thigh are tested in a seated position.[67,69] The rectal examination, along with a pelvic examination in the woman, is very important in the diagnosis. Tenderness of the lateral pelvic wall is often found, and this reproduces the patient's pain.[67] The sciatic notch may also be tender.[70]

No diagnostic laboratory tests assist with this diagnosis. The differential diagnosis includes other causes of low back, pelvic, hip, and leg pain. Unlike cases of spondylosis and radiculopathy, no neurological deficit is found in patients with the piriform syndrome despite the fact that the sciatic nerve may be irritated. Tenderness of the lateral pelvic wall, pain and weakness of resisted hip abduction and external rotation, and pain on internal rotation of the hip are clinical clues suggestive of the piriform syndrome.[67]

Neurogenic Claudication

Another cause of focal back and projected leg pain that does not have the typical features of a monoradiculopathy has been termed neurogenic claudication. This "specific" clinical syndrome is usually secondary to a narrowed lumbar spinal canal and is often due to lumbar spondylosis, with or without associated congenital spinal stenosis.[71,72] The major clinical features are pain, weakness, and numbness.[73] The clinical manifestations and laboratory studies found in spinal stenosis and neurogenic claudication are reviewed in the next chapter.

Spinal Instability

Two pain syndromes deserve special mention because of their clinical significance and risk of neurologic morbidity: pain arising from spinal instability and neural or dural sac compression.

Acute instability is associated with structural failure of the spine. It is a graded phenomenon. It can be separated into two subtypes: (1) overt and (2) limited. Overt instability is associated with a grossly unstable spine, such as a fracture or dislocation. In a patient with overt instability, an accompanying distortion of periosteum is common. It is associated with a circumferential disruption of bony and soft tissue elements (including the disc interspace). This, in turn, is associated with the stimulation of nociceptive nerve endings and the perception of pain.

Limited instability is similar in nature, but less extensive. Circumferential instability is not present. Usually, there is only ventral, or less commonly, dorsal spinal involvement. Nevertheless, distortion of the periosteum results in the perception of pain. This type of pain is aggravated by movement of the involved injured spinal segment(s). In addition, the pain is elicited by percussion over the injured segment(s).[42]

Neural or dural sac compression is associated with classical axial and radicular pain syndromes. Spinal cord compression may result in sharp lancinating axial or appendicular pain (Lhermitte's sign). Dural sac compression may result in a dull, aching pain that is usually midline and nonradiating (axial). Nerve root compression or distortion results in the sensation of pain in the distribution of the nerve's dermatomal distribution pattern. Sciatica is an example.[42]

CLINICAL ASSESSMENT OF THE PATIENT

This section discusses the more frequent clinical features of neck, back, and referred pain identified during the history and physical examination that may help distinguish among the various etiologies

(Table 3–2). These are general clinical features. Specific aspects of the history and physical examination may be misleading in the assessment of any individual patient. The clinical features should only be

Table 3–2. **Some Frequent Causes of Spinal Pain**[*]

TRAUMATIC OR MECHANICAL

Musculoligamentous strain
Myofacial pain syndrome
Herniated intervertebral disc
Spondylosis (osteoarthritis: usually lower cervical or lumbar)
Spinal stenosis
Vertebral fracture
Postoperative

METABOLIC

Osteopenia with vertebral collapse
Gout, Paget's disease, diabetic neuropathy

CONGENITAL

Spondylolysis/spondylolisthesis

NEOPLASMS (PRIMARY AND METASTATIC, MALIGNANT AND BENIGN)

Epidural
Extramedullary-intradural
Intramedullary
Leptomeningeal metastases

INFLAMMATORY DISEASES

Ankylosing spondylitis, rheumatoid arthritis
Arachnoiditis

INFECTIONS

Discitis, osteomyelitis, paraspinal and spinal abscess, zoster, meningitis

REFERRED PAIN

Visceral (e.g., neoplastic and inflammatory) and vascular lesions of chest, abdomen, and pelvis
Retroperitoneal lesions

PREGNANCY

NONORGANIC CAUSES

Psychiatric causes
Malingering
Substance abuse

*Adapted from Howell, DS,[149] p. 1955.

considered as a guide. Laboratory and imaging studies often must be used to confirm a clinical impression or reveal an unexpected diagnosis.

History

The medical history is often the most important component of the evaluation of back or neck pain. The most important historical features to record are the location, character, onset, duration, and aggravating and palliating features of the pain. These features help establish the pain's source and mechanism. The circumstances at or prior to the onset of pain may be helpful in establishing cause. The patient should be asked about a history of trauma and the occurrence of a similar pain in the past. A list of medications used for pain or other conditions should also be obtained.

Patients should be asked to describe the pain, initially in their own words. If the description provided by the patient is inadequate to help discriminate among the myriad etiologies, the physician should specifically ask about different clinical manifestations. Dull, aching pain has an entirely different significance than shooting or burning pain. Aching or boring pain usually arises from locally irritated tissues, but burning pain is most suggestive of neural injury. Sharp, stabbing pains are often observed in association with radiculopathies. Dysesthesias, and pain elicited by tactile stimulation of the skin, also implicate a neural cause.

In evaluating patients, the correct localization of pain is critical. Many patients identify the location of pain referral and consider it to be the site of pathology. For example, a patient may believe that he/she has a hip or knee problem and become surprised or annoyed when the physician seems more concerned with their lumbar spine. Rather than using anatomical terms that may prejudice the evaluation, it is preferable to ask the patient to point to the location and extent of pain. A pain diagram drawn by the patient may be helpful.

Most mechanical causes of pain are never elucidated but instead are attributed to muscle strain or unusual activity despite the fact that there may be no identifiable precipitating event. As mentioned earlier, pain due to muscle strain is usually dull and aching. It is typically exacerbated by activity and minimized by rest and mild analgesics. Individuals often awaken the morning after strenuous activity with stiffness of the neck or back accompanied by pain. When the pain has been recurrent over many years and is familiar to the patient, he/she does not usually seek medical attention. They frequently present to the physician when the pain is more severe than usual or when it is not identical to their previous complaint. In such cases, it is important to determine whether the other characteristics of their pain (location, type, and provocative and palliating features) are similar to those of the pain they have had in the past. As mentioned above, when the pain is exacerbated by bed rest, one should consider neoplasm or other more serious causes.

When the pain projects from the spine to other regions, associated symptoms and physical findings may help discriminate between referred and radicular pain. The patient should be queried regarding asso-ciated sensory loss, weakness, or sphincter disturbances. When the pain is associated with these abnormalities, a radicular component should be considered. When the patient reports that the pain is exacerbated by coughing, sneezing, or the Valsalva maneuver, it often signifies structural disease of the spine because the epidural venous plexus, a collateral site of blood flow from intrathoracic and intra-abdominal locations, becomes engorged. This further compromises the spinal canal.[74]

Pain secondary to cervical and lumbar spondylosis and intervertebral disc disease is common. In the cervical region, the lower cervical spine is most often affected. In such cases, the patient usually complains of a stiff neck and pain radiating into the shoulder and arm. The C5–6 and/or C6–7 levels are usually involved. Dorsolateral disc herniation causes compression of the nerve root (Fig. 3–4). In one series, the C7 nerve root was compressed in 69% of cases and the C6 root in 19%.[75] When the C6 nerve root is involved, pain and sensory loss typically radiate along the radial border of the forearm and hand and into the thumb. When the C7 nerve root is compressed, the sen-

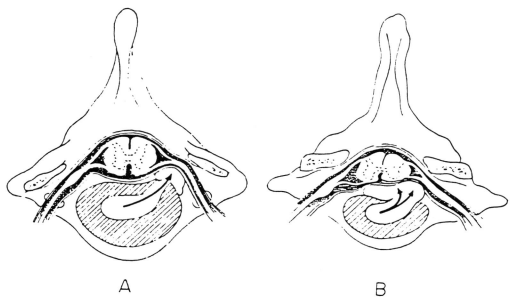

A   B

Figure 3–4. (A) Lateral cervical disc herniation causing nerve root compression. (B) Central cervical disc herniation casuing spinal cord and nerve root compression. (From Adams, RD and Victor, M,[146] with permission and adapted from Kristoff, FV and Odom, GL.[147])

sory disturbance is more medial and tends to involve the middle finger.

In the case of lumbar spondylosis and disc disease, the levels most commonly involved are L4–5 and L5–S1. In a study of single prolapsed lumbar intervertebral discs, the L4–5 and L5–S1 levels were involved in 97% of cases.[76] Among all lumbar levels, L4–5 and L5–S1 were the levels of symptomatic spondylosis causing single-level radiculopathy in 98% of cases.[76] Thinning of the posterior longitudinal ligament laterally along the dorsal surface of the vertebral bodies and the intervertebral discs makes dorsolateral herniation of the nucleus pulposus most common. In contrast to cervical roots, each lumbar nerve root exits above the corresponding intervertebral disc, so herniation of the disc most frequently compresses the exiting root just caudal to the level of disc herniation (Fig. 3–5). Consequently, with lumbar disc disease, a unilateral L5 or S1 radiculopathy most commonly arises from a disc herniation at L4–5 or L5–S1, respectively.

Patients with disc disease usually complain of pain in the low back and pain radiating in a sciatic distribution. When pain radiates down the dorsolateral aspect of the leg, the L5 nerve root is typically compressed, and pain radiates from the dorsal thigh and calf to the medial aspect of the foot. When the S1 nerve root is compressed, the pain usually radiates down the dorsolateral thigh and calf to the lateral aspect of the foot. As expected, such radicular pain is often provoked by coughing, sneezing, and Valsalva maneuvers.

Spondylolisthesis (subluxation of one vertebral body on another) in the lower lumbar region may be asymptomatic, but it may also clinically present with low back pain and pain radiating into the lower extremities. In some cases, spondylolisthesis is secondary to spondylolysis, a bony defect in the pars interarticularis (isthmic spondylolisthesis); however, it may also be classified as degenerative, traumatic, or pathologic. With ventral subluxation of one vertebral body on another, palpation of the spinous processes may reveal a "step." Since isthmic spondylolisthesis most commonly occurs at the L5–S1 level (less commonly at L4–L5), pain in the sciatic distribution and neurologic impairments referable to the compressed nerve

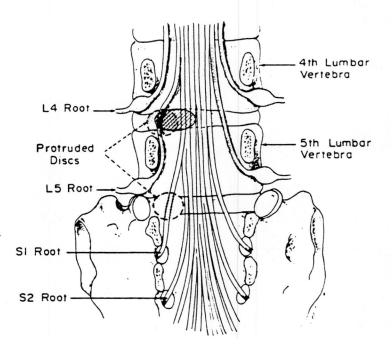

Figure 3–5. The mechanism of lateral disc herniation at L4–5 and L5–S1 causing L5 and S1 nerve root compression, respectively. A more medially placed disc protrusion may cause cauda equina compression. (From Adams, RD and Victor, M,[146] with permission.)

4th Lumbar Vertebra

L4 Root

Protruded Discs

5th Lumbar Vertebra

L5 Root

S1 Root

S2 Root

roots are commonly observed. They must be differentiated from sciatica secondary to herniated disc disease, spondylosis, and other causes. Spondylolisthesis may also cause spinal stenosis.

Spinal stenosis often occurs in conjunction with degenerative spondylolisthesis, in which there is an intact pars interarticularis. This is most common at the L4–5 segmental level. These "slips" rarely progress beyond 25% of the width of the vertebral body, whereas an L5–S1 isthmic spondylolisthesis commonly progresses beyond this extent.

In obtaining a pain history, it is imperative to review a patient's past medical history. A history of malignancy suggests the possibility of metastasis, even if the cancer has been considered cured for many years. A history of fever, chills, or recent infection should suggest the possibility of discitis and/or epidural abscess. Diabetics and patients with AIDS seem especially prone to such infections. In the young adult, an insidious onset and progression of stiffness and pain that are exacerbated by rest suggest a spondyloarthropathy such as ankylosing spondylitis. A family history of back pain early in life may also suggest the possibility of one of the spondyloarthropathies. Pain in the back, buttocks, and legs that is exacerbated by walking and relieved by lying down, sitting, or bending forward might implicate lumbar spinal stenosis.

It is important with regard to the diagnosis of back pain to consider visceral disease. This entity may project pain to the spine. The patient should be queried regarding a change in bowel habits, hematuria, pyuria, fever, and, in women, vaginal bleeding or discharge, because such pathologies may result in pain referred to the back. For example, back pain and tenderness in the costovertebral angle have been shown to be important findings in nearly one-third of women with urinary tract infections.[77] In addition, low back pain is present in 56% of women during pregnancy.[78] In 45% of such cases, the pain radiated into the lower extremities. Finally, intrathoracic pathology may also result in upper back pain via compression of paravertebral structures or via referred pain from visceral disease (see Chapter 2).

Physical Examination

To search for an undiagnosed systemic illness, the patient should undergo a thorough general physical examination. The abdominal examination may reveal evidence of an abdominal aortic aneurysm or other mass that may be the cause of back pain. A rectal examination, including stool guaiac test, should be performed to screen for cases of gastrointestinal cancer, ulcer disease, or other sources of bleeding that may relate to back pain. In women complaining of low back pain, a thorough pelvic examination is important because pathology of pelvic viscera is a common cause of such pain. The vascular examination should include palpation of peripheral pulses because back and lower-extremity pain may be due to vascular insufficiency.

The examination is then directed to the musculoskeletal system, including evaluation of posture and mobility. During this portion of the examination, the physician may be able to elucidate a mechanism provoking the pain. The posture and spontaneous movements of the patient are often best assessed prior to the initiation of a formal physical examination. At this time, one can often identify a limitation of neck or back movement (or normal mobility) due to pain and muscle spasm when the patient is unaware that he or she is being examined. If these findings are at variance with those found during the formal physical examination, they must be reconciled.

The formal physical examination of the musculoskeletal system begins by the examination of the patient in the standing position. In the presence of a herniated lumbar disc causing sciatica, the patient may maintain the affected leg in a flexed position at the hip, knee, and ankle, preventing the heel from reaching the ground. Such a leg posture releases the traction on the sciatic nerve root(s) that occurs when the leg is extended, as is demonstrated with the straight-leg-raising test. The spine tends to list to the side that places the least traction on the nerve root, resulting in a functional scoliosis. When the disc is lateral to the nerve root, the list is usually directed away from the side of herniation. When the disc is medial to the nerve root, the list is toward the side of herniation.[79] Although these findings are commonly observed in patients with lumbar disc disease, they are not specific for this etiology. They may also be found in patients with metastatic disease or other structural abnormalities of the spine.

Palpation of the entire spine and paravertebral structures is performed. Pain that can be elicited by palpation or percussion of the spine suggests structural disease at that site. In the cancer patient, it strongly suggests the possibility of metastasis. However, the absence of spine tenderness does not rule out the existence of spine metastasis. In one study, only 13 of 20 (65%) patients with epidural metastases had percussion tenderness at the time of diagnosis.[80]

The examination is then directed to identifying those positions or movements that provoke pain. This helps elucidate the mechanism, and often the source, of pain. As already mentioned, the movement of inflamed or irritated tissues generally causes pain. Even passive movements are prevented by muscle spasm and splinting. In patients complaining of neck or back pain, a gentle attempt to flex, extend, and rotate the neck should be made to determine if the pain arises from these structures. Passive extension of the cervical spine is especially helpful in evaluating patients with neck pain. Because cervical extension narrows the intervertebral foramina, patients with cervical radiculopathy due to foraminal compromise commonly complain of pain with cervical spine extension. If slow and gentle movement of the spine is associated with severe pain in the neck, one should consider the possibility of major structural pathology of the spine, such as fracture or dislocation (if the history is consistent).

The shoulder-abduction test has been cited as a reliable way to identify cervical monoradiculopathies secondary to extradural compressive disease such as cervical spondylosis, disc disease, and possibly

neoplasm in the lower cervical spine.[81] When shoulder abduction (with the elbow in flexion) results in pain relief, the patient is considered to have a positive result and a high probability of extradural compression of a cervical nerve root.[81] Alternatively, if the abducted arm is extended at the elbow and laterally rotated (Fig. 3–6), pain is usually increased in cases of cervical nerve root and brachial plexus disorders.[48] This latter maneuver is similar to the hyperabduction test, or Allen test, used in the diagnosis of thoracic outlet syndrome or scalenus anticus syndrome.[58] In the case of thoracic outlet syndrome, the patient experiences an increase in symptoms with this maneuver.

If neck flexion causes pain in the thoracic or lumbar region, especially if the pain is radicular, spinal cord compression should seriously be considered and excluded with alacrity. The following illustration demonstrates a case where the history initially suggested cranial disease, but maneuvers on physical examination led to the correct diagnosis of metastasis to the spinal column.

CASE ILLUSTRATION

A 42-year-old woman with known metastatic colon cancer was referred for evaluation of headaches. She was reported to have a normal neurological examination and negative head CT scan prior to neurological referral. Her headaches, primarily occipital in location, were worsened by sitting up or standing and relieved by lying down. Her neurological examination, including funduscopic examination, was normal. These maneuvers caused the patient severe limitation of neck movement and paravertebral cervical muscle spasm with exacerbation of her pain. Gentle downward compression of the head when she was sitting resulted in severe occipital pain.

Given the marked limitation of neck movement, a presumptive diagnosis of cervical spine metastasis was made. She was referred for cervical spine films, which demonstrated destruction of the C2 vertebral body by neoplasm. A CT scan with intravenous contrast through the area confirmed the diagnosis and demonstrated epidural extension of the metastasis

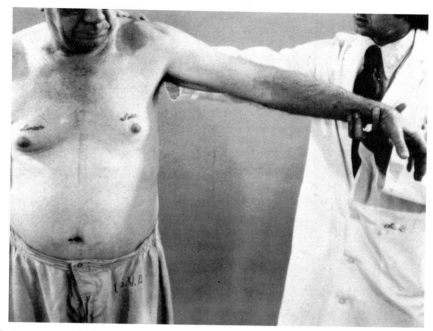

Figure 3–6. A maneuver which may produce radicular pain in a patient with cervical radiculopathy. The arm is abducted and laterally rotated, and the elbow is in extension. (From Waxman, SG,[48] with permission.)

without spinal cord compression. The patient was placed in a collar and underwent radiation therapy to the region, which led to improvement of her pain. Although she died several months later due to widespread metastatic disease, she never developed clinical signs of spinal cord compression.

The examination of the low back includes testing mobility by forward flexion, lateral bending, rotation, and hyperextension. In cases of herniation of a lumbar disc causing compression of a nerve root, the lumbar spine often assumes a protective posture to prevent further compression or stretch of the nerve root. As described above, the direction of the list is that which places the least traction on the nerve root.[79] Under these circumstances, lateral bending to the side away from the list is usually limited.

Most causes of low back pain limit forward flexion due to associated muscle spasm. Herniated lumbar discs and other causes of mass within the lumbar canal (e.g., metastatic cancer or spinal sepsis) may be associated with increased pain during maneuvers that increase the lum-bar lordosis such as hyperextension of the lumbar spine.

STRAIGHT-LEG-RAISING TEST

Several clinical tests have been developed over the last century to evaluate the patient with low back pain with or without radiation into the leg. The most well known is the straight-leg-raising test. Often referred to as the Lasegue sign, the test actually was described by Lasegue's student, Forst, in 1881.[82] The sciatic nerve is stretched over the ischial tuberosity, as the extended leg is flexed at the hip, so that pain is elicited or exacerbated in cases where the sciatic nerve or the affected nerve root is already compressed.[82] Forst proposed the test as a means of differentiating hip disease from sciatica. However, as noted below, this maneuver does not confidently accomplish this. The straight-leg-raising test is performed on the supine patient by flexing the thigh at the hip, with the knee extended (Fig. 3–7). If pain radiating down the leg in a sciatic distribution is provoked, the result is considered positive. If the foot is also

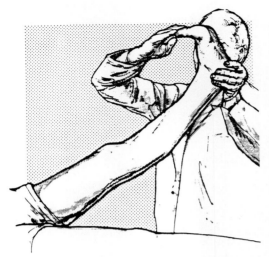

Figure 3–7. The straight-leg-raising test. (From DeJong, RN,[58] with permission.)

dorsiflexed during the straight-leg raising, the pain is often intensified.

Positive results with the straight-leg-raising test are often considered evidence for L5 or S1 nerve root compression. This often occurs with herniated discs at L4–5 and L5–S1, respectively. Falconer showed (during surgery) that the L5 nerve root moves 2–6 mm caudally during the act of straight-leg raising,[83,84] which supports this concept. However, positive results of the straight-leg-raising test may also be observed in diseases of the hip, thigh, and pelvis. They are therefore not specific for lumbar spine disease and radiculopathy. This impression was confirmed in a neurosurgical series[85] (intended to study patients with herniated discs and, therefore, excluding patients with spinal tumors) in which patients with low back pain, leg pain, or both were tested for straight-leg raising. Of 351 patients with positive results, only 64% proved to have a disc herniation. This underscores the lack of specificity of this sign. Moreover, positive results are not invariably present in cases of prolapsed lower lumbar intervertebral discs. One study found that only 80% of individuals with surgically proven herniated lower lumbar discs had positive results on straight-leg-raising tests.[86]

Occasionally, patients are reported to have sciatica, but their pain actually has a nonorganic component. In order to distinguish between organic and nonorganic pain, the "flip test" has been recommended.[87,88] This maneuver is a modification of the straight-leg-raising test which is usually performed with the patient supine. When the flip test is performed, to identify a nonorganic component to pain as described by Waddell and colleagues,[88] the patient is distracted during the maneuver. One method of performing the test involves extending the leg at the knee with the patient in a seated position in order to test the plantar reflex. The patient with a nonorganic component to sciatic-type pain may report pain with straight-leg raising in the supine position but no pain with the flip test in the seated position.[88] Waddell and colleagues have presented several nonorganic physical signs associated with low back pain that they recommend as part of the evaluation of these patients. Even so, the presence of such a nonorganic sign does not rule out the possibility of coexisting organic disease.

CROSSED-STRAIGHT-LEG RAISING TEST

Another helpful clinical test is the crossed-straight-leg-raising test. This test is performed in a manner similar to the straight-leg-raising test, but in this case positive results are defined as pain projected to the affected leg when the unaffected leg is raised. Positive results are explained by the observation that straight-leg raising causes the contralateral as well as the ipsilateral L5 and S1 roots to be pulled caudally.

Woodhall and Hayes[89] found that of 95 patients with positive results, 90 had a herniated disc demonstrated surgically. All but two of the herniated discs were at the L4–5 or L5–S1 level. In another study, 54 of 56 (97%) patients who had positive results were found to have a herniated disc.[85] These findings suggest that the test is highly specific for localizing disease to the spine. Although herniated discs were found in these two studies, spinal tumors in the same location also may give rise to positive results on this test. Thus, positive results more accurately indicate a compressive lesion in the lower lumbar spinal canal than do positive results with the straight-leg-raising test. When the subjective response has been accurately reported and interpreted, this sign is exceedingly reliable in localizing disease to the spine. In the authors' experience, cases in which the localization has been misleading have been those rare patients with severe metastatic disease to the pelvis. In this instance, any movement of one leg may cause pain in the contralateral leg as well.

REVERSED-STRAIGHT-LEG-RAISING TEST

A useful clinical test to evaluate patients with suspected upper lumbar spine disease and radiculopathies is termed the femoral-nerve-traction test[83,90,91] or the reversed-straight-leg-raising test. The test is not specific for spinal disease or a radiculopathy, since positive results are often observed with femoral neuropathy due to ischemia in diabetes mellitus or with retroperitoneal masses such as psoas hematoma or abscess.

The test may be performed with the patient lying on his/her painless side and with their neck flexed to increase tension on the cauda equina. The painful leg is then pulled back by the examiner to hyperextend it at the hip. The knee is then flexed, further stretching the upper lumbar nerve roots (Fig. 3–8). In an alternative technique, the test may be performed by flexing the knee of the patient, who is in a prone position. In cases of L3 radicu-

lopathy, pain often radiates to the ventral thigh. In cases of L4 radiculopathy, the pain is more apt to radiate below the knee. The results of this test are negative in cases of L5 and S1 radiculopathies[91] but positive in cases of upper lumbar radiculopathy.

PATRICK'S MANEUVER

Buttock, hip, and knee pain may arise from hip disease such as metastasis, osteoarthritis, or infection. The location and pattern of pain referral are often similar to those of radicular pain arising from the lumbar spine. When positive, the Patrick sign is often helpful in localizing the source of pain to the hip.[58,92]

This test is performed by placing the heel of the lower extremity being tested on the contralateral knee; downward and outward pressure is then exerted on the ipsilateral knee. The resultant movement is flexion, abduction, and external rotation of the involved hip. Flexion of the knee helps to relieve tension on the nerve roots. If the patient's pain complaint is reproduced in the hip or ipsilateral thigh, the hip may be the source of pain. Since stretch is not placed on the sciatic nerve with this test, Patrick's maneuver helps in distinguishing between sciatica and referred pain from the hip. Other lesions of the pelvis and lower extremity, such as metastases, may also give rise to a positive Patrick sign.

Hip pain may also, and perhaps more predictably, be elicited by extending the

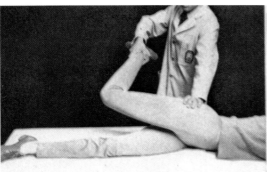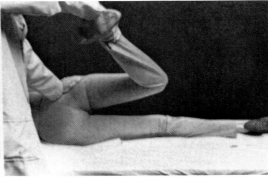

Figure 3–8. The reversed-straight-leg-raising test. Left, anterior view. Right, posterior view. (From Jabre, JF and Bryan, RW,[91] with permission.)

affected knee and flexing the hip, while at the same time percussing the calcaneus region of the foot. The "impulse" is transmitted to the hip joint, thus often resulting in hip region pain if "hip disease" is present.

Neurological Examination

When abnormalities are found when the neurological examination is performed, they may not only localize the level of the lesion but may also suggest the etiology. For example, as already mentioned, cervical disc disease most frequently occurs at the C5–6 and C6–7 levels, and lumbar disc disease most frequently involves the L4–5 and L5–S1 levels. Although metastases, infection, or other diseases may be responsible, when radicular signs place the lesion at these levels, spondylosis and disc disease are prominent considerations. When neurological signs localize the lesion to levels other than these, while spondylosis may be the cause, there is a greater likelihood of other causes. One of the most common sources of delay in diagnosis of metastatic cancer to the spine occurs when a physician attributes neurological abnormalities to spondylosis and disc disease in the upper lumbar region or thoracic area. These are levels that are rarely involved clinically with these disorders.

Deep tendon reflexes should be tested carefully to detect asymmetry. In the upper extremity, depressed or asymmetric reflexes at the biceps (C5, C6), brachioradialis (C5, C6), or triceps (C7) are often seen in association with cervical spondylosis at these levels. An asymmetrical Hoffmann's reflex suggests the presence of pathology at the C7–T1 level or the lower brachial plexus levels. This result is not common in patients with spondylosis but is frequently found in those with superior sulcus tumors.[93] In the lower extremity, an absent ankle jerk (S1) is a common finding in patients with lumbar spondylosis and disc disease. However, an absent knee reflex is an unusual sign of spondylosis because over 90% of herniated lumbar discs occur at the L4–5 or L5–S1 levels.[76]

Muscle strength, bulk, and tone are usually not severely affected in cases of mono-

radiculopathy. Some abnormalities may be found in cases of radiculopathy, however, when testing muscles that receive a preponderance of innervation from the affected nerve root. These segment "pointer" muscles[94] are presented in Chapter 2. Muscle spasm and guarding may also be responsible for abnormalities. If the abnormalities are thought to be related to pain, the examination should be repeated after the pain has been controlled with analgesics.

In patients with suspected spine disease, the sensory examination is performed to distinguish between a sensory level and a dermatomal sensory loss. When sensory testing is performed in patients suffering from peripheral neuropathy, decreased sensation distally in the lower extremities is often found. This distal type of sensory loss is not necessarily confined to the limbs. In many peripheral neuropathies, there is a relative invariance over the entire body surface regarding the distance from the spinal or cranial nerve root of origin to the border of normal sensation.[95] If the neuropathy is advanced, sensory loss over the distal aspect of the intercostal distribution in the midventral trunk may be observed in the context of sensory loss in the distal limbs.[96] This ventral distribution of truncal sensory loss widens with progression of the neuropathy (Fig. 3–9A and B). Ventral truncal sensory loss due to peripheral neuropathy can be mistakenly attributed to a spinal cord lesion. Confusion can be avoided if the sensory examination includes the back and buttocks, because the thoracic, lumbar, and sacral dermatomes are represented dorsally as well as ventrally.

The distinction between sensory loss due to peripheral neuropathy and that due to spinal cord pathology must often be made in cancer patients receiving vinca alkaloids who complain of numbness in their legs. These drugs commonly cause a peripheral neuropathy. Such patients may also have painful dysesthesias of the distal legs secondary to the peripheral neuropathy. If they complain of back, neck, or radicular pain, or if they have a sensory level on the trunk, their symptoms should not be attributed to peripheral neuropathy. These patients should be considered

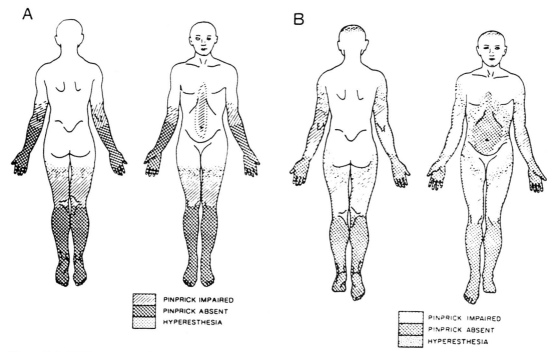

Figure 3–9. (A) Sensory map in patient with moderately advanced diabetic neuropathy. Note distal sensory loss in arms and legs and in the most distal part of the territory served by truncal nerves. (B) Sensory map in severe diabetic neuropathy. Sensory loss has progressed to include anterior thorax, in addition to the arms and legs, which show an advanced "glove-and-stocking" pattern. Note that unless the posterior thorax is examined, the pattern of sensory loss over the trunk can be confused with a sensory level due to spinal cord compression. (From Waxman, SG and Sabin, TD,[148] with permission.)

as candidates for the diagnosis of spinal disease.

Superficial reflexes are often abnormal in patients suffering from spinal cord or cauda equina disease. The pathophysiology and methods of obtaining the superficial abdominal, cremasteric, anal, and Babinski reflexes were reviewed in Chapter 2. It should be emphasized that in spinal cord disease involving descending pathways, there may be an increase in deep tendon reflexes, in conjunction with a diminution of superficial abdominal, anal, and cremasteric reflexes. This dissociation of reflexes should alert the physician to pathology of the pyramidal tracts.

Laboratory Studies

In most cases of acute low back or neck pain, where the history and physical examination do not lead to a suspicion of serious underlying disease, no laboratory investigations are required. The pain is typically due to musculoligamentous strain and is self-limited. However, these patients require close clinical observation before one can confidently exclude more serious underlying pathology.

In persistent or atypical cases, or if the history and physical examination lead to the suspicion of underlying systemic disease, a more thorough evaluation should be undertaken. Any relevant leads already uncovered should be pursued. In addition, a CBC, sedimentation rate, urinalysis, and serum chemistry profile may yield clues to the existence and identity of more serious disease. For example, acid phosphatase or prostatic specific antigen may be elevated in men with carcinoma of the prostate. If multiple myeloma is in the differential diagnosis, a serum and urine protein electrophoresis may be helpful. When inflammatory disease is suspected, a tuberculin test, antinuclear antibody, rheumatoid factor, human leukocyte antigen (HLA) B-27, and other screening studies for autoimmune and infectious causes may be helpful.

Imaging Studies

Imaging studies for pain of spinal origin are indicated to (1) determine neural compression and/or (2) establish a diagnosis for a mechanical origin of pain. One must clearly separate these indications so that an appropriate diagnostic scheme and management plan may be derived.

Imaging for neural or dural compression is relatively straightforward in most circumstances. Possible techniques include radiograph, CT, myelography, and MRI. Imaging to establish a mechanical origin of spinal pain is somewhat more controversial. Techniques include radiography, CT, MRI, and discography. Each is controversial in its own way. Radiography provides the most "surgically conservative" approach to the diagnosis of mechanical back pain, whereas CT and MRI are intermediate. Discography provides an increased sensitivity to disc degeneration, but because some degenerated discs are not clinically significant, it may (if read in isolation from the clinical findings) cause an "overreading" of the degenerated disc. Furthermore, its use must be employed with a provocation component for it to be clinically relevant. Provocation of symptoms during discography allows a clinical component of the test to be introduced; i.e., the combination of an imaging study with a study in which the pain of origin (patient's mechanical back pain) is reproduced.

Back pain is one of the most common symptoms associated with the use of radiography in ambulatory settings in the United States.[97] In most cases, the purpose of ordering such "plain films" is to detect serious underlying diseases such as cancer, fractures, infections, and spondyloarthropathies. Although compression fractures may be observed in 3% of cases, cancer has been reported to be found in approximately 6 per 1000 cases and vertebral osteomyelitis in 1 in 100,000 patients with acute low back pain in primary care

settings.[97–99] In an attempt to establish selective criteria for ordering radiological studies in the patient with acute low back pain, Deyo and Diehl[98] suggested in 1986 that spinal radiographs are indicated when the patient meets any of the following criteria:
1. When the patient is over 50 years of age
2. When there has been significant trauma
3. When a history or physical examination suggests ankylosing spondylitis or demonstrates a neuromotor deficit
4. When there is a history of drug or alcohol abuse, a history of treatment with corticosteroids, or a temperature over 37.8° C
5. When there is a history of cancer, pain at rest, or unexplained weight loss
6. When there has been a recent visit for the same problem, which has not improved
7. When the patient is seeking compensation

However, Frazier and colleagues[99] then concluded that adoption of these criteria would increase the use of roentgenographic studies. More recently, Suarez-Almazor and colleagues[100] reported that adoption of these guidelines would result in obtaining radiographs in 44% of patients with low back pain. Accordingly, the difficulty in establishing strict criteria for the use of roentgenographic studies for this problem remains.[97]

In cases of subacute or chronic neck or back pain, spine radiographs are often performed. Since radiographic studies often reveal cervical and/or lumbar spondylosis in asymptomatic individuals[4,9,19,101] the physician must be wary of attributing a patient's symptom or sign to a finding that may be incidental and asymptomatic.

In an epidemiological study of the frequency of abnormal spine radiographs, plain anteroposterior and lateral radiographs of the lumbar spine were taken in a randomly selected group of men between the ages of 18 and 55.[19] One group had a history of no low back pain, the second group had a history of moderate low back pain, and the third had severe low back pain. The authors found no difference among these groups in the incidence of transitional vertebrae, Schmorl's nodes, narrowing of the disc spaces between the third and fourth lumbar vertebrae and between the fifth lumbar and first sacral vertebrae, or of other abnormalities. Only the presence of traction spurs and/or disc space narrowing between the fourth and fifth lumbar vertebrae correlated with the symptoms of severe low back pain and numbness, weakness, and pain in the lower extremities. As in other studies,[19,102] these authors found a high degree of interobserver variation in the interpretation of conventional roentgenograms, which might have contributed to the lack of correlation between the patients' histories and the radiological studies. As noted below, similar findings have been reported with other imaging modalities.

In a study using CT of the lumbar spine in a group of asymptomatic adults, 35% were abnormal.[21] More than 50% of individuals over 40 years of age had abnormal scans. The most common abnormality in the entire group of asymptomatic subjects was a herniated nucleus pulposus, found in 20% of individuals.

Similarly, radiological evidence of cervical spondylosis has been reported in a large proportion of individuals without specific complaints.[103] Such evidence was found on the plain radiographs films of 50% of individuals over the age of 50 and on those of 75% of those over the age of 65; many of these individuals were asymptomatic.[104]

The abnormalities found on plain radiography and CT have been corroborated by findings on total spine myelography in asymptomatic patients. In a study of total myelograms incidentally performed for the evaluation of acoustic neuromas, 37% of 300 otherwise asymptomatic individuals with no history of neck, back, or radicular pain had spinal abnormalities.[20] The abnormalities ranged from deformed nerve root sleeves and ruptured discs to nearly complete obstruction. The defects were solitary in 19% of cases, and multiple in 18%. Lumbar abnormalities were present in 24% and cervical abnormalities in 21% of these asymptomatic individuals.

In a smaller study of patients with asymptomatic intervertebral disc protrusions, McCrae[105] performed postmortem myelograms and dissections of 18 complete spines in individuals over 30 years of age. He concluded that "nearly everybody, 40 years of age or older, has at least one posterior cervical and one posterior lumbar disc protrusion."[105] In a study of magnetic resonance imaging (MRI) of the lumbar spine in 96 asymptomatic people (mean age 42 years), Jensen et al.[106] found that 52% of subjects had disc bulges at at least one level, 27% had protrusions, and 1% had extrusions. (Rather than use the term herniation, these authors subdivided herniation into protrusion and extrusion of the nucleus pulposus.) Similarly, using MRI in 67 people without symptoms, Boden and colleagues found herniated discs in 20% of those less than 60 years of age and in 36% of those 60 years and over.[107]

These reports underscore the importance of making a correct clinical diagnosis and not relying exclusively on radiological studies in the absence of other clinical data. Radiographic studies in many cases demonstrate structural abnormalities that are not related to the patient's complaint.

MANAGEMENT

Neck and Back Pain

Neck and back pain affects nearly 80% of adults. It is the most common cause of disability in patients aged younger than 45 years.[8] It accounts for a large fraction of the U.S. health care budget ($25 billion a year). Although most adults experience low back and neck pain, only a small percentage require surgery.[108] Therefore, nonoperative management schemes are extremely valuable. The most clinically relevant of these are discussed below.

Acute low back pain and neck pain in which no specific pathoanatomic diagnosis can be made are usually self-limited disorders even without specific therapy. In these cases, the term muscle strain or spasm is often used. In some of these cases, however, the pain is sufficient to warrant the use of a brief period of bed rest, antiinflammatory agents, muscle re-laxers, or local heat. In a systematic review of randomized controlled trials of the most common interventions for acute back pain, van Tulder et al.[109] found strong evidence for the effectiveness of muscle re-laxers and nonsteroidal antiinflammatory drugs and for the ineffectiveness of exercise therapy. In the case of neck pain, a collar and cervical traction may be used effectively.

Based on national surveys, bed rest is the most frequently used treatment modality for neck and low back pain.[110] However, the efficacy of bed rest has not been proven. Although the direct costs of bed rest are small, the indirect costs may be excessive. Of note is that nearly half of patients with back pain reported only minimal relief with bed rest.[111] In the review cited above, van Tuler et al.[109] found that there was strong evidence that bed rest is not an effective treatment option for acute low back pain. Furthermore, there are significant disadvantages associated with bed rest, including the psychological association a patient may make between many days in bed and severe illness. This may lead to depression, exacerbation of pain, and a predisposition to diminished effort in an exercise program.[108] Deconditioning, with muscle atrophy (1%–1.5% per day[112]), cardiopulmonary function loss (15% in 10 days,[113]), and bone mineral loss, occurs relatively rapidly. Medical complications, including deep venous thrombosis and pneumonia, are more common with bed rest.[108]

A study of the duration of bed rest for acute mechanical low back pain without significant neurological deficit demonstrated that two days of bed rest were as effective as seven days.[12] Moreover, some patients with acute low back pain who continue ordinary activities "within the limits permitted by the pain" may do better than those who undergo bed rest or back-mobilizing exercises.[114] Although no consensus on bed rest has been reached, a brief period of bed rest (e.g., one or two days) is a reasonable strategy for many patients with acute back pain, followed by mobilization.[108]

Chiropractic or spinal manipulative therapy includes adjustment, manipulation, stimulation, and traction. Approximately 30% of patients with back pain seek chiropractic care. Carey et al. recently evaluated outcomes in patients treated for back pain by primary care physicians, chiropractors, and orthopedic surgeons.[115] They found that the outcomes were similar in all groups. The costs of orthopedic and chiropractic care were significantly greater those of primary care physicians. Patients expressed a greater overall satisfaction with chiropractic care; however, a long-term follow-up at 3 and 12 months did not demonstrate a significant difference. In a study of patients with low back pain, Cherkin and colleagues compared the clinical outcome and costs associated with the McKenzie method of physical therapy versus chiropractic manipulation versus provision of an educational booklet.[115a] These authors found that the physical therapy group and chiropractic manipulation group had similar clinical outcomes which were "marginally" better than the outcomes receiving the educational booklet. The treatment costs were significantly less in the booklet group compared to the other two groups.

For chronic low back pain, van Tulder et al.[109] found studies in the literature demonstrating strong evidence for the use of manipulation, back schools, and exercise therapy. After the acute bout of pain, exercise programs may be used to reduce the risk of recurrence.[3,116–118] Lahad et al.[119] have reviewed the effectiveness of exercise programs in the prevention of low back pain. Transcutaneous electrical nerve stimulation (TENS) for the treatment of chronic low back pain has not been found to be efficacious.[120] In addition, a controlled trial of corticosteroid injection into facet joints for chronic low back pain has found to be little more effective than saline injections.[121] While "back schools" (back schools include education in biomechanics) have been shown to be effective,[109] an educational program among postal workers that stressed lifting techniques to prevent low back injuries failed to show long-term benefits. Thus exercise programs may be needed to prevent recurrence of back pain and radicular pain. This has been the experience of the authors (see below).

Traditionally, the management of low back pain, with or without radicular pain due to a herniated lumbar disc, is similar to that of mechanical low back pain except that the necessary period of bed rest is usually longer. It may be important to reassure the patient that in the majority of cases of low back pain (with or without sciatica) due to a herniated lumbar disc, the pain will resolve with nonsurgical therapy.[108,122,123]

Nerve Root Compression

For patients with nerve root compression, bed rest, analgesics, antiinflammatory agents, muscle relaxants, and avoidance of activities that provoke leg pain are recommended by many clinicians. In most cases of severe pain, bed rest, except for bathroom privileges, may be used until there is significant improvement of pain. A gradual increase in activity is allowed, pain permitting. Activities that exacerbate the pain are usually avoided. In the majority of cases, the pain from a herniated disc improves with nonoperative treatment.

Recent data, however indicate, that bed rest provides no advantage or is worse than the continuation of normal activity in some patients with sciatica.[123a] Therefore, bed rest as a treatment for sciatica may be overrated.[108] Epidural steroid injection for sciatica due to herniated disc has been used since the 1950s. There have been contradictory reports of efficacy (reviewed by Carette et al.[124]). Recently, in a double-blind controlled trial, Carette et al.[124] found that epidural corticosteroid injections may offer short-term benefit for leg pain and sensory loss but do not offer significant functional benefit or reduce the need for surgery.

The need for surgical intervention in patients with sciatica secondary to herniated nucleus pulposus has been controversial. Operations on such patients occur ten times more frequently in the United States than in Great Britain[122,125] and several studies have demonstrated that in the majority of patients, nonsurgical therapy is successful. A few of these are cited below. There have been a number of studies, using chemonucleolysis, in which some patients underwent double-blind placebo injections. Generally, patients must have failed to respond to "conservative" therapy to enter the study. One such series[126] demonstrated that muscle weakness improved in 66% in the placebo group; in two other series, the placebo treatment was considered successful in approximately 50% of cases.[127,128]

Several recent studies utilizing CT and MRI to confirm the presence of herniated nucleus pulposus as the cause of sciatica have revealed that the great majority of patients with sciatica secondary to herniated nucleus pulposus can be managed without surgical intervention.[122,129–131] Bush and colleagues[122] reported the outcome of 165 patients with sciatica secondary to compression by disc material (bulging or herniated or sequestered disc) for an average of 4.2 months. These authors treated patients with epidural steroid injections, following patients clinically and with computed tomography. Patients who failed to respond to this regimen underwent surgical decompression. Among the 165 patients, 23 (14%) required surgical decompression. The remaining patients were assessed clinically and with follow-up CT scans at one year. All patients reevaluated at one year had returned to work and their usual recreational activities. Among this group, the average reduction in pain on the visual analog scale was 94%. Furthermore, follow-up CT scans showed 76% of disc herniations and 26% of disc bulges partially or completely resolved. Remarkably, among ten patients harboring sequestered discs, one returned to normal and eight (80%) improved without surgical intervention. The observation that the largest disc herniations and sequestrations have been those that have had the highest rate of spontaneous resolution has been reported in several other studies.[132–135] In another study utilizing MRI to follow patients with clinically symptomatic lumbar disc herniation managed nonsurgically, 63% of patients showed a reduction of disc herniation of more than 30% (48% had a reduction of more than 70%) whereas only 8% demonstrated worsening.[132] Therefore, the management of most patients includes a nonsurgical approach, supplemented when necessary with a multidisciplinary chronic pain management program.[108]

Exercises

Significant controversy exists regarding exercise type and efficacy. Aerobic exercise theoretically improves endurance, motor control, coordination, mechanical efficiency, and the strength of abdominal and paraspinous muscles. Additional benefits of aerobic exercise include weight loss, and the psychologic effects of improved mood and lessened anxiety. Some have suggested that particular types of high impact exercise should be avoided because of the potential for raising intradiscal pressure.[136] This stance, however, has not been supported by objective data.

Stretching (flexibility) exercises are occasionally advocated to improve the extensibility of muscles and other soft tissues and to reestablish normal joint range of motion.[108] Pain commonly limits mobility. Muscle spasm, or sprain, may also be present. Stretching is thought to maintain mobility and reduce spasm. Kraus reported a study of the effects of stretching exercises on back pain. He found that nearly 80% of people with chronic back pain who entered the program reported improvement at the end of a six-week training session.[137] The benefit of stretching exercises, however, may not persist.[120]

Isometric (strengthening) exercises have enjoyed significant popularity. Williams[138] suggested that isometric flexion exercises offered patients the best relief of pain. His rationale was that flexion (1) widened the intervertebral foramina and facet joints, reducing nerve root compression; (2) stretched hip flexors and back extensors; (3) strengthened abdominal and gluteus

muscles; and (4) reduced dorsal fixation of the lumbosacral junction. There has been concern over the use of flexion exercises specifically regarding substantial increases in intradiscal pressure that may aggravate bulging or herniation of an intervertebral disc.[4] Randomized controlled trials have shown conflicting results.[139–141]

More recently, McKenzie[142] has advocated extension exercises. These limit the risk of aggravating nerve root compression that may occur by extruding a disc fragment. McKenzie's program is complicated. Some investigations have suggested that it offers an advantage over the Williams method. However, there is a high noncompliance rate.[108]

Based on mounting evidence, weak paraspinous supporting muscles are associated with back and neck pain.[143–145] Therefore, strengthening exercises have more than a theoretical benefit. Activities that stress the spine without a simultaneous strengthening of muscles that support the spine could result in an imbalance of stress and muscle strength.

AN ALGORITHM FOR AGGRESSIVE NONSURGICAL MANAGEMENT OF BACK PAIN

An ideal exercise program should be efficacious and be associated with a high level of compliance. It should also be cost-effective. Similarly, it should incorporate a *lifestyle alteration* component (active rather than passive participation in the program). Finally, patient motivation should be assessed by monitoring compliance.[42,108]

The four-point management scheme outlined below may be individualized to "fit" specific clinical situations. It addresses many of the issues raised above.[42,108] The program can be useful in the nonsurgical management process associated with mechanical back pain: (1) **G**eneral sense of well-being augmentation (2) **A**erobic exercise, (3) **S**tretch exercises, and (4) **S**trengthening exercises (**GASS**). Each of these involves patient education, either on the part of the physician/surgeon, or other health care providers (e.g., nurse practitioners), or, more appropriately, both.[42,108]

General Sense of Well-being Augmentation

Sense of well-being augmentation causes the patient to improve *attitude* and simulta-neously become a better surgical candidate (if surgery, indeed, is deemed appropriate). The process can include a program for the cessation of smoking and weight loss. Tobacco use and obesity are associated with back and neck pain. Both can be objectively assessed and recorded on a periodic basis. If the patient cannot demonstrate progress

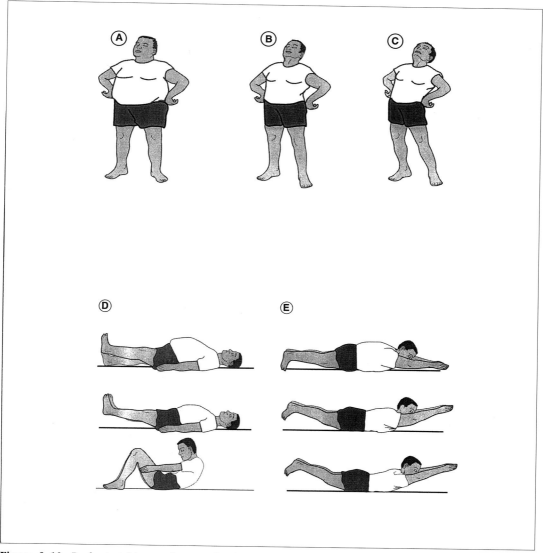

Figure 3–10. Back stretching and strengthening exercises. Progressive degrees of stretching (A–C) and strengthening (D and E) exercises are depicted. For stretching exercises, (A–C) the patient must hold the position for 10–20 seconds. For strengthening exercises, strength imbalances may increase pain. Both abdominal (D) and paraspinous (E) muscle strengthening are thus recommended. Progress may be measured in terms of duration and progression of complexity of exercises.

in these areas, their motivation may be insufficient to warrant surgery or even further nonoperative care.[42,108]

Aerobic Exercise

Aerobic exercise can be quantitated. The increased sense of well-being and accomplishment acquired from a planned aerobic exercise program (walking, running, swimming, cycling, etc.) can create a positive psychological as well as physiological milieu and can establish the extent of the patient's motivation.[42,108]

Stretching Exercise

The augmentation of flexibility is an integral component of the algorithm. Flexibility can be improved via stretching. Toe touching can be monitored by asking patients to reach for their toes with their knees locked and to hold the lowest position achievable for 20 seconds. The distance from the floor is measured and recorded. Bouncing is discouraged. Other exercises include *extension* and the *foot on stool* exercises. They, however, are not as easily quantitated and monitored (Fig. 3–10). Less aggressive exercises are appropriate initially, to be succeeded by more aggressive exercises with increasing stretch and duration.[42,108] Patients with sciatica perhaps should resrict or eliminate the use of this component of the program.

Strengthening Exercises

Much of the pain of spinal origin is associated with mechanical instability (dysfunctional segmental motion). This may be re-

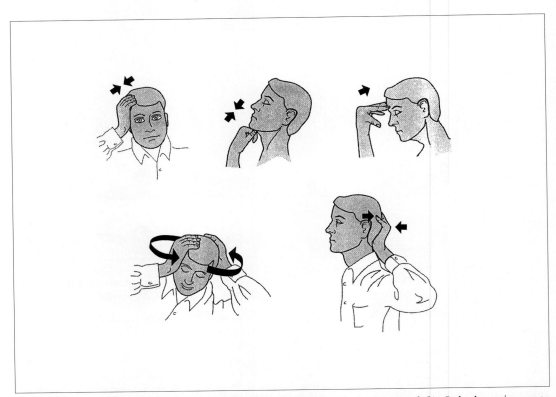

Figure 3–11. Neck strengthening resistance to lateral bending is depicted (upper left). Only the resistance to right lateral bending is demonstrated. However, both right and left exercises should be performed. Resistance to flexion by pressure on the chin and forehead exercises different muscle groups (upper middle and right). Right and left rotational resistance exercises are accomplished by resisting rotation in both directions (lower left). Resistance to extension (lower right).

duced by an appropriate strengthening program. The supporting muscles of the spinal column assist with normal motion, provide support, and prevent excessive spinal movement. If an asymmetry of muscle strength exists, excessive stresses may be placed on the spine or on its supporting muscles and ligaments. In this case strengthening the muscles that stress the spine such as by weight lifting or by running, without strengthening the muscles that support the spine (abdominal and paraspinous muscles), could result in an imbalance. This may aggravate the *dysfunctional motion segment*.[42,108]

Exercises for the dorsal paraspinous and abdominal muscles deserve specific attention. These include supine leg lifts (progressing to sit-ups) for abdominal muscle strengthening and prone leg lifts (progressing to the *airplane* or *rocking chair* exercise) for paraspinous muscle strengthening (Fig. 3–10). Similarly, strengthening exercises for cervical pain may be used (Fig. 3–11).[42,108]

Documentation and Patient Education

Patient education is essential. If patients understand the importance of their active participation in the program, achieving the goal is more likely. Documentation of progress (or lack thereof) can be very helpful.

SUMMARY

The clinical importance of back and neck pain is extraordinary. For example, after colds, back and neck pain are the second most common reasons for visits to primary care physicians (see text for references). Furthermore, back pain is reported to be the most expensive chronic illness among persons 30–60 years of age in our society. The number of individuals disabled by back pain was reported to have grown at a rate 14 times that of the population between 1971 and 1981. Therefore, it is important for all physicians seeing such patients to develop an understanding of the pathophysiology of spinal pain and its

treatment. Although spinal pain may afflict the majority of all individuals, it can usually be managed successfully with modest diagnostic and therapeutic interventions.

Alternatively, since back pain may be a sign of a serious underlying disease such as cancer, many physicians resort to noninvasive imaging such as CT and MRI in patients with back or neck pain. However, as discussed in this chapter and in Chapter 4, there is a high prevalence of asymptomatic disc herniations in middle-aged individuals (including asymptomatic volunteers who undergo imaging). Accordingly, it is imperative to correlate the patient's clinical history and physical examination with the imaging findings in order to avoid unnecessary further diagnostic tests and even surgery for asymptomatic disc disease.

This chapter has reviewed the classification of pain of spinal origin into local (axial) pain; referred, radicular, and funicular pain; pain secondary to muscle spasm; chronic pain; neurogenic claudication pain; and acute spinal instability pain. An approach to a careful history and physical examination was presented, followed by a discussion of the spectrum of laboratory and imaging tests available.

When no specific pathoanatomic diagnosis can be found, acute low back and neck pain is usually a self-limited disorder. When treatment is instituted it usually consists of nonoperative intervention including rest, antiinflammatory agents, and an exercise program. These approaches have been discussed in this chapter along with the many controversies surrounding each approach. Specific management approaches to disc herniation and other specific diseases of the spine are discussed elsewhere in this book.

REFERENCES

1. Cypress BK. Characteristics of physician visits for back symptoms: a national perspective. *Am J Public Health* 1983;73:389–95.
2. Bonica JJ. Historical, socioeconomic and diagnostic aspects of the problem. In Carron H, McLaughlin RE, editors. *Management of Low*

Back Pain. Bristol: The Stonebridge Press; 1982;pp. 1–15.

3. Frymoyer JW. Back pain and sciatica. *N Engl J Med* 1988;318:291–300.
4. Nachemson AL. The lumbar spine; an orthopaedic challenge. *Spine* 1976;1:59–71.
5. Reisbord LS, Greenland S. Factors associated with self-reported back pain prevalence: a population-based study. *J Chronic Dis* 1985;38:691–702.
6. Mooney V. Where is the pain coming from? *Spine* 1987;12:754–9.
7. Schwarzer A, Aprill C, Derby R, et al. The relative contributions of the disc and zygoapophyseal joint in chronic low back oain. *Spine* 1994;19:801–6.
8. Kelsey JL, White AA. Epidemiology and impact of low-back pain. *Spine* 1980;5:133–42.
9. Hall FM. Overutilization of radiological examinations. *Radiology* 1976;120:443–8.
10. Lippitt AB. The facet joint and its role in spine pain: management with facet joint injections. *Spine* 1984;9:746–50.
11. Simons DG, Travell JG. *Myofascial Pain and Dysfunction: The Trigger Point Manual*. Baltimore: William & Wilkins; 1983.
12. Deyo RA, Diehl AK, Rosenthal M. How many days of bed rest for acute low back pain? A randomized clinical trial. *N Engl J Med* 1986;315:1064–70.
13. Hadler N. Regional back pain. (editorial). *N Engl J Med* 1986;315:1090–2.
14. Schiff D, O'Neill B, Suman V. Spinal epidural metastasis as the initial manifestation of malignancy: clinical features and diagnostic approach. *Neurology* 1997;49:452–6.
15. Deyo RA, Diehl AK. Cancer as a cause of back pain: frequency, clinical presentation and diagnostic strategies. *J Gen Intern Med* 1988;3: 230–8.
16. Galasko CSB. The anatomy and pathways of skeletal metastases. In Weiss L, Gilbert HA, editors. *Bone Metastasis*. Boston: G.K. Hall; 1981;pp. 49–63.
17. Barron KD, Hirano A, Araki S, et al. Experiences with metastatic neoplasms involving the spinal cord. *Neurology* 1959;9:91–106.
18. Posner JB. Back pain and epidural spinal cord compression. *Med Clin North Am* 1987;71: 185–204.
19. Frymoyer JW, Newberg A, Pope MH, Wilder DG, Clements J, MacPherson B. Spine radiographs in patients with low-back pain. *J Bone Joint Surg* 1984;66A:1048–55.
20. Hitselberger WE, Witten RM. Abnormal myelograms in asymptomatic patients. *J Neurosurg* 1968;28:204–6.
21. Wiesel SW, Tsourmas N, Feffer HL, et al. A study of computer-assisted tomography 1. The incidence of positive CAT scans in an asymptomatic group of patients. *Spine* 1984;9:549–51.
22. Bogduk N. The innervation of the lumbar spine. *Spine* 1983;8:286–93.
23. Parke WW. Applied anatomy of the spine. In Rothman RH, Simeone FA, editors. *The Spine*. Philadelphia: W.B. Saunders; 1982; pp. 18–51.

24. Wiberg G. Back pain in relation to the nerve supply of the intervertebral disc. *Acta Orthop* 1947;19:211–21.
25. Edgar MA, Ghadially JA. Innervation of the lumbar spine. *Clin Orthop Rel Res* 1976;115: 35–41.
26. Sherman MS. The nerves of bone. *J Bone Joint Surg* 1963;45A:522–8.
27. Roofe PG. Innervation of annulus fibrosus and posterior longitudinal ligament. *Arch Neurol Psych* 1940;44:100–3.
28. McCall IW, Park WM, O'Brien JP. Induced pain referral from posterior lumbar elements in normal subjects. *Spine* 1979;4:441–6.
29. Edgar MA, Nundy S. Innervation of the spinal dura mater. *J Neurol Neurosurg Psychiatry* 1966; 29:530–4.
30. Kimmel D. Innervation of spinal dura mater and dura mater of the posterior cranial fossa. *Neurology* 1961;10:800–9.
31. Malinsky J. The ontogenetic development of nerve terminations in the intervertebral discs of man. *Acta Anat* 1959;38:96–113.
32. Bogduk N, Tynan W, Wilson AS. The nerve supply to the human lumbar intrvertebral discs. *J Anatomy* 1981;132:29–56.
33. Yoshizawa H, O'Brien JP, Smith WT, et al. The neuropathology of intervertebral discs removed for low back pain. *J Pathol* 1980;132: 95–104.
34. Hirsch C, Ingelmark B-E, Miller M. The anatomical basis for low back pain: studies on the presence of nerve endings in ligamentous capsular and intervertebral disc structures in the human lumbar spine. *Acta Orthop Scand* 1963; 33:1–17.
35. O'Brien JP. Mechanisms of spinal pain. In Wall PD, Melzak R, editors. *Textbook of Pain*. Edinburgh: Churchill Livingstone; 1984.
36. Hirsch C. An attempt to diagnose the level of a disc lesion clinically by disc puncture. *Acta Orthop Scand* 1948;18:132–40.
37. Cailliet R. *Low Back Pain Syndrome, 4th Edition*. Philadelphia: F.A. Davis; 1988.
38. Selby DK, Paris SV. Anatomy of facet joints and its clinical correlation with low back pain. *Contemp Orthopaedics* 1981;3:20–3.
39. Jackson HC, Winkelman RK, Bickel WH. Nerve endings in the human lumbar spinal column and related structures. *J Bone Joint Surg* 1966; 48A:1272–81.
40. Stillwell DL. The nerve supply of the vertebral column and its associated structures in the monkey. *Anat Rec* 1948;125:132–40.
41. Fielding JW, Burstein AH, Frankel VH. The nuchal ligament. *Spine* 1976;1:3–14.
42. Benzel E. *Biomechanics of Spine Stabilization: Principles and Clinical Practice*. New York: McGraw-Hill; 1995.
43. Rasmussen TB, Kernohan JW, Adson AW. Pathologic classification, with surgical consideration, of intraspinal tumors. *Ann Surg* 1940; 111:513–30.
44. Foley KM. Pain syndromes in patients with cancer. *Med Clin North Am* 1987;71:169–84.

45. Bernard TN, Kirkaldy-Willis WH. Recognizing specific characteristics of nonspecific low back pain. *Spine* 1987;217:266–80.
46. Fairbank JCT, Park WM, McCall IA, et al. Apophyseal injection of local anesthetic as a diagnostic aid in primary low-back pain syndromes. *Spine* 1981;6:598–605.
47. Mooney V, Robertson J. The facet syndrome. *Clin Orthop* 1976;115:149–56.
48. Waxman SG. The flexion-adduction sign in neuralgic amyotrophy. *Neurology* 1979;29: 1301–4.
49. Frykholm R. Cervical nerve root compression resulting from disc degeneration and root sleeve fibrosis. A clinical investigation. *Acta Chir Scand (Suppl)* 1951;160.
50. Booth RE, Rothman RH. Cervical angina. *Spine* 1976;1:28–32.
51. Brodsky A. Cervical angina: a correlative study with emphasis on the use of coronary arteriography. *Spine* 1985;10:699–709.
52. Guidetti B, Fortuna A. Differential diagnosis of intramedullary and extramedullary tumors. In Vinken PJ, Bruyn GW, editors. *Handbook of Clinical Neurology, Volume 19.* Amsterdam: North-Holland; 1975; pp. 51–75.
53. Austin GM. The significance and nature of pain in tumors of the spinal cord. *Surg Forum* 1959;10:782–5.
54. Shenkin HA, Alpers BJ. Clinical and pathological features of gliomas of the spinal cord. *Arch Neurol Psychiat* 1944;52:87–105.
55. Torma T. Malignant tumors of the spine and the spinal extradural space. *Acta Chir Scand Suppl* 1957;225:1–176.
56. Lhermitte J, Bollak NM. Les douleurs a type de decharge electrique consecutives a la flexion cephalique dans la sclerose en plaque. *Rev Neurol (Paris)* 1924;31:36–52.
57. Smith KJ, McDonald WI. Spontaneous and mechanically evoked activity due to central demyelinating lesions. *Nature* 1980;286:154–5.
58. DeJong RN. *The Neurologic Examination, 4th Edition.* Hagerstown: Harper & Row; 1979.
59. Walther PJ, Rossitch E, Bullard DE. The development of Lhermitte's sign during cisplatin chemotherapy: possible drug-induced toxicity causing spinal cord demyelination. *Cancer* 1987;60:2170–2.
60. Vollmer TL, Brass LM, Waxman SG. Lhermitte's sign in a patient with herpes zoster. *J Neurol Sci* 1991;106:153–7.
61. Word JA, Kalokhe UP, Aron BS, Elson HR. Transient radiation myelopathy (Lhermitte's sign) in patients with Hodgkin's disease treated by mantle radiation. *Int J Radiat Oncol Biol Phys* 1980;6:1731–3.
62. Sandyk R, Brennan MJW. Lhermitte's sign as a presenting symptom of subacute degeneration of the cord. *Ann Neurol* 1983;13:215–6.
63. Baldwin RN, Chadwick D. Lhermitte's "sign" due to thoracic cord compression (letter to the editor). *J Neurol Neurosurg Psychiatry* 1986;49:840–1.
64. Simons DG, Travell JG. Myofascial origins of low back pain. *Postgrad Med* 1983;73:66–108.
65. Simons DG, Travell JG. Myofascial pain syndromes. In Wall PD, Melzack R, editors. *Textbook of Pain.* Edinburgh: Churchill Livingstone; 1984; pp. 263–76.
66. Pace JB, Naghle D. Piriform syndrome. *West. J Med* 1976;124:435–9.
67. Pace JB. Commonly overlooked pain syndromes. *Postgrad Med* 1975;58:107–13.
68. Freiberg AH. Sciatic pain and its relief by operations on muscle and fascia. *Arch Surg* 1937;34:337–50.
69. Freiberg AH, Vinke TH. Sciatica and the sacroiliac joint. *J Bone Joint Surg* 1934;16: 126–36.
70. Robinson DR. Piriformis syndrome in relation to sciatic pain. *Am J Surg* 1947;73:355–8.
71. Verbiest H. Further experiences on the pathologic influence of a developmental narrowness of the bony lumbar vertebral canal. *J Bone Joint Surg* 1955;37:576–83.
72. Verbiest H. The significance and principles of computerized axial tomography in idiopathic developmental stenosis of the lumbar vertebral canal. *Spine* 1979;4:369–78.
73. Hall SH, Bartleson JD, Onofrio BM, et al. Lumbar spinal stenosis: clinical features, diagnostic procedures, and results of surgical treatment in 68 patients. *Ann Int Med* 1985;103:271–5.
74. Batson OV. The function of the vertebral veins and their role in the spread of metastases. *Ann Surg* 1940;112:138–48.
75. Yoss RE, Corbin KB, MacCarty CS, Love JG. Significance of symptoms and signs in localization of involved root in cervical disc protrusion. *Neurology* 1957;7:673–83.
76. Friis ML, Gulliksen GC, Rasmussen P. Distribution of pain with nerve root compression. *Acta Neurosurg* 1977;39:241.
77. Wigton RS, Hoellerich VL, Ornato JP, Leu V, Mazzotta LA, Cheng I-H. Use of clinical findings in the diagnosis of urinary tract infection in women. *Arch Intern Med* 1985;145:2222–7.
78. Fast A, Shapiro D, Ducommun EJ, et al. Low-back pain in pregnancy. *Spine* 1987;12:368–71.
79. Weitz EM. The lateral bending sign. *Spine* 1981;6:388–97.
80. O'Rourke T, George CB, Redmond J, others. Spinal computed tomography and computed tomographic metrizamide myelography in the early diagnosis of metastatic disease. *J Clin Oncol* 1986;4:576–83.
81. Davidson RI, Dunn EJ, Metzmaker JN. The shoulder abduction test in the diagnosis of radicular pain in cervical extradural compressive monoradiculopathies. *Spine* 1981;6:441–6.
82. Dyck P. Lumbar nerve root: the enigmatic eponyms. *Spine* 1984;9:3–6.
83. Estridge MN, Rouhe SA, Johnson NG. The femoral stretching test: a valuable sign in diagnosing upper lumbar disc herniations. *J Neurosurg* 1982;57:813–7.
84. Falconer M, McGeorge M, Begg A. Observations on the cause and mechanism of symptom production in sciatica and low back pain. *J Neurol Neurosurg Psychiatry* 1948;11:13–26.

85. Hudgins WR. The crossed straight leg raising test: a diagnostic sign of herniated disc. *J Occup Med* 1979;21:407–8.

86. Edgar MA, Park WM. Induced pain patterns on passive straight-leg raising in lower lumbar disc protrusion. *J Bone Joint Surg* 1974;56-B: 658–67.

87. Simpson JF. Meningeal signs. In Vinken PJ, Bruyn GW, editors. *Handbook of Clinical Neurology, Volume 1.* Amsterdam: North-Holland; 1969; pp. 546.

88. Waddell G, McCulloch JA, Kummel E, et al. Nonorganic physical signs in low-back pain. *Spine* 1980;5:117–25.

89. Woodhall B, Hayes GJ. The well-leg-raising test of Fajerstajn in the diagnosis of ruptured lumbar intervertebral disc. *J Bone Joint Surg* 1950; 32-A:786–92.

90. Dyck P. The femoral nerve traction test with lumbar disc protrusion. *Surg Neurol* 1976;6: 163–6.

91. Jabre JF, Bryan RW. Bent-knee pulling in the diagnosis of upper lumbar root lesions. *Arch Neurol* 1982;39:669–70.

92. Hoppenfeld S. *Physical Examination of Spine and Extremities.* New York: Appleton-Century-Crofts; 1976.

93. Pancoast HK. Superior pulmonary sulcus tumor: tumor characterized by pain, Horner's syndrome, destruction of bone and atrophy of hand muscles. *JAMA* 1932;99:1391–6.

94. Schliack H. Segmental innervation and the clinical aspects of spinal nerve root syndromes. In Vinken PJ, Bruyn GW, editors. *Handbook of Clinical Neurology, Volume 2.* Amsterdam: North-Holland; 1969; pp. 157–77.

95. Sabin TD, Geschwind N, Waxman SG. Patterns of clinical deficit in peripheral nerve disease. In Waxman SG, editor. *Physiology and Pathobiology of Axons.* New York: Raven Press; 1978; pp. 431–9.

96. Bolton B. Blood supply of the human spinal cord. *J Neurol Neurosurg Psychiatry* 1939;2: 137–48.

97. Deyo RA. Plain roentgenography for low-back pain: finding needles in a haystack (editorial). *Arch Intern Med* 1989;149:27–9.

98. Deyo RA, Diehl AK. Lumbar spine films in primary care: current use and effects of selective ordering criteria. *J Gen Intern Med* 1986;1: 20–5.

99. Frazier LM, Carey TS, Lyles MF, et al. Selective criteria may increase lumbosacral spine roentgenogram use in acute low-back pain. *Arch Intern Med* 1989;149:47–50.

100. Suarez-Almazor M, Belseck E, Russell A, et al. Use of lumbar radiographs for early diagnosis of low back pain. Proposed guidelines would increase utilization. *JAMA* 1997;277:1782–6.

101. Witt I, Vestergaard A, Rosenklint A. A comparative analysis of X-ray findings of lumbar the lumbar spine in patients with and without lumbar pain. *Spine* 1984;9:298–300.

102. Frymoyer JW, Phillips RB, Newberg AH, et al. A comparative analysis of teh interpretations

103. Freidenberg ZB, Miller WT. Degenerative disc disease of the cervical spine: a comparative study of asymptomatic and symptomatic patients. *J Bone Joint Surg* 1963;45A: 1171–8.

104. Pallis C, Jones AM, Spillane JD. Cervical spondylosis. *Brain* 1954;77:274–89.

105. McCrae DL. Asymptomatic intervertebral disc protrusions. *Acta Radiol* 1956;46:9–27.

106. Jensen M, Brant-Zawadzki M, Obuchowski N, et al. Magnetic resonance imaging of the lumbar spine in people without back pain. *N Engl J Med* 1994;331:69–73.

107. Boden S, Davis D, Dina T, et al. Abnormal magnetic resonance scans of the lumbar spine in asymptomatic subjects: a prospective investigation. *J Bone Joint Surg Am* 1990;72:402–8.

108. Adams M, Sypert G, Benzel E. The nonoperative management of neck and back pain. In Benzel E, editor. *Spine Surgery: Techniques and Complications and Avoidance.* New York: Churchill Livingstone; 1998.

109. vanTulder M, Koes B, Bouter L. Conservative treatment of acute and chronic nonspecific low back pain. *Spine* 1997;22:2128–56.

110. Deyo RA, Tsui-Wu Y-J. Descriptive epidemiology of low-back pain and its related medical care in the US. *Spine* 1987;12:264–8.

111. Waddell G. 1987 Volvo award in clinical sciences. A new clinical model for the treatment of low back pain. *Spine* 1987;12:632–44.

112. Muller E. Influence of training and inactivity on muscle strength. *Arch Phys Med Rehabil* 1970; 51:449–62.

113. Convertino V, Hung J, Goldwater D, DeBusk R. Cardiovascular responses to exercise in middle-aged men after 10 days of bed rest. *Circulation* 1982;65:134–40.

114. Malmivaara A, Hakkinen U, Aro T, et al. The treatment of acute low back pain—bed rest, exercises, or ordinary activity? *N Engl J Med* 1995; 315:1064–70.

115. Carey T, Garrett J, et al. The outcome and costs of care for acute low back pain among patients seen by primary care practitioners, chiropractors and orthopedic surgeons. *N Engl J Med* 1995;333:913–7.

115a. Cherkin D, Deyo R, Battie M, et al. A comparison of physical therapy, chiropractic manipulation, and provision of an educational booklet for the treatment of patients with low back pain. *NEJM* 1998;339:1021–9.

116. Frost H, KalberMoffet J, Moser J, et al. Randomised controlled trial for evaluation of fitness programme for patients with chronic low back pain. *BMJ* 1995;310:151–4.

117. Hansen F, Bendix T, Skov P, et al. Intensive dynamic back muscle exercises, conventional physiotherapy, or placebo-control treatment of low-back pain. *Spine* 1993;18:98–107.

118. Risch S, Norvell N, Pollock M, et al. Lumbar strengthening in chronic low back pain. *Spine* 1993;18:232–8.

119. Lahad A, Malter A, Berg A, et al. The effectiveness of four interventions for the prevention of low back pain. *JAMA* 1994;272:1286–91.

120. Deyo R, Walsh N, Martin D, et al. A controlled trial of transcutaneous electronic nerve stimulation (TENS) and exercise for chronic low back pain. *N Engl J Med* 1990;322:1627–34.

121. Carette S, Marcoux S, Truchon R, et al. A controlled trial corticosteroid injections into the facet joints for chronic low back pain. *N Engl J Med* 1991;325:1002–7.

122. Bush K, Cowan N, Katz D, Gishen P. The natural history of sciatica associated with disc pathology: a prospective study with clinical and independent radiologic follow-up. *Spine* 1992; 17:1205–12.

123. Rybock JD. Acute back pain and disc herniation. In Johnson RT, editor. *Current Therapy in Neurological Disease—2*. Toronto: B.C. Decker; 1987; pp. 48–50.

123a. Vroomen PCAJ, DeKrom MCTFM, Wilmink JT, et al. Lack of effectiveness of bed rest for sciatica. *N Engl J Med* 1999;340:418–23.

124. Carette S, Leclaire R, Marcoux S, et al. Epidural corticosteroid injections for sciatica due to herniated nucleus pulposus. *N Engl J Med* 1997;336:1634–40.

125. DIckson R. The surgical treatment of low back pain. *Curr Orthop* 1987;1:387–90.

126. Javid M, Nordby E, Ford L, et al. Safety and efficacy of chympapain (Chymodiactin) in herniated nucleus pulposus with sciatica: results of a randomized double blind study. *JAMA* 1983;249:2489–94.

127. Fraser R. Chymopapain for the treatment of intervertebral disc herniation: the final report of the double blind trial. *Spine* 1984;9: 815–18.

128. Diabezies E, Langford K, Morris J, et al. Safety and efficacy of chympapain in the treatment of sciatica due to herniated nucleus pulposus: results of a randomized double blind study. *Spine* 1988;13:561–5.

129. Saal J, Saal J. Non-operative treatment of herniated lumbar intervertebral disc with radiculopathy: an outcome study. *Spine* 1989;14: 431–7.

130. Saal J, Saal J, Herzog R. The natural history of lumbar disc extrusions treated non-operatively. *Spine* 1990;15:683–6.

131. Weber H. Lumbar disc herniation: a controlled prospective study with ten years of observation. *Spine* 1983;8:131–40.

132. Bozzao A, Gallucci M, Masciocchi C, Aprile I, Barile A, Passariello R. Lumbar disc herniation—MR-imaging assessment of natural history in patients treated without surgery. *Radiology* 1992;185:135–41.

133. Jensen R, Bliddal H, Hansen S, et al. Severe low back pain: changes in CT scans in the acute phase and after long term observation. *Scand J Rheumatol* 1993;22:30–4.

134. Maigne J, Rime B, Deligne B. Computed tomographic follow-up study of forty-eight cases of non-operatively treated lumbar intervertebral disc herniations. *Spine* 1992;17:1071–4.

135. Delauche J, Budot C, Laredo J, et al. Lumbar disc herniation: computed tomography scan changes after conservative treatment of nerve root compression. *Spine* 1992;17:927–33.

136. Nutter P. Aerobic exercises in the treatment and prevention of low back pain. *Occup Med* 1988;3: 137–45.

137. Kraus H, Melleby H, Gaston S. Back pain correction and prevention. National voluntary organizational approach. *NY State J Med* 1977; 77:1335–8.

138. Williams P. *The Lumbosacral Spine, Emphasizing Conservative Management*. New York: McGraw Hill; 1965.

139. Kendall P, Jenkins J. Exercises for backache: a double-blind controlled trial. *Physiotherapy* 1968;54:154–7.

140. Davies J, Gibson T, Tester L. The value of exercises in the treatment of low back pain. *Rheumatol Rehabil* 1979;18:243–7.

141. Gilbert J, Taylor D, Hildebrand A, Evans C. Clinical trial of common treatments for low back pain in family practice. *Br Med J* 1985; 291:791–4.

142. McKenzie R. *The Lumbar Spine, Mechanical Diagnosis and Therapy*. Waikenae, New Zealand: Spinal Publications; 1981.

143. Hultman G, Nordin M, Saraste H, et al. Body composition, endurance, strength, cross section of area and density of erector spinae muscles in men with and without low back pain. *J Spinal Disord* 1993;6:113–23.

144. Mayer T, Smith S, Keely J, Mooney V. Quantification of lumbar function. Plane trunk strength in chronic low back patients. *Spine* 1985;10:91–103.

145. Shirdo O, Kaneda K, Ito T. Trunk muscle strength during concentric and eccentric contraction: a comparison between healthy subjects and patients with low back pain. *J Spinal Disord* 1992;5:175–82.

146. Adams RD, Victor M. Diseases of the spinal cord. In Adams RD, Victor M, editors. *Principles of Neurology*. New York: McGraw-Hill; 1985; pp. 665–98.

147. Kristoff FV, Odom GL. Ruptured intervertebral disk in the cervical region. *Arch Surg* 1947;54:287–304.

148. Waxman SG, Sabin TD. Diabetic truncal polyneuropathy. *Arch Neurol* 1981;38:46–7.

149. Howell DS. The painful back. In Wyngaarden JB, Smith LH, editors. *Cecil Textbook of Medicine, 17th Edition* Philadelphia: W. B. Saunders; 1985; pp. 1955.

Chapter 4

DEGENERATIVE DISORDERS OF THE SPINE

Osteoarthritis and spondylosis, which are "normal" aging phenomena, are almost universally present by the time of late middle age and collectively are often referred to as degenerative disorders of the spine. While osteoarthritis refers to degenerative disease of the diarthrodial facet joints of the spine, spondylosis refers to degeneration of the fibrocartilagenous intervertebral disc joints. Osteoarthritis and spondylosis frequently coexist, because when the process begins in either the facet joint or the intervertebral disc joint, abnormal function (motion) of the affected joint transmits abnormal forces to the corresponding (intervertebral and/or facet) joints at the same and adjacent levels, resulting in additional degeneration. In practice, when referring to the spine, the terms osteoarthritis and spondylosis are often used interchangeably.

Spondylosis, a common cause of pain and disability in middle and later years, frequently occurs in the cervical and lumbar regions. In the cervical spine, it is a common cause of radiculopathy and/or myelopathy, and in the lumbar region, it commonly causes low back pain, radiculopathy, the cauda equina syndrome, and/or neurogenic claudication.

Stenosis of the spinal canal and intervertebral foramina is the mechanism whereby spondylosis causes most of its associated symptoms and signs.[1] The primary event in the development of spondylosis appears to be degeneration of the intervertebral disc. This results in disc space narrowing, allowing the disc to bulge centrifugally. In response to this narrowing of disc space, adjacent vertebral bodies produce osteophytes. This is a result of bone formation, the osteophytes, along with cartilaginous and fibrous tissue overgrowth, may combine to bulge dorsally into the spinal canal and intervertebral foramina, resulting in compression of the adjacent spinal cord and nerve root(s). Unlike acute prolapse of an intervertebral disc, which often occurs after trauma, there is usually no herniation of the nucleus pulposus in patients with spondylosis. Instead, an expansion of the circumference of the disc in association with osteophytic, cartilaginous, and fibrous growth is found.[2]

Although neurologic symptoms and signs may not occur in patients with spondylosis, the degenerative changes that cause progressive narrowing of the spinal canal and intervertebral foramina frequently give rise to myelopathy and radiculopathy in cases of cervical spondylosis, and to radiculopathy in cases of lumbar spondylosis. The clinical importance of cervical spondylosis is underscored by its frequency. According to Adams and Victor,[3] it is the most common cause of myelopathy found in patients in the general hospital population. In addition, many cases of low back pain and sciatica may be attributed to lumbar spondylosis.

PATHOPHYSIOLOGY OF DISC DEGENERATION AND THE SPONDYLOTIC PROCESS

Spondylosis is defined as "vertebral osteophytosis secondary to degenerative disc disease."[4] Spondylosis is not to be confused with inflammatory processes that are also associated with osteophyte formation. These are grouped together as inflammatory arthritides (e.g., rheumatoid arthritis and ankylosing spondylitis). The osteophytes of spondylosis are associated with degeneration of the intervertebral disc. The intervertebral disc is an amphiarthrodial joint that has no synovial membrane. The inflammatory arthritides, however, classically involve the diarthrodial joints that are lined with synovium; e.g., the facet joints. The presence of spondylosis is, therefore, defined by the presence of noninflammatory disc degeneration. It is a complex process that involves many alterations of normal physiology.[5]

Intradiscal Hydrostatic and Oncotic Pressure

Persistent elevation of intradiscal pressure causes a narrowing of the disc interspace. This results in distortion and stretching of the annulus fibrosus and the facet joint capsule, and an acceleration of the degeneration process. The degeneration process can be considered to be a manifestation of the normal aging process; however, its pathological acceleration is of obvious clinical significance.

The water content of the disc interspace and the vascularity of the disc gradually decrease throughout life so a well-vascularized disc at birth essentially has no vascular supply by age 30. These and other factors contribute to changes in the chemical and anatomical makeup of the disc. Fibroblasts begin to produce inferior-quality fibers and ground substance. The disc becomes dessicated and less able to function as a cushion. Fissures occur in the cartilaginous plates, with defects resulting in internal herniations (Schmorl's nodes).[6] Gas can accumulate in the disc (vacuum phenomenon). Mucoid degeneration, an ingrowth of fibrocartilage, and obliteration of the nucleus fibrosus, ensue. Generalized disc deterioration results in instability. This, in turn, results in annulus fibrosus tension, compression, and bulging, all of which result in pathological deformation.[5]

Disc Deformation

Bulging of the annulus fibrosus elevates the periosteum of adjacent vertebral bodies at the attachment site of Sharpy's fibers. Bony reactions (subperiosteal bone formation) occur, resulting in spondylotic ridge (osteophyte) formation (Fig. 4–1). This process most commonly results in spinal canal encroachment in the cervical and lumbar regions, with a relative sparing of the canal in the thoracic region. This is due to the fact that the natural lordosis in these spinal regions results in the concavity of the spinal curvature, and hence the tendency toward annular bulging occurs in the direction of the spinal canal. The spondylotic process is deterred or retarded by fusion or immobilization.[5,7]

Regarding a lateral bending deformity (scoliotic curvature), osteophyte formation predominantly occurs *on the concave side of a curve,* where annulus fibrosus bulging is similarly most significant (Fig. 4–2A and B). In the cervical and lumbar regions, the thin dorsal annulus fibrosus and relatively weak posterior longitudinal ligament (particularly laterally) combine with the migratory tendencies of the nucleus pulposus to encourage dorsolateral disc herniation (Fig. 4–3).

Many factors participate in inducing the dorsal and lateral locations of disc herniation. These include the migratory tendencies of the nucleus pulposus, the relatively weak lateral portion of the dorsal longitudinal ligament, and the thin lateral portion of the annulus fibrosus. Most disc herniations do not occur (or more appropriately do not become manifest) immediately following trauma. Laboratory investigations that attempt to determine the mechanism of disc herniation are lacking. This has hampered research in this area for years. Adams and Hutton, however, determined that a high percentage of lumbar discs in the laboratory could be encouraged to herniate if the disc (*1*) was degenerated and (*2*) a specific force pattern was acutely delivered to the motion segment. This force pattern includes (*1*) flexion (causing dorsal nucleus pulposus migration), (*2*) lateral bending away from the side of disc herniation (causing dorsal nucleus pulposus migration), and (*3*) the application of an axial load (causing an increase in intradiscal pressure).[8] As is portrayed in Figure 4–3, this complex loading pattern of the intervertebral disc results in (*1*) the application of tension on the weakest portion of the annulus fibrosus (dorsolateral position; the location of the herniation), (*2*) migration of the nucleus pulposus towards this position, and (*3*) and an increase in intradiscal pressure (asymmetric). A degenerated disc is a requisite for this process to occur. These factors, plus the increasing frequency of annulus fibrosus tears with age and the observation of peak nucleus fibrosus pressures in the 35–55 age group, are among the mitigating factors related to an increased incidence of disc herniation.[5]

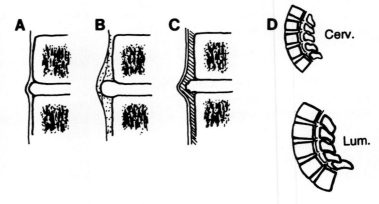

Figure 4–1. Osteophytes are caused by subperiosteal bone formation, which results from elevation of the periosteum by disc bulging (A). A spondylotic ridge then develops (B and C). This commonly encroaches upon the spinal canal in the cervical and lumbar regions, because the lordotic spinal curvature causes the disc bulging and osteophyte formation to occur toward the spinal canal (D). This is less common in the thoracic region, because the concavity is oriented away from the spinal canal. (From Benzel, EC,[5] with permission.)

Cerv.

Lum.

Extradiscal Soft Tissue Involvement

Soft tissue pathological processes, in addition to discogenic and facet joint degeneration, contribute to spondyliotic conditions. Hypertrophy and buckling of the ligamentum flavum is involved in the development of myelopathy in patients with cervical spondylotic myelopathy.[5]

The Degenerative Process

The degenerative process as a whole involves the disc interspace, facet joints, and intra- and paraspinal tissues. Degenerative changes of the intervertebral disc include one or a combination of four processes: (1) loss of disc interspace height, (2) irregularities in the disc end plate, (3) sclerosis of the disc margins, and/or (4) osteophyte formation. Soft tissue proliferation may accompany these processes as an associated phenomenon, or may be a primary process. *Degenerative disc disease* is defined by Kramer as *biomechanical and pathological conditions of the intervertebral segment caused by degeneration, inflammation, or infection.*[9] As with the changes associated with disc interspace degeneration, facet joint degenerative changes are also associated with an increased laxity in movement. As the degenerative process proceeds, however, an element of stability is often acquired (spinal restabilization).[15]

Intra- and paraspinal tissue changes including calcification, and hypertrophy are commonly associated with spondylosis (e.g., hypertrophy of the ligamentum flavum), rheumatoid arthritis (e.g., bursa inflammation and pannus formation), and OPLL (ossification and hypertrophy of the posterior longitudinal ligament) (Fig. 4–4A and B). Ankylosing spondylitis per se typically does not predispose to disc herniation. It, however, is associated with increased stability via decreased allowed motion.[5] (see chapter 9)

The pathogenesis of degenerative disc disease varies, depending upon the underlying disease process. Fundamentally,

aberrant physiological responses to stress placed upon the spine, and the resulting accelerated deterioration of the integrity of spinal elements, underlie the pathological process regardless of the disease entity or region of the spine involved. Before one can appreciate one of the degenerative processes and its accompanying pathology, one must appreciate the normal physiological processes involved with the disc interspace and related structures.[5]

Anatomy and Physiology of the Disc Interspace

A great deal of work has been done on the disc interspace.[9,10] The disc interspaces contribute approximately 20% to the height of the spine. The disc consists of an outer annulus fibrosus and an inner nucleus pulposus. It is bordered rostrally and caudally by a cartilaginous plate. The latter is part of the vertebral body and is composed of hyaline cartilage.

To retain water, fluid movement must occur against a very steep pressure gradient, since the pressure within a disc is much higher than that outside a disc. The mechanism through which this occurs is via osmotic pressure driven counter to hydrostatic pressure. In equilibrium, the following equation describes the case.[5]

$$\text{Extradiscal hydrostatic pressure} + \text{intradiscal oncotic pressure} = \text{Intradiscal hydrostatic pressure} + \text{extradiscal oncotic pressure}$$

The tissue pressure outside the disc plus the oncotic pressure within the disc equals the tissue pressure inside the disc plus the oncotic pressure outside the disc. Whenever one side of the equation outweighs the other side (e.g., secondary to weight bearing), equilibrium is disrupted and a movement of fluid across the disc's semipermeable membrane occurs. Increased weight bearing causes intradiscal fluid to escape via hydrostatic forces. This increases the concentration of macromolecules (long molecules that are contained within the disc because they cannot pass

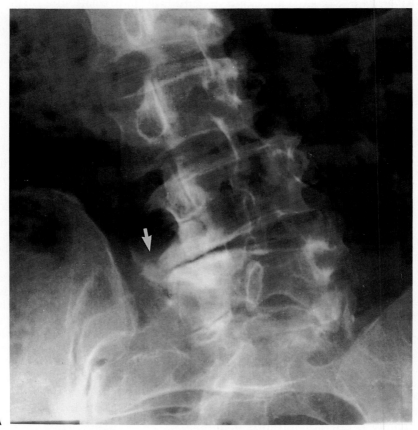

Figure 4–2. Spondylotic ridges (osteophyte formation), associated with scoliosis, predominantly occur on the concave side of a curve—i.e., on the side of chronic or long-term annulus fibrosus bulging (A). This is demonstrated at two separate levels, on opposite sides of the spine, in a patient with a biconcave curve (B). (From Benzel, EC,[5] with permission.)

through membranes) within the disc interspace, and results in an increase in intradiscal oncotic pressure. The macromolecules take up fluid due to their hydroscopic capacity. This, in turn, increases the absorption capacity of the disc.

In addition to the biomechanical effects, this fluid movement allows for nutrient and waste product passage across the membrane. Therefore, the greater the activity of the patient, the more active this form of transport. Traction is obviously a

mechanism by which the intradiscal pressure can be reduced, thus causing an increase in intradiscal water content and an increase in disc height. These points are summarized in Figure 4–5.[5]

Biomechanics of the Intervertebral Motion Segment

During the axial loading of a disc interspace, the intradiscal pressures are sym-

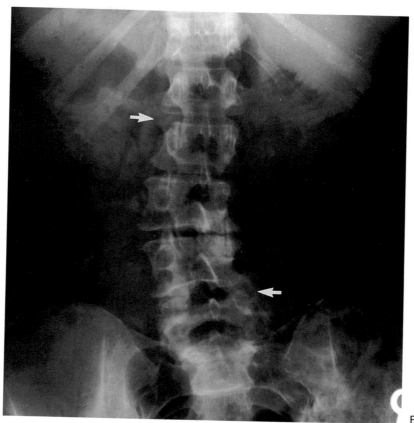

B

Figure 4–2.—Continued

metrically distributed. Eccentrically placed loads, however, result in the asymmetric distribution of pressures within the disc. This, in turn, causes the nucleus pulposus to move within the disc from a region of high pressure (high load) to a region of low pressure (low load); e.g., forward flexion results in the dorsal migration of the nucleus pulposus. Conversely, the annulus fibrosus responds to asymmetric force application to the disc interspace by bulging on the side of the of the disc with the greatest stress applied; i.e., the annulus fibrosus bulges on the side opposite the direction of migration of the nucleus pulposus (Fig. 4–6).[5] Although these concepts

were discussed and illustrated earlier in this chapter, their importance makes them worthy of reiteration here.

Spinal Configuration

Surgical approaches to both decompression and stabilization of degenerative diseases of the spine often include a combination of decompression, fusion, and instrumentation, performed from either or both of a combination of ventral or dorsal exposures. The most appropriate surgical approach utilized for any given spinal disorder, including the application of an in-

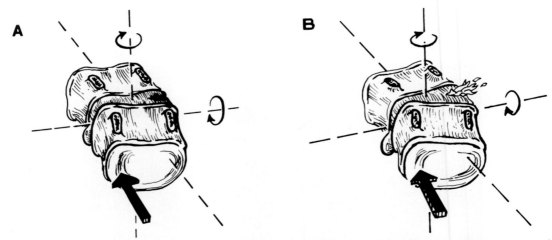

Figure 4–3. Dorsal view of the intervertebral segment with pedicles and laminae removed. The application of an axial load, lateral bending, and flexion causes the nucleus pulposus to migrate in the direction of the region of the annulus fibrosus that is under tension and prone to tearing (A). This may result in disc herniation in the dorsal paramedian location if the disc is degenerated (and thus predisposes it to pathological migration) (B). (From Benzel, EC,[5] with permission.)

strumentation construct, should be determined, at least in part, by considering the intrinsic curvature of the spine.[5]

THE CERVICAL SPINE

In the cervical spine, the spondylotic degenerative process results in a loss of height, predominantly of the disc inter-

space. This loss of height begins in the ventral aspect of the disc. Initially, the disc space is thicker ventrally than dorsally. This contributes to the normal cervical lordosis. As the ventral height of the disc interspace decreases, the lordotic posture is diminished, and eventually is lost. This "straightening" of the spine then increases the forces placed on the ventral aspects of

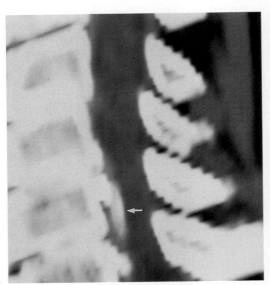
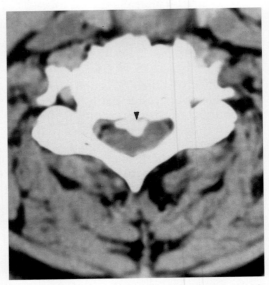

A   B

Figure 4–4. CT scan of the cervical spine showing ossification of the posterior longitudinal ligament (arrows). (A) Sagittal view. (B) Axial view. (Courtesy of Dr. Richard Becker.)

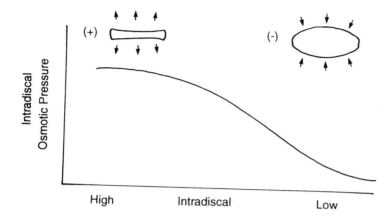

Figure 4–5. Osmotic and hydrostatic factors affecting the disc interspace (after Kramer[9]). Note that an increased intradiscal pressure, resulting from an increase in weight-bearing, causes fluid to migrate out of the intradiscal space (arrows). This, in turn, increases the concentration of macromolecules and the oncotic pressure within the disc space (+). Hence the absorption capacity of the disc is increased. Decreasing intradiscal pressure has the opposite effect. (From Benzel, EC,[5] with permission.)

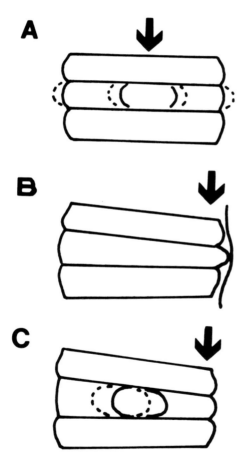

Figure 4–6. An axial load causes an equally distributed force application to the disc (A). An eccentric force application results in annulus fibrosus bulging on the side of the greatest force application—i.e., the concave side of the bend (B). The nucleus pulposus moves in the opposite direction (C). Dashed lines indicate the positions of structures during force application. (From Benzel, EC,[5] with permission.)

the vertebral bodies by increasing the length of the moment arm through which the forces are applied. This exposes the ventral aspect of the vertebral body to increasing stresses and to a tendency to develop compression fractures. As the loss of lordosis progresses and the kyphosis-producing forces placed on the spine increase, the vertebral bodies begin to lose height ventrally more than dorsally, via "compression fractures" (Fig. 4–7). This process is "encouraged" by the gradual loss of calcium in patients with osteoporosis. The collapse of the disc interspace and the vertebral body results in a forward bending of the dural sac and spinal cord, which contributes to the overall pathological relationship between the neural elements and the surrounding bony and soft tissues (Fig. 4–7B and C).[5]

Since the assessment of the curvature of the spine is imperative regarding appropriate decision making, a precise definition of curvature types is important. An *effective cervical kyphosis* is defined as a configuration of the cervical spine in which any part of the dorsal aspect of any of the C3–7 vertebral bodies crosses a line drawn in the midsagittal plane (on a lateral cervical spine tomogram, myelogram, or MRI) from the dorsocaudal aspect of the vertebral body of C2 to the dorsocaudal aspect of the vertebral body of C7. Conversely, an *effective cervical lordosis* is a configuration of the cervical spine in which no part of the dorsal aspect of any of the C3–7 vertebral bodies crosses this line. The definition of

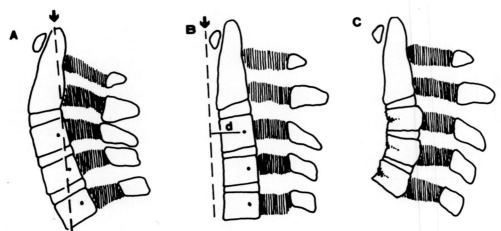

Figure 4–7. In a nonpathological situation, where the dorsal intervertebral disc height is less than the ventral height, normal lordotic curvature in the cervical spine results (A). Ventral disc interspace height loss (via the typical degeneration process) results in the loss of the nonpathological lordotic posture (B). This elongates the moment arm applied to the spine, d, leading to ventral vertebral body compression. A further exaggeration of a pathological kyphotic posture may then ensue (C). (From Benzel, EC,[5] with permission.)

this "imaginary" line is associated with a zone of uncertainty ("gray zone") within which surgeon bias and clinical judgment play a role in the determination of whether lordosis or kyphosis is the predominant spinal configuration in the midsagittal section (Fig. 4–8). If, in the opinion of the surgeon, there is no gray zone (i.e., only an "effective" kyphosis or an "ef-

fective" lordosis is possible), then surgical decision making is simpler. On the other hand, if a gray zone exists, the decision-making process is more complex. Patients whose spinal configuration falls in the gray zone, should perhaps be defined as having a "straightened" spine.[5]

The surgical indications for myelopathy associated with degenerative diseases

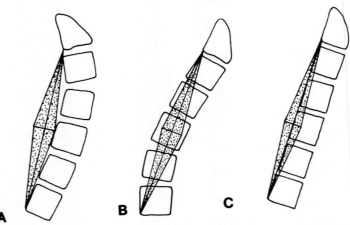

Figure 4–8. A midsagittal section of a cervical spine (as observed by MRI or myelography) configured in lordotic posture ("effective" cervical lordosis). A line has been drawn from the dorsocaudal aspect of the vertebral body of C2 to the dorsocaudal aspect of the vertebral body of C7 (solid line). The gray zone is outlined by dotted lines (A). A midsagittal section of a cervical spine that is configured in kyphosis ("effective" cervical kyphosis) (B). Note that portions of the vertebral bodies are located dorsal to the gray zone. (C) A midsagittal section of a "straightened" cervical spine. Note that the most dorsal aspect of a cervical vertebral body is located within, but not dorsal to, the gray zone. (From Benzel, EC,[5] with permission.)

vary.[5,11–13] Ventral as well as dorsal decompressive approaches to degenerative and inflammatory diseases of the spine should be used in patients in whom the given approach to spinal decompression (and stabilization) is associated with a high probability of success.[12,14–17] Spinal geometry is an important determinant of the appropriateness of either the ventral or the dorsal approach in individual situations.[14,15] The presence of an "effective" lordosis may be a relative indication for a dorsal approach, whereas the presence of an "effective" kyphosis may be a relative indication for a ventral approach to the pathology.

THE THORACIC SPINE

In the thoracic spine, disc height loss (predominantly ventral disc height loss) results in progression of kyphotic deformity that can be superimposed upon a pre-existing kyphotic deformity. Therefore, there is progressive exaggeration of the deformity. This is, in part, the case in Sheuermann's disease.

The stability conferred by the rib cage to the thoracic spine minimizes the progression of the thoracic kyphosis due to degenerative changes.[5] This stability is predominantly related to the rib's attachment to the vertebral and costovertebral joints, and particularly to the sternum.[9,10]

THE LUMBAR SPINE

The lumbar spine is not protected by the rib cage like the thoracic region is. Furthermore, the coupling response to movements is opposed to those observed in the cervical region. Coupling is defined here as the obligatory movement along or about one axis in response to movement along or about another axis (Fig. 4–9). Degenerative rotatory scoliosis is an example of the coupling phenomenon. This is attributed to the absence of the uncovertebral joints and the different orientation of the facet joints. These factors all contribute to the progression of lateral bending deformities in the lumbar spine, rather than the kyphotic deformities observed in the cervical and thoracic spine. An asymmetric loss of height of the lumbar intervertebral disc may progress to an asymmetric collapse of the vertebral body. If this lateral bending (scoliotic deformity) occurs and progresses, it is associated with an obligatory rotation of the spine that is caused by the coupling characteristics of the lumbar spine. Similarly, osteophytes occur on the concave side of the curvature (Figs. 4–1 and 4–2).[5]

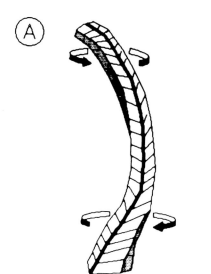

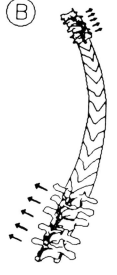

Figure 4–9. Perhaps the most important manifestation of the coupling phenomenon is the relationship between lateral bending and rotation in the cervical and lumbar regions. This is depicted diagramatically (A) and anatomically (B). Note that the coupling phenomenon results in rotation, in opposite directions, in these two regions. Also note that the thoracic spine does not exhibit significant coupling. (From Benzel, EC,[5] with permission.)

The obligatory association of a rotatory deformity with a lateral bending deformity (coupling) makes lumbar spinal instrumentation surgery more difficult and dangerous. Lateral transverse process dissection can result in injury to the nerve roots because of their relatively dorsal location with respect to the transverse processes, while deformity correction by distraction of the concave side of the spine may result in the stretching of shortened and tethered nerve roots. Proximal (intradural) nerve roots are much less tolerant of stretching because of their lack of perineurium compared to their more peripheral nerve counterparts.[5]

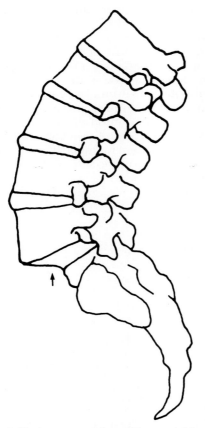

Figure 4–10. An exaggeration of the normal lumbar lordosis places excessive translational stresses on the lumbosacral junction when the patient is upright. This may result in a parallelogram-like translational deformation at the lumbosacral junction (arrow) (From Benzel, EC,[5] with permission.)

Normal Posture

The cervicothoracic and thoracolumbar junctions are transition zones between kyphotic and lordotic postures. The lumbar spine again assumes a lordotic posture, much like that of the cervical spine. The clinical impact of degenerative changes on spinal curvature in the thoracic and lumbar spine is not as evident as it is in the cervical spine. Normal thoracic kyphosis can be exaggerated in the degenerated spine. This occasionally causes or contributes to spinal cord compressive processes and predisposes the spine to further deformation. Lumbar lordosis can precipitate or exaggerate sagittal plane translation deformities (Fig. 4–10).[5]

CERVICAL SPONDYLOSIS AND CERVICAL SPONDYLOTIC MYELOPATHY (CSM)

In 1911, Bailey and Casamajor[18] reported on a series of patients with cervical spondylosis. They speculated on the pathogenesis of the disorder suggesting that a thinning of the intervertebral disc was the primary pathological event leading to trauma of the adjacent vertebral bodies and bony overgrowth. This disease mechanism for spondylosis is still favored today (see above). The authors further suggested that dorsally placed osteophytes could cause spinal cord compression. Some years later, Stookey[19,20] classified extradural cervical chondromas into three clinical groups: (1) midline ventral lesions compressing both sides of the spinal cord; (2) lesions just lateral to the midline that compress only one half of the spinal cord, producing a Brown-Séquard syndrome; and (3) lesions that are laterally placed that compress only the cervical nerve root. Thus the protean clinical manifestations of cervical spondylosis were recognized in the first decades of this century. It was not until 1934, though, that the chondromata, which had previously been considered neoplastic in origin, were recognized as protrusions of intervertebral discs.[21–23] Interested readers may wish to read more about the history of cervical spondylotic myelopathy.[24,25]

A study from 1954[26] found that among individuals without neurologic complaints, there was radiological evidence of cervical spondylosis in 50% of individuals over the age of 50 years and in 75% of those over 65. Limitation of neck movement was found in 40% of those over 50. Furthermore, 60% had some neurologic abnormality referable to cervical spondylosis.

Pathogenesis

Although no portion of the cervical spine is immune to the development of spondylosis, the lower cervical spine is most vulnerable. The reason is uncertain but has been considered to be due to its extensive mobility.[3,27] During flexion and extension, the vertebral bodies "roll" on one another, with the nucleus pulposus of each intervertebral disc acting as a ball bearing.[28] As discussed above, the water content of the intervertebral disc declines with age, and the nucleus pulposus becomes replaced with fibrocartilage, resulting in narrowing of the disc space. This process is superimposed upon the spinal configuration changes that frequently accompany the degenerative process (see above). Degeneration of the annulus fibrosus results in tears that allow bulging or frank herniation of disc material into the spinal canal.

With this change in architecture, the ball-bearing movement at the intervertebral joint is lost and is replaced by a sliding motion that places stress on the anterior and posterior longitudinal ligaments and vertebrae, resulting in osteophyte formation.[27] Most commonly, disc degeneration occurs at multiple levels with aging. Therefore, spondylosis is typically observed at more than a single level. However, when a single intervertebral disc herniates, the spondylotic process may proceed at that level without involvement elsewhere, via a similar mechanism.[29]

Although there has been controversy surrounding the pathogenesis of CSM, the most important factors appear to be spinal canal size, impairment of blood supply to the spinal cord, and mechanical factors.[30,31] The observation that the anteroposterior diameter of the spinal canal of patients with CSM is, on average, smaller than that of patients without myelopathy suggests that simple compression should in part explain the myelopathy.[32–34] In an anatomicopathological study of the cervical spines of patients with myelopathy secondary to cervical spondylosis, Payne and Spillane[33] found that the average anteroposterior diameter of the spinal canal at the C4–7 levels was smaller in those with myelopathy. Although spondylosis reduced the diameter of the vertebral canal of all patients, those patients with CSM had congenital spinal canal diameters that were smaller than those with spondylosis, but without myelopathy. As the degenerating cervical disc narrowed, the resulting apposition of the vertebral bodies caused deformity of the uncovertebral joints, narrowing of the intervertebral foramen, and formation of an osteophytic bar along the ventral spinal canal wall. Although in population studies there is a correlation between a narrow sagittal diameter of the spinal canal and CSM, there is a considerable degree of overlap between the frequency histograms for the minimum anteroposterior diameter of the asymptomatic population and those with CSM.[31]

Brain suggested that interfering with the blood supply to the spinal cord is a probable cause of spondylotic myelopathy.[35] Pathological studies have supported this hypothesis,[36,37] and Allen's observation of blanching of the spinal cord with neck flexion during laminectomy further corroborates this ischemic explanation.[38] It has been noted however, that the temporal profile of patients with CSM is unlike that of other ischemic disorders.[27] In addition, anterior spinal artery thrombosis has only rarely been verified pathologically.[39]

An alternative hypothesis for CSM pathogenesis that has found considerable support is as follows. As the neck naturally moves, the spinal cord is intermittently compressed and injured.[3,27,30,40,41] When the neck is flexed and extended, the spinal cord moves rostrally and caudally in the spinal canal.[42–44] During hyperextension, the ligamenta flava bulge, thereby compressing the spinal cord dorsally.[45] Given the triangular anatomical configuration of the cervical spinal canal, a hypertrophied and bulging ligamenta flava compress the posterior and lateral columns and the dorsal root entry zone.[46] In addition, during extension, the cross-sectional area of the cervical spinal cord has been found to enlarge.[42,47] These findings may explain the occasional exacerbation of symptoms and myelographic and manometric block that are encountered in patients with hyperextension of the cervical spine and the clinical improvement that is often observed when the neck is immobilized with a collar.[27,43] Symptoms and signs may also be exacerbated with neck flexion. In this case, the spinal cord is injured as it is stretched over a ventral osteophytic bar during flexion.[29,42–44]

The pathogenesis of radiculopathy secondary to cervical spondylosis is usually considered to be due to compression of the nerve root, arising from adjacent osteophytes.[26] However, patients may have narrowed intervertebral foraminae without associated radiculopathy, or radiculopathy without radiographic signs of narrowing of the intervertebral foramen.[48] Imaging studies of the intervertebral foraminae, with the spine in a neutral position, may not reveal narrowing that may be present when the neck is extended.[47,49] Such narrowing may contribute to nerve root compression with extension and thus also explain the improvement observed, at times, when the neck is immobilized with a collar or surgical foraminotomy. Furthermore, radiculopathy might be aggravated during flexion of the neck secondary to stretching of the nerve root.[43]

Pathology

While any level may be involved, cervical spondylosis occurs most frequently at the interspaces C3–4 to C6–7. The C5–6 level is the most commonly affected. The most easily recognized pathologic finding is osteophytes at the level of the affected intervertebral joint space. Such osteophytes form transverse bars that may extend the entire width of the spinal canal or involve only a portion of it. Laterally placed bulging soft tissue and osteophytes may narrow the adjacent intervertebral foramina. The dura may be thickened and adherent to the adjacent bone.[2]

The spinal cord is often indented at the level of the offending osteophytes and may show a broad range of pathology, from minor changes to severe destruction (Fig. 4–11). The spinal cord is usually flattened in an anteroposterior direction. Hughes[2] has classified the changes into four groups: (1) dorsal long tract degeneration that is more prominent at the C1 level than the T1 level; (2) lateral tract degeneration that is more prominent at the T1 level than the C1 level; (3) white matter destruction, for example, myelin pallor or necrosis; and (4) gray matter destruction, for example, ischemic changes or neuronal loss.

The pathological findings in patients with cervical spondylotic radiculopathy appear to be even more sparse than those in patients with CSM.[27] The uncovertebral osteophyte is often responsible for the foraminal narrowing.[2] Because on pathological examination spondylotic radiculopathy and myelopathy are often seen together the findings secondary to radi-culopathy alone can be obscured. Nevertheless, because spondylotic radiculopathy typically involves part of the root proximal to the dorsal root ganglion, Wallerian degeneration may be observed in the posterior columns rostral to the root compression.

Clinical Features

The clinical features of cervical spondylotic radiculopathy and CSM are presented together because they are often found simultaneously. Symptoms may begin in either the upper or lower extremities. As in other forms of spinal cord compression, the symptoms and signs may include pain and motor, sensory, or sphincter disturbances.

Symptoms most frequently begin between 50 and 70 years of age but may occur earlier or in advanced years. Men are affected more frequently than women.[50]

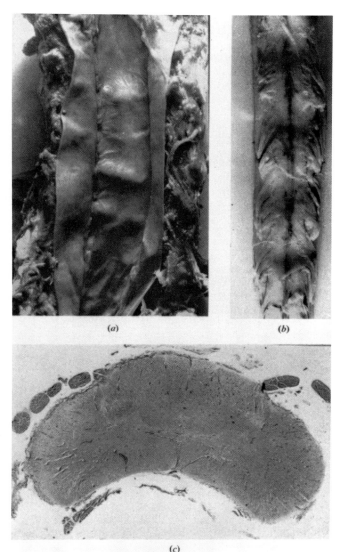

(a)   *(b)*

(c)

Figure 4–11. (A) The spinal canal is shown following a laminectomy in a case of cervical spondylosis. The spinal cord has been removed and spondylotic bars are seen bulging into the spinal canal. (B) The anterior aspect of the spinal cord is seen to contain indentations which have occurred secondary to the spondylotic bars. (C) A transverse section through the C6 level of the spinal cord has been indented. Leptomeningeal fibrosis and vascular proliferation within the cord is seen. Hematoxylin and Van Giesen, × 8. (From Hughes, JT,[2] with permission.)

The clinical history typically is one or two years but may extend over only weeks or date back over more than a decade. The symptoms may develop progressively or in a stepwise fashion, with remissions between periods of deterioration. Symptoms and signs may develop for the first time or be aggravated following injuries such as a fall, motor vehicle accident, or hyperextension of the neck (Fig. 4–12).

Pain in the neck, shoulder, and/or arm is a common presenting complaint. Pain may radiate in a radicular distribution and is usually dermatomal. However, it occasionally may occur in the distribution of the affected myotome. Muscle spasm usually occurs, resulting in a tilted and rotated posture, and pain which can arise from spasm. Paresthesias, fasciculations, and muscle weakness in the distribution of the affected nerve roots are often encountered. Reduction in the biceps (C5, C6, brachioradialis [C5, C6], or triceps [C7]) reflexes may be observed. These depressed deep tendon reflexes may be associated with hyperactive reflexes caudal to

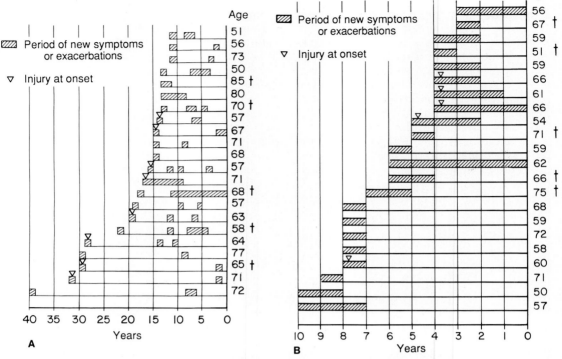

Figure 4–12. Clinical course of cervical spondylotic myelopathy. (A) Pattern of disease in 22 patients who had symptoms for more than 10 years. (B) Pattern of disease in 22 patients who had symptoms for 10 years or less. Each "block" represents the initial symptom or an exacerbation of symptoms. Between blocks, the horizontal lines represent periods in which no new symptoms or signs of myelopathy developed; the patients were stable or improving. The vertical line on the right represents the last follow-up or death (indicated by cross at far right). (From Lees, F and Turner, JWA,[78] with permission.)

the level of spondylosis, when radiculopathy and myelopathy simultaneously occur. When a depressed brachioradialis reflex is associated with hyperactivity of the finger flexors, the resulting reflex on stimulation of the brachioradialis is termed inverted finger flexors and may be a valuable localizing finding. Radicular symptoms and signs may be observed at levels of myelomalacia a few segments above and below the level of the spondylotic osteophyte. These areas, which may be secondary to ischemic changes, may create a perplexing clinical picture by causing lower motor neuron signs at multiple levels above and below the level of spondylosis.[51]

The symptoms and signs of myelopathy include spasticity, weakness, sensory findings, and bowel and bladder complaints. Often, the earliest findings of CSM are reduced distal vibratory sensation with ex-

aggeration of deep tendon reflexes and, occasionally, Babinski signs.[50] Although the patient may complain only of unilateral lower extremity symptoms, the neurologic examination usually reveals signs of bilateral disturbance of long tract function. Spasticity is an especially prominent sign, and jumping legs may be reported. Sensory complaints in the lower extremities often are not prominent. When sensory abnormalities are found in the lower extremities, vibratory sensation usually is more impaired than position sense. Pain and temperature are typically unimpaired unless spinal damage is advanced.[50] Lhermitte's sign is often reported. Disturbances of sphincter function are late phenomena and generally do not occur in the absence of advanced spinal cord dysfunction, which manifests itself earlier by dysfunction of other modalities.

Laboratory and Imaging Studies

Laboratory studies are usually unremarkable in patients with cervical spondylosis. Cerebrospinal fluid examination is typically normal or shows a nonspecific elevation in protein concentration.[52] Manometric testing may demonstrate a block, especially when the neck is extended.

Plain radiographs of the cervical spine most frequently show narrowing of the intervertebral disc space(s), with adjacent osteophytes narrowing the spinal canal and/or the intervertebral foramina, and sclerosis of the vertebral endplates, but of course they do not image the spinal cord or nerve roots directly. Osteophytes may develop on the facet joints and uncovertebral joints as well.[53] A range of normal dimensions of the sagittal diameter of the cervical spinal canal have been reported elsewhere.[33,53,54] Although there is not a good correlation between specific findings on plain radiographs and the clinical manifestations,[50] it has been suggested that if the anteroposterior dimension is greater than 13 mm, spinal cord compression from spondylotic changes alone is unlikely.[55] Plain radiographs may also serve as a valuable adjunct to MRI (see below). A frequent clinical pitfall lies in erroneously attributing neurologic symptoms to spondylosis in cases where these common radiological findings are incidental and asymptomatic.

In the setting of cervical spondylosis, myelography may show any of the following, alone or in combination: (*1*) extradural defects from osteophytes, disc material, ligamenta flava and other associated spondylotic changes protruding into the spinal canal; (*2*) nonfilling of nerve root sleeves; (*3*) flattening and widening of the spinal cord (that may simulate an intramedullary mass lesion, especially when viewed in the anteroposterior projection alone); and (*4*) obstruction to the flow of contrast, that may be exacerbated by extension of the neck.[53] Others have also emphasized that myelography has been valuable in demonstrating a functional or dynamic relationship between the osteophytes and spinal cord in that flexion–extension views may reveal changing cord compression that may not be evident on static views.[56,57]

A CT may demonstrate the dimensions of the spinal canal and reveal the location of osteophytes in relation to the intervertebral foramina and spinal cord. In patients with cervical radiculopathy due to spondylosis, CT may confirm the presence of the offending osteophyte.[58,59] A CT-assisted myelography was compared to myelography, CT, and MRI by Brown and colleagues in a group of preoperative patients.[60] These authors found that CT-assisted myelography provided better image resolution than myelography or CT scanning alone. The CT-assisted myelography was equivalent to MRI in revealing most herniated discs but was superior to MRI in detecting osteophytes adjacent to herniated discs. Plain films were helpful in identifying osteophytes when correlated with the MR images. The rapid evolution in MRI technology will hopefully bring with it an enhanced ability to distinguish bone from soft tissue.

The combination of plain radiographs of the cervical spine with flexion–extension views, read in conjunction with MRI, has been found to be more sensitive and specific for a diagnosis of causes of spinal canal, stenosis, herniated discs, and intradural lesions than observed in most patients undergoing CT-assisted myelography alone.[56] Given the additional benefit that MRI is noninvasive, it is has been recommended that for the initial evaluation of patients suspected of having cervical spondylotic myelopathy, MRI should be performed first with plain radiographs if needed. Following these studies, if the information obtained is suboptimal or inadequate, CT and/or CT-assisted myelography may be helpful in selected patients.[53,56,61–63]

In cases of CSM, CT may demonstrate hypodense intramedullary cavitations of the spinal cord that extend above and below the levels of spondylotic cord compression.[64] Following the intrathecal administration of contrast material, many patients have delayed enhancement of the gray matter at and near the level of the spondylotic bar.[65,66] These lesions have been described as looking like snake eyes or fried eggs when visualized in the axial projection. These abnormalities correlate with the histological finding of necrosis in the central gray matter in cases of CSM.[67] Extending several levels from the spondylotic bar, pencil-shaped softenings reported to occur in cases of spinal cord compression and ischemia[68] have been visualized with CT.[66] Snake eyes and pencil-shaped zones have been observed on MRI of the spinal cords of CSM patients.[69] These findings may explain the neurologic changes that occur distant from the level of spondylosis, such as atrophy, and fasciculations of the hand muscles with spondylosis at the midcervical levels.[51,70]

Magnetic resonance imaging is an excellent modality for the visualization of a narrowed spinal canal associated with thecal compression due to cervical spondylosis and degenerative disc disease.[56,71] Additionally, herniated discs and their relationship to the cord and neural foramina can be visualized. The MRI can reveal cord signal abnormalities on T_2-weighted images at the site of compression which may signal evidence for edema, demyelination, gliosis, or myelomalacia (Fig. 4–13).[72] Braakman[56] has advocated surgical decompression in patients with minimal clinical findings but with appreciably abnormal T_2 signal change.

Matsuda and colleagues[73] have studied the preoperative and postoperative MRI appearance of cord abnormalities in patients with cervical spondylotic myelopathy. In their study, the severity of preoperative T_2-weighted cord signal abnormaities correlated with the degree of clinical impairment. Postoperatively, the cord signal abnormality again tended to parallel the clinical evolution of the patient. Thus T_2-signal abnormalities generally improved in patients with clinical recovery and tended to not improve or worsen in those who did not improve clinically or actually worsened. Postoperatively, the cord diameter may increase following successful decompression.[56,73,74] Alternatively, postoperative MRI may demonstrate that the reason for poor clinical outcome is inadequate decompression or cord atrophy, as reported by Clifton et al.[75]

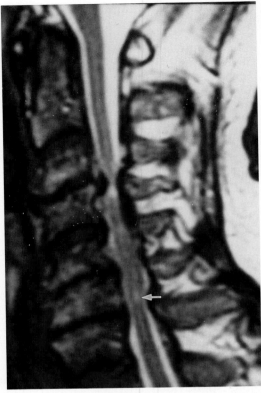

Figure 4–13. An MRI revealing cervical spondylosis resulting in spinal stenosis and cord compression. Focal cord signal abnormality (arrow) is seen within the spinal cord secondary to compression. (Courtesy of Dr. Richard Becker.)

Differential Diagnosis

In its complete form, CSM is usually readily recognized as consisting of neck pain and brachialgia, radicular motor–sensory–reflex signs in the upper extremities, and myelopathy. However, other causes of spinal cord compression, such as neoplasms and syringomyelia, may cause symptoms and signs that are difficult to differentiate from cervical spondylosis on the basis of the clinical history and physical examination alone. This problem is compounded by the fact that an erroneous clinical diagnosis of CSM might be supported by the presence of coincidental and asymptomatic spondylosis observed on imaging studies. It is wise to remember that cervical spondylosis most commonly involves the lower cervical spine. Clinical manifestations that point to other cervical levels or, certainly, to thoracic levels, are atypical of spondylosis.

Extradural spinal neoplasms are usually associated with a more rapid temporal clinical evolution than spondylosis. In addition, there is often (although not invariably) a history of prior malignancy, and imaging studies generally show signs of neoplasm. Similar to spondylosis, intradural–extramedullary neoplasms may have a very long clinical history. Imaging studies may show widening of the spinal canal rather than narrowing. Intramedullary neoplasms and syringomyelia most frequently occur in younger age groups than is typical for cervical spondylosis. Furthermore, these intramedullary processes often give rise to dissociated sensory disturbances (loss of pain and temperature function with preservation of vibration and position sensation) in a cape-like distribution. Cervical spine plain radiographs usually show widening of the spinal canal rather than narrowing. The MRI has been useful in identifying intramedullary mass lesions.

Noncompressive forms of myelopathy such as multiple sclerosis (MS), subacute combined degeneration, and amyotrophic lateral sclerosis (ALS) may rarely present as clinical syndromes similar to CSM. With MS there is often a history, or findings on examination, of disease above the foramen magnum such as optic neuritis, nystagmus, or internuclear ophthalmoplegia. Although progressive spinal forms do occur (especially in middle-aged individuals), MS is typically a disease with remission and exacerbations that occurs most frequently in younger individuals.[76,77] Early impairment of sphincter function also is often observed, whereas it is atypical with CSM. Localized nerve root signs in the upper extremities are very unusual in patients with MS. The CSF, evoked potentials, and MRI usually differentiate demyelinating disease from CSM.

Motor neuron disease or ALS produces motor disturbances without sensory findings. Unlike spondylosis, pain is not typical, and eventually signs of lower motor neuron disease are observed in muscles above the foramen magnum. The CSF

and spine imaging studies are not revealing in ALS.

Subacute combined degeneration secondary to vitamin B_{12} deficiency has protean clinical manifestations. Unlike spondylosis, however, neck pain is not characteristic. Signs of peripheral neuropathy are often present. Loss of position sense in the lower extremities is more often observed with this kind of combined systems disease than in cervical spondylosis. Laboratory studies are usually diagnostic.

Natural History

There are few studies of the natural history of CSM. Lees and Turner[78] reported their findings on the long-term follow-up of 44 patients who had CSM at the time they first visited the Neurology Department of St. Bartholomew's Hospital. Only eight of these patients underwent surgical intervention. The clinical course of CSM in these patients is shown in Figure 4–12. The maximal disability and disability at follow-up among the same patients is shown in Table 4–1. The authors concluded that in most patients, CSM is a chronic disorder characterized by long periods of nonprogressive disability interrupted by shorter periods of exacerbation of myelopathy. Disability may improve with conservative management alone (Table 4–1). In a minority of patients, these authors found that the course of CSM is characterized by progressive deterioration.

In another study of the long-term prognosis of CSM, Epstein and associates[79] found that among 114 nonsurgical patients culled from the literature, 36% improved, 38% remained stable, and 26% deteriorated. They found that when progressive myelopathy does occur, it may show a pattern of stepwise worsening interrupted by long periods of stability, improvement, or slow deterioration; the intervals of stability or improvement may last for many years. Alternatively, deterioration may be slow and steady, without remissions or stabilization. LaRocca concluded that it is not possible to predict the

Table 4–1. **Disability and Employment of Patients with Cervical Spondylotic Myelopathy***

Duration of Symptoms	Maximum Disability			Disability at Follow-up				Unemployed
	Mild	Moderate	Severe	Nil	Mild	Moderate	Severe	
More than 10 years	1				1			0
		6				6		0
			15	1		5	9	3
10 years or less	3			1	2			0
		9				8	1	0
			10			2	8	3
Totals	4	15	25	2	3	21	18	6

*From Lees, F and Turner, JWA.[78] p. 1608, with permission.

clinical course precisely in an individual patient.[80] Unfortunately, this variability in prognosis jeopardizes the assessment of therapy and leads to controversy in the management of CSM.

Management

In general, the neck pain of cervical spondylosis can be successfully managed with rest, local heat, collar, antiinflammatory agents, and analgesics. Surgery is considered for patients with progressive, major neurologic impairment due to spondylotic radiculopathy unresponsive to optimal conservative management.

Management of patients with CSM includes both nonsurgical and surgical means. In patients without major neurological deficits or signs of progression, a conservative approach including rest and stabilization of the neck with a collar or neck strengthening exercises is often successful. Alternatively, if the patient is moderately or severely disabled from progressive CSM, surgery may be considered. Surgery should also be considered if the patient develops signs of progressive myelopathy despite conservative management.[80] Surgical approaches include diskectomy and stabilization via a ventral approach,[81] or laminectomy.[82]

The management of CSM has been complicated, somewhat by an inconsistent application of terminology among physi-

cians, particularly with regard to the term cervical spondylotic radiculomyelopathy.[83] Cervical spondylotic radiculomyelopathy is a "catchall" term that encompasses all neural compressive phenomena related to cervical spondylosis. Management issues are confused by the implication that radiculopathy and myelopathy are intimately interrelated and that they are thus treated similarly. This is, perhaps, inappropriate. It may be better to consider myelopathy, radiculopathy, and combined symptomatic myelopathy and radiculopathy as three separate entities. The rationale for this is based on the differing clinical manifestations (e.g., myelopathy versus radiculopathy) and surgical approaches (e.g., spinal cord versus nerve root decompression) associated with each. Usually, cervical spondylotic myelopathy (CSM) encompasses three or more spinal levels (at least two motion segments),[84–87] and cervical radiculopathy is most often single level in origin and multifactorial in nature (e.g., soft versus hard disc).[88]

The discussion here is limited to the surgical treatment of the most disabling and significant aspect of cervical spondylosis, CSM, and does not include a discussion of radiculopathy. The surgical approaches for CSM include (1) multiple level ventral corpectomies with interbody fusion, (2) multiple single level discectomies and dural sac decompressions with accompanying multiple single level interbody fusions, (3) utilization of either of the prior two with ventral spinal instrumentation techniques, (4) spinal fusion without decompression, (5) cervical laminectomy, and finally (6) laminectomy with an accompanying dorsal fusion.[88]

Selecting appropriate treatment is critical for the surgical management of CSM. First, it involves the selection of surgical candidates. Second, it involves the selection of the most appropriate operation. Surgical failures may be secondary to either.

Dorsal surgical approaches to spinal canal decompression have been clearly established as safe and efficacious[83,89–102] While ventral and ventrolateral decompression operations have been strongly recommended for the treatment of CSM,[103–110], some have found the ventrally oriented approaches to CSM to be less than satisfactory[111]. Significant neurological and nonneurological complications associated with ventral surgical approaches to CSM have been reported[103,106,108,109,111]. These may be related to the complexity and degree of difficulty of the operation. Since all ventral operations for CSM require spine fusion, one must consider the long-term complications of spinal fusion as well, such as increased spinal laxity and accelerated degenerative changes immediately above and below the fusion levels.[5] One must also consider the patient's increased chance of neural injury, infection (by virtue of the obligatory increased operation time), and donor site complications.[88]

Primary considerations in selecting of surgical candidates include the extent to which the patient's symptoms and physical disability impact upon lifestyle and the level of confidence the physician has that these symptoms and disabilities are secondary to spinal cord compression. Symptoms and degree of disability can be readily quantitated.[83,85,112,113] Their impact on the patient's lifestyle can only be addressed by careful and honest assessment by the patient and the physician. The question must be asked: "Is it worth the risk of surgery to try to alleviate the patient's symptoms and disability?"[88] Ball and Saunders make a compelling case for surgical intervention even in less severely involved patients.[88,112]

But we may not always be certain that it is the spinal cord compression (determined by imaging studies) that is causing the symptoms and disability. Central nervous system degenerative disorders that are included in the differential diagnosis of cervical myelopathy, such as ALS and multiple sclerosis, can complicate the decision-making process. These factors must be considered during surgical candidate selection.[88,112]

Prophylaxis against sudden catastrophic neurologic deterioration[114] may be indicated in some patients with mild symptomatic disease and significant neural encroachment. The risks of the prophylactic surgery must be weighed against the chance of catastrophe associated with untreated cervical stenosis.

One must keep an open mind regarding surgical approaches to the treatment of CSM. Both ventral and dorsal approaches are indicated in specific situations. Some clinicians suggest that patients with an "effective" kyphosis (in the opinion of the surgeon) and with symptoms of CSM be treated with a ventral decompressive operation and that patients with an "effective" lordosis (in the opinion of the surgeon) be treated with a posterior decompressive operative approach. Patients with "straightened" spines may be treated either way. Surgeon bias regarding the management approach to the "straightened" spine, as well as its definition, are cruxes in the ongoing controversy regarding surgical approach selection.[88]

SPINAL STENOSIS AND NEUROGENIC CLAUDICATION

Intermittent claudication, a clinical syndrome first described in humans by Charcot in 1858, refers to the onset of discomfort and weakness in the lower extremities while walking. These symptoms progressively worsen to a point at which walking becomes impossible; then they disappear when the patient stops walking. Although intermittent claudication is commonly recognized as occurring secondary to ischemia of the muscles of the lower extremities and is considered to be a cardinal symptom of peripheral vascular disease, intermittent neurogenic claudication refers to a similar functional disturbance of the lower extremities that occurs secondary to disturbances of function of the spinal cord or cauda equina.[115] Distinguishing claudication due to peripheral vascular disease from that of a neurogenic etiology is a common clinical problem.

Although ischemia of the spinal cord and cauda equina were originally considered the cause of neurogenic claudication, some authors[116–118] consider compression of these neural structures due to spinal stenosis to be primarily responsible. Recently, these two hypotheses have been reconciled by a proposed pathophysiological mechanism that includes both compressive and ischemic elements.[119] The following discussion reviews the classification of spinal stenosis and presents the pathogenesis, symptoms, and signs of neurogenic claudication.

Types of Spinal Stenosis

In anatomical or imaging terms, spinal stenosis refers to a reduction in the cross-sectional area of the spinal canal. It may be classified as congenital, acquired, or due to a combination of both.[120] Table 4–2 lists examples of causes of spinal stenosis.

CONGENITAL SPINAL STENOSIS

The congenital and developmental forms of spinal stenosis are usually idiopathic, associated with Klippel-Feil syndrome[121–123] or with achondroplasia.[124,125] At the craniocervical junction, stenosis may be secondary to developmental anomalies of the foramen magnum, atlas, and axis.[124] Patients with developmental stenosis may be asymptomatic until superimposed acquired lesions such as spondylosis, trauma, or disc disease occur. Spinal stenosis may be familial.[126] Spondylolysis resulting in spondylolisthesis, malalignment of adjacent vertebrae, may cause lumbar stenosis with nerve root compression.[126]

In patients with developmental stenosis, the spinal canal tends to be uniformly

Table 4–2. Classification of Spinal Stenosis*

CONGENITAL-DEVELOPMENTAL
Idiopathic
Achondroplastic
Morquio's disease
Klippel-Feil

ACQUIRED
Degenerative
Spondylolisthetic
Postsurgical
Posttraumatic
Paget's disease
Acromegaly
Steroid-induced lipomatosis
Fluorosis
Ossification of posterior longitudinal ligament
Ossification of the ligamenta flava

COMBINED (ACQUIRED SUPERIMPOSED ON CONGENITAL)

*Adapted from Kricun, R and Kricun, ME,[62] p. 398.

stenotic along a region that can extend several levels along the spinal axis.[127] In addition, the pedicles are usually short (short pedicle syndrome), which decreases the anteroposterior diameter of the canal. Acquired stenosis, on the other hand, usually is segmental, with areas of normal spinal canal dimensions apart from stenotic regions.

In cases of achondroplasia, early fusion of the neurocentral synchondroses occurs, resulting in spinal stenosis.[128,129] The thoracolumbar spine is the region that most commonly becomes symptomatic. The stenosis usually becomes symptomatic after degenerative changes develop that further compromise the spinal canal.[62,128,129] Other bony abnormalities such as scoliosis or gibbus deformity are common in conjunction with achondroplasia and may aggravate symptoms. Cervical spinal stenosis and deformities at the craniocervical junction are also common.[129,130]

ACQUIRED SPINAL STENOSIS

As noted, narrowing of the spinal canal in cases of acquired spinal stenosis is not uniform throughout the spinal axis, but rather is segmental. Although spondylosis is the most common cause, it may be post-traumatic, be caused by spondylolisthesis, or be secondary to a number of other conditions (Table 4–2).

When spondylosis is the cause, narrowing is typically found at the disc and facet levels,[131] and the anteroposterior diameter of the spinal canal is often normal between the discrete levels of narrowing. The stenosis arises secondary to a combination of factors that include hypertrophy of the facet joints, vertebral osteophytes, hypertrophy of the ligamentum flavum,

and bulging of the annulus fibrosus.[62,124,132] (Figs. 4–14 and 4–15).

In the cervical spine, spondylotic stenosis usually occurs between the C4 and C6 levels.[128] In the thoracic spine, it is usually secondary to generalized metabolic, rheumatologic, or orthopedic disorders, or it is posttraumatic.[133,134] It rarely occurs in the absence of these. When it does, it most commonly is due to hypertrophy of the ligamentum flavum and articular processes in the lower thoracic spine.[133,135] The more frequent involvement of the

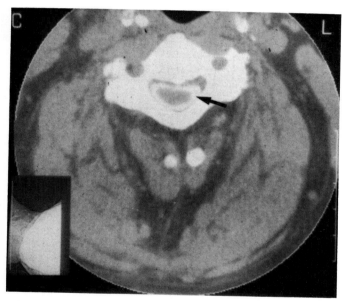

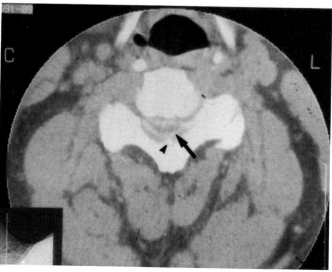

Figure 4–14. A CT scan demonstrating acquired cervical spinal stenosis due to cervical spondylosis. The upper panel shows intrathecal contrast material (arrow) without spinal cord compression (normal). The lower panel demonstrates uncovertebral spondylosis, partial calcification of the ligamentum flavum (arrowhead), and secondary thecal and spinal cord compression (arrow). (Courtesy of Dr. Helmuth Gahbauer)

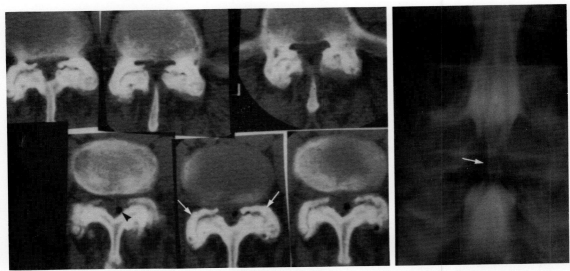

Figure 4–15. Myelogram and CT scan demonstrating acquired lumbar stenosis due to lumbar spondylosis. Note the air (black arrowhead) in the degenerated facet joint (white arrows) shown on the CT scan. The myelogram demonstrates a stenosis in the form of an hourglass deformity (white arrows) secondary to severe spondylosis. (Courtesy of Dr. Helmuth Gahbauer.)

lower thoracic spine, rather than at higher levels, may be related to the greater mobility of the lower segments.[136]

Lumbar stenosis secondary to spondylosis involves the lower lumbar spine more commonly than the more rostral lumbar levels.[62,124] Among patients with cervical or lumbar stenosis, 5% have been reported to have symptoms secondary to stenosis at both levels.[137] This clinical constellation has been termed tandem lumbar and cervical stenosis.[3,138]

Pathogenesis of Intermittent Neurogenic Claudication

The pathogenesis of neurogenic claudication has been debated as being secondary to either ischemia or mechanical compression.[118] In some cases, arteriosclerotic vascular disease or vascular malformations have been found to be the cause.[115,119,139] More commonly, however, neurogenic claudication is secondary to compression of the spinal cord or cauda equina due to spinal stenosis.

Blau and Logue[140] have suggested that the increase in metabolic demand of neural tissue that occurs with exercise can-

not be met by an increase in blood flow due to compression of blood vessels. Others[115,118] have shown that in many patients with claudication involving cauda equina dysfunction, symptoms correlate with posture and do not require exercise. In such patients, the lumbar lordosis alone is sufficient to provoke symptoms that are alleviated by flexing the lumbar spine. These findings suggest that mechanical compression of the cauda equina is more important than ischemic factors in the pathogenesis of clinical manifestations. A clinical study of lumbar stenosis[117] also suggests that mechanical factors are more important than primary vascular causes in the pathogenesis of the disorder.

Madsen and Heros[119] postulated a pathogenesis of neurogenic claudication that may reconcile the vascular and mechanical-compressive hypotheses. These investigators have considered the potential role of venous hypertension in the development of neurogenic claudication (Fig. 4–16). Although arteriovenous malformations that may cause a rise in venous pressure were present in their two cases, they suggest that degenerative changes, such as osteophytes, annular bulging, and hypertrophy of ligaments may compress both neural elements and the draining

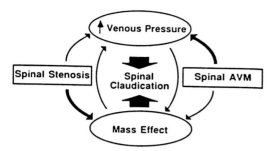

Figure 4–16. Proposed pathophysiological mechanism for the development of neurogenic claudication in patients with either spinal stenosis or a spinal arteriovenous malformation (AVM). Either lesion alone may contribute to mass effect or increase venous pressure, and these in turn complicate one another, leading to neurogenic claudication. When spinal stenosis and spinal AVM coexist, they may further exacerbate one another. (From Madsen, JR and Heros, RC,[119] with permission.) (From Lees, F and Turner, JWA,[78] with permission.)

veins that exit the canal with the spinal roots. Lordotic postures, such as those assumed with ambulation, further narrow the spinal canal and intervertebral foramina. They therefore further compress both nerves and veins. The resulting increased venous pressure could cause ischemia of the spinal cord or cauda equina and result in neurogenic claudication. According to this hypothesis, a positive feedback loop would be created in which increases in venous pressure cause a greater compressive effect on neural elements. This, in turn, further increases venous pressure. Progressive neurogenic claudication is the outcome. It is relieved only by maneuvers that interrupt this cycle. Although their hypothesis arose from observations related to spinal arteriovenous malformations and spinal stenosis, spinal stenosis alone can potentially cause neurogenic claudication through a similar mechanism.

Intermittent Neurogenic Claudication of Spinal Cord Origin

Neurogenic claudication shares many features with, and must be distinguished from claudication due to peripheral vascular disease.

CLINICAL FEATURES

Originally described by Dejerine,[141] claudication due to spinal cord dysfunction is characterized by progressive weakness of the lower extremities that occurs during walking. It is relieved by rest. The weakness may initially be unilateral, but it usually progresses to become bilateral. Sensory complaints may consist of paresthesias or dysesthesias. Unlike claudication due to cauda equina dysfunction, spinal cord claudication rarely causes severe pain, although cramps may occur.[115] With progression of the clinical syndrome, the amount of walking required to cause symptoms decreases.

The clinical hallmark of neurogenic claudication of spinal cord origin is the change in the neurologic examination following exercise. After a period of rest, the patient's neurologic examination may be entirely normal, but after a period of exercise, there may be spasticity and hyperreflexia of the lower extremities, in association with Babinski signs that have been described as "afternoon Babinskis."[115] These abnormal signs often resolve with rest.

As noted above, the lower cervical spine is the most common site of compression. Patients may, therefore, have symptoms and signs of radiculopathy at these levels in addition to intermittent claudication. When the thoracic spine is the site of stenosis, most often the lower thoracic spine is involved.[133,135] These patients may present with symptoms and signs suggestive of either spinal claudication or cauda equina claudication, since both upper and lower motor neurons are located at this level.[71,133,135]

IMAGING

Radiographic studies of patients with spinal cord claudication often show signs of spinal stenosis. In cases of developmental stenosis, the spine imaging studies may reveal uniform stenosis. In patients with acquired stenosis, abnormalities suggestive of the diseases shown in Table 4–2 may be seen. The anteroposterior diameter of the stenotic cervical spinal canal is usually equal to or less than 10 mm.[137,138,142] CT-myelography typically shows evidence of a partial or complete block of contrast material at several levels. (Figs. 4–13 and 4–14) Compression of the spinal cord is usually observed on these imaging studies and MRI.[137,138]

Intermittent Neurogenic Claudication Due to Cauda Equina Compression

As with neurogenic claudication due to spinal cord disease, neurogenic claudication from cauda equina compression may mimic claudication due to peripheral vascular disease.

CLINICAL FEATURES

The clinical syndrome of intermittent neurogenic claudication due to cauda equina dysfunction is typically characterized by back and leg pain, weakness, and numbness precipitated by walking (or standing) and alleviated by rest.[118,120] Because it shares many of the features of claudication due to vascular insufficiency of the lower extremities, it has been termed pseudoclaudication or intermittent claudication of neurogenic origin.[118]

Claudication due to cauda equina dysfunction may be secondary to vascular malformations[119] and other vascular diseases of the cauda equina. However, it is most commonly secondary to lumbar spinal stenosis,[115,118] which may be developmental (congenital) in origin,[125,131,143] due to acquired disease such as spondylosis,[117,124,140] or due to acquired stenosis superimposed on a developmentally narrow canal.[144]

Originally described by Van Gelderen in 1948,[145] the clinical syndrome and pathophysiology of intermittent claudication secondary to lumbar stenosis have been studied extensively by Verbiest[143,144,146] and others.[140,147–149] The principal clinical features are listed in Table 4–3.

Pseudoclaudication, considered to be any discomfort in the buttock(s), thigh(s), or leg(s) that develops with walking or standing and is relieved by rest, is the most common symptom. The discomfort is often described as pain, numbness, or weakness. A combination of these complaints is frequent (Table 4–3). Sensory symptoms may ascend from the distal lower extremities to the buttocks or, alternatively, descend to the lower extremities. Such a "sensory march" is considered common in cauda equina claudication but unusual for claudication due to peripheral vascular disease.[118,149] Low back pain is a frequent complaint, and is present in 65% of the patients in the Mayo Clinic series depicted in Table 4–3. Although the symptoms are generally bilateral, they may not be symmetrical. The entire limb or only part may be affected. Radicular pain alone is unusual, in contrast to the pain of a herniated disc.

Intermittent dysfunction of autonomic fibers has also been found. For example, Ram and colleagues[150] reported on a 70-year-old man who developed priapism and urinary incontinence along with sen-

Table 4–3. Symptoms and Signs of Lumbar Spinal Stenosis in 68 Patients*

Symptom or Sign	Prevalence (%)
Pseudoclaudication	94
Standing Discomfort	94
Description of Discomfort	
Pain	93
Numbness	63
Weakness	43
Bilateral Symptoms	69
Site	
Whole limb	78
Above knee alone	15
Below knee alone	7
Radicular Pain Only	6
Ankle Reflex Decreased or Absent	43
Knee Reflex Decreased or Absent	18
Objective Weakness	37
Positive Straight-Leg-Raising Sign	10

*From Hall, SH, et al,[117] p. 272, with permission.

sory disturbances and leg weakness while walking. Following decompressive lumbar surgery, the patient's exercise tolerance returned to normal, as did his erectile and urinary symptoms.

Symptoms of neurogenic claudication due to cauda equina dysfunction are typically relieved by lying with the legs flexed, sitting, flexing the waist, or squatting. Thus patients may not become symptomatic if they lean forward to push a cart, climb a hill, or ride a bicycle. However, descending a hill may exacerbate symptoms because this activity usually increases lumbar lordosis. Such a response to change in posture is atypical for claudication due to peripheral vascular disease.[118]

Although abnormal neurologic signs may be present in patients with neurogenic claudication (Table 4–3), the neurologic examination may be entirely normal, particularly after a period of rest. A paucity of neurologic findings, despite a history of severe disability, is typical of spinal stenosis.[118] Characteristic of lumbar stenosis, however, is the development of neurologic signs when the patient is symptomatic after a period of walking.[118] In such cases, deep tendon reflexes may be lost and weakness and sensory loss may develop. The straight-leg-raising test is rarely positive.

Recently, a series of seven patients with thoracic spinal stenosis was reported with symptoms of pseudoclaudication resembling the syndrome of lumbar stenosis. Pain radiating down the legs, however, was not present.[135] The stenosis was in the low thoracic spine and was caused by thickening of the laminar arch and facet joints. The authors noted that a compressive lesion between T10 and T12 caused a mixture of upper and lower motor neuron symptoms and signs in the lower extremities. It should be recalled, however, that thoracic spinal stenosis may also present with intermittent neurogenic claudication in which the spinal cord, not the cauda equina, is the primary site of involvement (see above).

In summary, in differentiating claudication due to cauda equina dysfunction from claudication secondary to peripheral vascular disease, the following features may

be considered that are more suggestive of cauda-equina-related claudication:[118]

1. Worsening neurologic symptoms and signs following ambulation or accompanying an increase of the lordotic posture of the lumbar spine
2. A "march" of symptoms through the lower extremities
3. Relief of symptoms with a change in posture alone while exercise continues (e.g., flexion of the lumbar spine while walking)
4. Symptoms not relieved after a few minutes of rest[118]

LABORATORY AND IMAGING STUDIES

Laboratory findings, including neurophysiologic and imaging investigations, can be very helpful with the diagnosis of lumbar spinal stenosis.[151] In the Mayo Clinic study cited above, the electromyogram (EMG) was abnormal in 34 of the 37 patients in whom it was performed. This test was considered to be more sensitive than the neurologic examination.[117] The EMG abnormalities consisted of denervation in muscles innervated by lumbosacral nerve roots. The findings from the Mayo Clinic study are often bilateral and are located in the paraspinal areas.[117] The CSF usually shows a normal cell count, but the protein concentration is often elevated.[118]

Although plain radiographs of the lumbar spine may be normal, they usually show evidence of degenerative disc disease, osteoarthritis of the facet joints, or other abnormalities.[117] Lumbar spinal stenosis most frequently involves the lower lumbar spine, especially the L4–5 level.[124,127] The laminae may be hypertrophied. Although controversial (see below), a midsagittal diameter of the lumbar canal less than 15 mm radiographically identifies patients who are at risk for the development of symptoms, whereas those with a diameter greater than 20 mm have much lower risk.[152] Other abnormalities often associated with lumbar spinal stenosis include Paget's disease, synovial cysts, spondylolisthesis, acromegaly, ankylosing spondylitis, trauma, and congenital/developmental abnormalities (Fig. 4–17).[117,118,127,153] Myelog-

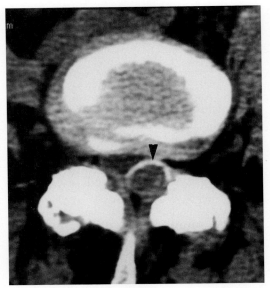

Figure 4–17. A CT scan showing a synovial cyst (arrowhead) arising from a degenerated facet joint which caused symptoms of spinal stenosis. (Courtesy of Dr. Richard Becker.)

raphy has been considered valuable in confirming the diagnosis of lumbar stenosis. It may show compression of the dural sac during extension, which improves with flexion (Fig. 4–18). These anatomical findings correlate with the clinical presentation.

A CT may demonstrate the short, thickened pedicles and decreased interpedicular distance often observed in patients with developmental lumbar stenosis. An anteroposterior diameter of less than 10 mm has been considered evidence of spinal stenosis, according to one study.[143] Alternatively, in degenerative cases, the anteroposterior dimensions have been found to be abnormal in only a minority of patients. In one study,[154] only 20% of patients had an anteroposterior posterior diameter less than 13 mm. For this reason, in cases of degenerative lumbar stenosis, some investigators have suggested that the cross-sectional area of the thecal sac

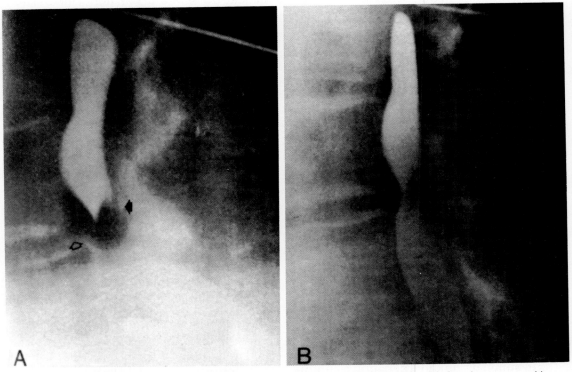

Figure 4–18. Myelograms showing lumbar spinal stenosis. (A) During extension, the dural sac is compressed by ligamentum flavum with obstruction (solid arrow). Note the spondylolisthesis of L4 on L5 (open arrow) with an intact neural arch. (B) With mild flexion, the stenosis at L4 due to a bulging annulus anteriorly and thickened ligamentum flavum posteriorly is decreased. (From Hall, SH, et al,[117] with permission.)

should be considered a more accurate indicator of spinal stenosis. A normal cross-sectional area of the lumbar thecal sac has been reported to be 180 mm^2 ± 50 mm^2; an area of less than 100 mm^2 was considered evidence of stenosis. Other authors[62] have suggested that the dimensions of the spinal canal are not necessary to make a CT diagnosis. Rather, the characteristic CT features, including segmental stenosis at disc and facet levels, hypertrophy of the ligamentum flavum and articular processes, bulging of an annulus fibrosus, and obliteration of epidural fat, may be sufficient to confirm the presence of lumbar spinal stenosis.[62] An MRI has been reported to be valuable in assessing spinal stenosis, although osteophytes and facet hypertrophy generally may be better visualized with CT.[71] In patients with combined spinal stenosis secondary to developmental disturbances and superimposed degenerative disease, the CT and MRI findings demonstrate features of both conditions. Compared to CT, MRI has the advantage of being multiplanar and the conus and intraspinal tumors can be more readily seen.

Management

The only truly effective management of neurogenic claudication of both spinal cord and cauda equina origin is surgical decompression. For patients with neurogenic claudication due to lumbar stenosis, the results of surgery can be gratifying. For example, in one study, the mean distance of ambulation at which claudication developed increased from 180 m preoperatively to 2.4 km postoperatively.[117] After a period of follow-up (mean 4 years), 62% of patients reported that laminectomy (often multilevel) gave good to excellent results. Nonoperative management strategies are often essentially ineffective.

Controversy in surgical circles surrounds the most appropriate surgical option for lumbar stenosis.[155–158] Decompressive surgery in and of itself is almost certainly destabilizing. Therefore, some surgeons suggest the use of a fusion procedure, with or without instrumentation, in conjunction with laminectomy for the management of this problem. However, most surgeons recommend laminectomy alone, unless a preexisting tendency toward instability is present—e.g., excessive mobility or spondylolisthesis. This discussion is amplified below.

PREEXISTING SPINAL DEFORMITY

The presence of a preexisting translational deformity is somewhat controversial as an indicator for fusion (with or without instrumentation) to supplement a dorsal decompressive procedure. It should, however, be kept in mind that degenerative lumbar spondylolisthesis rarely progresses beyond a 30% vertebral body translational deformation.[159] Therefore, the virtue of *routine* fusion and instrumentation following spinal canal decompression, as is commonly advocated,[160–162] must be questioned. This is particularly so if a careful decompression is performed in which care is taken to adequately decompress the lateral recesses and neuroforaminae, while minimally disrupting facet joint integrity.[5,163–169]

The combination of a vertically oriented facet joint[170,171] and an exaggerated lordotic posture predisposes the spine to translation deformation. In contrast to more rostral spine levels, the relative vertical orientation of the disc interspace causes an applied axial load to result in the application of a shear-deforming force to the spine and the disc interspace. In addition, vertically (sagittally) oriented facet joints are in a biomechanically disadvantageous position to inhibit this translational deformation. It is these patients who may benefit from fusion and instrumentation if laminectomy is performed, particularly if further facet joint disruption is surgically created.[164]

THE PREDICTION OF POSTOPERATIVE INSTABILITY

Patients with lumbar spondylosis and lumbar stenosis commonly complain of both neurologic (neurogenic claudication, radicular, or myelopathic) complaints and axial back pain. The latter is often of a *mechanical nature*, although neural (dural) compression may, indeed, cause a similar pain syndrome. Most patients who undergo dorsal decompressive surgery for lumbar stenosis have predominantly neurologic complaints. Mechanical back pain may suggest a fusion procedure to some surgeons. Furthermore, most patients undergoing surgery for lumbar stenosis are older than 50 years and are beginning, or are well into, the spine restabilization process. The latter involves the narrowing of the disc interspace, the formation of spurs, and the calcification of spinal ligaments, and results in a stiffening of the spine. *The fact that most patients undergoing surgery for lumbar stenosis for neurologic reasons already have a stable spine, and are simultaneously at high risk for complication after complicated and extensive operations, makes a simple laminectomy the most appealing operative procedure for the vast majority of these patients.* In most circumstances, the management of the back pain component of the pain syndrome is best accomplished with nonoperative measures.[164,172] Matsunaga et al. described four radiographic risk factors that predispose a patient with degenerative spondylolisthesis to subluxation after laminectomy. Postoperative (postlaminectomy) instability is uncommon if the patient does not harbor these risk factors. These risk factors are (*1*) loss of disc interspace height; (*2*) spur formation; (*3*) end plate sclerosis; and (*4*) spinal ligament calcification.[173] In addition to Matsunaga's risk factors, advancing age provides the advantage of accelerating the spine restabilization process. Additional risk factors include preexisting appendicular joint laxity and sagittally oriented facet joint angle.[164]

According to a Mayo Clinic series, the most common causes of postoperative (postlaminectomy) failure for the management of lumbar stenosis were the absence of a preoperative complaint of neurogenic claudication coupled with the absence of severe stenosis on preoperative imaging studies.[174] In addition, the most common technical error was an inadequate decompression. In other words, the most common causes for failure of laminectomy are (*1*) absence of surgically treatable pathology and (*2*) performance of an inadequate

operation. In the Mayo Clinic series, only three patients had nonobvious causes of their failure to respond to surgery pain. Only this small fraction of patients could have even been remotely considered as candidates for fusion at the time of their initial operation. Predicting the identity of this group of patients accurately would be nearly impossible.[164]

INTERVERTEBRAL DISC HERNIATION

Intervertebral disc herniation refers to a condition in which a portion of an intervertebral disc herniates beyond the confines of the surrounding annulus fibrosus.[2,71] Although herniation into the adjacent vertebral body is very common (Schmorl's node), it has no clinical significance. On the other hand, herniation of disc material dorsally into the spinal canal or intervertebral foramen may cause spinal cord or nerve root compression.

Using CT criteria, degenerative disc disease has been classified as (*1*) annular bulge, (*2*) herniation, or (*3*) sequestration or free fragment.[71] Bulging of the annulus is frequently observed in association with spondylosis. In this condition, the nucleus pulposus does not extend beyond the confines of the intact annulus fibrosus. Such a bulging disc usually suggests no focal nerve root compression.[71] A herniated disc refers to a focal extension of the nucleus pulposus beyond the outer margin of the annulus fibrosus. When herniation occurs into the spinal canal or intervertebral foramen, neural compression may ensue. A sequestered disc or free fragment refers to a herniated nucleus pulposus that has lost continuity with the original nucleus pulposus. When the free fragment is within the spinal canal, it may migrate rostrally or caudally under the posterior longitudinal ligament, lateral to the posterior longitudinal ligament, or rupture through the posterior longitudinal ligament. In the present context, the term herniated disc includes all forms of symptomatic extension of the nucleus pulposus beyond its normal boundaries.

In 1934, Mixter and Barr[22] surgically removed herniated cervical and lumbar disc material from a series of patients, establishing the relationship between disc herniation and neural compression. Kristoff and Odom[175] found a much higher frequency of nerve root compression than spinal cord compression and suggested that cervical disc protrusion should be divided into three stages: (*1*) nerve root compression, (*2*) unilateral spinal cord compression, and (*3*) bilateral spinal cord compression. It is now recognized that spinal cord compression due to herniated intervertebral discs may occur without radicular symptoms or signs.[116] Although intervertebral disc protrusion may coexist with spondylosis, whenever possible, disc protrusion without spondylosis should be distinguished from that with spondylosis, since the etiologies, pathogeneses, and results of diagnostic studies usually differ.

Pathology

Herniation of an intervertebral disc is defined in pathological terms as an extension of the fluid nucleus pulposus through a tear in the annulus fibrosus.[2] This protrusion usually occurs through the dorsal region of the annulus fibrosus, which is thinnest.

Although the herniated nucleus pulposus may return to its normal position, it usually remains extruded, and often becomes calcified. However, there is no osteophyte formation unless secondary spondylosis develops.[40,176] In some cases, the annulus fibrosus does not tear but rather bulges into the spinal canal or adjacent intervertebral foramina.[2] Such cases may be difficult to differentiate from those that occur in patients with spondylosis.

Clinical Features

Although severe trauma may cause symptomatic protrusion of an intervertebral disc, more commonly, minor repeated trauma from activities of daily living is found in the clinical history.[177] Occasion-

ally cervical discs and rarely thoracic discs may protrude to compress the spinal cord to cause myelopathy. In the lumbar region, intervertebral discs occasionally herniate dorsally to cause cauda equina dysfunction. This section outlines the clinical features of herniated intervertebral discs in each region.

CERVICAL DISC HERNIATION

Although herniation of cervical intervertebral discs typically causes symptoms and signs of radiculopathy, it may occasionally cause a painless myelopathy that mimics a degenerative disease of the spinal cord.[116] In such cases, the disc is often centrally herniated and does not cause a radiculopathy. The most common levels for herniated discs in the cervical spine are at the C5–6 and C6–7 levels.[116,177,178]

Cervical disc herniation occurs much more commonly in men than in women.[178] Most patients are middle-aged. In a series of 100 patients, their age at the time of operation ranged from 30 to 65 years, with a median of 46.[178] Symptoms and signs of myelopathy, including motor, sensory, and sphincter disturbances, are similar to other extrinsic lesions compressing the spinal cord. However, as in cases of cervical spondylosis, patients with herniated cervical discs may demonstrate evidence of both radicular and myelopathic signs in the arms and myelopathic signs in the lower extremities.

The diagnosis of a herniated cervical disc causing myelopathy is confirmed by CT and/or MRI. Because the cervical spine lacks the large amount of epidural fat observed in the lumbar spine, cervical CT has some limitations.[179] For CT evaluation of cervical disc disease and spondylosis, some investigators advocate the use of intravenous or intrathecal contrast material (Fig. 4–19), while others prefer conventional CT scans.[58,61,62] A CT scan with intrathecal contrast material is often able to differentiate a soft herniated disc from spondylosis.[62] In the presence of myelopathy, MRI or CT-myelography has been recommended over CT because they have the advantage of being able to examine large areas of the spinal axis.[62]

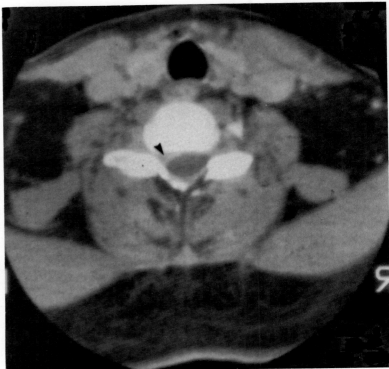

Figure 4–19. Cervical spine CT scan following intravenous contrast enhancement demonstrating intervertebral disc herniation on the left. Note the enhancing epidural venous plexus on the left (arrowhead) displaced posteriorly by the disc herniation. (Courtesy of Dr. Helmuth Gahbauer.)

In cases of cervical radiculopathy, T_2 and gadolinium enhanced MRI has been compared to CT-myelography recently.[180] Among 20 patients with cervical radiculopathy, gadolinium-enhanced 2D T_1 images did not confer any benefit over three-dimensional (3D) T_2 images. The 3D T_2 white cerebrospinal fluid images had an accuracy of close to 90% for the diagnosis of foraminal encroachment. The authors concluded that when the findings are incompatible with the clinical symptomatology, CT-myelography is still indicated (Fig. 4–20).

THORACIC DISC HERNIATION

Herniation of thoracic discs is an unusual clinical problem and thus may not be readily recognized. Surgery for thoracic disc herniations represents only three to five cases per 1000 disc operations.[181] In a surgical series at the Mayo Clinic,[182] 69% of cases of thoracic disc herniation were located at the last four interspaces, with the T11 space most commonly involved. Other studies have shown a similar predilection for the lower thoracic spine.[183] Herniation

is more likely to occur in the midline than laterally. Therefore, the spinal cord is jeopardized, especially given the narrow diameter of the spinal canal in this region.[181]

Thoracic disc herniations most commonly occur at ages 30 to 55; both sexes appear to be affected equally. Pain in the back or radicular pain or both are the most common presenting manifestations. Occasionally, spinal cord symptoms and signs without pain herald the onset of thoracic disc herniation.[182,184] In one review,[181] pain or dysesthesias were the presenting complaint in 80% of cases and paresis in 15%. Sphincter disturbances were observed in 22 of the 61 cases reported from the Mayo Clinic.[182] This high frequency of sphincter disturbance may be due to the proximity in many cases to the conus medullaris. Thoracic discs also may cause compression of the artery of Adamkiewicz, causing ischemia of the caudal spinal cord.[185]

Conventional radiographs of the thoracic spine are frequently normal, but calcification within the spinal canal at the level of intervertebral disc space narrow-

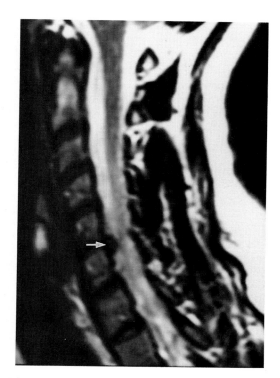

Figure 4–20. An MRI of the cervical spine revealing a C5–6 disc herniation (arrow) of the right side. The patient complained of right arm numbness in the radial aspect of the arm and had a depressed brachioradialis reflex. (Courtesy of Dr. Richard Becker.)

ing may be observed in approximately 55% of cases.[186] A CT may be very helpful in demonstrating herniation of a calcified thoracic disc.[187–189] However, the relative paucity of epidural fat in the thoracic spine and the difficulty in defining the segmental level of involvement limit the value of CT in the diagnosis of this disorder.[62] Lee and associates[71] recommend MRI as the initial diagnostic imaging procedure of choice for thoracic disc pathology. However, it should be emphasized that asymptomatic thoracic disc herniations commonly occur in the thoracic spine. Wood et al.[190] reported the thoracic spine MRI findings of 90 asymptomatic individuals. Among these, herniated thoracic discs were found in 37%, bulging of a disc in 53%, annular tear in 58%, deformation of the spinal cord in 29%, and Scheuerman end plate irregularities or kyphosis in 38% (see below).

LUMBAR DISC HERNIATION

Herniation of a lumbar disc usually causes low back pain and symptoms and signs of radiculopathy. Much less frequently, such herniation may result in a cauda equina syndrome. In this situation, paralysis of both legs and sphincters and sensory loss may develop acutely or subacutely. The sensory level and the distribution of weakness are usually determined by the level of disc herniation.

Lumbar disc disease more commonly affects males than females,[191] and most frequently affects young and middle-aged adults. According to Gathier,[192] 70% of individuals are between 20 and 40 years of age. Some authors, however, have found a greater frequency in those 40 to 49. Most emphasize the rarity of the disorder among individuals less than 20 years of age (Table 4–4).[192]

The most frequent levels of involvement are L4–5 and L5–S1. Although there are differences among various series, these two levels appear to account for 90%–98% of surgically treated lumbar disc herniations.[192] Furthermore, according to surgical series, the L4–5 and L5–S1 levels are approximately equally involved.[191,193] The levels of involvement, as found on CT scanning, are shown in Table 4–5.[62] The clinical manifestations of pain, sensory complaints, reflex changes, and weakness generally follow the patterns predicted by the segmental level involved. Nonradicular referred pain, such as myofascial pain syndromes and the facet syndrome, must also be considered.[194] In general, sensory, motor, and reflex dysfunction are rarely

Table 4–4. **Frequency of Age (Years) at Operation for Lumbar Disc Disease**[*]

<20	1%
20–29	16%
30–39	39%
40–49	31%
50–59	11%
>60	3%

[*]From Harkelius, A and Hindmarch, J,[191] p. 234, with permission.

Table 4–5. **Frequency of Lumbar Disc Herniation by Disc Level as Demonstrated on CT**[*]

L5–S1	35%–40%
L4–5	50%–60%
L3–4	5%–10%
L1–2, L2–3	<1%

[*]From Kricun, R and Kricun, ME,[62] p. 391, with permission.

prominent in such cases, and radicular pain is more sharp and localized than nonradicular referred pain.[194] Furthermore, signs of nerve root compression on physical examination (such as a positive straight-leg-raising test) are much more prominent in radicular pain syndromes.

Imaging modalities for evaluating lumbar disc disease are rapidly evolving. Many abnormalities in patients with back pain are similarly found among those without symptoms and thus do not necessarily confirm the diagnosis of symptomatic lumbar disc disease.[195] Studies using myelography[196,197] and CT[198] and MRI[199] have shown a high incidence of protruding or herniated discs among the asymptomatic population. Nevertheless, imaging of lumbar disc disease has been exceptionally helpful (Fig. 4–21). CT has been sensitive in diagnosing the axial location of lumbar disc herniations, which have been found to occur with the following frequency: dorsolaterally, 60%–85%; centrally, 5%–35%; and laterally, 5%.[62] CT has been reported to be more accurate than myelography in detecting: (1) a herniated disc at the L5–S1 level and (2) lateral disc herniation.[62,200,201] CT also may be valuable in recognizing a herniated nucleus pulposus that extends through the posterior longitudinal ligament[202] and the rarely found condition in which it has traversed the dura mater.[203,204] It may be useful in differentiating between a soft disc herniation and a hard disc, which may be a calcified herniated disc or an osteophyte secondary to spondylosis. The use of intravenous contrast enhancement with CT also helps to distinguish recurrent disc herniation from postoperative scar formation.[205]

An MRI in the evaluation of lumbar disc disease has been exceptionally sensitive in identifying herniated lumbar discs (Fig. 4–22A and B).[206,207] An MRI may reveal both disc bulges and disc herniations, often in asymptomatic patients or at levels that are asymptomatic.[199] Thus the challenge with MRI is often to confirm clinically that the disc pathology seen is responsible for the symptoms and signs. For example, Jensen and colleagues found that among 98 asymptomatic subjects undergoing lumbar spine MRI, only 36% had normal discs at all levels. Fifty-two percent had a bulge at at least one level, 27% had a disc protrusion, and 1% had a disc extrusion. Schmorl's nodes (disc herniations into the vertebral bodies) were seen in 19% of subjects. The findings were similar for both men and women, and the frequency of abnormalities increased with age.

Management

The treatment of herniated discs, also discussed in Chapter 3, is controversial. As in spondylosis, most patients will respond to bed rest, antiinflammatory agents, and muscle relaxants. In the case of cervical disc disease, in addition to these measures, a cervical collar and traction are often helpful. Following the acute phase of pain, a course of physical therapy and an exercise program are often useful in preventing recurrence.[208] If during recuperation or later the patient experiences pain (especially radicular pain) reminiscent of that associated with the herniated disc, he or she should be advised that this is a warning and that activities should be modified to reduce the risk of further injury.[209] Lumbar disc herniation has been shown by MR imaging to improve in symptomatic patients not undergoing surgical intervention.[210] Bozzao and colleagues[210] performed follow-up MR scans in 69 symptomatic patients with herniated lumbar discs on MRI. On follow-up imaging (average 11 months post initial imaging) 63% of the patients showed a reduction in disc herniation of more than 30% (48% had a reduction of more than 70%). Fur-

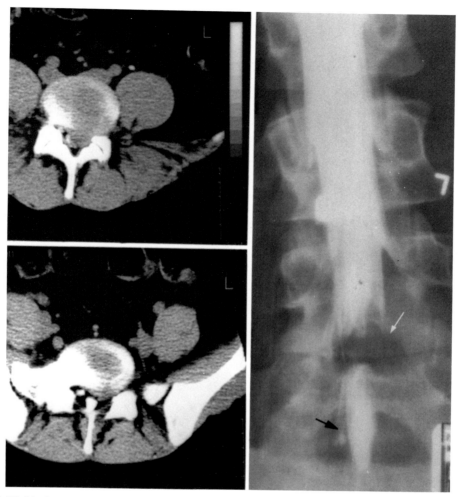

Figure 4–21. Myelogram (right) and postmyelogram CT scan (left) of lumbar spine demonstrating disc hernia-tions at L4–5 and L5–S1. At L4–5, there is a large disc herniation effacing the intrathecal contrast material seen on the myelogram (white arrow) and CT scan (upper left panel). On the myelogram, the normal right S1 nerve root is shown (black arrow); alternatively, the left S1 nerve root sleeve is compressed by the L5–S1 disc and therefore is not visualized on the myelogram and CT scan (lower left panel). (Courtesy of Dr. Helmuth Gah-bauer.)

thermore, the largest disc herniations were found to decrease in size the most. There was a good clinical outcome in 71% of patients. These authors concluded that in many cases lumbar disc herniation can be managed successfully without surgical intervention and that follow-up MR imaging reveals reduction in the size of disc herniation without surgical intervention.

Occasionally, patients with a herniated disc require surgical intervention. When a sufficient trial of conservative manage-ment fails to relieve incapacitating pain, surgery is often beneficial. Alternatively, urgent surgical consultation is recom-mended in the following: (*1*) acute cervical or thoracic disc herniation that causes sig-nificant myelopathy, (*2*) lumbar disc herni-ation causing cauda equina dysfunction (such as impaired bowel or bladder control due to cauda equina compression), and (*3*) major neurological deficit (for example, foot drop) that is severe or progresses, de-spite conservative management.[209]

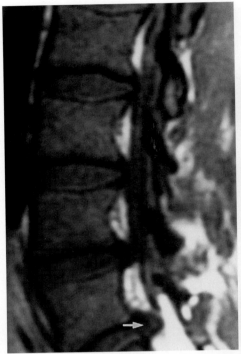
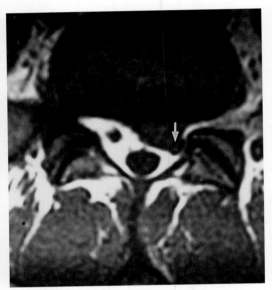

Figure 4–22. An MRI of the lumbar spine shows an L5–S1 disc herniation with S1 root compression (arrow) in a patient with sciatica. (A) Sagittal view. (B) Axial view. (Courtesy of Dr. Richard Becker.)

SCHEUERMANN'S DISEASE

In the developing spine, the intradiscal oncotic pressure is normally relatively high. This can result in focal sites of penetration of the end plate (Schmorl's nodes) with a resulting destruction of the growth plate. The preexisting thoracic kyphosis, which is associated with asymetrically high ventral intradiscal pressures, may lead to the exaggeration of focal end plate penetration in this circumstance. This phenomenon is known as Scheuermann's disease (osteochondrosis). It is associated with a disproportional loss of ventral vertebral body height, Schmorl's nodes (predominantly ventrally located), irregularities of the vertebral endplates, and narrowing of the disc interspaces (predominantly ventrally).[211] As stated by Kramer, *the developmental disorder of Scheuermann's disease involves secondary changes. These are caused by increased pressure of the developing disc tissue on the ventral parts of the intervertebral segments in the kyphotic area of the spine.*[5] Because of the increased focal pressures exerted, degeneration of the disc is accelerated. Fibrous and, ultimately, bony fusion occurs.[5] This results in a fused, kyphotic spine.

OSTEOPOROSIS

Osteoporosis, the most common metabolic bone disorder to involve the spine, is a condition in which bone density is less than optimal.[127] It may be associated with a variety of metabolic diseases but is most commonly found in the elderly, especially postmenopausal women. As osteoporosis progresses, vertebral collapse may occur, causing back and/or flank pain.

Although vertebral collapse due to osteoporosis is a common cause of complaint in the elderly, spinal cord compression appears to be a rarely reported complication. A report[212] of two cases of spinal cord compression due to osteoporosis (confirmed at necropsy) noted the clinical and radiographic findings. In both cases, back pain, leg weakness, sensory loss, and sphincter disturbance evolved over several days. Myelography demonstrated a complete block due to an extradural mass at the level of a collapsed vertebral body that was considered secondary to metastatic disease on the basis of the radiographic findings. In both cases, however, necropsy revealed only an osteoporotic compression fracture, with secondary spinal cord compression. This report emphasized the rarity of this complication, as well as the need to consider osteoporosis in the differential diagnosis of spinal cord compression.

SUMMARY

Degenerative disease of the spine including osteoarthritis, spondylosis, and disc disease occurs in essentially all individuals by late middle age. Accordingly, it is the most common disorder of the spine and is one of the most common reasons for patients to see physicians.

This chapter first reviewed the pathogenesis of disc degeneration and the spondylotic process. Subsequently, the clinical presentation of disc degeneration and spondylosis were discussed. The most common initial clinical presentation of degenerative disease of the spine is pain and limitation of motion. However, because the pathologic hallmark of spondylosis is the development of osteophytes, compression of nerve roots or the spinal cord may cause neurologic dysfunction. This is the most serious complication and, when present, usually dominates the clinical picture.

The current ready availability of imaging with CT and MRI has expedited the evaluation of these patients but also brings to clinical attention a large number of patients with asymptomatic disease such as herniated discs. Thus, in some instances, rather than assisting the clinician in managing the patient, modern imaging modalities may create the quandary of radiographic diagnoses which have no clinical symptomatology. It is imperative, therefore, to develop the clinical skills needed in order to make clinical–radiologic correlations in order to manage patients appropriately. This chapter has endeavored to show the common neurologic presentations associated with spondylosis and degenerative disc disease.

Cervical spondylotic myelopathy is a common condition arising from spinal cord compression due to osteophytes in the cervical spine encroaching on the spinal canal and spinal cord. The clinical presenation and management of cervical spondylotic myelopathy are reviewed. Neurogenic claudication which arises from spinal stenosis due to spondylosis may be difficult to clinically distinguish from claudication secondary to peripheral vascular disease. Neurogenic claudication may occur due to compression of the cauda equina or, less commonly, the spinal cord. The clinical manifestations and management options of neurogenic claudication are also presented. Finally, intervertebral disc herniations which may be present and asymptomatic in about one-quarter of individuals over the age of 40 may also cause serious neurologic injury. The clinical and radiologic evaluation and management of these patients have been discussed.

Since back and neck pain are such common ailments, patients present to physicians in a variety of specialties. Often physicians are seeking an algorithm or rational approach to these problems. This chapter has attempted to provide such an approach to the management of these endemic disorders.

REFERENCES

1. Lestini WF, Wiesel SW. The pathogenesis of cervical spondylosis. *Clin Orthop* 1989;239:69–93.
2. Hughes JT. *Pathology of the Spinal Cord* Philadelphia: W.B. Saunders; 1978.
3. Adams RD, Victor M. Diseases of the spinal cord. In Adams RD, Victor M, editors. *Principles of Neurology.* New York: McGraw-Hill; 1985; pp. 665–98.
4. Weinstein PR, Ehni G, Wilson CB. Lumbar spondylosis. Diagnosis, management and surgical treatment. Chicago: Year Book Medical; 1977.
5. Benzel EC. *Biomechanics of Spine Stabilization: Principles and Clinical Practice.* New York: McGraw-Hill; 1994.
6. Resnick D, Niwayama G. Intravertebral disc herniations: cartilaginous (Schmorl's) nodes. *Radiology* 1978;126:57–65.

7. Baker WC, Thomas TG, Kirkaldy-Willis WH. Changes in the cartilage of the posterior intervertebral joints after anterior fusion. *J Bone Joint Surg* 1969;51B:736–46.

8. Adams MA, Hutton WC. Prolapsed intervertebral disc. A hyperflexion injury. *Spine* 1982;8:184–91.

9. Kramer J. Intervertebral Disc Disease. Causes, Diagnosis, Treatment, and Prophylaxis, 2nd Edition. New York: George Thieme Verlag Stuttgart; 1990.

10. White AA, Panabi MM (eds.). *Clinical Biomechanics of the Spine*, 2nd Edition. Philadelphia: J.B. Lippincott; 1990.

11. Ball PA, Saunders RL. The subjective myelopathy. In Cervical Spondylotic Myelopathy. Saunders RL, Bernini PM, editors. Boston: Blackwell Scientific; 1992; pp. 48–55.

12. Carol MP, Ducker TB. Cervical spondylitic myelopathies: surgical treatment. *J Spinal Disord* 1988;1:59–65.

13. Crandall PH, Batzdorf U. Cervical spondylotic myelopathy. *J Neurosurg* 1966;25:57–66

14. Batzdorf U, Batzdorff A. Analysis of cervical spine curvature in patients with cervical spondylosis. *Neurosurgery* 1988;22:827–36.

15. Benzel EC. Cervical spondylotic myelopathy: posterior surgical approaches. In Cooper PR, editor. *Degenerative Disease of the Cervical Spine*. Park Ridge, Illinois: AANS; 1993.

16. Mann KS, Khosla VK, Gulati DR. Cervical spondylotic myelopathy treated by single-stage multilevel anterior decompression. *J Neurosurg* 1984;60:80–7.

17. Mayfield FH. Cervical spondylosis: a comparison of the anterior and posterior approaches. *Clin Neurosurg* 1965;13:181–8.

18. Bailey P, Casamajor L. Osteo-arthritis of the spine as a cause of compression of the spinal cord and its roots. *J Nerv Ment Dis* 1911;38:588–609.

19. Stookey B. Compression of the spinal cord due to ventral extradural cervical chondromas. Diagnosis and surgical treatment. *AMA Arch Neurol Psychiat* 1928;20:275–91.

20. Stookey B. Compression of spinal cord and nerve roots by herniation of the nucleus pulposus in the cervical region. *Arch Surg* 1940;40:417–32.

21. Mixter WJ, Ayer JB. Herniation or rupture of the intervertebral disc into the spinal canal. Report of thirty-four cases. *N Engl J Med* 1935;213:385–93.

22. Mixter WJ, Barr JS. Rupture of the intervertebral disc with involvement of the spinal canal. *N Engl J Med* 1934;211:210–5.

23. Peet MM, Echols DH. Herniation of the nucleus pulposus. A cause of compression of the spinal cord. *Arch Neurol Psychiat* 1934;32:924–32.

24. Hastings DE, Macnab I, Lawson V. Neoplasms of the atlas and axis. *Can J Surg* 1968;11:290–6.

25. Gowers WR. *Diseases of the Nervous System. Volume I, Spinal Cord and Nerves, 1st Edition*. London: J. and A. Churchill; 1886.

26. Pallis C, Jones AM, Spillane JD. Cervical spondylosis. *Brain* 1954;77:274–89.

27. Adams C. Cervical spondylotic radiculopathy and myelopathy. In Vinken PJ, Bruyn GW, editors. *Handbook of Clinical Neurology, Volume 26*. Amsterdam: North-Holland; 1976; pp. 97–112.

28. Keyes DC, Compere EL. The normal and pathological physiology of the nucleus pulposus of the intervertebral disc. An anatomical, clinical, and experimental study. *J Bone Joint Surg* 1932;14:897–939.

29. O'Connell JEA. Cervical spondylosis. *Proc R Soc Med* 1956;49:202–8.

30. Bohlman HH, Emery SE. The pathophysiology of cervical spondylosis and myelopathy. *Spine* 1988;13:843–6.

31. Nurick S. The pathogenesis of the spinal cord disorder associated with cervical spondylosis. *Brain* 1972;95:87–100.

32. Ogino H, Tada K, Okada K, et al. Canal diameter, anteroposterior compression ratio, and spondylotic myelopathy of the cervical spine. *Spine* 1983;8:1–15.

33. Payne EE, Spillane JD. Cervical spine. An anatomico-pathological study of 70 specimens using a special technique with particular reference to the problem of cervical spondylosis. *Brain* 1957;80:571–96.

34. Veidlonger OF, Colwill JC, Smyth HS, Turner D. Cervical myelopathy and its relationship to cervical stenosis. *Spine* 1981;6:550–2.

35. Brain WR. Rupture of the intervertebral disc in the cervical region. *Proc R Soc Med* 1948;49:509–11.

36. Mair WGP, Folkerts JF. Necrosis of the spinal cord due to thrombophlebitis (subacute necrotic myelitis). *Brain* 1953;76:563–75.

37. Taylor AR. Vascular factors in the myelopathy associated with cervical spondylosis. *Neurology* 1964;14:62–8.

38. Allen KL. Neuropathies caused by bony spurs in the cervical spine with special reference to surgical treatment. *J Neurol Neurosurg Psychiatry* 1952;15:20–36.

39. Hughes JT, Brownell B. Cervical spondylosis complicated by anterior spinal artery thrombosis. *Neurology* 1964;14:1073–7.

40. Wilkinson M. The morbid anatomy of cervical spondylosis and myelopathy. *Brain* 1960;83:589–617.

41. Wilkinson M. *Cervical Spondylosis. Its Early Diagnosis and Treatment*. London: Heinemann; 1970.

42. Adams CBT, Logue V. Studies in cervical spondylotic myelopathy. I. Movement of the cervical roots, dura and cord and their relation to the course taken by extrathecal roots. *Brain* 1971;94:557–68.

43. Adams CBT, Logue V. Studies in cervical spondylotic myelopathy. II. Observations on the movement and contour of the cervical spine in relation to the neural complications of cervical spondylosis. *Brain* 1971;94:569–86.

44. Adams CBT, Logue V. Studies in cervical spondylotic myelopathy. III. Some functional effects of operations for cervical spondylotic myelopathy. *Brain* 1971;94:587–94.

45. Taylor AR. The mechanism of injury to the spinal cord in the neck without damage to the

vertebral column. *J Bone Joint Surg* 1951;33-B:543–7.

46. Elster AD, Challa VR, Gilbert TH, et al. Meningiomas: MR and histopathological features. *Radiology* 1989;170:857–62.

47. Waltz TA. Physical factors in the production of the myelopathy of cervical spondylosis. *Brain* 1967;90:395–404.

48. Brooker AE, Barter AW. Cervical spondylosis. Clinical study with comparative radiology. *Brain* 1965;88:925–36.

49. Hadley LA. *The Spine: Anatomico-radiographic Studies, Development and the Cervical Region.* Springfield, IL: Charles C. Thomas; 1956.

50. Plum F, Olson ME. Myelitis and myelopathy. In: Baker AB, Baker LH, editors. *Clinical Neurology.* Hagerstown: Harper & Row; 1973; pp. 1–52.

51. Good DC, Couch JR, Wacasar L. "Numb, clumsy hands" and high cervical spondylosis. *Surg Neurol* 1984;22:285–91.

52. Clarke E, Robinson PK. A complication of cervical spondylosis. *Brain* 1956;79:483–507.

53. Banna M. *Clinical Radiology of the Spine and Spinal Cord.* Rockville: Aspen Systems; 1985.

54. Kuhn RA. Functional capacity of the isolated human spinal cord. *Brain* 1950;73:1–51.

55. Brain WR, Wilkinson M. *Cervical Spondylosis and Other Disorders of the Cervical Spine.* London: Heinemann; 1967.

56. Braakman R. Management of cervical spondylotic myelopathy and radiculopathy. *J Neurol Neurosurg Psychiatry* 1994;37:257–63.

57. Fukui K, Kataoka O, Sho T, et al. Pathomechanism, pathogenesis and results of treatment in cerviacl spondylotic myelopathy caused by dynamic canal stenosis. *Spine* 1990;15:1148–52.

58. Badami JP, Norman D, Barbaro NM, et al. Metrizamide CT myelography in cervical myelopathy and radiculopathy: correlation with conventional myelography and surgical findings. *Am J Roentgenol* 1985;144:675–80.

59. Coin CG, Coin JT. Computed tomography of cervical disk disease: technical considerations with representative case reports. *J Comput Assist Tomogr* 1981;5:275–80.

60. Brown B, Schwartz R, Frank E, et al. Preoperative evaluation of cervical radiculopathy and myelopathy by surface-coil MR imaging. *Neuroradiology* 1988;9:859–66.

61. Daniels DL, Grogan JP, Johansen JG, et al. Cervical radiculopathy: Computed tomography and myelography compared. *Radiology* 1984;151:109–13.

62. Kricun R, Kricun ME. Computed tomography. In Kricun ME, editor. *Imaging Modalities in Spinal Disorders.* Philadelphia: W.B. Saunders; 1988; pp. 376–467.

63. Scotti G, Scialfa G, Pieralli S, et al. Myelopathy and radiculopathy due to cervical spondylosis: Myelographic–CT correlations. *AJNR* 1983;4:601–3.

64. Lucci B, Reverberi S, Greco G. Syringomyelia and syringomyelic syndrome by cervical spondylosis. Report of three cases presenting with neurogenic osteoarthropathies. *J Neurosurg Sci* 1981;25:169–72.

65. Iwasaki Y, Abe H, Isu T, et al. CT myelography with intramedullary enhancement in cervical spondylosis. *J Neurosurg* 1985;63:363–6.

66. Jinkins JR, Bashir R, Al-Mefty O, et al. Cystic necrosis of the spinal cord in compressive cervical myelopathy: demonstration by iopamidol CT-myelography. *AJNR* 1986;7:693–701.

67. Al-Mefty O, Harkey LH, Middleton TH, Smith RR, Fox JL. Myelopathic cervical spondylotic lesions demonstrated by magnetic resonance imaging. *J Neurosurg* 1988;68:217–22.

68. Hashizume Y, Iljima S, Kishimoto H, Hirano A. Pencil-shaped softening of the spinal cord: pathologic study in 12 cases. *Acta Neuropathol (Berl)* 1983;61:219–24.

69. Al-Mefty O, Harkey LH, Middleton TH, et al. Myelopathic cervical spondylotic lesions demonstrated by magnetic resonance imaging. *J Neurosurg* 1988;68:217–22.

70. Brain WR, Northfield D, Wilkinson M. The neurological manifestations of cervical spondylosis. *Brain* 1952;75:187–225.

71. Lee SH, Coleman PE, Hahn FJ. Magnetic resonance imaging of degenerative disk disease of the spine. *Radiol Clin North Am* 1988;26:949–64.

72. Takahashi M, Sakamoto Y, Miyawaki M, et al. Increased MR signal intensity secondary to chronic cervical cord compression. *Neuroradiology* 1987;29:550–6.

73. Matsuda Y, Mitazaki K, Tada K, et al. Increased MR signal intensity due to cervical myelopathy. Analysis of 29 surgical cases. *J Neurosurg* 1991;74:887–92.

74. Harada A, Mimatsu K. Postoperative changes in the spinal cord in cervical myelopathy demonstrated by magnetic resonance imaging. *Spine* 1992;17:1275–80.

75. Clifton A, Stevens J, Whitear P, et al. Identifiable causes for poor outcome in surgery for cervical spondylosis. *Neuroradiology* 1990;32:450–5.

76. Lehtinen K, Kaarela K, Antilla P, et al. Sacroilitis in inflammatory joint diseases. *Rheumatology* 1984;52:19–22.

77. Poser S, Hermann-Gremmeis I, Wikstrom J, Poser W. Clinical features of the spinal form of multiple sclerosis. *Acta Neurol Scand* 1978;57:151–8.

78. Lees F, Turner JWA. Natural history and prognosis of cervical spondylosis. *Br Med J* 1963;2:1607–10.

79. Epstein JA, Janin Y, Carras R, Lavine LS. A comparative study of the treatment of cervical spondylotic myeloradiculopathy. *Acta Neurochir* 1982;61:89–104.

80. LaRocca H. Cervical spondylotic myelopathy: natural history. *Spine* 1988;13:854–5.

81. Whitecloud TS. Anterior surgery for cervical spondylotic myelopathy. Smith-Robinson, Cloward, and vertebrectomy. *Spine* 1988;13:861–3.

82. Epstein JA. The surgical management of cervical spinal stenosis, spondylosis, and myeloradiculopathy by means of the posterior approach. *Spine* 1988;13:864–9.

83. Benzel EC, Lancon J, Kesterson L, Hadden T. Cervical laminectomy and dentate ligament sec-

tion for cervical spondylotic myelopathy. *J Spin Disord,* In press.

84. Epstein BS, Epstein JA, Jones MD. Cervical spinal stenosis. *Radiol Clin North Am* 1977;15: 215–26.
85. Nurick S. The pathogenesis of the spinal cord disorder associated with cervical spondylosis. *Brain* 1972;95:87–100.
86. Payne EE, Spillane JD. The cervical spine. An anatomico-pathological study of 70 specimens (using a special technique) with particular reference to the problem of cervical spondylosis. *Brain* 1957;80:571–96.
87. Wilkinson AH, LeMay ML, Ferris EJ. Clinical-radiographic correlations in cervical spondylosis. *J Neurosurg* 1969;30:213–18
88. Benzel EC. Cervical spondylotic myelopathy: posterior surgical approaches. In Cooper PR, editor. *Degenerative Disease of the Cervical Spine.* Park Ridge, IL: AANS; 1993.
89. Batzdorf U, Batzdorff A. Analysis of cervical spine curvature in patients with cervical spondylosis. *Neurosurgery* 1988;22:827–36
90. Carol MP, Ducker TB. Cervical spondylitic myelopathies: surgical treatment. *J Spinal Disord* 1988;1:59–65.
91. Crandall PH, Batzdorf U. Cervical spondylotic myelopathy. *J Neurosurg* 1966;25:57–66.
92. Cusick JF, Ackmann JJ, Larson SJ. Mechanical and physiological effects of dentatotomy. *J Neurosurg* 1977;46:767–75.
93. Dolan EJ, Tator CH, Endrenyi L. The value of decompression for acute experimental spinal cord compression injury. *J Neurosurg* 1980;53: 749–55.
94. Doppman JL, Girton M. Angiographic study of the effect of laminectomy in the presence of acute anterior epidural masses. *J Neurosurg* 1976;45:195–202.
95. Fager CA. Reversal of cervical myelopathy by adequate posterior decompression. *Lahey Clin Found Bull* 1969;18:99–108.
96. Fager CA. Results of adequate posterior decompression in the relief of spondylotic cervical myelopathy. *J Neurosurg* 1973;38:684–92.
97. Kahn EA. The role of the dentate ligaments in spinal cord compression and the syndrome of lateral sclerosis. *J Neurosurg* 1947;4:191–9.
98. Keegan JJ. The cause of dissociated motor loss in the upper extremity with cervical spondylosis; a case report. *J Neurosurg* 1965;23:528–36.
99. Piepgras DG. Posterior decompression for myelopathy due to cervical spondylosis: laminectomy alone versus laminectomy with dentate ligament section. *Clin Neurosurg* 1977; 24:508–15.
100. Reid JD. Effects of flexion-extension movements of the head and spine upon the spinal cord and nerve roots. *J Neurol Neurosurg Psychiatry* 1960;23:214–21.
101. Rogers L. The surgical treatment of cervical spondylotic myelopathy. Mobilisation of the complete cervical cord into an enlarged canal. *JBJS* 1961;43-B:3–6.
102. Rogers L. The treatment of cervical spondylitic myelopathy—mobilisation of the cervical cord into an enlarged spinal canal. *J Neurosurg* 1961; 18:490–2.

103. Guidetti B, Fortuna A. Long-term results of surgical treatment of myelopathy due to cervical spondylosis. *J Neurosurg* 1969;30:714–21.
104. Hanai K, Fujiyoshi F, Kamei K. Subtotal vertebrectomy and spinal fusion for cervical spondylotic myelopathy. *Spine* 1986;11:310–5.
105. Irvine GB, Strachan WE. The long-term results of localized anterior cervical decompression and fusion in spondylotic myelopathy. *Paraplegia* 1987;25:18–22.
106. Kadoya S, Nakamura T, Kwak R. A microsurgical anterior osteophytectomy for cervical spondylotic myelopathy. *Spine* 1984;9:437–41.
107. Magnaes B, Hauge T. Surgery for myelopathy in cervical spondylosis: safety measures and preoperative factors related to outcome. *Spine* 1980;5:211–3.
108. Mann KS, Khosla VK, Gulati DR. Cervical spondylotic myelopathy treated by single- stage multilevel anterior decompression. *J Neurosurg* 1984;60:80–7.
109. Saunders RL, Bernini PM, Shirreffs TG, et al. Central corpectomy for cervical spondylotic myelopathy: a consecutive series with long-term follow-up evaluation. *J Neurosurg* 1991;74:163–70.
110. Verbiest H, Paz y Guese HD. Anterolateral surgery for cervical spondylosis in cases of myelopathy or nerve-root compression. *J Neurosurg* 1966;25:611–22
111. Lunsford LD, Bissonette DJ, Zorub DS. Anterior surgery for cervical disc disease. *J Neurosurg* 1980;53:12–9.
112. Ball PA, Saunders RL. The subjective myelopathy. In Saunders RL, Bernini PM, editors. *Cervical Spondylotic Myelopathy.* Blackwell Scientific; Park Ridge. Chapter 4. 1992; pp. 48–55.
113. Yonenobu K, Okada K, Fuji T, Fujiwara K, Yamashita K, Ono K. Causes of neurologic deterioration following surgical treatment of cervical myelopathy. *Spine* 1985;11:818–23.
114. White AA, Johnson RM, Panjabi MM, Southwick WO. Biomechanical analysis of clinical stability in the cervical spine. *Clin Orthoped Rel Res* 1975;109:85–96
115. Verbiest H. Neurogenic intermittent claudication—lesions of the spinal canal and cauda equina, stenosis of the vertebral canal, narrowing of intervertebral foramina and entrapment of peripheral nerves. In Vinken PJ, Bruyn GW, editors. *Handbook of Clinical Neurology, Volume 20.* Amsterdam: North-Holland; 1976; pp. 611–804.
116. Adams RD, Victor M. Pain in the back, neck, and extremities. In Adams RD, Victor M, editors. *Principles of Neurology.* New York: McGraw-Hill; 1985; pp. 149–72.
117. Hall SH, Bartleson JD, Onofrio BM, et al. Lumbar spinal stenosis: clinical features, diagnostic procedures, and results of surgical treatment in 68 patients. *Ann Int Med* 1985;103:271–5.
118. Jellinger K, Neumayer E. Claudication of the spinal cord and cauda equina. In Vinken PJ, Bruyn GW, editors. *Handbook of Clinical Neurology, Volume 12.* Amsterdam: North-Holland; 1972; pp. 507–47.

119. Madsen JR, Heros RC. Spinal arteriovenous malformations and neurogenic claudication. Report of two cases. *J Neurosurg* 1988;68:793–7.

120. Arnoldi CC, Brodsky AE, Cauchoix J, et al. Lumbar spinal stenosis and nerve root entrapment syndromes: definition and classification. *Clin Orthop* 1976;115:4–5.

121. Elster AD. Quadriplegia after minor trauma in the Klippel-Feil syndrome: a case report and review of the literature. *J Bone Joint Surg* 1984; 66A:1473–4.

122. Epstein NE, Epstein JA, Zilkha A. Traumatic myelopathy in a seventeen year-old child with cervical spinal stenosis (without fracture or dislocation) and a C2–C3 Klippel-Feil fusion: a case report. *Spine* 1984;9:344–7.

123. Prusick VR, Samberg LC, Wesolowski DP. Klippel-Feil syndrome associated with spinal stenosis. A case report. *J Bone Joint Surg* 1985;67:161–4.

124. Epstein B, Epstein JA, Jones MD. Lumbar spinal stenosis. *Radiol Clin N Am* 1977;15: 227–39.

125. Kikaldy-Willis WH, Paine KWE, Cauchoix J, et al. Lumbar spinal stenosis. *Clin Orthop* 1974;99: 30–50.

126. Postacchini F, Massobrio M, Ferro L. Familial lumbar stenosis: case report of three siblings. *J Bone Joint Surg* 1985;67A:321–3.

127. Kricun ME. Conventional radiography. In Kricun ME, editor. *Imaging Modalities of Spinal Disorders*. Philadelphia: W.B. Saunders; 1988; pp. 59–288.

128. Alexander EJr. Significance of the small lumbar spinal canal: cauda equina compression syndromes due to spondylosis: achondroplasia. *J Neurosurg* 1969;31:513–9.

129. Morgan DF, Young RF. Spinal neurological complications of achondroplasia: results of surgical treatment. *J Neurosurg* 1980;52:463–72.

130. Naidich TP, McLone DG, Harwood-Nash DC. Systemic malformations. In Newton TH, Potts DG, editors. *Computed Tomography of the Spine and Spinal Cord*. San Anselmo: Clavadell Press; 1983; pp. 367–81.

131. Epstein BS, Epstein JA, Lavine L. The effect of anatomic variations in the lumbar vertebrae and spinal canal on cauda equina and nerve root syndromes. *Am J Roentgenol* 1964;91:1055–63.

132. Freidenberg ZB, Miller WT. Degenerative disc disease of the cervical spine: a comparative study of asymptomatic and symptomatic patients. *J Bone Joint Surg* 1963;45A:1171–8.

133. Barnett GH, Hardy RW, Little JR, Bay JW, Sypert GW. Thoracic spinal canal stenosis. *J Neurosurg* 1987;66:338–44.

134. Parfitt AM, Duncan H. Metabolic bone disease affecting the spine. In Rothman RH, Simeone FA, editors. *The Spine*. Philadelphia: W.B. Saunders; 1982; pp. 775–905.

135. Yamamoto I, Matsumae M, Ikeda A, et al. Thoracic spinal stenosis: experience with seven cases. *J Neurosurg* 1988;68:37–40.

136. White AA, Panjabi MM. The basic kinematics of the human spine. A review of past and current knowledge. *Spine* 1978;3:12–20.

137. Epstein NE, Epstein JA, Carras R, et al. Coexisting cervical and lumbar spinal stenosis: diagnosis and management. *Neurosurgery* 1984;15: 489–96.

138. Eaton LM, Craig WM. Tumor of the spinal cord: sudden paralysis following lumbar puncture. *Proc Staff Meet Mayo Clin* 1940;15:170–2.

139. Wyburn-Mason R. *Vascular Abnormalities and Tumors of the Spinal Cord and Its Membranes*. London: Kimpton; 1943.

140. Blau JN, Logue V. The natural history of intermittent claudication of the cauda equina. *Brain* 1978;101:211–22.

141. Dejerine J. Sur la claudication intermittente de la moelle epiniere. *Rev Neurol* 1906;14: 341–50.

142. Harsh GR, Sypert GW, Weinstein PR, et al. Cervical spine stenosis secondary to ossification of the posterior longitudinal ligament. *J Neurosurg* 1987;67:349–57.

143. Verbiest H. The significance and principles of computerized axial tomography in idiopathic developmental stenosis of the bony lumbar vertebral canal. *Spine* 1979;4:369–78.

144. Verbiest H. Results of surgical treatment of idiopathic developmental stenosis of the lumbar vertebral canal. *J Bone Joint Surg* 1977;59-B: 181–8.

145. Gelderen CV. Ein orthotisches (lordotisches) Kaudasyndrom. *Acta Psychiat Scand* 1948;23:57–68.

146. Verbiest H. A radicular syndrome from developmental narrowing of the lumbar vertebral canal. *J Bone Joint Surg* 1954;26-B:230–7.

147. Brish A, Lerner MA, Braham J. Intermittent claudication from compression of cauda equina by a narrowed spinal canal. *J Neurosurg* 1964; 21:207–11.

148. Paine KWE. Clinical features of lumbar spinal stenosis. *Clin Orthop* 1976;115:77–82.

149. Wilson CB. Significance of the small lumbar spinal canal. Cauda equina compression syndromes due to spondylosis. 3. Intermittent claudication. *J Neurosurg* 1969;31:499–506.

150. Ram Z, Findler G, Spiegelman R, et al. Intermittent priapism in canal stenosis. *Spine* 1987; 12:377–8.

151. Johnsson K-E, Rosen I, Uden A. Neurophysiologic investigation of patients with spinal stenosis. *Spine* 1987;12:483–7.

152. Edwards WC, LaRocca SH. The developmental segmental diameter in combined cervical and lumbar spondylosis. *Spine* 1985;10:42–9.

153. Sabo R, Tracy P, Weinger J. A series of 60 juxtafacet cysts: clinical presentation, the role of spinal instability and treatment. *J Neurosurg* 1996;85:560–5.

154. Bolender NF, Schonstrom NSR, Spengler DM. Role of computed tomography and myelography in the diagnosis of central spinal stenosis. *J Bone Joint Surg* 1985;67A:240–6.

155. Fischgrund J, Mackay M, Herkowitz H, et al. 1997 Volvo Award winner in clinical studies. Degenerative lumbar spondylolisthesis with spinal stenosis: a prospective, randomized study comparing decompressive laminectomy

and arthrodesis with and without spinal instrumentation. *Spine* 1997;22:2807–12.

156. Hanley E. The indications for lumbar spinal fusion with and without instrumentation. *Spine* 1995;20(24 Suppl):143S–53S.

157. Sonntag V, Marciano F. Is fusion indicated for lumbar spinal disorders? *Spine* 1995;20(24 Suppl):138S–42S.

158. Zdeblick T. The treatment of degenerative lumbar disorders. A critical review of the literature. *Spine* 1995;20(24 Suppl):126S–37S.

159. Rosenberg NJ. Degenerative spondylolisthesis: surgical treatment. *Clin Orthop* 1976;117:112–20.

160. Feffer NB, Wiesel SW, Cuckler JM, et al. Degenerative spondylolisthesis. To fuse or not to fuse. *Spine* 1985;10:287–9.

161. Herkowitz HN, Kurz LT. Degenerative lumbar spondylolisthesis with spinal stenosis: a prospective study comparing decompression with decompression and intratransverse process arthrodesis. *J Bone Joint Surg* 1991;73A:802–8.

162. Lombardi JS, Wiltse LL, Reynolds J, et al. Treatment of degenerative spondylolisthesis. *Spine* 1985;10:821–7.

163. Alexander E, Kelly DL, Davis CH, et al. Intact arch spondylolisthesis. J Neurosurg 1985;63:840–4.

164. Benzel EC. Surgery for the Back Pain Associated With Degenerative Spondylolisthesis. In press.

165. Dall BE, Rowe DE. Degenerative spondylolisthesis: its surgical management. *Spine* 1985;10:668–72.

166. Epstein JA, Epstein BS, Lavine LS, et al. Degenerative lumbar spondylolisthesis with an intact neural arch (pseudospondylolisthesis). *J Neurosurg* 1976;44:139–47.

167. Herron LD, Trippi AC. Degenerative spondylolisthesis. The results of treatment by decompressive laminectomy without fusion. *Spine* 1989;14:534–8.

168. Salibi BS. Neurogenic intermittent claudication and stenosis of the lumbar spinal canal. *Surg Neurol* 1976;5:269–72.

169. Shenkin HA, Hash CJ. Spondylolisthesis after multiple bilateral laminectomies and facetectomies for lumbar spondylosis. Follow-up review. *J Neurosurg* 1979;50:45–7.

170. Atkinson R, Ghelman B, Tsairis P, et al. Sarcoidosis presenting as cervical radiculopathy: a case report and literature review. *Spine* 1982;7:412–6.

171. Cinotti G, Postacchini F, Fassari F, Urso S. Predisposing factors in degenerative spondylolisthesis. A radiographic and CT study. *Int Orthop* 1997;21:337–42.

172. O'Sullivan P, Phyty G, Twomey L, Allison G. Evaluation of specific stabilizing exercise in the treatment of chronic low back pain with radiologic diagnosis of spondylolysis or spondylolistheseis. *Spine* 1997;22:2959–67.

173. Matsunaga S, Sakou T, Morizono Y, et al. Natural history of degenerative spondylolisthesis. Pathogenesis and natural course of the slippage. *Spine* 1990;15:1204–10.

174. Deen HG, Zimmerman RS, Lyons MK, et al. Analysis of early failures after lumbar decompressive laminectomy for spinal stenosis. *Mayo Clin Proc* 1995;70:33–6.

175. Kristoff FV, Odom GL. Ruptured intervertebral disk in the cervical region. *Arch Surg* 1947;54:287–304.

176. O'Connell JEA. Involvement of the spinal cord by intervertebral disk protrusions. *Br J Surg* 1955;43:225–47.

177. Mulder DW, Dale AJD. Spinal cord tumors and disks. In Baker AB, Baker LH, editors. *Clinical Neurology*. Hagerstown: Harper & Rowe; 1975; pp. 1–28.

178. Yoss RE, Corbin KB, MacCarty CS, Love JG. Significance of symptoms and signs in localization of involved root in cervical disc protrusion. *Neurology* 1957;7:673–83.

179. Haughton VM, Williams AL. *Computed Tomography of The Spine*. St. Louis: C.V. Mosby; 1982.

180. Bartlett R, Hill C, Gardiner E. A comparison of T2 and gadolinium enhanced MRI with CT myelography in cervical radiculopathy. *Br J Radiol* 1998;71:11–19.

181. Dreyfus P, Six B, Dorfman H, Seze SD. Thoracic disc hernia. In Vinken PJ, Bruyn GW, editors. *Handbook of Clinical Neurology, Volume 20*. Amsterdam: North-Holland; 1976; pp. 565–71.

182. Love JG, Schorn VS. Thoracic disc protrusions. *JAMA* 1965;191:627–31.

183. Arce CA, Dohrmann GJ. Thoracic disc herniation: improved diagnosis with computerized tomographic scanning and a review of the literature. *Surg Neurol* 1985;23:356–61.

184. Arseni C, Nash F. Protrusion of thoracic intervertebral discs. *Acta Neurochir (Wien)* 1963;31:3–33.

185. Caron JP, Djindjian R, Julian H, et al. Les hernies discales dorsales. *Ann Med* 1971;6–7:675–88.

186. McCallister VL, Sage MR. The radiology of thoracic disc protrusion. *Clin Radiol* 1976;27:291–9.

187. Hochman MS, Pena C. Calcified herniated thoracic disc diagnosed by computerized tomography: case report. *J Neurosurg* 1980;52:722–3.

188. Schmiel S, Deeb ZL. Herniated thoracic intervertebral disks. *J Comput Tomogr* 1985;9:141–3.

189. Duym FCvAv, Wiechen PJ. Herniation of calcified nucleus puposus in the thoarcic spine: Case report. *J Comput Assist Tomogr* 1983;7:1122–3.

190. Wood K, Garvey T, Gundry C, Heithoff K. Magnetic resonance imaging of the thoracic spine. Evaluation of asymptomatic individuals. *J Bone Joint Surg (Am)* 1995;77:1631–8.

191. Harkelius A, Hindmarsh J. The comparative reliability of preoperative diagnostic methods in lumbar disc surgery. *Acta Orthop Scand* 1972;43:234–8.

192. Gathier JC. Radicular disorders due to lumbar discopathy (hernia nuclei puplosi). In Vinken PJ, Bruyn GW, editors. *Handbook of Clinical Neurology, Volume 20*. Amsterdam: North-Holland; 1976; pp. 573–604.

193. Dinakar I, Balaparameswararao I. Lumbar disc prolapse. Study of 300 surgical cases. *Int Surg* 1972;57:299–302.

194. Bernard TN, Kirkaldy-Willis WH. Recognizing specific characteristics of nonspecific low back pain. *Spine* 1987;217:266–80.

195. Frymoyer JW, Newberg A, Pope MH, Wilder DG, Clements J, MacPherson B. Spine radiographs in patients with low-back pain. *J Bone Joint Surg* 1984;66A:1048–55.

196. Hitselberger WE, Witten RM. Abnormal myelograms in asymptomatic patients. *J Neurosurg* 1968;28:204–6.

197. McRae DL. Bony abnormalities in the region of the foramen magnum: correlation of the anatomic and neurologic findings. *Acta Radiol* 1953;40:335–54.

198. Wiesel SW, Tsourmas N, Feffer HL, et al. A study of computer-assisted tomography 1. The incidence of positive CAT scans in an asymptomatic group patients. *Spine* 1984;9:549–51.

199. Jensen M, Brant-Zawadzki M, Obuchowski N, et al. Magetic resonance imaging of the lumbar spine in people without back pain. *N Engl J Med* 1994;331:69–73.

200. Godersky JC, Erickson DL, Seljeskog EL. Extreme lateral disc herniation: diagnosis by computed tomographic scanning. *J Neurosurg* 1984;14:549–52.

201. Shapiro R. *Myelography, 4th Edition*. Chicago: Year Book Medical; 1984.

202. Williams AL, Haughton VM, Daniels DL, et al. Differential CT diagnosis of extruded nucleus puplosus. *Radiology* 1983;146:141–6.

203. Ciapetta P, Delfini R, Cantore GP. Intradural lumbar disc hernia: description of three cases. *Neurosurgery* 1981;8:104–7.

204. Dillon WP, Kaseff LG, Knackstedt VE, et al. Computed tomography and differential diagnosis of the extruded lumbar disc. *J Comput Assist Tomogr* 1983;7:969–75.

205. Braun IF, Hoffman JC, Davis PC, et al. Contrast enhancement in CT differentiation between recurrent disc herniation and post-operative scar: prospective study. *Am J Roentgenol* 1985;145:785–90.

206. Chafetz N, Genant HK, Gillespy T, Winkler M. Magnetic resonance imaging. In Kricun ME, editor. *Imaging Modalities in Spinal Disorders*. Pjiladelphia: W.B. Saunders; 1988; pp. 478–502.

207. Modic MT, Masaryk T, Boumphrey F, et al. Lumbar herniated disk disease and canal stenosis: prospective evaluation by surface coil MR, CT, and myelography. *Am J Roentgenol* 1986; 147:757–65.

208. Frymoyer JW. Back pain and sciatica. *N Engl J Med* 1988;318:291–300.

209. Rybock JD. Acute back pain and disc herniation. In Johnson RT, editor. *Current Therapy in Neurological Disease—2*. Toronto: B.C. Decker; 1987; pp. 48–50.

210. Bozzao A, Gallucci M, Masciocchi C, Aprile I, Barile A, Passariello R. Lumbar disc herniation—MR-imaging assessment of natural history in patients treated without surgery. *Radiology* 1992;185:135–41.

211. Stoddard A, Osborn JF. Scheuermann's disease of spinal osteochondrosis. Its frequency and relationship with spondylosis. *J Bone J Surg* 1979; 61b:56–8.

212. Taggart HMcA, Tweedyie DR. Spinal cord compression: remember osteoporosis. *Br Med J* 1987;294:1148–9.

Chapter 5

EPIDURAL TUMORS

Neoplasms not originating from spinal structures differ in their propensity to metastasize to the spine. However, any malignancy with metastatic potential may appear in the spine and cause epidural spinal cord compression (ESCC). (The term spinal cord compression is used to include cauda equina compression unless otherwise noted.)

Epidural neoplasms can be classified as either metastatic or primary. Since metastatic tumors are far more common, they will be discussed extensively in this chapter. Among primary epidural neoplasms, several different benign or malignant tumors may arise from those cells that form the vertebral column and its associated supporting structures. The most common are osteogenic, chondrogenic, vascular, fibrous, hematopoietic, lipomatous, and undifferentiated mesenchymal elements and these are discussed at the end of this chapter.

The diagnosis of epidural neoplasms can be difficult. Pain is usually the first symptom of both primary and metastatic epidural spinal tumors.[1-3] However, as discussed in Chapter 3, pain is a common manifestation of many nonneoplastic spinal disorders as well, which makes clinical history alone rarely sufficient to establish a cause with certainty. Rather, a meticulous history and physical examination, supplemented when indicated, with appropriate laboratory and diagnostic imaging studies, often are necessary to identify the cause.

Even when diagnostic imaging studies demonstrate an epidural neoplasm, one still must distinguish between a primary and a metastatic tumor. If there is a history of malignancy with a propensity to metastasize to the spine, the epidural tumor is usually considered metastatic; rarely, a metastasis from a second unknown primary or even a primary spinal tumor may be the cause. When a malignancy has not been previously diagnosed, one must still consider the possibility of a metastasis from an unknown primary source, since metastatic epidural spinal tumors are much more frequent than primary tumors of the spine. Certain clues can help the physician locate a primary tumor:

1. The patient's gender and age may suggest the most likely histological types to consider. For example, whereas breast, lung, and prostate cancers are frequent sources of spinal metastases in adults,[4–7] sarcomas and neuroblastoma are common causes in children.[8]
2. The general physical examination and laboratory screening may help in establishing leads.
3. The frequency with which certain primary tumors in adults metastasize to the spine often guides the workup for a primary tumor. For example, prostate, lung, and breast cancer are among the most common primary tumors.

There are two reasons to search for a nonspinal primary tumor. First, metastases (even from occult primary tumors) are much more common than primary spinal tumors. Second, an accurate diagnosis of the neoplasm causing ESCC is necessary for most effective treatment. Histological confirmation may be essential for further management if the diagnosis is in doubt.

This chapter first reviews in detail the clinical features and imaging studies frequently encountered in the evaluation of metastatic spinal neoplasms. A brief review of some of the clinical features of primary epidural tumors follows.

METASTATIC NEOPLASMS

Epidemiology

Much of the epidemiological information on spinal tumors is obtained from neurosurgical series. These series often underrepresent the frequency of metastatic cancer because many of these patients may not be considered good surgical candidates, and therefore may not be referred for surgical management. One review[9] cites several neurosurgical studies that report that extramedullary–intradural tumors (e.g., neurofibroma and meningioma) are the most common tumor type. Spinal metastases from systemic cancer were excluded from the analysis.

When epidural tumors are considered alone, metastatic tumors are found to be more common than primary spinal neoplasms. This has been the experience even in some neurosurgical series.[1,10] For example, in one study of vertebral tumors,[1,11] 66% of 350 tumors were metastatic, whereas only 30% were primary. The remaining 4% were paravertebral tumors that invaded the spinal column. An extensive review of the literature on primary and secondary tumors of the vertebral column[10] concludes that metastatic tumors are three to four times more frequent than primary malignant neoplasms. In a neurosurgical series of 413 solitary tumors of the vertebral column,[2] 121 were metastatic in origin, thus emphasizing that even apparently solitary vertebral lesions are often metastatic.

The enormous clinical impact of cancer that metastasizes to the vertebral column and epidural space in the general population is supported by several large autopsy series[10,12–14] that report vertebral metastases in 15% to 41% of patients dying of cancer. Furthermore, the frequency of skeletal metastases is much higher for some specific tumor types: 84% of prostatic cancer cases and 74% of breast cancer cases. Moreover, among patients with skeletal metastases, the vertebral column has been found to be the most common site.[15,16] A review of the pathophysiology and management of bone metastases has been published.[17]

All patients with vertebral metastasis are at potential risk of developing spinal cord compression. The frequency of spinal cord compression from metastases to the vertebral column is unknown, but one autopsy study[4] estimated that approximately 5% of patients dying of cancer have spinal cord compression, the great majority of which is caused by vertebral metastases.

Thus, of the nearly 400,000 individuals dying of cancer annually in the United States, between 60,000 and 160,000 have spinal metastases, and 20,000 of these individuals develop ESCC. These figures, although only estimates, underscore the magnitude of the clinical problem of spinal metastases in the cancer population. It must be emphasized that vertebral metastases are not confined to patients dying of cancer; this treatable complication occurs even in patients whose primary malignancy is also treatable, and in about 8% of patients, it may be the only symptom.

Mechanisms of Cancer Metastasis

Cancer metastasis implies the release of cells from one primary site and passage of these cells through lymphatics or blood vessels to a distant site where there is invasion and growth of a secondary neoplasm.[18] The mechanism of passage of these "shed" cancer cells has been a source of debate.[19] Although both organ and tumor cell properties are probably important in the initiation of metastatic cascade,[20] the predominant view has been that anatomic and hemodynamic factors play a primary role in the dissemination of cancer.

Hemodynamic theory explains the metastatic cascade on the basis of the anatomy of draining veins. In a series of elegant experiments using human cadavers, Batson[21] showed that injection of radiopaque material into the dorsal vein of the penis and the draining breast veins resulted in opacification of the vertebral venous system. Furthermore, in living primates, abdominal straining augmented venous flow from the pelvic viscera to the vertebral veins (Fig. 5–1). Batson demon-

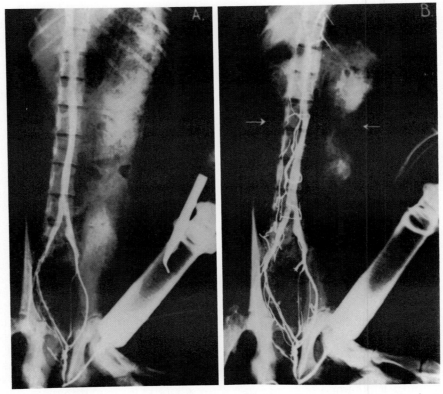

Figure 5–1. The roentgenogram of a living monkey injected with radiopaque material in the deep dorsal vein of the penis. (A) The injected material passes into the inferior vena cava without entering the vertebral veins. (B) The same animal is shown, but the abdomen has been compressed with a towel, mimicking a Valsalva maneuver. The contrast material passes upward through the vertebral venous system. (From Batson, OV,[21] with permission.)

strated that because the vertebral venous system is valveless and of low intraluminal pressure, coughing, sneezing, and straining allow venous effluent from the breast, intrathoracic, intra-abdominal, and pelvic organs to enter and move unimpeded in a rostral or caudal direction.

Batson noted in 1956 that he had rediscovered this plexus of veins, which was first described by Breschet in the first half of the 19th century and then overlooked for over a century.[22] In recognition of Breschet's contribution, Batson generously stated, "Eponymically, the veins in the vault of the skull are known as Breschet's veins. We commonly forget that the veins in the bodies of the vertebrae are likewise Breschet's veins." Figure 5–2

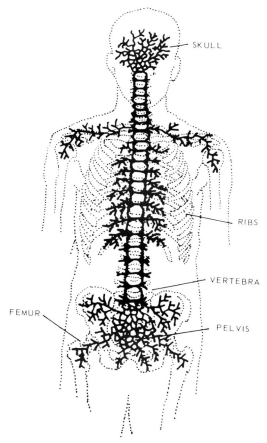

Figure 5–2. Neoplasms from the pelvis, abdomen, breast, and elsewhere show collaterals with the vertebral venous system. (From del Regato, JA,[214] with permission.)

illustrates some of the pathways available for metastatic spread to the axial skeleton from pelvic, abdominal, thoracic, and breast malignancies.

In a series of experiments supporting this hemodynamic approach,[23] suspensions of tumor cells were injected into the veins of rats and rabbits. The pattern of metastases in animals (experimental group) in which intra-abdominal pressure was elevated transiently during the injection was compared with the pattern in which there was no increase in pressure (control group). The results of these studies confirmed Batson's hypothesis. In nearly all of the control animals, the metastases were localized to the lungs alone. The majority of experimental animals, however, demonstrated spinal metastases. Furthermore, the spinal metastases arose from emboli to the thin-walled vertebral veins, not the arterial system.

Although the system of vertebral veins that has come to be called Batson's plexus can explain many cases of aberrant metastasis, it is now recognized that patterns of metastases are not explained by hemodynamic factors alone. Although the hemodynamic model may explain the arrest of tumor embolus in a specific organ, it may not predict the ultimate pattern of metastasis, which requires invasion and growth of the tumor cells.[24] Thus ultimately both Paget's seed-and-soil hypothesis[20] and Ewing's anatomic and hemodynamic factors[25] may also have a role in explaining the metastatic spread of cancer.[19]

Location of Epidural Tumor in Relation to Spinal Cord

Spinal metastases may be intramedullary, leptomeningeal or epidural in location (Fig. 5–3). Intramedullary and leptomeningeal neoplasms are discussed elsewhere in this book. Epidural metastases and resulting ESCC can occur in to one of three sites: the vertebrae, the paravertebral tissues, or the epidural space itself (Fig. 5–3 C, D, and E). By extending into the adjacent vertebral canal, a tumor in any of these locations may impinge on the neural structures. An understanding

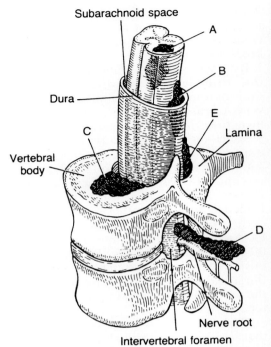

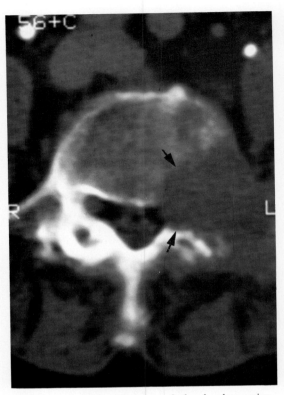

Figure 5–3. Locations of metastases to the spine are shown. Intramedullary metastases are located within the spinal cord (A). Leptomeningeal metastases are in the subarachnoid space (B) and are extramedullary and intradural. Epidural metastases arise from the extension of metastases located in the adjacent vertebral column (C), in the paravertebral spaces through the intervertebral foramina (D), or rarely, in the epidural space itself (E). As these epidural metastases grow, they compress adjacent blood vessels, nerve roots, and spinal cord, resulting in local and referred pain, radiculopathy, and myelopathy. (From Byrne, TN,[215] with permission.)

Figure 5–4. This CT scan of the lumbar spine demonstrates a metastasis from lung cancer (arrows) to a pedicle, which extends into the vertebral body, vertebral canal, and paravertebral tissues.

of these different mechanisms of compression is helpful in recognizing the pathogenesis of spinal cord compression and interpreting imaging studies.

The vertebral column is the most frequent site from which metastases may cause ESCC. The regions involved most often are the vertebral body (especially subchondral areas) and the pedicles (Fig. 5–4), probably because of the extensive vascular supply to these areas.[26,27]

In one study, 85% of patients with metastatic ESCC at Memorial Sloan-Kettering Cancer Center (MSKCC) were found to have vertebral column involvement.[28] In a neurosurgical series,[29] review of the radiological findings of 600 cases of

spinal cord compression from metastatic cancer showed the vertebral column was involved in 94% of cases. Of those with vertebral metastases, 86% showed more than one involved vertebral body. Isolated bone lesions without extension of tumor into the epidural space were found in 10% of the 600 cases; in this setting, vertebral body collapse with resulting cord compression was considered responsible for neurologic abnormalities. These findings not only explain the pathogenesis of many cases of metastatic ESCC (vertebral involvement leads to cord compression) but also place in perspective the value of performing radiological procedures on the vertebral column. One must conclude that a negative plain radiograph of the spine or a negative radionuclide bone scan does not entirely exclude metastatic ESCC, because a few patients will have no vertebral involvement. Although radionuclide bone scanning is far more sensitive than plain radiographs in the detection of bone metastases,[30,31] false-negative radionuclide bone scans remain a problem.[32]

Paravertebral tumors that extend into the vertebral canal through the intervertebral foramina constitute another important cause of ESCC. Plain radiographs of the spine and radionuclide bone scan are often unrevealing if the vertebrae are not involved by tumor. While any paravertebral neoplasm may be responsible, this phenomenon seems to be most commonly observed in patients with renal cell cancer, superior sulcus tumors (Pancoast syndrome[33]), neuroblastoma, and lymphoma, especially if the paravertebral regions are not included in the radiotherapy port (Fig. 5–5A).[5] Lymphoma is considered a neoplasm especially prone to cause spinal cord compression by invading the epidural space through the intervertebral foramina from paravertebral lymph nodes rather than via the more commonly encountered vertebral metastasis (Fig. 5–5B).[28] Among all cases of metastatic ESCC, exactly how often paravertebral tumors are responsible is unknown, but one estimate is approximately 10%.[28] With the advent of high-resolution CT scanning and MRI that can adequately study the paravertebral soft tissues, these lesions may be more frequently recognized.

Pure epidural lesions alone are rare. In the neurosurgical series referred to above,[29] the incidence of epidural tumor alone was 5% (Fig. 5–6).

Pathology

The evolution of spinal cord symptoms and signs may be better appreciated in light of the pathological findings within the spinal cord, including areas of demyelination, infarction, and cystic necrosis.

Over 30 years ago, McAlhany and Netsky[34] performed a clinicopathological study on a series of patients with extramedullary spinal cord compression. Of

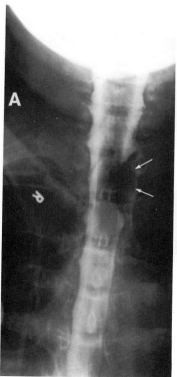
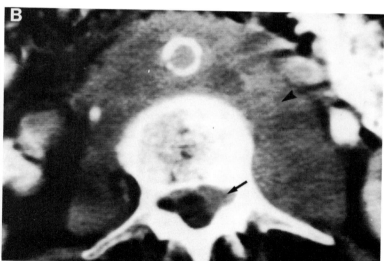

Figure 5–5. Paravertebral neoplasms with epidural extension through intervertebral foraminae without bone involvement. (A) This myelogram demonstrates an epidural metastatic breast cancer at the T1–2 level. The bone scan and plain films were negative. The tumor had extended from a paravertebral mass through the intervertebral foramen. (B) This upper lumbar spine CT scan demonstrates a paravertebral lymphoma (arrowhead) extending into the epidural space (arrow).

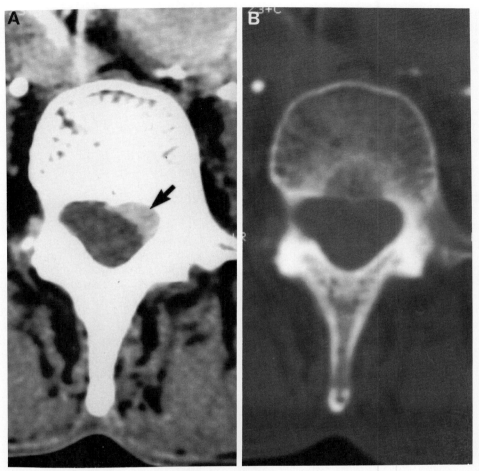

Figure 5–6. A CT scan of the lumbar spine of an 82-year-old woman with rectal carcinoma who complained of radiating pain into the left anterolateral thigh. Her left knee deep tendon reflex was absent. (A) CT scan of the lumbar spine using soft-tissue windows demonstrates a metastasis in the epidural space. (B) CT scan at the same level using bone windows shows no vertebral involvement.

the 19 cases reported, 15 were epidural, predominantly from metastatic cancer; the remaining 4 were intradural–extramedullary meningiomas. These authors found no correlation between the location of the neoplasm in the transverse plane of the spinal cord and the presenting neurologic complaint of their patients. For example, in a patient with a laterally placed epidural mass, corticospinal dysfunction was not ipsilateral to the lesion initially, nor was the loss of pain and temperature contralateral. This clinical observation was explained by the fact that both the ipsilateral and/or contralateral areas were demyelinated. At times, the contralateral damage was more marked than the ipsilateral injury. Furthermore, the white matter tended to be more severely affected than the gray matter. The white matter of the anterior funiculus was relatively spared in comparison to that of the lateral and posterior columns, even in ventrally placed epidural masses. Thus the authors rejected the previously held belief that the dentate ligaments, which anchor the spinal cord in the vertical plane, play a significant role in the evolution of spinal cord compression.[35] Moreover, distribution of pathology in the transverse plane did not reveal areas of demyelination that conformed to the arterial supply. In addition to demyelination, areas of infarction were also found, but the regions of infarction did not conform to the vascular distribution of any major radicular or sulcal blood vessel.

Pathologists have also reported pencil-shaped softenings of the spinal cord at the level of epidural tumors.[36] These softenings may extend longitudinally over several segments of the spinal cord in a cephalad or, less frequently, caudad direction. The necrotic cavity that forms the pencil-shaped softening is usually located in the ventral portion of the posterior column or posterior horn. This region, which corresponds to the region involved in cases of venous infarction,[37,38] is also considered to be a watershed zone for arterial circulation.[37] Although circulatory disturbances are important in the development of pencil-shaped softenings,[39] mechanical factors also have been cited.[36] These cystic necrotic lesions have been imaged using delayed CT myelography and MRI.

Pathophysiology of Neurologic Signs and Symptoms in Spinal Cord Compression

The mechanism by which epidural tumors induce spinal cord injury is complex and probably multifactorial. Neurosurgical experience has shown that venous engorgement and diminished arterial pulsation both play a role.[40] Tarlov[41,42] undertook a series of experiments to produce acute or chronic ESCC in dogs. He inflated a balloon in the spinal canal for varying periods of time. When the balloon was rapidly inflated to a pressure just sufficient to produce motor paralysis and complete sensory loss below the compression, recovery ensued if the compression was relieved within two hours. However, when the balloon was slowly inflated over a 48-hour period, a pressure just sufficient to cause complete paralysis and a sensory level at the level of compression could be maintained for one week before paralysis was irreversible. Tarlov considered that, rather than ischemia, this type of mechanical pressure on nervous tissue was primarily responsible for paralysis.[43]

Several authors have studied the sequence of vascular, biochemical, pathological, and neurophysiological changes in experimental ESCC under conditions that simulate those of neoplastic cord compression. Ushio and colleagues[44] injected Walker 256 carcinoma cells into the epidural space of the rat and demonstrated that vasogenic edema of the spinal cord is an early pathological finding. A marker normally excluded from the spinal cord entered the cord at the site of compression, suggesting the breakdown of the blood–spinal cord barrier as a cause of edema. As vasogenic edema developed, animals manifested increasing hindlimb weakness. Improvement in spinal cord function following the administration of corticosteroids to the animals was paralleled by improvement in vasogenic edema.

These findings have been extended and confirmed.[45,46] The pathophysiology of circulatory disturbances secondary to ESCC appears to follow a stepwise progression: (1) Compression of Batson's plexus by tumor causes venous congestion, white matter edema, and axonal swelling and is associated with the clinical evidence of early myelopathy. Experimentally, these changes may occur in the absence of tumor within the spinal canal, suggesting that paravertebral masses may disturb venous drainage in the spinal cord, resulting in neurologic symptoms. At this early stage of spinal cord compression, spinal cord blood flow is not diminished.[46] (2) In the middle stage, direct tumor compression of the spinal cord is added to venous congestion of the cord. White matter edema progresses, and spinal cord blood flow becomes altered at the level of compression and caudal to compression in response to carbon dioxide inhalation. Clinical evidence of myelopathy also progresses. During this period when the spinal cord edema is vasogenic, the edema and clinical signs of myelopathy may be improved by the administration of corticosteroids.[44,47] (3) In the final stage of spinal cord compression, the tumor compresses the spinal cord further, blood flow drops precipitously, and irreversible spinal cord damage occurs.

Several recent studies have attempted to identify the biochemical processes involved in the pathophysiology of neurologic dysfunction. Confirming an earlier report,[48] Siegal and colleagues[49] found abnormalities in spinal somatosensory-evoked responses preceding neurologic signs of myelopathy. In an experimental model, they studied prostaglandins and cord edema. Myelin destruction was caused by both mechanical compression and ischemia as demonstrated by electron-microscopic studies. Subsequently, these authors conducted a series of investigations studying the roles of prostaglandin E_2, serotonin, and glutamate in the pathophysiology of neoplastic spinal cord compression.[49–53] These studies demonstrated an increase in prostaglandin E_2 and an increased metabolism of serotonin. In a previous study, prostaglandin E_2 had been reported to promote vasodilatation and plasma exudation in parallel with the development of spinal cord edema.[54] Furthermore, Siegal and colleagues reported that serotonin antagonists, such as cyproheptadine, improve spinal cord function in experimental animals.[51,52] In addition, the glutamate antagonists ketamine and MK-801 diminish spinal cord edema.[52] These studies are of interest, but their clinical implications are as yet unknown. Because glutamate does not trigger calcium-mediated injury of white matter axons,[55] and several alternative pathways involving the $Na^+–Ca^{2+}$ exchanger[56,57] and calcium channels[58] are involved in this process, it seems likely that treatment with multiple physiological agents will be necessary for protection of the spinal cord in ESCC.

Mechanical compression of spinal axons per se may also interfere with conduction. It is well established that focal compression of myelinated fiber tracts can cause damage to myelin[59] and the conduction block.[60] As would be expected from a biomechanical perspective, larger fibers are more susceptible to the effects of compression.[61,62] On the basis of careful morphological study, it is now clear that demyelination can occur at sites of spinal cord compression[63–65] (Fig. 5–7). There is, moreover, some evidence for remyelination after transient compression of the spinal cord,[66] providing a possible morphological correlate for recovery of function following prompt surgical relief of spinal cord compression.

Types of Primary Neoplasms Metastasizing to the Spine

Several studies report the relative frequency of primary tumors that metastasize to the spine and cause ESCC.[1,2,4,5,7,10,29,67] As discussed earlier, such reports from neurosurgical series select patients who are considered candidates for surgical procedures. If patients who are not surgical candidates are excluded, the epidemiological data are subject to bias. In an attempt to overcome a selection bias, the studies reviewed in Table 5–1 and cited below are those that attempted to include all patients that presented to reporting institutions, irrespective of the therapy chosen.[4–7]

The often-quoted autopsy study of 127 cases exhibiting symptomatic spinal cord compression by Barron and colleagues[4] provides a basis for epidemiological analysis of metastatic ESCC. A review of their findings indicates that epidural metastasis was found in all but three patients (two with intramedullary metastases and one with leptomeningeal metastases) whose primary tumor types were also recorded. Thus, the risk of developing spinal cord compression with each individual tumor type could be determined. Over ten different primary tumors were found to be responsible for ESCC. In descending frequency, the five most common malignancies were lung ($n = 31$; 24%), breast (20; 16%), lymphoma (20; 16%), kidney (12; 9%), and myeloma (9; 7%). Recognizing a changing pattern of primary malignancies, these authors noted that neither the earlier series of Neustaedter[68] nor that of Elsberg[69] reported a case of lung cancer as a cause of spinal cord compression. Also, unlike an earlier series[70] in which spinal metastasis from prostate cancer was considered a rarity, Barron and colleagues[4] found it to be the fifth most common cause

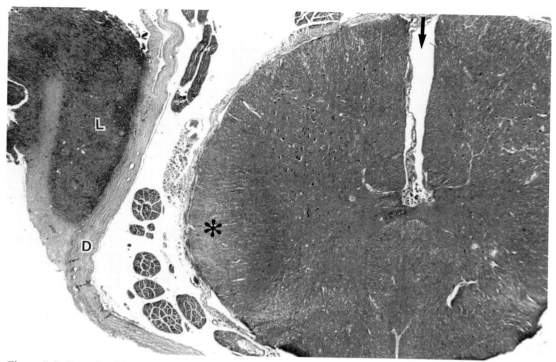

Figure 5–7. Extradural lymphoma (L) abutting the spinal dura (D). The adjacent lateral column shows a poorly defined area of subtle demyelination (asterisk). Arrow: Anterior median fissure. Luxol fast blue stain. Magnification ×14. (Courtesy of Dr. Jung Kim.)

in males. The increasing frequency of spinal metastases from prostate cancer is discussed below.

Gilbert and colleagues[5] found breast, lung, and prostate cancers to be the most frequent primary tumors causing ESCC, comprising over 40% of the total cases (see Table 5–1). The relative frequencies of these primary tumors reflected those commonly observed at MSKCC, except that

Table 5–1. Types of Primary Tumors Causing Metastatic Epidural Spinal Cord Compression in Various Series (%)

Primary Tumor	Barron et al.[4]	Gilbert et al.[5]	Stark et al.[7]	Rodichok et al.[6]
Lung	24	13	33	31
Breast	16	20	28	24
Prostate	4	9	4	8
Kidney	9	7	3	1
Myeloma	7	4	Excluded	1
Lymphoma	16	11	Excluded	6
Melanoma	—*	3	1	4
Sarcoma	6	9	1	4
Female reproductive	—	2	3	6
GI	5	4	5	9
Miscellaneous	13	18	22	8

*— = insufficient data.

gastrointestinal tumors did not cause spinal cord compression as frequently as would have been expected based on their relative incidence. A similar experience was reported by Barron and colleagues.[4] Of further interest, Gilbert and associates[5] found lymphomas less frequently represented in the later years of their study. They attributed this change to modified therapy that includes total nodal irradiation including the paravertebral regions.

The London Hospital study by Stark and colleagues[7] (see Table 5–1) reports a ten-year experience of spinal metastases from solid tumors (hematological malignancies were excluded). Although there are some differences in the relative frequencies of primary tumors in these various series, lung, breast, and prostate cancers are generally the most frequent offenders. Furthermore, lung cancer is much more likely to present initially as a spine metastasis than breast cancer; the latter usually causes spinal cord compression after the diagnosis of cancer is already established.[7] Although not a common cause of ESCC, leukemia is an occasional offender.

Table 5–2 demonstrates the relative frequency of primary malignancies causing

Table 5–2. Types of Primary Tumors Causing Metastatic Epidural Spinal Cord Compression in Men and Women (%)

	Stark et al.[7]		Barron et al.[4]	
	Male	Female	Male	Female
Lung	53	12	32	14
Breast	0	59	0	39
Prostate	8	N/A	8	N/A
Kidney	3	3	12	6
Myeloma	Excluded		8	6
Lymphoma	Excluded		20	9
Melanoma	0	1	—	—
GI	5	3	5	5
Female reproductive	N/A	6	N/A	6
Miscellaneous	31	16	15	15

ESCC for men and women separately.[7] This information is important in evaluating the patient who presents with the clinical and radiographic constellation of malignant ESCC.

As noted above, by comparing the number of autopsied cases of spinal cord compression secondary to a specific tumor with the total number of autopsied cases with the same neoplasm, Barron and colleagues[4] were able to estimate the risk of developing spinal metastasis with individual neoplasms. Multiple myeloma and prostate cancer had the highest risks, 14% and 10%, respectively; ovarian (0%) and stomach cancer (1%) were the least likely to cause spinal cord compression. The commonly encountered breast and lung malignancies had frequencies of approximately 5% each. The authors noted that these frequency figures should be considered as minimums since some patients with spinal cord compression may not have been recognized clinically.

The changing pattern of spinal metastasis from prostate cancer deserves further comment. Barron and associates[4] noted that the incidence of spinal cord compression in their patients with prostate cancer was significantly higher than that found in an earlier study.[70] They speculated that the increasing frequency of spinal metastases could be due to the advent of hormonal manipulation, which might prolong life and could, thereby, increase the risk of metastases (hormones = improved therapy = longer life = more time to develop complications). Although some recent studies continue to show a low frequency of spinal metastasis from prostate cancer,[71] others have found that 80% of men dying of prostate cancer demonstrate vertebral metastases,[72] although in one recent series spinal cord compression was found in only 7%.[73] A similar experience of increasing neurologic involvement, as more effective controls of systemic malignancy evolve, has been reported for other types of malignancy such as leukemia,[74–77] lymphoma,[78,79] small-cell bronchogenic carcinoma,[80] and others.[81]

Interval From Primary Tumor Diagnosis to Epidural Spinal Cord Compression

The interval between the diagnosis of cancer and the development of spinal cord compression is extremely variable. In the series from MSKCC, it was zero to 19 years.[5] While only ten patients in this series presented with cord compression as the initial manifestation of their malignancy, this may be explained by the fact that most patients in a cancer hospital already carry a diagnosis of malignancy. Alternatively, in the study from the London Hospital,[7] 62 of 131 patients had spinal cord compression as the presenting manifestation of cancer. The series reported by Barron and colleagues[4] from a general hospital similarly concluded that lung cancer often presents with spine metastasis, whereas this mode of presentation is atypical with breast cancer. These factors probably explain the greater frequency of breast cancer than lung primaries in the MSKCC series.[5]

Age and Gender Distribution

The age of patients with spinal metastases reflects the age at which the respective primary neoplasms occur. In many series, incidence rates peak at 50–70 years.[5–7,67] Similarly, the sex ratio is dependent on the underlying neoplasms. Breast cancer has been much more frequently observed than lung cancer in women, but this is expected to change as lung cancer becomes more common.

Level of Spinal Cord Compression

Most studies agree that the thoracic spine is the most frequent site of spinal cord compression.[4,5,7,73,82,83] In the MSKCC series,[5] the cervical spine was the site of epidural tumor in 15% of cases, the thoracic spine in 68%, and the lumbosacral spine in 16%. Lung and breast cancer tended to metastasize to the thoracic spine, whereas the spread of colon cancer was disproportionately more frequent to the lumbosacral spine.[5] In two other studies[71,73] of genitourinary tumors alone, the thoracic spine was the most common site, followed by the lumbar and then the cervical spinal regions.

In the London Hospital study,[7] breast metastases showed no predisposition to any single area of the spine. Pelvic tumors more often spread to the lumbar spine than tumors from elsewhere. Lung cancer demonstrated a slight tendency to spread to the thoracic spine.

Clinical Presentation of Epidural Metastasis

The dominant presenting clinical signs and symptoms of ESCC are pain, weakness, sensory loss, and autonomic disturbance; on rare occasions, ataxia is found. This pattern is similar among patients with different primary tumors.[7] The time course of these signs and symptoms is important for diagnosis as well as for predicting outcome.

PAIN

Pain is the most common initial complaint of both vertebral metastasis and ESCC. In cancer patients with symptoms and signs of spinal metastases, it is often difficult to distinguish those patients with vertebral metastasis alone from those with spinal cord compression. In a study of patients with symptoms of spinal metastases who were suspected of ESCC,[84] no single clinical symptom or sign, or index of symptoms and signs, could accurately distinguish between patients with metastatic cord compression and those with vertebral metastasis alone. Thus each patient with symptoms or signs of spinal metastases must be viewed as at risk for ESCC.

Pain generally occurs at the stage of irritation of the innervated spinal structures, before spinal cord or cauda equina compression occurs. The prognosis for continued ambulation is optimal if the diagnosis is made at this stage.

In their autopsy study, in which the patients were not examined directly by the authors, Barron and colleagues[4] reported back pain, radicular pain, or both as preceding signs of neurologic deficit in 82% of patients. Chade[67] reported radicular pain in 96% of 172 cases with ESCC referred to a neurosurgical clinic. In the London Hospital,[7] a somewhat lower incidence of pain was reported as the presenting manifestation, with 69% describing this complaint preceding neurological deficit. However, at the time of diagnosis of spinal cord compression, only 14% of patients denied pain. When pain was reported, it was described as axial (local) in 72% of cases, and radicular in 41%. There was no significant difference in the prevalence of pain between groups of patients with different primary tumor types.

In the MSKCC series,[5] pain was the presenting symptom in 96% of 130 cases of ESCC (Table 5–3). Pain was of an axial and/or radicular type. Radicular pain was found in 79% of cervical lesions, 55% of thoracic lesions, and 90% of lumbosacral lesions and was typically bilateral when it occurred in the thoracic region. Occasionally, local and radicular pain were misleading in localizing the level of spinal involvement. Of particular note, vertebral tenderness was reported in only 42 of 130 patients.[5] The London Hospital study[7] found no spinal tenderness in over 25% of

cases. These results are comparable to another study[85] in which findings on physical examination were correlated with spinal CT scanning. No spinal percussion tenderness was reported in seven of 20 patients with epidural extension of tumor from a vertebral metastasis. Thus, although it is often sought by clinicians, spinal tenderness is absent in many patients ultimately proven to have ESCC.

Pain of epidural spinal metastasis is often reported to be exacerbated by the Valsalva maneuver, neck flexion, and, less commonly straight-leg raising.[5] In addition, recumbency provokes pain in many patients.[4,5,86] At times, because the pain appears intermittent and exacerbated by activity, it may be considered secondary to a musculoligamentous strain or bony instability. Often the diagnosis of spinal cord compression is delayed because the complaint of pain, in the absence of other neurological signs, is attributed to arthritis, rheumatism, or neurosis.[1,4,10] As emphasized in Chapter 3, the finding of incidental osteoarthritis or degenerative joint disease on radiographs of the spine can be interpreted as confirming the incorrect clinical impression in these cases and can result in a delay in diagnosis of several months.[10]

The duration of pain prior to diagnosis of the spinal cord compression from different primary tumors had been analyzed in the London Hospital series.[7] On average, pain was present for 5 months (range 3 days to 3.8 years) prior to diagnosis. This duration was significantly shorter for spine metastases from lung cancer (mean, 4 months) than for metastases secondary to breast cancer (mean, 7 months). In the MSKCC series,[5] the median duration of pain was 2 months for all patients irrespective of their primary tumor. Similar results have been reported by others.[10]

Table 5–3. **Signs and Symptoms of Epidural Spinal Cord Compression in 130 Patients***

Sign/Symptom	First Symptom		Symptoms at Diagnosis	
	No.	%	No.	%
Pain	125	96	125	96
Weakness	2	2	99	76
Autonomic dysfunction	0	0	74	57
Sensory complaints	0	0	66	51
Ataxia	2	2	4	3
Herpes zoster	0	0	3	2
Flexor spasms	0	0	2	1

*From Gilbert, RW, et al.,[5] p. 42, with permission.

MOTOR LOSS

Although weakness may be the presenting complaint in some patients with metastatic ESCC, it much more commonly follows pain. For example, as shown in Table 5–3, only two of 130 patients in the MSKCC series[5] had weakness as the initial manifestation of cord compression. However, at the time of diagnosis, these authors reported subjective weakness in over 76% of patients and objective signs of weakness in 87%.

In the London Hospital series,[7] leg weakness was reported in 82% of patients at the time of diagnosis. According to the Medical Research Council scale, 24% of all patients were graded as 0–1/5 strength. Among patients with spinal metastasis from lung cancer, 40% were grade 0–1/5, compared with 16% of those with metastasis secondary to breast cancer. As the severity of neurological deficit at the time of diagnosis affects outcome, this difference may account for the worse prognosis experienced by patients with spine metastases from lung cancer than from breast cancer.

SENSORY LOSS

Although often present at the time of diagnosis, sensory loss is rare as a sole presenting manifestation of metastatic ESCC; it was not the presenting manifestation in any of the 600 patients with spinal metastasis reported by Constans and colleagues.[29] Although sensory disturbance was not the presenting complaint in any of the 130 patients from MSKCC,[5] numbness and paresthesias were reported at the time of diagnosis by 51% of patients (Table 5–3). On examination, sensory loss was found in 78% of the MSKCC group. Loss of pinprick sensibility was as frequent as loss of vibration and position sense.

In the London Hospital series,[7] sensory symptoms were present in the form of radicular complaints in 17% of patients. Numbness or tingling below the level of the lesion was present in 44%. A sensory level was found on physical examination in 72%. No difference was found in sensory symptoms or signs among patients with different primary tumors metastatic to the spine. Although generally there was a good correlation between the sensory level and the level of cord compression, misleading sensory levels were observed in this study and have been reported by others. For example, Barron and colleagues[4] reported cases of sacral sensory sparing

associated with extramedullary tumors, perhaps due to the collapse of intramedullary blood vessels as the tumor enlarges, causing patchy areas of infarction and demyelination, as has been shown pathologically.[34] The lamination of the lateral spinothalamic tracts is often responsible for an apparent ascending sensory level in patients with extramedullary neoplasms.

AUTONOMIC DISTURBANCES

As an initial and isolated finding, sphincter disturbances are infrequently the presenting manifestation of ESCC, unless the lesion is located at the conus medullaris or cauda equina.[5,87–90] Among the series of 600 patients reported by Constans and colleagues,[29] sphincter disturbances were the sole presenting complaint in only 2% of patients. Similarly, one of 127 patients reported by Barron and colleagues[4] presented with isolated incontinence several weeks in duration.

In the MSKCC series,[5] no patients presented with sphincter dysfunction alone. At the time of diagnosis, however, sphincter disturbances were present in 57% (Table 5–3). The only patients with sphincter disturbances without motor or sensory loss were those with lesions at T10–12 vertebral bodies. Sphincter disturbance was a poor prognostic indicator for continued ambulation after therapy.

Alternatively, patients with caudal tumors may present with bladder difficulties and impotence.[87,88] Large volumes of urine may be retained, with secondary overflow incontinence.

UNUSUAL CLINICAL MANIFESTATIONS

The Brown-Séquard syndrome (ipsilateral weakness and position/vibration loss and contralateral pain, and temperature dysfunction) is rare among patients with metastatic ESCC.[67] Only 2% of cases in the London Hospital series had a true Brown-Séquard syndrome.

Herpes zoster is commonly observed in patients suffering from cancer. Some authors have claimed that an eruption of zoster frequently will presage an episode of spinal cord compression at the same level. Among the 127 patients reported by Barron and colleagues,[4] seven had an eruption at the level of cord compression. In another series,[5] three of 130 patients were similarly affected. Others have not commented on the association.[7,29] Some authors consider that the virus in the dorsal root ganglion is activated by tumor invasion.[4,5]

Gait ataxia[91] and truncal ataxia[92] have been reported as rare presenting manifestations. Ataxia was the sole presenting symptom in 2% of cases in the MSKCC series and was present in an additional seven patients on examination.[5] The mechanism of gait ataxia was not secondary to position sense abnormalities; these were not significantly impaired. It may be secondary to compression of the spinocerebellar tracts and, when not associated with pain or signs of myelopathy, may suggest cerebellar or cerebral disease.

Laboratory Studies

CEREBROSPINAL FLUID ANALYSIS AND LUMBAR PUNCTURE

There is no specific information to be gained from CSF analysis that assists in the diagnosis of malignant ESCC. Therefore, lumbar puncture should not be performed to rule in or rule out this diagnosis. If infectious or neoplastic meningitis is suspected, CSF analysis is indicated, with close neurological observation following lumbar puncture and neurosurgical consultation when indicated.

Abnormalities in CSF in cases of malignant ESCC are nonspecific. Because the tumor is epidural, and not within the central nervous system per se, CSF findings differ from those in leptomeningeal cancer, in which malignant cells are present within the subarachnoid space. The CSF may be obtained from patients at the time of myelography. The protein content is typically elevated, as expected in cases of partial or complete spinal block. In the detailed London Hospital report,[7] of 56 CSF analyses the protein was below 40 mg per

dl in 9 cases, between 41 and 100 mg per dl in 11 cases, and above 100 mg per dl in 36 cases. In the study of Barron and colleagues,[4] the lowest CSF protein in the setting of a complete manometric block was 48 mg per dl. The highest protein levels were found in cases of epidural tumor in the region of the cauda equina, with one case showing a protein level greater than 2000 mg per dl. At higher spinal levels, the CSF protein did not correlate with the level of spinal cord compression or the primary tumor type.

The CSF cell count is usually normal; Barron and colleagues[4] found CSF pleocytosis in only one case, in a patient with an associated carcinomatosis of the leptomeninges. In the London Hospital[7] experience, CSF pleocytosis occurred in 7 of 56 patients, but only 2 had over 10 cells. This mild CSF pleocytosis may reflect inflammation from a parameningeal tumor or concomitant metastases involving the leptomeninges. Although these authors did not find malignant cells in the CSF of their patients, it is well known that the CSF cytology is positive in approximately 60% of patients with leptomeningeal invasion on the initial lumbar puncture.[93,94] The CSF glucose is typically normal in cases of malignant ESCC.

Lumbar puncture in the presence of increased intracranial pressure secondary to mass lesions may result in a cerebral and cerebellar herniation.[95,96] Similar risk of spinal herniation is a concern in patients harboring spinal tumors. Although not all investigators have had similar experiences,[4] some reports suggest that lumbar puncture may result in neurological deterioration in patients with extramedullary neoplasms.[97,98] For instance, Elsberg[40] believes that radicular pain and neurological disturbances worsen after the removal of spinal fluid in some patients with spinal tumors. He particularly notes that occasionally an indefinite sensory level becomes distinct after lumbar puncture is performed.[40]

A recent study[98] reviewed the risk of neurological deterioration below the level of a complete spinal subarachnoid block after lumbar puncture for myelography. In this retrospective series, 14% of 50 patients had significant neurological deterioration after lumbar puncture. No deterioration was observed in patients undergoing myelography via a cervical (C1–2) puncture. The mechanism for neurological deterioration following lumbar puncture is uncertain but is thought to be secondary to impaction of the spinal cord tumor, also known as spinal coning.[99] Elsberg[40] attributed it to removal of CSF, which acted as a buffer between the tumor and the spinal cord.

Despite these occasional reports, the risk is difficult to establish. There were no cases of clinical worsening that could be attributed to lumbar puncture in 72 patients reported in the series of Barron and colleagues.[4] No neurological worsening was reported after myelography in several series[5–7] composed of an accumulated several hundred patients. The advent of MRI precludes the need for myelography in most patients.

Diagnostic Imaging Studies

Radiological evaluation of patients with suspected spinal cord compression is changing because of rapid advances in imaging techniques. Plain radiography, radionuclide bone scanning, and myelography have been the standard techniques reported in large clinical studies, which form the basis of our current understanding of the problem. Both CT and MRI have now emerged as important imaging modalities for the evaluation of these patients.[11,85,100,101]

This section reviews selected reports concerning the value of various imaging techniques in the evaluation of metastatic spinal cord compression. Myelography was historically considered to be the gold standard; however, it has been replaced by less invasive MRI in most cases. Nevertheless, in those patients who cannot undergo MRI (such as those with aneurysm clips or pacemakers, those who cannot remain still during the procedure, or those patients in hospitals where MRI is not available), myelography remains a procedure of choice.

PLAIN RADIOGRAPHY

Plain radiography of the spine often is performed as an initial screening test in patients who may have metastatic ESCC, because epidural metastases usually extend from metastasis in the vertebra. Some of the abnormalities observed in patients with metastatic disease include osteolytic and/or osteoblastic lesions and collapse of vertebrae. Paravertebral soft tissue masses are also occasionally observed.

Plain radiographs of bone are very insensitive to the presence of metastatic disease because at least 50% of bone must be destroyed before a lesion is identified.[102] In a postmortem study of spinal metastases, Wong et al.[103] found that approximately 25% of lesions were not identified on plain radiographs. Furthermore, the radiological manifestations of metastatic disease are protean and require the interpretation of a skilled radiologist. The physician who has examined the patient should review the radiographs with the radiologist to provide clinical–radiological correlation.

The Barron series[4] provides information regarding the findings on plain radiographs of the spine in an era prior to the development of many of the newer imaging modalities. Overall, these authors found that 83% of patients with spine metastases complaining of back or radicular pain alone had roentgenographic signs of metastatic disease. The frequency of roentgenographic involvement varied among different primary tumors. In cases of spine metastasis secondary to carcinoma of the prostate, breast cancer, and multiple myeloma, abnormal plain radiographs were generally present even at the stage of pain before the development of neurological signs. Such was not the case, however, with lung cancer, lymphoma, and renal cancer, where normal plain radiographs, although still in the minority, were more common.

In the same series,[4] among patients with different primary tumor types, the frequency of solitary spinal metastasis was compared with multiple metastases. Carcinoma of the breast and multiple myeloma invariably were associated with several vertebral levels of involvement, whereas lung cancer, renal cancer, and lymphoma often demonstrated only a single level of metastasis on plain radiographs. Of the 109 cases available for plain radiograph analysis, the test did not accurately predict the level of involvement in 15 patients (14%); in eight, the epidural lesion was distant from the site of metastasis observed on plain radiograph; and in seven patients, the spine was too diffusely involved to define a level of epidural disease.

normal in patients with epidural spinal metastases, they cannot be relied upon confidently to rule in or rule out the presence of epidural tumor, or to design the radiation treatment port.

RADIONUCLIDE BONE SCANNING

Radionuclide bone scanning is more sensitive than plain radiography for visualizing skeletal metastases.[15] This additional sensitivity is gained at the expense of specificity, because other skeletal conditions such as degenerative joint disease may also cause abnormal scans. In patients with metastatic disease, this results in a false-positive rate of spine metastasis that has been reported to range from 20% to 74%;[109] plain radiographs, CT, or other techniques often are necessary to differentiate among these diagnoses. Occasionally, false-negative radionuclide scans also occur.[110]

In a series of patients with suspected vertebral column metastases,[6] an abnormal myelogram was found in 65% of those with abnormal bone scans, while an abnormal myelogram was found in 32% of those with normal bone scans. This study concluded that radionuclide bone scanning does not improve the accuracy of predicting the presence or absence of epidural tumor over that obtained by plain radiographs alone.

In a study[105] of patients with suspected spinal cord compression from breast cancer, radionuclide bone scans were positive in 100% of patients with myelographically proven epidural metastases; but in 90% of these cases, there were multiple levels of involvement. Among patients with negative myelograms, positive radionuclide bone scans were found in 47%. These studies indicate that radionuclide bone scanning, although more sensitive than plain radiographs of the spine, is inadequate to confirm or exclude the presence and level(s) of epidural spinal cord metastases.

MYELOGRAPHY

Although myelography has been largely superseded by magnetic resonance imaging for visualization of the spinal canal, the importance of imaging the spinal canal in patients at risk for harboring epidural tumor was established during the era of myelography. Since many of the same clinical principles apply in establishing indications for MRI, lessons learned from myelography studies will be presented.

The historical importance of myelography in evaluating and managing patients with suspected metastatic spinal cord compression already has been noted.[4,5,7,29,67,86] The arguments for myelography as outlined by Barron and colleagues[4] were as follows: (1) Plain radiographs may be normal in the presence of epidural tumor; (2) abnormalities on plain radiographs may be confused with osteoporosis or Paget's disease; and (3) other sites of epidural involvement may be present aside from those shown on plain radiographs.

These arguments have been supported by other clinical studies. In the MSKCC study,[5] myelography identified a complete block, or high-grade partial block in the absence of bony involvement, on routine studies in 15% of cases. Although myelography was performed in only 52% of cases reported from London Hospital,[7] it showed multiple levels of epidural involvement in 10% of all cases and 29% of cases secondary to breast cancer. Another study[111] showed that myelography may reveal the presence of spinal cord compression in the face of a normal neurological examination. Of 59 patients with radicular pain but no neurological deficit, 15 (25%) were found to have a complete spinal subarachnoid block on myelography.

Other studies[6,112,113] quantified the value of myelography in patients with suspected metastatic spinal cord compression. In a study by Rodichok et al.,[113] plain radiography correctly identified the level of spinal cord compression in only 13 of 18 (72%) patients presenting with myelopathy.[113] In a follow-up study, it was found that those patients diagnosed at an early stage of epidural disease were much more likely to remain ambulatory until death, compared with those diagnosed later in their course. These findings resulted in a subsequent detailed study of the role of myelography in cancer patients at risk for ESCC.[6] Patients were divided into five groups: group 1—myelopathy; group 2—radiculopathy; group 3—plexopathy; group 4—back pain with normal neurological examination and abnormal plain spine radiograph or bone scan; group 5—back pain with normal neurological examination and normal radiological studies.

Of 26 patients in group 1, 20 (77%) had abnormal myelograms. Of these 20, 19 had abnormal plain radiographs at the site of epidural tumor. Of the remaining six patients with negative myelograms, abnormal plain radiographs were found in two that could have resulted in radiation therapy of asymptomatic sites. The authors believed this to be potentially important because three of the six were thought to have radiation myelopathy that could have been exacerbated by further irradiation.

Of 43 patients with radiculopathy but no signs of spinal cord involvement (group 2), 27 (63%) had positive myelograms. When the plain radiographs were positive for metastatic disease at the clinical level of radiculopathy, the chance of epidural disease was 91%. When the plain radiographs were negative at the level of radiculopathy, 33% had evidence of epidural neoplasm on myelography. Of seven myelograms performed in group 3, one had an epidural defect.

Among 43 patients in group 4 (back pain with normal neurological examination and abnormal plain radiograph or bone scan), 63% had epidural tumor on myelogram. Of patients in group 5 (back pain, normal neurological examination, and normal plain radiographs/bone scan), none showed evidence of epidural tumor. Combining groups 4 and 5 yields a cohort of cancer patients presenting to their physician with nonradicular back pain and normal neurological examinations; based on the above data, of this large cohort 44% can be expected to have epidural tumor. Similarly, prior to radiological studies, the overall risk of epidural disease in those complaining of radicular pain with a normal neurological examination is 63%.

This detailed analysis underscores the importance of early diagnostic evaluation of cancer patients complaining of back pain and radicular pain. Given the above findings, the authors of the study[6] concluded that most cancer patients with back pain require myelography; prompt myelography was particularly recommended in patients with myelopathy and radiculopathy associated with normal plain radiographs or diffuse spinal metastases.

The above conclusions were supported by another study of the impact of myelography on radiotherapy of malignant spinal cord compression.[112] Patients with neurological deficits due to spinal cord compression were seen in consultation by a neurosurgeon, and plain radiographs of the spine were obtained. A mock radiation therapy port was then designed using clinical and plain radiography information. Additional information obtained by myelography was then used to evaluate the adequacy of the mock radiation therapy ports. They were found inadequate in 69% of cases.

When myelography is performed in patients suspected of ESCC, the entire spinal axis should be examined unless there is a contraindication. (The same is true for MRI.)[28,83,89] This approach permits the rostral and caudal extent of the block to be visualized and establishes whether multiple levels of metastatic involvement are present. This information is of value in determining radiation therapy ports and surgery, if planned.

COMPUTERIZED TOMOGRAPHY

Computed tomography has been demonstrated to be more sensitive and specific for identifying neoplasms of the vertebral column and paravertebral structures than bone scanning plain radiographs.[83,85,114–116] When used following myelography with water-soluble contrast material, CT has helped to locate an extension of tumor from vertebrae and paravertebral structures to the epidural space. For example, using spinal CT-myelograms in 30 patients harboring epidural metastases at[87] vertebral levels, Weissman and associates[116] have demonstrated that epidural tumor extension occurs via three mechanisms: (*1*) direct extension from metastasis to the adjacent vertebra (81%); (*2*) craniocaudal extension from tumor arising in vertebrae at rostral or caudal levels (17%); and (*3*) epidural extension from paravertebral tissues through the intervertebral foramina (2%).

Conversely, in one study 85 of 109 (78%) vertebrae with cortical disruption from tumor invasion extended epidurally as well.[116] However, the absence of cortical disruption at a single vertebral level could not exclude the presence of epidural disease at that level, since epidural tumor was observed in 21 of 183 vertebral levels at which no cortical disruption was present. In all but one of these cases, the epidural tumor was due to extension from craniocaudal levels or paravertebral tissues. The risk of craniocaudal extension in the epidural space was significant, with 20% of patients studied showing this phenomenon; 10% of patients with epidural tumor demonstrated craniocaudal extension of more than two vertebral levels. This is important therapeutically because standard radiotherapy ports using plain radiographs include two vertebral levels above and below the spinal metastasis. In this 10% of patients, however, the radiotherapy port would have been inadequate to encompass the entire epidural tumor. The authors stated, "This, coupled with our findings of a 38 percent incidence of synchronous noncontiguous epidural deposits, emphasizes the need for careful myelographic documentation of the extent of the tumor before instituting therapy."[116]

Despite the excellent bony detail afforded by spinal CT, the same authors found limitations in identifying the presence or absence of vertebral cortical disruption from tumor invasion, especially in cases of severe osteoporosis, which may make cortical margins indistinct, and in cases of osteoblastic metastases arising from carcinoma of the prostate. They suggested that in cases of suspected epidural tumor, patients with back pain, normal neurological examination, and evidence of metastases on plain radiographs should undergo myelography. In similar cases with normal or equivocal plain radiographs, they recommended spinal CT scanning. If evidence of vertebral cortical disruption is found on the CT scan, then the patient is referred for myelography. Due to its sensitivity in demonstrating paravertebral soft tissues, spinal CT may be the initial diagnostic study of choice in patients suspected of harboring paravertebral metastases with epidural extension.

In a later study, O'Rourke and colleagues[85] studied the value of spinal CT and spinal CT metrizamide myelography in detecting metastases in cancer patients with new spinal lesions on radionuclide bone scanning. Patients with an abnormality on bone scanning underwent plain radiographs of the spine. Group 1 consisted of patients with normal plain radiographs. Group 2 consisted of those with compression fracture on plain radiograph. Group 3 consisted of those with evidence of metastasis on plain radiographs.

Patients in group 1 underwent spinal CT. CT-myelography was performed in all patients in groups 2 and 3, and those in group 1 with cortical bone discontinuity. Using this algorithm, it was found that CT scanning of the spine could differentiate benign from malignant disease in most cases and that the presence of cortical bone discontinuity was associated with epidural tumor in 20 of 31 (64%) of cases. Unlike the previous study noted,[116] no mention was made of epidural tumor at levels other than those with cortical bone destruction.

O'Rourke and colleagues[85] recommended the following algorithm for the evaluation of spinal metastasis: Patients with abnormal bone scan or back pain and no neurological findings undergo plain spine radiographs and then spinal CT. If no metastases are found, no further workup is needed at that time; if spinal metastases are found but the cortical bone is intact, then a follow-up CT scan is performed in one month or as clinically indicated. If spinal metastasis with cortical bone discontinuity or soft tissue mass is observed, CT-myelography is recommended

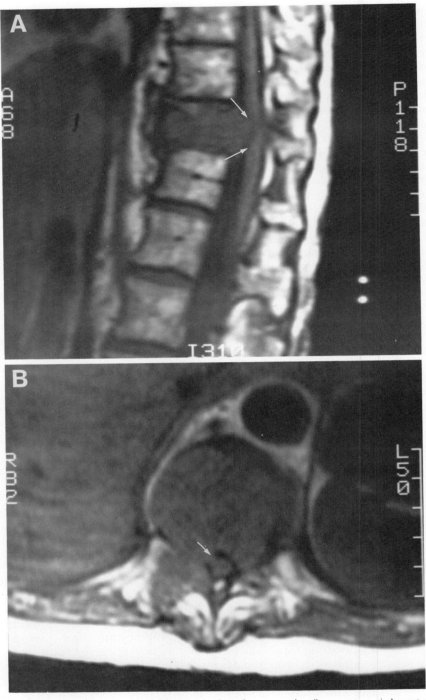

Figure 5–8. An MRI scan demonstrating epidural spinal cord compression from metastatic breast cancer to the vertebral column and epidural extension. (A) Sagittal view. (B) Axial view.

to rule out spinal cord compression. The authors indicate that cases of benign and malignant disease would be differentiated using this protocol. The authors did not address the issue of therapy in this study[85] but validated the usefulness of their clinical approach in a follow-up study.[117]

MAGNETIC RESONANCE IMAGING

Magnetic Resonance Imaging has become the procedure of choice for evaluating patients with suspected neoplastic epidural spinal cord compression.[118–121] Several studies have shown the advantage of MRI over myelography.[118,120–123] and CT.[119,124] Magnetic resonance imaging has been reported to be more sensitive than plain films and CT scanning in detecting vertebral metastases.[119] With the advent of contrast-enhanced MRI with gadolinium, its role and value in the evaluation and management of these patients are further increased.[125,126] The principles in the section on myelography above apply to the use of MRI to image the spinal canal directly in evaluating patients with suspected metastatic disease. Figures 5–8 and 5–9 provide examples of the excellent imaging potential of MRI for ESCC.

In an early study of noncontrast MRI of the spine, MRI appeared more sensitive than radionuclide bone scanning in the detection of vertebral metastases.[101] In another study[124] of tumors involving the osseous spine, MRI was compared to CT scanning in defining the anatomic relationships of the tumor, vertebral column, spinal canal, paravertebral tissues, and vascular involvement; MRI was found superior to CT without intrathecal contrast injection and equal to CT with contrast. The CT without contrast was found superior to MRI in detecting cortical bone destruction due to the poor signal intensity of cortical bone with MRI.[127]

In another study, spinal MRI was performed in 58 patients with epidural metastases and compared with myelography in 22 of these patients.[123] In 60 of 64 studies performed in 58 patients, MRI was found to be diagnostic. In the 22 patients undergoing both procedures, myelography was diagnostic in 20 studies and MRI yielded the same diagnosis in 19 of 22 cases. The authors concluded that when a technically satisfactory MRI study can be obtained, it is equivalent to myelography or CT-myelography in detecting clinically significant epidural disease. In the same

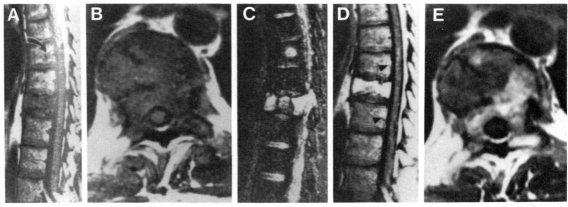

Figure 5–9. Gadolinium-enhanced MRI of the spine of a 36-year-old patient with a plasmacytoma. (A) and (B) Sagittal (A) and axial (B) images showing partial collapse of the T10 vertebral body and replacement of normal high-intensity bone marrow with low-intensity tumor. In addition, a poorly defined hypointense focus is seen in the T8 vertebral body (arrow, A). (C) T_2-weighted images show both lesions. (D) and (E) After the administration of contrast, the T_1-weighted sagittal (D) and axial (E) images show enhancement of the T10 vertebral body. The previously prominent hypointense region of tumor in T8 is not easily seen, due to the fact that it is isointense with the remainder of the vertebral body on this enhanced study. The axial scan (E) shows greater enhancement on the left than the right side of the vertebral body. Although tumor may permeate the entire vertebral body, results of multiple biopsy attempts on the right side were negative, whereas results of biopsy attempts on the left revealed tumor. (From Sze, G, et al,[126] with permission.)

study, the authors found T_1-weighted images optimal for demonstrating spinal cord compression, whereas T_2-weighted images were best for identifying subarachnoid space compression without cord impingement. Furthermore, paravertebral masses that would have been missed on myelography were recognized with MRI. Finally, because a spinal MRI requires 60–90 minutes, compared with the two hours required for myelography or CT myelography, patients seemed to tolerate the MRI better. It should be recognized, however, that movement artifact degrades the quality of MRI images; because patients with spinal metastases are often in pain, especially when lying supine, pain control as well as claustrophobia remains problematic with MRI. Finally, the authors note that the cost of a spinal MRI examination in most institutions is equal to or less than a myelogram followed by CT.

In a comparison study of myelography and MRI among 36 patients, three patients were found to have metastatic deposits on myelography that were not seen on MRI.[120] There were no metastases seen with MRI that were not identified with myelography. However, this study did not use contrast-enhanced MRI, and it was a relatively early study during the MRI era. Accordingly, with the refinements in MRI since its publication in 1992, it is difficult to conclude from this study that myelography is superior to MRI.

With the advent of contrast-enhanced MRI with gadolinium-DTPA, the value of MRI is further increased.[125,126] Sze and colleagues have reported that some regions of epidural tumor demonstrate marked enhancement, while other areas show minimal or no enhancement.[126] These authors[126] conclude that contrast-enhanced MRI is helpful in delineating and characterizing some epidural neoplasms when compared with precontrast MRI scans. However, in some cases, lesions that are hypointense on noncontrast MRI become isointense with surrounding bone following the administration of gadolinium-DTPA, decreasing the ability to detect these epidural metastases (Fig. 5–9).

Although the detection of vertebral and epidural neoplasms may be obscured by contrast administration, contrast-enhanced MRI scans may be very useful in the evaluation of patients with suspected epidural tumor. Gadolinium administration may help differentiate epidural tumor from disc herniation because herniated disc material should not enhance immediately following contrast administration, unlike tumor.[125] Furthermore, contrast-enhanced scans may demonstrate areas of active tumor involvement more readily than noncontrast studies. In patients with diffuse metastases, biopsy of enhancing areas of vertebral involvement resulted in a greater yield than biopsy of nonenhancing abnormal regions.[125] Gadolinium also may reveal specific areas of spinal cord compression more readily than noncontrast studies alone.[125,126] In addition, contrast administration may have a role in evaluating response to therapy. Preliminary studies suggest that successfully treated bone metastases do not enhance with gadolinium, whereas unresponsive metastases continue to enhance.[125,126]

Clinical Approach to the Patient Suspected of Spinal Metastasis

Cancer patients with clinical evidence of spinal metastases fall into three groups: (1) patients with back or neck pain with or without referred or radicular pain; (2) those with mild, stable, or equivocal evidence of spinal cord compression; and (3) patients with new or rapidly progressive symptoms and/or signs of spinal cord compression (As elsewhere in this chapter, the terms myelopathy and spinal cord compression include cauda equina dysfunction and compression). The goal of diagnosis is to recognize those patients with spinal metastases before neurological abnormalities arise, because the outcome of therapy is so much more favorable in the first two groups.[5,128] No single approach or algorithm can apply to all patients or supersede clinical judgment;[129] because circumstances often require that the approach be modified for individual cases, the following is only a guide to the workup.

In cancer patients with back or neck pain and normal neurologic examinations who are not suspected of harboring ESCC, many physicians initially obtain a radionuclide bone scan and plain spine radiograph. If these studies reveal findings that explain the patient's symptoms (e.g., vertebral metastasis at the level of pain), many medical oncologists and radiotherapists treat with systemic agents and/or radiotherapy without further diagnostic studies. In such cases, it must be recognized that clinically unsuspected epidural metastases may be present at the level of the known vertebral metastasis, adjacent to it, or at a distant vertebral level. Therefore, it is important to follow the patient's clinical course carefully and proceed with MRI or, if MRI is unavailable, myelography if neurological signs consistent with spinal cord compression develop.

Alternatively, because many cancer patients with back and/or projected pain and normal neurological examinations harbor clinically unsuspected ESCC, many physicians recommend spinal MRI in planning therapy.[83] If MRI is unavailable or cannot be performed, a plain radiograph of the spine may identify vertebral metastases. According to one study, if the plain radiograph shows greater than 50% collapse of the vertebra due to metastasis, there is a nearly 90% risk of epidural tumor; if there is pedicle erosion, epidural tumor may be found in approximately 30% of patients; only 7% had epidural tumor if the metastasis was restricted to the vertebral body without collapse.[130] Thus, MRI (or myelography, if MRI is unavailable) may be selected in those patients with a positive plain radiograph or in those who have a significant risk of epidural extension. If a radiograph is negative for metastases or shows limited involvement, spinal CT scanning of the symptomatic areas may be performed next. Those patients with CT scans that are negative for metastases and in whom there is a low clinical suspicion for epidural tumor are next considered for lumbar puncture to evaluate for leptomeningeal metastases. Alternatively, MRI is still recommended in cancer patients with a negative CT scan for metastasis but in whom there is a high clinical suspicion for epidural tumor, or for those with CT scans that are positive for vertebral metastases with cortical disruption bordering the vertebral canal or paraspinal mass.[117] All patients with spine metastases should undergo careful follow-up to identify neurological deterioration that might lead to consideration of other options for treatment.

For cancer patients with mild, stable, or equivocal symptoms and/or signs of spinal cord compression, a total spine MRI (if available) is performed. If MRI is unavailable, then an immediate radiograph of the spine is performed, followed by total spine myelography by the next day. Total spine studies are performed because some patients will have unsuspected metastases at multiple levels. During their evaluation, patients in this group should be closely observed to identify progressive myelopathy. Cancer patients with new or rapidly progressive signs of spinal cord compression should be given high-dose intravenous dexamethasone[116] (see page 190) to reduce spinal cord edema[44] and reduce the risk of spinal coning.[98] Then an immediate total spine MRI or myelogram is performed.

Because spinal MRI and myelography occasionally yield false-negative results in cases of spinal cord compression, the physician often must consider other diagnostic studies following a negative MRI or myelogram in the cancer patient with a myelopathy. For example, if the noncontrast spinal MRI is negative, the physician should consider a contrast-enhanced spinal MRI and CSF analysis to identify leptomeningeal metastases (see Chapter 7). Myelography should still be considered when clinical suspicion of a compressive lesion remains but none is identified on the spinal MRI; in such cases, CSF may be obtained for analysis at the time of myelography. Because neurologic deterioration may occur following myelography, neurosurgical consultation should be available.[98] Finally, contrast-enhanced MRI may demonstrate intramedullary metastases not observed on either myelography or plain MRI.

Therapy

CORTICOSTEROIDS AND RADIATION THERAPY

Metastatic epidural spinal cord compression is most commonly treated with corticosteroids and radiation therapy; selected patients undergo surgical decompression.[83] Corticosteroids have been found to reduce vasogenic spinal cord edema[44] and to usually help control pain and improve neurological function. The dosage and form of corticosteroid vary.[131] A randomized trial of high-dose corticosteroids, using 96 mg of dexamethasone daily (compared to placebo), demonstrated improved neurologic outcome in patients receiving the high-dose corticosteroid.[132] This improved efficacy may, however, be accomplished with a higher incidence of corticosteroid side effects. In a single institution historical case–control study comparing high-dose dexamethasone with moderate-dose dexamethasone, serious side effects were reported among 14% of the high-dose group compared to 0% in the moderate-dose group (total side effects were 29% and 8%, respectively.[133] Loblaw and Laperriere[134] evaluated the literature and found good evidence for the use of high-dose dexamethasone in treating patients with clinical signs of neurological dysfunction secondary to metastatic epidural spinal cord compression undergoing radiation therapy. A trial directly comparing high- and moderate-dose dexamethasone does not exist. Accordingly, doses of 10–100 mg of dexamethasone IV (intravenously) given immediately, followed by 4–24 mg qid, are often used. The lower doses are used for patients with mild pain and no, or equivocal, signs of myelopathy; the highest doses are used in patients with prominent, or rapidly progressive, myelopathy. Occasional patients will report pain or burning in the perineal region when high-dose corticosteroids are administered intravenously.

In general, the tapering of high-dose steroids is begun within 48–72 hours, and patients are followed closely for signs of steroid-induced complications such as glucose intolerance and infection. As the steroids are tapered, patients are observed for deterioration in neurological function, and the dose is increased if this occurs. Many patients can be tapered off steroids within two to three weeks.[116]

Radiation therapy has become the primary mode of treatment of metastatic ESCC because patients often harbor widespread metastatic disease and are poor surgical candidates. When radiotherapy is selected for treatment, it should commence as soon as the diagnosis of metastatic ESCC is established. The upper and lower extent of the epidural neoplasm should be defined by imaging studies so that the entire area of cord compression and epidural tumor can be treated. Because epidural metastases may occur at multiple levels, the entire rostrocaudal spinal axis is usually imaged with MRI (or myelography). In addition to identifying all levels of ESCC, this strategy allows the design of radiotherapy ports that include adjacent asymptomatic metastatic epidural deposits. If these adjacent epidural metastases are not included in the original treatment field and later require radiotherapy, the amount of radiation tolerated may be limited by overlapping spinal radiotherapy ports.

The prognosis for patients undergoing radiotherapy for metastatic ESCC depends upon their neurological function at the time treatment begins. In a study of metastatic spine disease with radiographic spinal cord compression but no clinical signs of myelopathy, Maranzano et al.[135,136] found that all patients remained ambulatory following treatment. Patients with neurological signs but who are ambulatory at the time of diagnosis usually retain this ability following radiotherapy. However, only about half of patients who are paraparetic at presentation regain ambulation, and paraplegic patients rarely are restored to ambulation with radiotherapy.[5]

SURGERY

Surgical decompression of metastatic ESCC has, until recently, consisted of laminectomy. However, several retrospective stud-

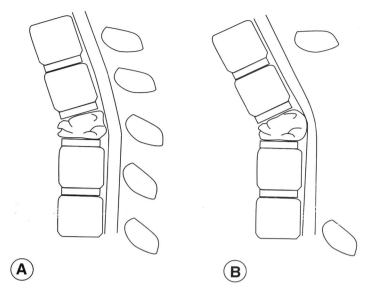

Figure 5–10. Resection of the lamina spinous processes and intervening ligaments (all are components of the spine that function as a tension band, preventing kyphosis in a checkrein manner) via laminectomy in the face of a ventral tumor (A) may result in further spinal cord compression or distortion. Kyphotic spinal deformation (kyphosis) is also a possible result. (B). Spinal stability may, therefore, be significantly threatened as well.

ies and one prospective study have shown that laminectomy followed by radiation therapy is not superior to radiation therapy alone.[5,137,138] Alternatively, because the metastatic tumor is usually ventral to the spinal cord in the vertebral body, a surgical approach consisting of vertebral body resection followed by stabilization has been reported with promising results.[135,139,140] Carefully selected paraparetic and paraplegic patients have been reported to ambulate following this surgical approach.[141,142] There have been no randomized controlled studies to compare

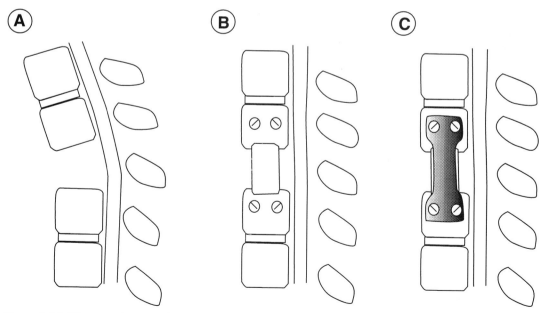

Figure 5–11. The ventral approach to a vertebral body lesion can achieve a ventral decompression (A) and augment stability. Stability and deformity correction were achieved following placement of a screw (for distraction and extension) and an interbody strut (B), followed by a plate (C).

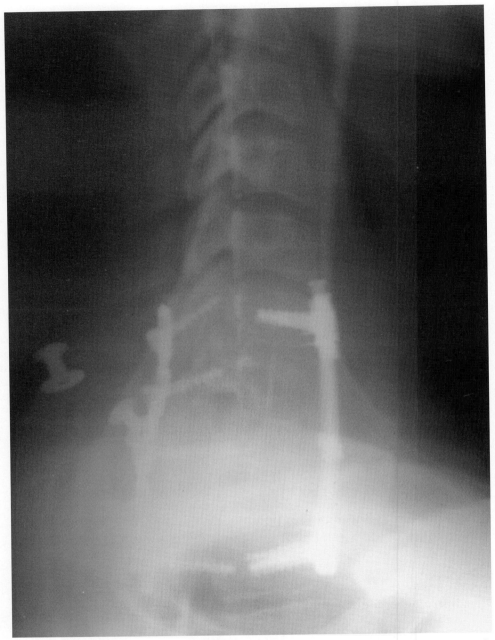

Figure 5–12. Spinal stability may be so inadequate that a combination ventral and dorsal operation may be warranted for stability purposes alone. Long instrumentation constructs (as depicted) provide multiple sites for attachment to the spine, as well as long lever arms that facilitate the acquisition of stability (also see Fig. 5–14).

ventral vertebral body resection with radiotherapy alone.

The indications for surgical decompression of metastatic ESCC are evolving and are case-dependent.[134] Surgical decompression should be considered in (*1*) patients without a diagnosis; (*2*) patients who are neurologically deteriorating due to spinal cord compression, who have been previously irradiated at the site of spinal cord compression, and whose medical condition permits surgery; and (3) those with progressive neurological deterioration during radiation therapy. Surgery is also considered for patients in whom the tumor is restricted in location and considered resectable or when the spine is unstable.[135,143–147] In addition, intractable pain and radio-resistant tumors are considered indications for surgical decompression in selected cases.

The unique nature of each individual case cannot be overemphasized. The studies that have been unable to demonstrate an advantage following surgical decompression[5,137,138] have used a dorsal approach (laminectomy) for their surgical paradigm. Although dorsal approaches may be appropriate in select cases, their utility is greatest in dorsal tumors without instability. This type of tumor is, indeed, an uncommon occurrence. Most compressive lesions are ventrally situated with respect to the dural sac. Furthermore, spinal stability is often suspect. When this is the case, laminectomy may further exacerbate the stability problem by removing dorsal elements that normally function as a tension band, preventing kyphotic deformation. In this situation, lack of neurologic improvement can be theoretically attributed to (1) ineffective decompressions and/or (2) exaggerated instability associated with kyphotic deformation (Fig. 5–10).

Ventral decompression with stabilization (interbody strut with instrumentation), in turn, can accomplish an effective decompression, as well as spinal stabilization (Fig. 5–11). In cases where significant instability exists, combination ventral and dorsal procedures may be warranted. Finally, long instrumentation constructs may be warranted if significant instability exists or if bony instrumentation purchase sites have been rendered ineffective via tumor involvement (Fig. 5–12).

It is clear that the decision-making process for spinal metastasis must be patient-specific. The aforementioned considerations, as well as results of the neurologic exam, life expectancy, and medical considerations, must be carefully taken into account.

PRIMARY EPIDURAL TUMORS

As indicated earlier, primary epidural spinal tumors arise from cellular elements that normally form the vertebral column and supporting structures. Their frequency is estimated to be approximately three times less than that of spinal metastases.[10] Their neurological presentation is similar to that of metastatic neoplasms: Pain is the prominent first complaint, followed by symptoms and signs of neural compression. The more common primary epidural spinal tumors are briefly reviewed (Table 5–5).

Multiple Myeloma

Multiple myeloma, a plasma cell neoplasm that proliferates in bone marrow, is the most common primary tumor of bone.[3] The neoplastic cells usually secrete an immunoglobulin protein. The disease is often associated with skeletal destruction, hypercalcemia, immunodeficiency, and impaired renal function. It generally affects older individuals (median age, seventh decade) but may affect those much younger.[148] Osteosclerotic myeloma, a rare variant, may be associated with polyneuropathy, organomegaly, endocrinopathy, and M protein and skin changes (POEMS syndrome).[149,150]

Epidural spinal cord compression is the most common neurological complication of multiple myeloma; it occurs in approximately 10% to 15% of cases.[4,151] The clinical presentation is similar to that of metastatic deposits.[4] In addition to ESCC,

Table 5–5. **Selected Primary Epidural Spinal Tumors**

Multiple myeloma
Osteogenic sarcoma
Chordoma
Chondrosarcoma
Ewing's sarcoma
Fibrous histiocytoma
Giant cell tumor
Benign tumors

neurological involvement[151] includes a variety of different forms of peripheral neuropathy[149,152] that may, at times, be difficult to differentiate from spinal root involvement.

The myeloma cell causes bone resorption through an osteoclast-activating factor.[126] Vertebral bodies often demonstrate osteolytic defects without reactive bone formation.[3,153] Vertebral body involvement typically occurs before the pedicles are invaded because there is normally less red marrow in the pedicles.[154,155] Radiographs may show a solitary sclerotic vertebra (ivory vertebra). Radionuclide bone scans are often unremarkable; conventional radiographs have been found to be more sensitive.[153,156] Computed tomography, myelography, and MRI may show the spinal and epidural involvement by tumor.

Multiple myeloma is usually radiosensitive and most patients with ESCC can be treated with corticosteroids and radiotherapy, as in the therapy of metastatic epidural tumors. Its diagnosis by history, laboratory, and imaging studies is, therefore, of extreme importance. Risky surgical procedures may be appropriately avoided.

Osteogenic Sarcoma

Osteogenic sarcoma is the second most common primary bone tumor. It usually occurs in childhood and adolescence. But it has a second peak of incidence in later life, often occurring in association with Paget's disease, previously irradiated bone, or other predisposing factors.[157-161] It may arise from transformation of an osteoblastoma or osteochondroma.[3,162]

The spine is a rare site of primary involvement, but it is a frequent site of metastatic spread from a primary osteogenic sarcoma elsewhere.[3,159,163-165] Pain is the most common initial complaint; in the Mayo Clinic series,[2] pain was usually present for several months, but ranged from 2 1/2 weeks to 2 years. Neurological signs of spinal cord compression were often found. Serum alkaline phosphatase is elevated in approximately one-

half of all patients.[158] Among other abnormalities, radiographic studies often demonstrate both lytic and blastic changes of bone.[3,158] The histological appearance can be variable and correlation of the clinical history, physical examination, and radiographic features can be very helpful in diagnosis and treatment planning.[2,3]

The treatment of osteogenic sarcoma has undergone major advances in recent years. In addition to surgery, developments in radiation therapy and chemotherapy have altered the management of this disease. There are several chemotherapy protocols that have been used for primary and metastatic disease.[158]

Chordoma

A chordoma is a rare neoplasm that arises from notochordal remnants of the spine and shows a predilection for the sacrococcygeal area (50%) and base of the skull (35%); the remaining cases are found elsewhere in the vertebral column.[158,166,167] Patients are usually over 30 years old. Although chordomas may metastasize, the high morbidity and mortality of this neoplasm are due to frequent local recurrence, the most common cause of death.[168,169] One review of the literature[170] found only 1% of 222 patients disease-free at ten years.

The most common early symptom is pain. As the tumor grows, neural structures are involved; when it occurs in the sacrococcygeal region, bowel and bladder symptoms and saddle anesthesia may occur. The duration of symptoms varies between two weeks and nine years and averages more than one year.[171] With sacrococcygeal chordomas, a presacral mass may be palpable on rectal examination. When the tumor occurs at other levels of the spine, it causes radicular and spinal cord symptoms and signs similar to those of other epidural tumors. Radiographically, there are a variety of different appearances.[172] The lesion may be osteolytic, osteoblastic, or contain both elements, or, at times, plain radiographs may show no abnormalities.[2] Diagnosis is established by biopsy.

Surgery is the primary therapy for chordomas. Many patients benefit from repeated surgical resections that are performed because the tumor recurs. In addition, radiation therapy may cause tumor regression that lasts for many years.[173] Proton beam radiation therapy may be especially effective in controlling local disease.[158] Postoperative radiation therapy has been recommended in many cases of incomplete surgical resection.[173]

Chondrosarcoma

Chondrosarcomas are cartilaginous neoplasms that arise in bone but lack direct osteoid formation.[158] Chondrosarcomas may arise de novo in bone, follow irradiation of bone, or develop in patients with preexisting Paget's disease or who have benign cartilage tumors such as osteochondroma or endochondromas.[3,174] They generally occur in individuals over 30 years of age; fewer than 5% occur in patients under 30.[2,130,167,175,176]

Chondrosarcomas typically occur in long bones or the pelvis but may occur in the vertebral column. Initially, they tend to involve the vertebral bodies more frequently than the vertebral arch.[3] The initial symptom of spinal chondrosarcoma is usually pain; in the Mayo Clinic series, the period of pain ranged from 2 weeks to 11 years, but symptoms often persisted for 4–5 years prior to diagnosis.[2] As the epidural tumor grows, neural compression develops, and symptoms and signs of radiculopathy and myelopathy referable to the level occur. Although they are highly unpredictable in their biological behavior, chondrosarcomas may become quite extensive locally before metastases appear. Radiographically, the lesions may appear as lytic lesions associated with lobular calcifications, but other appearances have been described[3,158]

Surgical resection is the treatment of choice for chondrosarcoma. Repeated surgical resections are often helpful for recurrent disease.[3] These tumors are relatively radioresistant, but radiotherapy may delay progression of the disease.[158]

Ewing's Sarcoma

Ewing's sarcoma is a rare, primitive round-cell tumor of bone usually occurring in childhood, adolescence, or early adult life.[177] This tumor usually arises in long bones, but it also may (rarely) originate in the vertebral column. Since it frequently metastasizes to bone, spinal involvement more often is due to a metastasis from a primary site elsewhere than to a primary Ewing's sarcoma of the spine.[175,178] When the tumor arises in the axial skeleton, the sacrum is the most common site of origin.[179]

Pain is the most frequent initial complaint and often may be present for a few months, although much shorter courses have also been noted.[2,3] Neurological abnormalities referable to radicular and spinal cord dysfunction usually follow. Imaging studies may reveal a variety of different appearances (Fig. 5–13).[2,172,180] On histological study, a variety of patterns may be observed.[2,181] The use of radiation therapy and chemotherapy has dramatically improved the prognosis for patients with Ewing's sarcoma.[177]

Benign Tumors and Tumor-like Conditions

Symptomatic primary benign bone tumors of the spine are unusual and are rare causes of spinal cord compression. For example, vertebral hemangiomas have been found in approximately 10% of routine autopsies,[2,3,182,183] but they are rarely symptomatic. However, when benign vertebral tumors do become symptomatic, they often present with pain and thus must be considered in the differential diagnosis of patients with axial and radicular pain. The more common neoplasms and tumor-like conditions include osteochondroma or exostosis,[184–187] osteoid osteoma,[188–190] osteoblastoma (Fig. 5–14),[188,189,191] giant-cell tumors,[192–194] fibrous dysplasia,[195] eosinophilic granuloma,[196] hemangioma, and aneurysmal bone cysts[197,198] (Fig. 5–15). In addition, spinal cord compression secondary to ex-

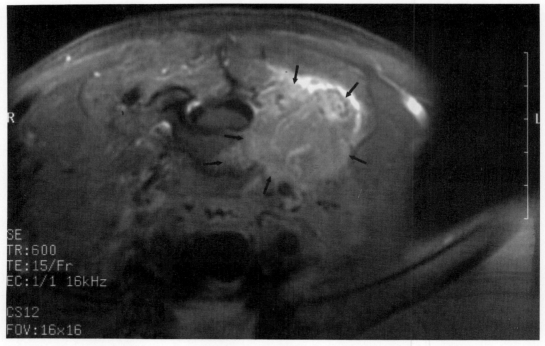

Figure 5–13. A cervicothoracic junction axial T_1-weighted MRI demonstrating a recurrent Ewing's sarcoma in a teenager who had previously undergone a laminectomy. The invasive nature of the tumor is seen.

tramedullary hematopoiesis[199–201,202] has been described in cases of myelofibrosis, sideroblastic anemia, sickle cell anemia, thalassemia, and other myeloproliferative disorders. Furthermore, epidural lipomatosis in the setting of Cushing's disease or corticosteroid administration also may cause spinal cord compression.[203–205]

The radiographic appearance may suggest the diagnosis, as in the case of osteochondroma[206] or hemangioma.[3,207] Tissue confirmation may be necessary in some cases. When neural compression occurs secondary to an expanding mass or collapse of the vertebral body, the symptoms and signs are similar to those of other epidural tumors.

Lipoma

Spinal lipomas are primary tumors of the spinal canal that may be part of the dysraphic state (developmental). Less commonly, they may exist as an isolated neoplasm. The former exist as an element of multiple congenital anomalies and may be associated with a subcutaneous palpable soft-tissue mass and abnormal fusion of the vertebrae (Fig. 5–16).[208–210] Those lipomas that occur as isolated tumors may be either intradural or extradural; they are discussed in more detail in Chapter 6. Such isolated intradural and extradural lipomas account for approximately 1% of all primary spinal neoplasms.[211] One study[212] found that of nondevelopmental spinal lipomas, two-fifths were epidural and three-fifths were intradural.

Extradural lipomas affect both sexes equally and may present at any age.[211] Unlike intradural lipomas, which typically have a prolonged history of symptoms prior to diagnosis, extradural lipomas usually have a duration of symptoms lasting less than one year.[211] Although any segmental level may be involved, the thoracic spine appears to be the most common site.[211] There is no characteristic constellation of clinical symptoms or signs that distinguishes epidural spinal lipomas

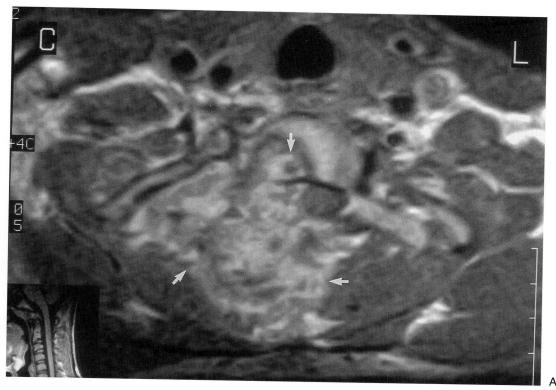

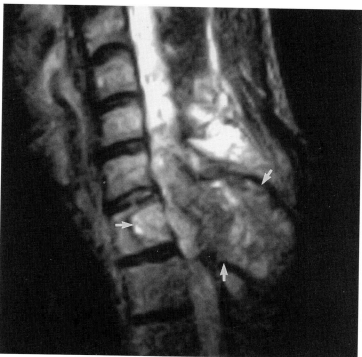

Figure 5–14. A 19-year-old male presented with progressive myelopathy and left arm pain. An MRI demonstrated both ventral and dorsal spinal column involvement with a tumor that was confined to the bony vertebral body in the cervicothoracic region. Axial (A) and sagittal (B) views demonstrate the extent of involvement (arrows). The lesion was resected via a staged dorsal and ventral operation (see Fig. 5–12). The tumor was very vascular and was shown to be an osteoblastoma histologically.

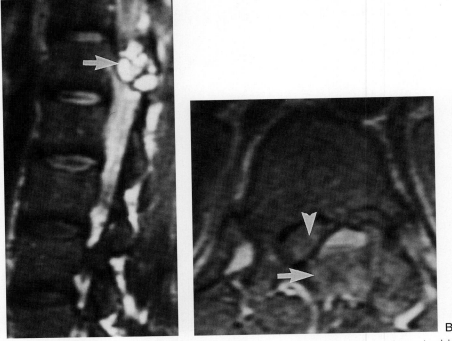

Figure 5–15. An MRI of the thoracolumbar spine demonstrating an aneurysmal bone cyst (arrow) arising from the T12 pedicle and causing spinal cord compression (arrowhead). (A) Sagittal view. (B) Axial view.

from many other epidural tumors. In one review,[211] no bony changes were observed on plain radiographs in two-thirds of cases. Surgery is the treatment of choice.[210, 211] Epidural lipomas must be differentiated from steroid-induced lipomatosis, which may cause spinal cord compression.[203,204,213]

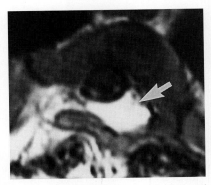

Figure 5–16. An MRI of the upper thoracic spine reveals an epidural lipoma (arrow) posterior to the spinal cord and associated with a vertebral anomaly.

SUMMARY

Metastatic epidural tumors compressing the spinal cord or cauda equina are one of the most frequent spinal diseases and neurologic complications of cancer encountered in practice. Metastatic epidural tumors typically begin as metastases to the vertebral column with secondary extension into the epidural space that causes neural compression. As discussed in this chapter, of the approximate 400,000 individuals dying from cancer each year in the United States, it is estimated that between 60,000 and 160,000 develop vertebral column metastases. Of this group approximately, 20,000 develop spinal cord or cauda equina compression. If these individuals are diagnosed and treated before they develop neurologic signs, most will enjoy continued ambulation. Alternatively, if the diagnosis and treatment do not begin until they lose the ability to ambulate only a minority will ever walk again.

This chapter has reviewed the mechanisms of cancer metastasis, including the propensity of some tumors to metastasize to the spine through Batson's plexus. The most common tumors, including lung, breast, and prostate cancer, are also discussed, which may help the clinician workup a primary tumor when confronted with a patient with an epidural neoplasm as an initial manifestation of malignancy.

Most importantly, the clinical presentation, which nearly always includes pain before the development of neurologic signs, is discussed. The symptom of increased pain on recumbency, which is common with epidural tumors and yet atypical of degenerative disc disease, is noted. A diagnostic imaging approach is presented for patients at risk for epidural metastases, and MRI is the imaging test of choice. Decisions regarding the length of spine which requires imaging are discussed in detail in the section on the clinical approach to the the patient suspected of spinal metastases. Finally, management issues once the diagnosis is confirmed, including corticosteroids, radiation therapy, and surgery, are presented.

Primary epidural spinal tumors, which are far less frequent than metastatic disease, are briefly reviewed at the end of the chapter. Since these tumors generally present with spine disease, they usually require open surgery or biopsy for diagnosis, unlike cases of metastatic disease where the histologic diagnosis is often already established. Decisions regarding radiation therapy and chemotherapy are beyond the scope of this book and the reader is referred to appropriate oncologic texts and journals.

REFERENCES

1. Arseni CN, Simionescu MD, Horwath L. Tumors of the spine: a follow-up study of 350 patients with neurosurgical considerations. *Acta Psychiat Scand* 1959;34:398–410.
2. Cohen DM, Dahlin DC, MacCarty CS. Apparently solitary tumors of the vertebral column. *Mayo Clin Proc* 1964;39:509–28.
3. Friedlander GE, Southwick WO. Tumors of the spine. In Rothman RH, Simeone FA, editors. *The Spine* Philadelphia: W.B. Saunders; 1982; pp. 1022–40.
4. Barron KD, Hirano A, Araki S, et al. Experiences with metastatic neoplasms involving the spinal cord. *Neurology* 1959;9:91–106.
5. Gilbert RW, Kim JH, Posner JB. Epidural spinal cord compression from metastatic tumor: diagnosis and treatment. *Ann Neurol* 1978;3:40–51.
6. Rodichok LD, Ruckdeschel JC, Harper GR, et al. Early detection and treatment of spinal epidural metastases: the role of myelography. *Ann Neurol* 1986;20:696–702.
7. Stark RJ, Henson RA, Evans SJW. Spinal metastases: a retrospective survey from a general hospital. *Brain* 1982;105:189–213.
8. Lewis DW, Packer RJ, Raney B, et al. Incidence, presentation, and outcome of spinal cord disease in children with systemic cancer. *Pediatrics* 1986;78:438–42.
9. Alter M. Statistical aspects of spinal cord tumors. In Vinken PJ, Bruyn GW, editors. *Handbook of Clinical Neurology, Volume 19*. Amsterdam: North-Holland; 1975; pp. 1–22.
10. Paillas J-E, Alliez B, Pellet W. Primary and secondary tumours of the spine. In Vinken PJ, Bruyn GW, editors. *Handbook of Clinical Neurology, Volume 20*. Amsterdam: North-Holland; 1976; pp. 19–54.
11. Graif M, Steiner RE. Contrast-enhanced magnetic resonance imaging of tumours of the central nervous system: a clinical review. *Br J Radiol* 1986;59:865–73.
12. Abrams HL, Spiro R, Goldstein N. Metastases in carcinoma. Analysis of 1000 autopsied cases. *Cancer* 1950;3:74–85.
13. Stein RJ. "Silent" skeletal metastases in cancer. *Am J Clin Pathol* 1943;13:34–41.
14. Young JM, Funk FJ. Incidence of tumor metastasis to the lumbar spine: a comparative study of roentgenographic changes and gross lesions. *J Bone Joint Surg* 1953;35-A:55–64.
15. Galasko CSB. The development of skeletal metastases. In Weiss L, Gilbert HA, editors. *Bone Metastasis* Boston: G.K. Hall; 1981; pp. 83–113.
16. Miller F, Whitehall R. Carcinoma of the breast metastatic to skeleton. *Clin Orthop* 1984;184:121–7.
17. Nielsen O, Munro A, Tannock J. Bone metastases: pathophysiology and management policy. *J Clin Oncol* 1991;9:509–24.
18. Onuigbo WIB. Historical concepts of cancer metastasis with special reference to bone. In Weiss L, Gilbert HA, editors. *Bone Metastasis* Boston: G.K. Hall; 1981; pp. 1–10.
19. Berretoni BA, Carter JR. Mechanisms of cancer metastasis to bone. *J Bone Joint Surg* 1986;68A:308–12.
20. Paget S. The distribution of secondary growths in cancer of the breast. *Lancet* 1889;1:571–3.
21. Batson OV. The function of the vertebral veins and their role in the spread of metastases. *Ann Surg* 1940;112:138–48.
22. Batson OV. The vertebral vein system. Caldwell Lecture, 1956. *Am J Roentgenol Rad Ther Nucl Med* 1957;78:195–212.

23. Coman DR, DeLong RP. The role of the vertebral venous system in the metastasis of cancer to the spinal column. *Cancer* 1951;4:610–8.

24. Fidler IJ, Hart IR. Principles of cancer biology: cancer metastasis. In DeVita VT, Hellman S, Rosenberg SA, editors. *Cancer: Principles and Practice of Oncology* Philadelphia: J.B. Lippincott; 1985; pp. 113–24.

25. Ewing J. *Neoplastic Diseases, 3rd Edition.* Philadelphia: W. B. Saunders; 1928.

26. Hashimoto M. Pathology of bone marrow. *Acta Haematol* 1962;27:193–216.

27. Kikaldy-Willis WH, Paine KWE, Cauchoix J, et al. Lumbar spinal stenosis. *Clin Orthop* 1974;99:30–50.

28. Posner JB. Spinal metastases: diagnosis and treatment. In Posner JB, editor. *Neuro-Oncology Course at Memorial Sloan-Kettering Cancer Center.* New York; 1981; pp. 42–54.

29. Constans JP, Divitiis ED, Donzelli R, et al. Spinal metastases with neurological manifestations: review of 600 cases. *J Neurosurg* 1983;59:111–18.

30. Citrin DL, Bessent RG, Greig WR. A comparison of the sensitivity and accuracy of TC-99 phosphate bone scan and skeletal radiograph in the diagnosis of bone metastases. *Clin Radiol* 1977;28:107–17.

31. McNeil BJ. Value of bone scanning in neoplastic disease. *Semin Nucl Med* 1984;14:277–86.

32. Covelli HD, Zaloznik AJ, Shekitka KM. Evaluation of bone pain in carcinoma of the lung: role of the localized false-negative scan. *JAMA* 1980;244:2625–7.

33. Pancoast HK. Superior pulmonary sulcus tumor: tumor characterized by pain, Horner's syndrome, destruction of bone and atrophy of hand muscles. *JAMA* 1932;99:1391–6.

34. McAlhany HJ, Netsky MG. Compression of the spinal cord by extramedullary neoplasms: a clinical and pathological study. *J Neuropathol Exp Neurol* 1955;14:276–87.

35. Kahn E. The role of the dentate ligaments in spinal cord compression and the syndrome of lateral sclerosis. *J Neurosurg* 1947;4:191–9.

36. Hashizume Y, Iljima S, Kishimoto H, Hirano A. Pencil-shaped softening of the spinal cord: pathologic study in 12 cases. *Acta Neuropathol (Berl)* 1983;61:219–24.

37. Henson RA, Parsons M. Ischaemic lesions of the spinal cord: an illustrated review. *Q J Med* 1967;36:205–22.

38. Hughes JT. Venous infarction of the spinal cord. *Neurology* 1971;21:794–800.

39. Nakashima K, Shimamine T. Anatomo-pathologic study of pencil-shaped softening of the spinal cord. *Adv Neurol Sci (Tokyo)* 1974;18:153–66.

40. Elsberg CA. *Surgical Diseases of the Spinal Cord, Membranes and Nerve Root.* New York: Hoeber; 1941.

41. Tarlov IM, Klinger H. Spinal cord compression studies II. Time limits for recovery after acute compression in dogs. *AMA Arch Neurol Psychiat* 1954;71:271–90.

42. Tarlov IM, Klinger H, Vitale S. Spinal cord compression studies I. Experimental techniques to produce acute and gradual compression. *AMA Arch Neurol Psychiat* 1953;70:813–19.

43. Tarlov IM. Spinal cord compression studies III. Time limits for recovery after gradual compression in dogs. *Arch Neurol* 1953;71:588–97.

44. Ushio Y, Posner R, Posner JB, et al. Experimental spinal cord compression by epidural neoplasms. *Neurology* 1977;27:422–9.

45. Ikeda H, Ushio Y, Hayakawa T, et al. Edema and circulatory disturbance in the spinal cord compressed by epidural neoplasms in rabbits. *J Neurosurg* 1980;52:203–9.

46. Kato A, Ushio Y, Hayakawa T, et al. Circulatory disturbance of the spinal cord with epidural neoplasm in rats. *J Neurosurg* 1985;63:260–5.

47. Delattre JY, Arbit E, Thaler HT, et al. A dose-response study of dexamethasone in a model of spinal cord compression caused by epidural tumor. *J Neurosurg* 1989;70:920–5.

48. Schramm J, Shigeno T, Brock M. Clinical signs and evoked response alterations associated with chronic experimental cord compression. *J Neurosurg* 1983;58:734–41.

49. Siegal T, Siegal TZ, Sandbank U, et al. Experimental neoplastic spinal cord compression: evoked potentials, edema, prostaglandins, and light and electron microscopy. *Spine* 1987;12:440–8.

50. Siegal T, Shohani F, Shapira Y, et al. Indomethacin and dexamethasone treatment in experimental neoplastic spinal cord compression. Part 2. Effect on edema and prostaglandin synthesis. *Neurosurgery* 1988;22:334–9.

51. Siegal T, Siegal Tz. Participation of serotonergic mechanisms in the pathophysiology of experimental neoplastic spinal cord compression. *Neurology* 1991;41:574–80.

52. Siegal T, Siegal T, Lossos F. Experimental neoplastic spinal cord compression: effect of antiinflammatory agents and glutamate receptor antagonists on vascular permeability. *Neurosurgery* 1990;26:967–70.

53. Siegal T, Siegal T. Serotonergic manipulations in experimental neoplastic spinal cord compression. *J Neurosurg* 1993;78:929–37.

54. Johnson M, Carey F, McMillan RM. Alternative pathways of arachidonate metabolism: prostaglandins, thromboxane and leukotrienes. *Essays Biochem* 1983;19:41–141.

55. Ranson B, Waxman S, Davis P. Anoxic injury of CNS white matter: protective effect of ketamine. *Neurology* 1990;40:1399–404.

56. Stys P, Waxman S, Ransom B. Ionic mechanisms of anoxic injury of CNS white matter: role of Na^+ channels and Na^+-Ca^{2+} exchanger. *J Neurosci* 1992;12:430–9.

57. Imaizumi T, Kocsis J, Waxman S. Anoxic injury in the rat spinal cord: pharmacological evidence for multiple steps in Ca^{2+}-dependent injury of the dorsal columns. *J Neurotrauma* 1997;14:293–312.

58. Fern R, Ransom B, Waxman S. Voltage-gated calcium channels in CNS white matter: role in anoxic injury. *J Neurophysiol* 1995;74:369–77.

59. Ochoa J, Fowler TJ, Gilliatt RW. Anatomical changes in peripheral nerves compressed by a pneumatic tourniquet. *J Anat (Lond)* 1972;113: 433–5.

60. Rudge P, Ochoa J, Gilliatt RW. Acute peripheral nerve compression in the baboon. *J Neurol Sci* 1974;23:403–20.

61. Blight A. Cellular morphology of chronic spinal cord injury in the cat: analysis of myelinated axons by live sampling. *Neuroscience* 1983;10: 521–43.

62. MacGregor RJ, Sharpless SK, Luttges M. A pressure vessel model of nerve compression. *J Neurol Sci* 1975;24:295–304.

63. Blight A. Delayed myelination and macrophage invasion: a candidate for secondary damage in spinal cord injury. *Central Nervous System Trauma* 1985;2:299–315.

64. Blight A. Morphometric analysis of experimental spinal cord injury in the cat: relation of injury intensity to survival of myelinated axons. *Neuroscience* 1986;19:321–41.

65. Waxman SG. Demyelination in spinal cord injury. *J Neurol Sci* 1989;91:1–15.

66. Gledhill RF, McDonald WI. Morphological characteristics of central demyelination and remyelination: a single-fiber study. *Ann Neurol* 1977;1:552–60.

67. Chade HO. Metastatic tumours of the spine and spinal cord. In Vinken PJ, Bruyn GW, editors. *Handbook of Clinical Neurology, Volume 20.* Amsterdam: North-Holland; 1976; pp. 415–33.

68. Neustaedter M. Incidence of metastases to the nervous system. *AMA Arch Neurol Psychiat* 1944; 51:423–5.

69. Elsberg CA. Extradural spinal tumors: primary, secondary, metastatic. *Surg Gynecol Obst* 1928; 46:1–20.

70. Bumpus HC. Carcinoma of the prostate. *Surg Gynecol Obst* 1926;43:150–5.

71. Liskow A, Chang CH, DeSanctis P, et al. Epidural cord compression in association with genitourinary neoplasms. *Cancer* 1986;58:949–54.

72. Rubin J, Lome LG, Presman D. Neurological manifestation of metastatic prostatic carcinoma. *J Urol* 1974;111:799–802.

73. Kuban DA, El-Mahdi AM, Sigfred SV, et al. Characteristics of spinal cord compression in adenocarcinoma of prostate. *Urology* 1986;28: 364–9.

74. Moore EW, Freireich EJ, Shaw RK, Thomas LB. The central nervous system in acute leukemia. *Arch Int Med* 1960;105:451–67.

75. Price RA, Johnson WW. The central nervous system in childhood leukemia: I. The arachnoid. *Cancer* 1973;31:520–33.

76. Rogalsky RJ, Black B, Reed MH. Orthopedic manifestations of leukemia in children. *J Bone Joint Surg* 1986;68A:494–501.

77. Yuill GM. Leukemia: neurological involvement. In Vinken PJ, Bruyn GW, editors. *Handbook of Clinical Neurology, Volume 39.* Amsterdam: North-Holland; 1980; pp. 1–25.

78. Bunn PA, Schein PS, Banks PM, DeVita VT. Central nervous system complications in patients with diffuse histiocytic and undifferentiated lymphoma: leukemia revisited. *Blood* 1976; 47:3–10.

79. Cairncross JG, Posner JB. Neurological complications of malignant lymphoma. In Vinken PJ, Bruyn GW, editors. *Handbook of Clinical Neurology, Volume 39.* Amsterdam: North-Holland; 1980; pp. 27–62.

80. Pedersen AG, Bach F, Melgaard B. Frequency, diagnosis, and prognosis of spinal cord compression in small cell bronchogenic carcinoma. *Cancer* 1985;55:1818–22.

81. Posner JB. Neurologic complications of systemic cancer. *Dis Mon* 1978;25:1–60.

82. Boland PJ, Lane JM, Sundarasen N. Metastatic disease of the spine. *Clin Orthop* 1982;169: 95–102.

83. Posner JB. Back pain and epidural spinal cord compression. *Med Clin North Am* 1987;71:185–204.

84. Bernat JL, Greenberg ER, Barrett J. Suspected epidural compression of the spinal cord and cauda equina by metastatic carcinoma. *Cancer* 1983;51:1953–7.

85. O'Rourke T, George CB, Redmond J, et al. Spinal computed tomography and computed tomographic metrizamide myelography in the early diagnosis of metastatic disease. *J Clin Oncol* 1986;4:576–83.

86. Rasmussen TB, Kernohan JW, Adson AW. Pathologic classification, with surgical consideration, of intraspinal tumors. *Ann Surg* 1940; 111:513–30.

87. Levitt P, Ransohoff J, Spielholz N. The differential diagnosis of tumors of the conus medullaris and cauda equina. In Vinken PJ, Bruyn GW, editors. *Handbook of Clinical Neurology, Volume 19.* Amsterdam: North-Holland; 1975; pp. 77–90.

88. Norstrom CW, Kernohan JW, Love JG. One hundred primary caudal tumors. *JAMA* 1961; 178:1071–7.

89. Rodriguez M, Dinapoli RP. Spinal cord compression: with special reference to metastatic epidural tumors. *Mayo Clin Proc* 1980;55:442–8.

90. Schliack H, Stille D. Clinical symptomatology of intraspinal tumors. In Vinken PJ, Bruyn GW, editors. *Handbook of Clinical Neurology Volume 19.* Amsterdam: North-Holland; 1975; pp. 23–49.

91. Karp SJ, Ho RTK. Gait ataxia as a presenting symptom of malignant epidural spinal cord compression. *Postgrad Med J* 1986;62:745–7.

92. Gudesblatt M, Cohen JA, Gerber O, Sacher M. Truncal ataxia presumably due to malignant spinal cord compression (letter). *Ann Neurol* 1987;21:511–2.

93. Wasserstrom WR, Glass JP, Posner JB. Diagnosis and treatment of leptomeningeal metastases from solid tumors: experience with 90 patients. *Cancer* 1982;49:759–72.

94. Young RC, Howser DM, Anderson T, et al. Central nervous system complications of non-Hodgkin's lymphoma. *Am J Med* 1979;66: 435–43.

95. Cushing H. Some experimental and clinical observations concerning states of increased intracranial tension. *Am J Med Sci* 1902;124:375–400.

96. Meyer A. Herniation of the brain. *Arch Neurol Psychiat* 1920;4:387–400.
97. Eaton LM, Craig WM. Tumor of the spinal cord: sudden paralysis following lumbar puncture. *Proc Staff Meet Mayo Clin* 1940;15:170–2.
98. Hollis PH, Malis LI, Zappulla RA. Neurological deterioration after lumbar puncture below complete spinal subarachnoid block. *J Neurosurg* 1986;64:253–6.
99. Jooma R, Hayward RD. Upward spinal coning: impaction of occult spinal tumors following relief of hydrocephalus. *J Neurol Neurosurg Psychiatry* 1984;47:386–90.
100. Modic MT, Masaryk T, Paushter D. Magnetic resonance imaging of the spine. *Radiol Clin North Am* 1986;24:229–45.
101. Sarpel S, Sarpel G, Yu E, et al. Early diagnosis of spinal-epidural metastasis by magnetic resonance imaging. *Cancer* 1987;59:1112–6.
102. Edelstyn GA, Gillespie PJ, Grebbell FS. The radiological demonstration of skeletal metastases. *Clin Radiol* 1967;18:158–62.
103. Wong D, Fornasier V, MacNab I. Spinal metastases: the obvious, the occult and the impostors. *Spine* 1990;15:1–4.
104. Liu CN, Chambers WW. An experimental study of the corticospinal system in the monkey (Macaca mulatta). The spinal pathways and preterminal distribution of degenerating fibers following discrete lesions of the pre- and post-central gyri and bulbar pyramid. *J Comp Neurol* 1964;123:257–84.
105. Harrison KM, Muss HB, Ball M, et al. Spinal cord compression in breast cancer. *Cancer* 1985;55:2839–44.
106. Selwood RB. The radiologic approach to metastatic cancer of the brain and spine. *Br J Radiol* 1972;45:647–51.
107. Grem JL, Burgess J, Trump DL. Clinical features and natural history of intramedullary spinal cord metastasis. *Cancer* 1985;56:2305–14.
108. Haddad P, Thaell JF, Kiely JM, et al. Lymphoma of the spinal extradural space. *Cancer* 1976;38:1862–6.
109. Kori SH, Krol G, Foley KM. Computed tomographic evaluation of bone and soft tissue metastases. In Weiss L, Gilbert HA, editors. *Bone Metastasis*. Boston: G.K. Hall; 1981; pp. 245–57.
110. Thrupkaew A, Henken R, Quinn JL. False negative bone scans in disseminated metastatic diseases. *Radiology* 1975;113:383–6.
111. Longeval E, Holdebrand J, Vollont GH. Early diagnosis of metastases in the epidural space. *Acta Neurochir* 1975;31:177–84.
112. Calkins AR, Olson MA, Ellis JH. Impact of myelography on the radiotherapeutic management of malignant spinal cord compression. *Neurosurgery* 1986;19:614–6.
113. Rodichok LD, Harper GR, Ruckdeschel JC, et al. Early diagnosis of spinal epidural metastases. *Am J Med* 1981;70:1181–8.
114. Braunstein EM, Kuhns LR. Computed tomographic demonstration of spinal metastases. *Spine* 1983;8:912–5.
115. Hermann G, Hermann P. Computerized tomography of the spine in metastatic disease. *Mt Sinai J Med (NY)* 1982;49:400–5.
116. Weissman DE, Gilbert M, Wang H, et al. The use of computed tomography of the spine to identify patients at high risk for epidural metastases. *J Clin Oncol* 1985;3:1541–4.
117. Redmond J, Freidl KE, Cornett P, Stone M, O'Rourke T, George CB. Clinical usefulness of an algorithm for the early diagnosis of spinal metastatic disease. *J Clin Oncol* 1988;6:154–7.
118. Sze G. Magnetic resonance imaging in the evaluation of spinal tumors. *Cancer* 1991;67(Suppl 4):1229–41.
119. Ludwig H, Fruhwald F, Tscholakoff D, et al. Magnetic resonance imaging of the spine in multiple myeloma. *Lancet* 1987;2:364–6.
120. Helweg-Larsen S, Wagner A, Kjaer L, et al. Comparison of myelography combined with post-myelographic spinal CT and MRI in suspected metastatic disease of the spinal canal. *J Neurooncol* 1992;13:231–7.
121. Li M, Holtas S, Larsson E-M. MR imaging of spinal lymphoma. *Acta Radiol (Diag) (Stockh)* 1992;33:338–12.
122. Masaryk TJ, Modic MT, Geisinger MA, et al. Cervical myelopathy: a comparison of magnetic resonance and myelography. *J Comput Assist Tomogr* 1986;10:184–94.
123. Smoker WRK, Godersky JC, Knutzon RK, Keyes WD, Norman D, Bergman W. The role of MR imaging in evaluating metastatic spinal disease. *AJR Am J Roentgenol* 1987;149:1241–8.
124. Beltran J, Noto AM, Chakeres DW, et al. Tumors of the osseous spine: staging with MR imaging versus CT. *Radiology* 1987;162:565–9.
125. Sze G. Gadolinium-DTPA in spinal disease. *Radiol Clin North Am* 1988;26:1009–24.
126. Sze G, Krol G, Zimmerman RD, Deck MDF. Gadolinium-DTPA: malignant extradural spinal tumors. *Radiology* 1988;167:217–23.
127. Einsiedel HGv, Stepan R. Magnetic resonance imaging of spinal cord syndromes. *Eur J Radiol* 1985;5:127–32.
128. Tang SG, Byfield JE, Sharp TR, Utley JF, Quinol L, Seagren SL. Prognostic factors in the management of metastatic epidural spinal cord compression. *J Neurooncol* 1983;1:21–8.
129. Blois MS. Medicine and the nature of vertical reasoning. *N Engl J Med* 1988;318:847–51.
130. Browne TR, Adams RD, Robertson GH. Hemangioblastoma of the spinal cord. *Arch Neurol* 1976;33:435–41.
131. Vecht ChJ, Haaxma-Reiche H, Putten WLJv, et al. Initial bolus of conventional versus high-dose dexamethasone in metastatic spinal cord compression. *Neurology* 1989;39:1255–7.
132. Sorensen S, Helweg-Larsen S, Mouridsen M, Hansen H. Effect of high-dose dexamethasone in carcinomatous metastatic spinal cord compression treated with radiotherapy: a randomized trial. *Eur J Cancer* 1994;30A:22–7.
133. Heimdal K, IHirschberg H, Slettebo H, et al. High incidence of serious side effects of high-dose dexamethasone treatment in patients with

epidural spinal cord compression. *J Neurooncol* 1994;12:141–4.

134. Loblaw D, Laperiere N. Emergency treatment of malignant extradural spinal cord compression: an evidence-based guideline. *J Clin Oncol* 1998;16:1613–24.

135. Maranzano E, Latini P. Effectiveness of radiation therapy without surgery in metastatic spinal cord compression: final results from a prospective trial. *Int J Radiat Biol Phys* 1995;32: 959–67.

136. Maranzano E, Latini P, Checcaglini F, et al. Radiation therapy in spinal cord compression: a prospective analysis of 105 consecutive patients. *Cancer* 1991;67:1311–7.

137. Findlay GFG. Adverse effects of the management of malignant spinal cord compression. *J Neurol Neurosurg Psychiatry* 1984;47:761–8.

138. Young RF, Post EM, King GA. Treatment of spinal epidural metastases: randomized prospective comparison of laminectomy and radiotherapy. *J Neurosurg* 1980;53:741–8.

139. Cooper P, Errico T, Martin R, et al. A systematic approach to spinal reconstruction after anterior decompression for neoplastic disease of the thoracic and lumbar spine. *Neurosurgery* 1993;32: 1–8.

140. Arbit E, Galicich J. Vertebral body reconstruction with a modified Harrington rod distraction system for stabilization of the spine affected by metastatic disease. *J Neurosurg* 1995;83:617–20.

141. Harrington KD. Anterior cord decompression and spinal stabilization for patients with metastatic lesions of the spine. *J Neurosurg* 1984; 61:107–17.

142. Siegal T, Tiqva P, Siegal T. Vertebral body resection for epidural compression by malignant tumors. *J Bone Joint Surg* 1985;67-A:375–82.

143. Galasko C. Spinal instability secondary to metastatic cancer. *J Bone Joint Surg (Br)* 1991;73: 104–8.

144. Cooper P, Errico T, Martin R, et al. A systematic approach to spinal reconstruction after anterior decompression for neoplastic disease of the thoracic and lumbar spine. *Neurosurgery* 1993;32: 1–8.

145. Perrin R, McBroom R. Spinal fixation after anterior decompression for symptomatic spinal metastasis. *Neurosurgery* 1988;22:324–7.

146. Posner J. *Neurologic Complications of Cancer* Philadelphia: FA Davis; 1995; Contemporary Neurology Series.

147. Scarantino C. Metastatic spinal cord compression: criteria for effective treatment. *Int J Radiat Oncol Biol Phys* 1995;32:1259–60.

148. Bergsagel DE, Rider WD. Plasma cell neoplasms. In DeVita VT, Hellman S, Rosenberg SA, editors. *Cancer: Principles and Practice of Oncology*. Philadelphia: J.P. Lippincott; 1985; pp. 1753–95.

149. Kelly JJ, Kyle RA, Miles JM, Dyck PJ. Osteosclerotic myeloma and peripheral neuropathy. *Neurology* 1983;33:202–10.

150. Resnick D, Greenway GD, Bardwick PA, et al. Plasma-cell dyscrasia with polyneuropathy, organomegaly, endocrinopathy, M-protein and skin changes: the POEMS syndrome. *Radiology* 1981;140:7–22.

151. Camacho J, Arnalich F, Anciones B, et al. The spectrum of neurologic manifestations in myeloma. *J Med* 1985;16:597–611.

152. Kelly JJ, Kyle RA, Miles JM, O'Brien PC, Dyck PJ. The spectrum of peripheral neuropathy in myeloma. *Neurology* 1981;31:24–31.

153. Grossman CB, Post MJDonovan. The adult spine. In Gonzalez CF, Grossman CB, Masdeau JC, editors. *Head and Spine Imaging*. New York: John Wiley; 1985; pp. 781–858.

154. Jacobson G, Poppel MH, Shapiro JH, et al. The vertebral pedicle sign. A roentgen finding to differentiate metastatic carcinoma from multiple myeloma. *AJR Am J Roentgenol* 1958;80: 817–21.

155. Kricun ME. Red-yellow marrow conversion: its effects on the location of some solitary bone lesions. *Skeletal Radiol* 1985;14:10–19.

156. Ludwig H, Kumpan W, Sinzinger H. Radiography and bone scintigraphy in mutiple myeloma: a comparative analysis. *Br J Radiol* 1982;55: 173–81.

157. Dowdle JA, Winter RB, Dehner LP. Postradiation osteosarcoma of the cervical spine in childhood. A case report. *J Bone Joint Surg* 1977;59A: 969–71.

158. Malawer MM, Abelson HT, Suit HD. Sarcomas of bone. In DeVita VT, Hellman S, Rosenberg SA, editors. *Cancer: Principles and Practice of Oncology*. Philadelphia: J.B. Lippincott; 1985; pp. 1293–342.

159. Shives TC, Dahlin DC, Sim FH, et al. Osteosarcoma of the spine. *Skeletal Radiol* 1986;68A: 660–8.

160. Smith J. Radiation-induced sarcoma of bone: clinical and radiographic findings in 43 patients irradiated for soft tissue neoplasms. *Clin Radiol* 1982;33:205–21.

161. Sundarasen N, Huvos AG, Rosen G, et al. Postradiation osteosarcoma of the spine following treatment of Hodgkin's disease. *Spine* 1986; 11:90–2.

162. Doron Y, Gruszkiewicz J, Gelli B, Peyser E. Benign osteoblastoma of the vertebral column and skull. *Surg Neurol* 1977;7:86–90.

163. Fielding JW, Fietti VG, Hughes JE, Gabrielian JC. Primary osteogenic sarcoma of the cervical spine. *J Bone Joint Surg* 1976;58A:892–4.

164. Ogihara Y, Sekiguchi K, Tsuruta T. Osteogenic sarcoma of the fourth thoracic vertebra: long-term survival by chemotherapy only. *Cancer* 1984;53:2615–8.

165. Patel DV, Hammer RA, Levin B, et al. Primary osteogenic sarcoma of the spine. *Skeletal Radiol* 1984;12:276–9.

166. Eriksson B, Gunterberg B, Kindblom L-G. Chordoma: a clinicopathologic review of 48 cases of chordoma. *Cancer* 1985;56:182–7.

167. Huvos AG. *Bone Tumors: Diagnosis, Treatment and Prognosis*. Philadelphia: WB Saunders; 1979.

168. Mindell ER. Current concept review: chordoma. *J Bone Joint Surg* 1981;63:501–5.

169. Rich TA, Schiller A, Suit HD, et al. Clinical and pathologic review of 48 cases of chordoma. *Cancer* 1985;56:182–7.

170. Gray SW, Singhabhandu B, Smith RA, et al. Sacrococcygeal chordoma: report of a case and review of the literature. *Surgery* 1975;78:573–82.

171. Stillwell DL. The nerve supply of the vertebral column and its associated structures in the monkey. *Anat Rec* 1956;125:139–69.

172. Kricun ME. Conventional radiography. In Kricun ME, editor. *Imaging Modalities of Spinal Disorders*. Philadelphia: W.B. Saunders; 1988; pp. 59–288.

173. Kornblith PL, Walker MD, Cassady JR. *Neurologic Oncology* Philadelphia: J.B. Lippincott; 1987.

174. Aprin H, Riseborough EJ, Hall JE. Chondrosarcoma in children and adolescents. *Clin Orthop* 1982;166:226–32.

175. Dahlin DC. *Bone Tumors: General Aspects and Data on 6,221 cases, 3rd Edition*. Springfield: Charles C. Thomas; 1978.

176. Hirsch LF, Thanki A, Spector HB. Primary spinal chondrosarcoma with eighteen-year follow up: case report. *Neurosurgery* 1984;14:747–9.

177. Pizzo PA, Miser JS, Cassady JR, Filler RM. Solid tumors of childhood. In DeVita VT, Hellman S, Rosenberg SA, editors. *Cancer: Principles and Practice of Oncology*. Philadelphia: J.B. Lippincott; 1985; pp. 1511–89.

178. Subbaro K, Jacobson HG. Primary malignant neoplasms. *Semin Roentgenol* 1979;14:44–57.

179. Whitehouse GH, Griffiths GJ. Roentgenologic aspects of spinal involvement by primary and metastatic Ewing's tumor. *J Can Assoc Radiol* 1976;27:290–7.

180. Vanel D, Contesso G, Couanet D, et al. Computed tomography in the evaluation of 41 cases of Ewing's sarcoma. *Skeletal Radiol* 1982;9:8–13.

181. Llombart-Bosch A, Blache R, Peydro-Olaya A. Ultrastructural study of 28 cases of Ewing's sarcoma: typical and atypical forms. *Cancer* 1978;41:1362–73.

182. Ghormley RK, Adson AW. Hemangioma of vertebrae. *J Bone Joint Surg* 1941;39:887–95.

183. Schnyder P, Fankhauser H, Mansouri B. Computed tomography in spinal hemangioma with cord compression: report of two cases. *Skeletal Radiol* 1986;15:372–5.

184. Buur T, Morch MM. Hereditary multiple exostoses with spinal cord compression. *J Neurol Neurosurg Psychiatry* 1983;46:96–7.

185. Carmel PW, Cramer FJ. Cervical cord compression due to exostosis in a patient with hereditary multiple exostoses. *J Neurosurg* 1968;28:500–3.

186. Esposito PW, Crawford AH, Vogler C. Solitary osteochondroma occurring on the transverse process of the lumbar spine: a case report. *Spine* 1985;10:398–400.

187. Karian JM, DeFillip G, Buchheit WA, et al. Vertebral osteochondroma causing spinal cord compression: case report. *Neurosurgery* 1984;14:483–4.

188. Janin Y, Epstein JA, Carras R, et al. Osteoid osteomas and osteoblastomas of the spine. *Neurosurgery* 1981;8:31–8.

189. Kirwan EOG, Hutton PAN, Pozo JL, et al. Osteoid osteoma and benign osteoblastoma of the spine. *J Bone Joint Surg* 1984;66B:21–6.

190. Swee RG, McLeod RA, Beabout JW. Osteoid osteoma. Detection, diagnosis and localization. *Radiology* 1979;130:117–23.

191. Omojola MF, Fox AJ, Vinuela FV. Computed tomographic metrizamide myelography in the evaluation of thoracic spinal osteoblastoma. *AJNR Am J Neuroradiol* 1982;3:670–3.

192. Dahlin DC. Giant cell tumor of the vertebrae above the sacrum: a review of 31 cases. *Cancer* 1977;39:1350–6.

193. DiLorenzo N, Spallone A, Nolletti A, et al. Giant cell tumors of the spine: a clinical study of six cases with emphasis on the radiological features. *Neurosurgery* 1980;6:29–34.

194. Schwimer DC, Bassett LW, Mancuso AA, et al. Giant-cell tumor of the cervicothoracic spine. *AJR Am J Roentgenol* 1981;136:63–7.

195. Garfin SR, Rothman RH. Fibrous dysplasia (polyostotic): case report. *Skeletal Radiol* 1986;15:72–6.

196. Sanchez RL, Llovet J, Moreno A, et al. Symptomatic eosinphilic granuloma of the spine: report of two cases and review of the literature. *Spine* 1984;7:1721–6.

197. Shacked I, Tadmor R, Wolpin G, et al. Aneurysmal bone cyst of a vertebral body with acute paraplegia. *Paraplegia* 1981;19:294–8.

198. Stillwell WT, Fielding JW. Aneurysmal bone cyst of the cervicodorsal spine. *Clin Orthop* 1984;187:144–6.

199. Heffez DS, Sawaya R, Udvarhelyi GB, Mann R. Spinal epidural extramedullary hematopoiesis with cord compression in a patient with refractory sideroblastic anemia. *J Neurosurg* 1982;57:399–406.

200. Lewkow LM, Shah I. Sickle cell anemia and epidural extramedullary hematopoiesis. *Am J Med* 1984;76:748–51.

201. Oustwani MB, Kurtides ES, Christ M, Ciric I. Spinal cord compression with paraplegia in myelofibrosis. *Arch Neurol* 1980;37:389–90.

202. Stahl SM, Ellinger C, Baringer JR. Progressive myelopathy due to extramedullary hematopoiesis: case report and review of the literature. *Ann Neurol* 1979;5:485–9.

203. Arroyo IL, Barron KS, Brewer EJ. Spinal cord compression by epidural lipomatosis in juvenile rheumatoid arthritis. *Arthritis Rheum* 1988;31:447–51.

204. Jungreis CA, Cohen WA. Spinal cord compression induced by steroid therapy: CT findings. *J Comput Assist Tomogr* 1987;11:245–7.

205. Lipson SJ, Naheedy MH, Kaplan MH. Spinal stenosis caused by epidural lipomatosis in Cushing's syndrome. *N Engl J Med* 1980;302:36.

206. Sinclair DC, Feindel WH, Falconer MA. The intervertebral ligaments as a source of segmental pain. *J Bone Joint Surg* 1948;30-B:515–21.

207. Laredo J-D, Reizine D, Bard M, Merland J-J. Vertebral hemangiomas: radiological evaluation. *Radiology* 1986;161:183–9.
208. Chapman PH. Congenital intraspinal lipomas: anatomical considerations and surgical treatment. *Child's Brain* 1982;9:37–47.
209. Emery JL, Lendon RG. Lipomas of the cauda equina and other fatty tumors related to neurospinal dysraphism. *Dev Med Child Neurol* 1969;2(Suppl 20):62–70.
210. Thomas JE, Miller RH. Lipomatous tumors of the spinal canal. *Mayo Clin Proc* 1973;48:393–400.
211. Giuffre R. Spinal lipomas. In Vinken PJ, Bruyn GW, editors. *Handbook of Clinical Neurology, Volume 20*. Amsterdam: North-Holland; 1976; pp. 389–414.
212. Ehni G, Love JG. Intraspinal lipomas. Report of cases; review of the literature, and clinical and pathologic study. *Acta Neurol Psychiat* 1945;53:1–28.
213. George WE Jr, Wilmot M, Greenhouse A, et al. Medical management of steroid induced epidural lipomatosis. *N Engl J Med* 1983;308:316–9.
214. del Regato J. Pathways of metastatic spread of malignant tumors. *Semin Oncol* 1977;4:33–8.
215. Byrne TN. Spinal cord compression from epidural metastases. *N Engl J Med* 1992;327:614–9.

Chapter 6

INTRADURAL–EXTRAMEDULLARY AND INTRAMEDULLARY TUMORS AND VASCULAR MALFORMATIONS

INTRADURAL-EXTRAMEDULLARY
 TUMORS
Meningioma
Nerve Sheath Tumors
VASCULAR MALFORMATIONS AND
 VASCULAR TUMORS
Vascular Malformations
Spinal Vascular Neoplasms
EPIDERMOID AND DERMOID CYSTS AND
 TERATOMAS
LIPOMA
INTRAMEDULLARY TUMORS
Ependymoma
Astrocytoma
Intramedullary Metastasis

Neoplastic disease involving the spine may be classified according to the location of the tumor: epidural, intradural–extramedullary, or intramedullary (Fig. 6–1). As reviewed in Chapter 5, most epidural neoplasms are metastatic. Intradural-extramedullary tumors and intramedullary tumors, on the other hand, are often primary tumors of the spine. Their clinical importance is demonstrated by the fact that among neurosurgical series, which tend to exclude cases of metastatic disease, intradural–extramedullary and intramedullary tumors compose the majority of spinal tumors.[1,2]

In some cases, a definite distinction cannot be made between an intramedullary and intradural–extramedullary location because the tumor may extend into both locations. In the present chapter, tumors are grouped according to where they most frequently occur.

INTRADURAL–EXTRAMEDULLARY TUMORS

Many intradural–extramedullary neoplasms are histologically benign tumors. If the condition is diagnosed and treated early in its course, neurological function is often preserved and the tumor is usually cured. However, if not recognized and surgically resected, these benign neoplasms generally cause progressive neurological dysfunction, and ultimately the loss of spinal cord and cauda equina function (As in other chapters, the term spinal cord compression includes cauda equina compression unless otherwise indicated). As reported in 1888, the first successful surgical removal of a spinal neoplasm was that of an intradural–extramedullary tumor.[3] Thus, it has been recognized for more than a century that there is a great premium on the early diagnosis and treatment of these benign neoplasms.

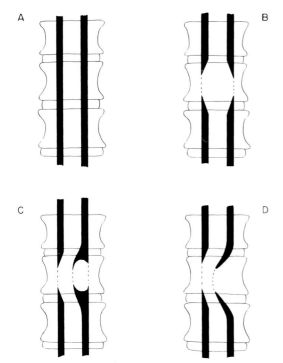

Figure 6–1. Masses within the spinal canal may be classified according to location relative to the spinal cord and dura mater. (A) Normal. (B) Intradural–intramedullary. (C) Intradural–extramedullary. (D) Epidural. (From Leeds, NE, et al.,[184] p. 350, with permission.)

In most neurosurgical series, intradural–extramedullary neoplasms are primarily histologically benign meningiomas and nerve sheath tumors.[1,2,4–6] For example, in one review,[1] nerve sheath tumor and meningioma were responsible for 52% to 72% of all spinal tumors among the four neurosurgical series cited. However, as discussed in Chapter 5, these series are biased in that patients selected for inclusion in neurosurgical series are more apt to have benign localized growths than metastatic disease. In addition to meningiomas and nerve sheath tumors, vascular neoplasms and malformations, epidermoids, and lipomas also are found in this location (intradural–extramedullary).

Leptomeningeal metastases from systemic cancer or central nervous system malignancies also may present as intradural–extramedullary neoplasms. Among the cancer population, this complication is fre-quent. For example, it has been estimated that approximately 5% of patients dying of systemic cancer develop leptomeningeal metastases.[7,8] Furthermore, in some forms of non-Hodgkin's lymphoma, the prevalence of leptomeningeal metastases may range from 5% to 29%.[9–14] The clinical manifestations of leptomeningeal metastases are protean, and the diagnostic evaluation is often different from that of other intradural–extramedullary tumors. For these reasons, leptomeningeal metastases are reviewed separately in Chapter 7.

Meningioma

Among primary neoplasms of the spine, meningiomas vie with nerve sheath tumors as the most common.[1,6] For example, meningiomas were found to compose approximately 25% of 1322 primary spinal tumors in a large Mayo Clinic series.[2] In other series,[15,16] meningiomas were responsible for 33% and 47% of primary spinal tumors.

Meningiomas may arise from any of the cell elements that form the meninges, but the majority stem from arachnoid cells.[17] Although over 90% of cases are purely intradural in location,[18,19] the remaining 7% to 10% may be extradural.[5,18,19] In many of the latter cases, the tumor may extend from an intradural to an extradural location.[19] Extradural meningiomas are considered more biologically aggressive than those in the intradural location and have been associated with a shorter clinical history.[18,19]

LOCATION

Meningiomas may occur at any level along the spinal axis, but the cervical and thoracic regions are more commonly involved than the lumbar region. In a review of the literature,[5] among a total of 705 reported spinal meningiomas, 17% of cases were in the cervical spine, 81% in the thoracic spine, and 2% in the lumbar region. In a series from the Cleveland Clinic[19] consisting of 97 spinal meningiomas, the cervical spine was the site of involvement in 17%, the thoracic spine in 75%, and the lumbar spine in only 7% of cases.

Of further clinical importance, the Cleveland Clinic study examined the relationship between sex and location.[19] Among women, 83% of the meningiomas were found in the thoracic region. Men had a nearly equal frequency of cervical (41%) and thoracic (47%) lesions. The reason for this predilection for the thoracic spine in women is unknown.

The location of meningiomas in the transverse plane of the vertebral canal also has been studied. Most meningiomas attach to the insertion of the dentate ligament, and they may extend ventrally or dorsally.[5] Thus they may be classified as ventral or dorsal to the dentate ligament, or may be lateral. Among 179 cases from the literature,[5] 61% were posterior to the dentate ligament, 28% were anterior, and the remaining 11% extended too far to classify. The ventral–dorsal location of meningiomas was analyzed with respect to their vertebral level of involvement in the Cleveland Clinic series[19] (Fig. 6–2). Eleven of 13 meningiomas above C7 were in the ventral location. Alternatively, at and be-

low the level of C7, there were 22 anterior and 45 dorsal meningiomas.

PATHOLOGY

In the Cleveland Clinic series,[19] 59% of meningiomas of the spinal canal were meningothelial, and 21% were psammomatous. Another study[20] found psammomatous tumors to be the most frequent histologically, followed by meningothelial tumors. Fibroblastic, angioblastic, and transitional tumors were less frequent in both series.[19,20] Although invasive tumors are occasionally observed, malignant meningiomas appear rarely. Calcium may be observed histologically, and occasionally on radiographs (Fig. 6–3).[18]

Multiple meningiomas are occasionally encountered (Fig. 6–4). Multiple spinal meningiomas may occur in patients with von Recklinghausen's disease in association with other forms of neoplasia or as an isolated event. Multiple spinal meningiomas rarely occur in isolation.[5] In one series,[20] multiple meningiomas occurred in

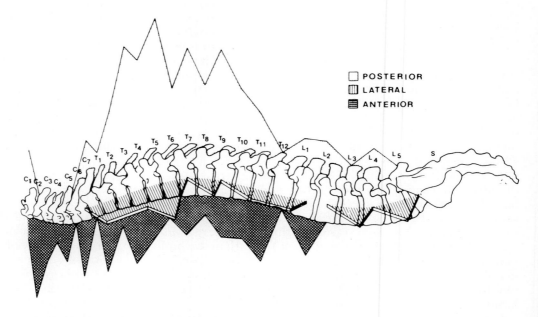

POSTERIOR
LATERAL
ANTERIOR

	C1	C2	C3	C4	C5	C6	C7	T1	T2	T3	T4	T5	T6	T7	T8	T9	T10	T11	T12	L1	L2	L3	L4	L5	SACRUM
POSTERIOR	2	0	0	0	0	0	2	1	3	6	5	6	3	5	3	5	3	2	0	1	1	0	1	0	0
LATERAL	0	0	0	0	0	0	0	1	1	1	1	2	1	0	1	0	1	1	1	0	0	1	0	1	0
ANTERIOR	1	4	2	1	2	0	3	0	3	1	3	2	1	2	1	2	2	3	0	2	0	0	0	0	0

Figure 6–2. Distribution of meningiomas relative to the spinal cord along the spinal axis in a series of 97 cases. (From Levy, WJ, et al.,[19] with permission.)

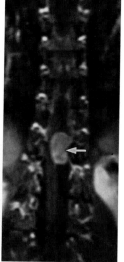

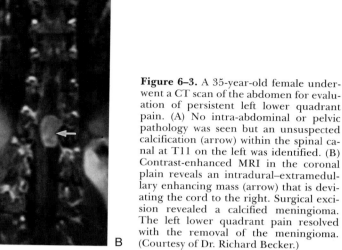

A

B

Figure 6–3. A 35-year-old female underwent a CT scan of the abdomen for evaluation of persistent left lower quadrant pain. (A) No intra-abdominal or pelvic pathology was seen but an unsuspected calcification (arrow) within the spinal canal at T11 on the left was identified. (B) Contrast-enhanced MRI in the coronal plain reveals an intradural–extramedullary enhancing mass (arrow) that is deviating the cord to the right. Surgical excision revealed a calcified meningioma. The left lower quadrant pain resolved with the removal of the meningioma. (Courtesy of Dr. Richard Becker.)

7% of 45 patients. They were found in only 2% of the Cleveland Clinic series of 97 patients.[19]

CLINICAL FEATURES

Gender and Age

Spinal meningiomas are much more frequently encountered in women than in men. In many series, approximately 80% of cases occur in women.[4,5,19,20] In Rand's series,[16] 95% of patients were women. As mentioned previously, in women the thoracic spine is disproportionately more involved than the cervical spine, whereas in men, meningiomas are more evenly distributed in the cervical and thoracic region.[5,19]

Spinal meningiomas have a peak incidence between the ages of 40 and 70 years. Symptoms develop under 30 years of age in only 10% of cases, and the tumor infrequently occurs under the age of 15.[4,5] The average age of males (51 years) and females (54 years) was not significantly different in the series from the Cleveland Clinic.[19]

Symptoms and Signs

Spinal meningiomas may represent a difficult diagnostic problem; in one series,[19] one-third of patients had been previously misdiagnosed. As in most other types of spinal tumor, pain is the most common presenting complaint.[19] Oddsson[15] reported the occurrence of pain in 85% of cases; in the Cleveland Clinic series,[19] it was a presenting complaint in 72% of cases. Pain may be axial or radicular in nature; Nittner[5] reported radicular pain as a major complaint in 50% of cases.

Sensory disturbances in the form of paresthesias, cold and hot sensations, and numbness have been reported in approximately one-third of cases at the time of diagnosis.[5,19] Sensory disturbances may be of a radicular nature or may be due to ascending tract dysfunction. They may ascend as the more peripheral spinothalamic fibers are compressed before central fibers. Dissociated sensory disturbances and the Brown-Séquard syndrome are infrequent.[4,5,19] Sensory disturbances including a sensory level were found in over three-quarters of patients in a recent series.[19]

Subjective motor weakness is frequently observed in patients with spinal meningiomas and is usually bilateral. Hemiparesis is uncommon but may occur with meningiomas in the region of the craniocervical junction.[5] Usually motor symptoms begin ipsilateral to the side of the tumor but occasionally they may begin contralaterally, with progression to in-

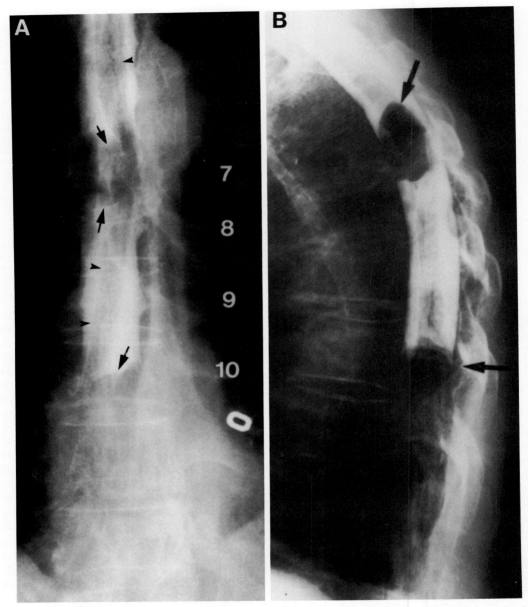

Figure 6–4. Two meningiomas demonstrated on myelography. (A) The meningioma (arrows) on the right side of the vertebral canal at T7 displaces the spinal cord (arrowhead) to the left. The meningioma (arrow) on the left at T10 displaces the cord (arrowheads) to the right. (B) This lateral view shows the two meningiomas (arrows) at T7 and T10. (Courtesy of Dr. Helmuth Gahbauer.)

clude both sides;[4] this clinical presentation may be due to contrecoup compression.[21] Although weakness was a subjective complaint in 66% of cases in the Cleveland Clinic series,[19] objective signs of paresis and reflex changes were present in approximately 80% of patients at diagnosis.

Sphincter dysfunction is a less frequent, albeit important, presenting complaint.[19,20] No patients in one series[20] presented with sphincter disturbance; 40% of the patients in the Cleveland Clinic series complained of bowel or bladder disturbance, while only 15% had objective evidence of sphincter dysfunction.

The duration of symptoms in patients with spinal meningiomas is quite variable. Occasional patients have abrupt onset of symptoms, often precipitated by trauma.[19] More frequently, symptoms begin insidiously and progress over several months. In one series,[20] 75% of patients had symptoms for 6 months or more, whereas in the Cleveland Clinic series[19] the average duration was 23 months prior to diagnosis; in one case, the symptoms were present for 20 years. Occasionally, symptoms may appear to have remissions and exacerbations and thus suggest demyelinating disease.[4]

LABORATORY AND DIAGNOSTIC IMAGING STUDIES

Diagnostic Imaging Studies

Abnormalities on plain spine radiographs suggesting tumor occur in approximately 10% of patients with spinal meningiomas.[5,18,22] These abnormalities include widening of the interpedicular distance at the level of the tumor, bony erosion, and calcification. Enlargement of an intervertebral foramen may occur if the tumor grows in an hourglass shape. This finding is more frequently observed with nerve sheath tumors.[5] Plain radiographs are not usually helpful in distinguishing intradural meningiomas from extradural meningiomas because both infrequently may cause bony erosion.[5,18] An increase in the interpedicular distance is not specific for meningiomas because nerve sheath tumors, intramedullary tumors, and other intraspinal masses may similarly widen the spinal canal. The relatively nonspecific findings of kyphosis and scoliosis may be observed in up to one-third of patients.[5]

Although calcification of spinal meningiomas is not often observed on plain radiographs, CT occasionally will demonstrate calcification of the tumor and hyperostosis of adjacent bones.[23] Scanning by CT following intravenous contrast administration may demonstrate dense enhancement of the tumor.[24] Extradural extension of meningiomas also may be observed on CT.

Intradural–extramedullary neoplasms have a rather characteristic pattern on myelography (Fig. 6–4). The spinal cord is displaced away from the mass and the subarachnoid space above and below the tumor is enlarged. In epidural and intramedullary neoplasms, the subarachnoid space is narrowed adjacent to the tumor. Differentiation of an intradural nerve sheath tumor from a meningioma based on myelography alone may be difficult.[22] Postmyelographic CT may better define the anatomical relationship between the spinal cord and the meningioma.

Although noncontrast MRI has been found to be less sensitive for the diagnosis of intradural–extramedullary tumors than of epidural tumors, it has been used in the localization of spinal meningiomas.[25,26] The spinal cord may appear displaced with enlargement of the subarachnoid space as observed by myelography. The transverse anatomical relationship of the meningioma to the spinal cord also may be demonstrated (Fig. 6–5). The administration of contrast agents with MRI has been shown to improve its sensitivity to intradural–extramedullary spinal tumors.[27–29] Because of its ability to image noninvasively in multiple projections and to demonstrate the spinal cord and paravertebral structures, MRI has become the imaging test of choice for evaluating spinal meningiomas.

Cerebrospinal Fluid

The CSF usually shows the nonspecific finding of elevated protein. Nittner's review[5] reports that the lumbar CSF protein was elevated in 76% to 90% of cases. There may be a slight degree of pleocytosis, but there is albumino-cytologic dissociation in 85% of cases.[5]

THERAPY

Surgery is the treatment of choice for spinal cord compression from meningioma. Laminectomy is usually performed. Rarely, a ventral approach is safer than laminectomy. This, however, necessi-

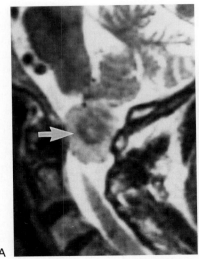
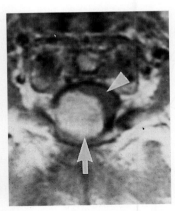

A   B

Figure 6–5. A 67-year-old woman with a chief complaint of bilateral hand numbness was referred for MR imaging of the cervical spine. (A) A sagittal nonenhanced MRI reveals a mass (arrow) within the spinal canal at the level of C1. (B) An axial contrast-enhanced MRI reveals a large contrast enhancing mass (arrow) posterolateral to the spinal cord (arrowhead). The mass is occupying most of the spinal canal and the spinal cord is severely compressed. Surgical removal of the mass revealed a meningioma. (Courtesy of Dr. Richard Becker.)

tates vertebral body resection, fusion, and usually instrumentation. Complete removal with the attached dura is usually followed by no recurrence, but incomplete removal of spinal meningiomas may also have an excellent prognosis, with no recurrence, or recurrence delayed by several years.[19] Epidural meningiomas and calcified meningiomas, however, often do not have such an excellent prognosis.[19]

As with other slow-growing mass lesions, an excellent recovery often occurs following surgery even if there is a severe neurological deficit at the time of diagnosis. In the Cleveland Clinic series,[19] 85% of patients had a favorable result with surgical removal. Thus patients with spinal meningioma are usually restored to ambulation unless they are paraplegic preoperatively; some paraplegic patients even become ambulatory in long-term follow-up.

Nerve Sheath Tumors

Nerve sheath tumors arise from cells that surround the axons of the peripheral nervous system. Such tumors may occur on spinal nerve roots, and may thereby cause spinal cord compression. The cells surrounding axons include Schwann cells, fibroblasts, and perineurial fibroblasts.[17] There has been considerable debate among pathologists as to the cell of origin of nerve sheath tumors, resulting in the use of several terms to describe such tumors, including schwannoma, neurofibroma, neurinoma, perineurofibroblastoma, and neurilemoma.[17]

PATHOLOGY

Rubinstein[17] classified nerve sheath tumors as schwannomas and neurofibromas. Schwannomas are typically solitary tumors composed of Schwann cells, and they are far more frequently found on sensory nerve roots than on motor roots (Fig. 6–6). When they are a manifestation of von Recklinghausen's neurofibromatosis, schwannomas may be multiple and associated with gliomas, meningiomas, and other neoplasms. Alternatively, neurofibromas arise from both Schwann cells and fibroblasts. In the setting of von Recklinghausen's neurofibromatosis, they are often multiple (Fig. 6–7) and may undergo malignant change, developing into neurofibrosarcomas.[17] Despite these pathological and biological differences, clinical series of spinal

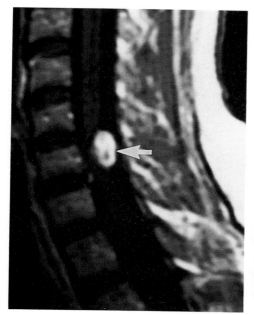
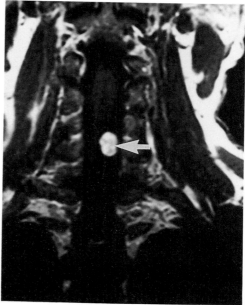

A

B

Figure 6–6. An MRI of the cervical spine, revealing a schwannoma. A 47-year-old man presented with neck and radicular pain initially suspected to be due to cervical spondylosis. When it did not improve with antiinflammatory agents and physical therapy an MRI was performed. (A) Sagittal image reveals a contrast enhancing extramedullary lesion in the posterior aspect of the spinal canal (arrow). (B) Coronal image demonstrates the tumor to be extramedullary and lateral to the cord (arrow). Following removal of the schwannoma, the patient had no neurologic impairment. (Courtesy of Dr. Richard Becker)

tumors[1,5,6,16,18,30] often do not distinguish between schwannomas and neurofibromas when nerve sheath tumors are being discussed. Therefore, in this text, "nerve sheath tumor" refers to both schwannomas and neurofibromas unless otherwise stated. It should be recognized, however, that a neurofibroma (or, less commonly, a schwannoma) in the setting of von Recklinghausen's disease has very different implications for clinical evaluation and management than does a solitary schwannoma.

Nerve sheath tumors have been considered to be among the most common primary spinal tumors. In one extensive series of spinal tumors,[2] they constituted 29% of all cases. In a review of 4885 histologically proven spinal tumors culled from the literature,[5] nerve sheath tumors accounted for 23% and meningiomas for 22%.

LOCATION

Nerve sheath tumors are more evenly distributed along the spinal axis than menin-

giomas. Among three series[30–32] with a total of 322 cases, 26% were cervical, 41% were thoracic, 31% were lumbar, and 2% were sacral. In the setting of von Recklinghausen's disease, multiple spinal nerve sheath tumors which may be associated with other neoplasms and pigmented skin lesions are frequently encountered.[5]

In relation to the meninges, nerve sheath tumors may be totally intradural, completely extradural, or extend both intradurally and extradurally. Among 163 cases,[32] 67% were intradural, 16.5% were intradural and extradural, and 16.5% were extradural. Intradural tumors are nearly always juxtamedullary; rarely, they may be intramedullary.[2,5]

Many nerve sheath tumors form dumbbell-shaped masses that extend through the intervertebral foramen. In one series,[30] 19% of nerve sheath tumors were dumbbell shaped. The extraspinal extension of such tumors can be massive and may, at times, be observed on chest radiograph or palpated on physical examination of the neck or abdomen. Although in

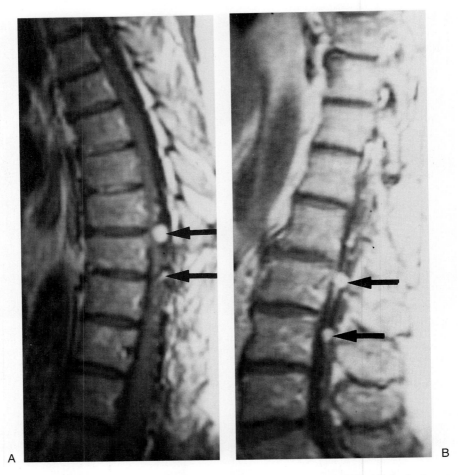

Figure 6–7. An MRI revealing multiple neurofibromas in neurofibromatosis (NF1). (A) Sagittal contrast-enhanced MRI of the thoracic spine demonstrates two neurofibromas (arrows). (B) An MRI of the lumbar spine reveals two more enhancing neurofibromas in the same patient (arrows). (Courtesy of Dr. Richard Becker.)

the transverse plane they may occur in any anatomical position in relation to the spinal cord, more tumors are located in the dorsal and lateral locations than ventrally.[30]

CLINICAL FEATURES

Gender and Age

Nerve sheath tumors affect both sexes equally.[5,30,31] They may occur in individuals ranging from childhood to the very elderly, but most are found in the middle-age years. Although one author reported that significant numbers were found between ages 11 and 70, more than 60% of cases were encountered from age 31 through 60.[30] In his series, the average age was 43.5 years (compared with 53 years as the average age of patients with spinal meningiomas[19]).

Symptoms and Signs

In an extensive literature review,[5] pain was the initial symptom in 74% of cases. The pain may be axial, radicular, and/or remote (referred lower in the spine or legs in cases of cervical or thoracic neoplasms). It is often exacerbated by Valsalva maneuvers, coughing, sneezing, and recumbency.[32,33] When symptoms and signs were analyzed according to level of spinal involvement, pain was the presenting complaint in 49% of cervical, 68% of thoracic, and 91% of lumbosacral tumors.[30]

Motor and sensory symptoms and signs are occasional presenting complaints, and are frequently found at the time of diagnosis. These neurological disturbances may be of radicular and/or funicular origin. In one series,[5] the presenting complaint was motility disturbance in 15% and sensory abnormalities in 9% of cases. However, by the time of diagnosis, motor disturbances were present in 85% of cases and sensory abnormalities in 70%. A similarly high incidence of motor and sensory symptoms and signs has been found at the time of diagnosis in other series.[30]

Sphincter disturbance and sexual dysfunction form the fourth principal symptom. Such disturbances were found to be the presenting complaint in only 2.5% of Nittner's published experience,[5] but at the time of diagnosis, approximately 54% of patients had such vegetative disturbances.

Out of the four principal clinical features (pain, motor disorder, sensory abnormalities, and sphincter dysfunction) most patients are found to have a combination of at least two of them at diagnosis. For example, more than 97% of cases cited by Nittner[5] had two abnormalities and 93% had three such clinical abnormalities at diagnosis;[34] 65% had all four. A similar experience was reported by another author.[30]

The duration of symptoms prior to diagnosis of a spinal nerve sheath tumor averages one to four years. The shortest average course of symptoms is observed in cervical lesions, and the longest is seen among lumbar neoplasms.[30] Occasionally, the duration of symptoms may be only weeks in length, and in exceptional cases, it may persist for decades. The longest reported course was over 28 years.[5]

LABORATORY AND DIAGNOSTIC IMAGING STUDIES

Diagnostic Imaging Studies

As in many clinical series, neurofibromas and schwannomas are often grouped to-gether as nerve sheath tumors in the radiological literature.[23,26] Abnormalities on plain radiographs are often encountered in contradistinction to the experience with spinal meningiomas. In three series, the incidence of abnormalities on plain radiograph in cases of spinal nerve sheath tumors ranged from 43% to 52%.[18,30,31] Those abnormalities most commonly encountered include widening of the intervertebral foramen, erosion of the pedicle or vertebral body, and widening of the interpedicular distance. In the case of large extradural thoracic tumors, the mass may be evident on chest radiograph. Spinal nerve sheath tumors associated with normal plain radiographs were more likely to be completely intradural, whereas those with extension into the extradural space are characteristically associated with plain radiograph abnormalities and are often of the dumbbell variety.[18]

Prior to the advent of CT and MRI, myelography was essential for the diagnosis of most cases of spinal nerve sheath tumor. In cases of intradural tumor, a mass is usually observed displacing the cord with widened subarachnoid space just above and below the lesion. Although such neoplasms arise from nerve sheath elements, they occasionally demonstrate no anatomical contact with a nerve root on myelography.[31] Although criteria have been proposed to distinguish nerve sheath tumors from meningiomas on myelography, they may be difficult to differentiate.[5,18,30] As in the case of any intraspinal neoplasm, lumbar puncture below a compressing lesion occasionally may be associated with neurological deterioration, and appropriate treatment must be undertaken urgently to prevent permanent neurological damage.[35]

Computed tomography is a sensitive technique for evaluating nerve sheath tumors if the spinal segment affected by the tumor is imaged.[36] Noncontrast CT often demonstrates a mass slightly more dense than the spinal cord.[37] With intravenous contrast, uniform tumor enhancement is typical.[37-39] The relationship of the tumor to the spinal cord may be identified by CT following the intrathecal administration of contrast material.[40]

Magnetic resonance imaging is a superb technique for identifying nerve sheath tumors and may demonstrate both the intaspinal and paraspinal extent of the tumor.[26,28,29] Commonly these tumors show bright peripheral contrast enhancement.[41,42] It has been reported that malignant lesions can sometimes be differentiated from benign lesions by using MR criteria. Irregular infitrating margins in the malignant lesions and differences in the intensity of the central regions of the tumor may be observed.[43]

Cerebrospinal Fluid

The cerebrospinal fluid in cases of spinal nerve sheath tumor usually shows no signs of pleocytosis, but typically it reveals an increase in protein. Of 98 CSF analyses,[30] only 12 patients had an elevated CSF white cell count. Some of the CSF analyses were bloodstained. In patients with CSF pleocytosis, the tumors were intradural.

The CSF protein content was elevated in 82% (82/98) of cases, and it was higher in cases of intradural tumor than when the tumor was totally extradural. As expected, it appeared also to be higher in those with higher-grade blocks than in those with smaller lesions.

THERAPY

Surgery (usually laminectomy) is the optimal therapy for spinal cord compression resulting from nerve sheath tumors. Resection often leads to an excellent recovery of neurological function even if the patient has signs of severe neurological dysfunction at the time of diagnosis. This is apparently due to the ability of the spinal cord to adapt to compression from these slow-growing lesions.[44]

With total removal of these lesions, recurrence is rare. However, because these tumors often are intimately attached to nerve roots, complete resection may not be possible without sacrificing the root. In the setting of neurofibromatosis, multiple nerve sheath tumors may be present. Some may not be surgically resectable, or it may be impractical or unwise to surgically address multiple lesions. Neurofibro-

mas often are dumbbell in shape; the hourglass waist is caused by the confines of the neuroforamina through which it passes.[45] Their location along nerve roots should warrant extra concern on the part of the surgeon due to the possibility of injury to a major radicular vessel, such as the radiculomedullary artery of Adamkiewicz during the surgical procedure, resulting in paralysis.

CASE ILLUSTRATION

A 30-year-old businessman presented with right-sided weakness and gait difficulty. He had noted progressive weakness of his right arm over a period of 18 months. In addition, he observed weakness and stiffness of the right and, more recently, the left lower extremities. His disability, however, did not prevent him from engaging in athletics. One week before neurological evaluation, he developed transient right hemiplegia after being struck on the head with a soccer ball. On neurological examination, there were no café au lait spots. Cranial nerves and funduscopic examinations were normal. He had disuse atrophy of the right upper extremity associated with spastic weakness. There was spastic weakness of both lower extremities, with the right more affected than the left. The left upper extremity motor examination was normal. Sensory examination was unremarkable. Jaw jerk was normal, deep tendon reflexes were increased throughout, and plantar responses were flexor bilaterally. Gait was slightly ataxic.

The clinical impression was a high cervical or foramen magnum neoplasm. An MRI was performed (Fig. 6–8). Severe spinal cord compression from an extra-axial mass was observed to the left of and anterior to the spinal cord. The patient underwent complete resection of the C1–2 mass, which was found to be a neurofibroma. He had a complete return of neurological function several months after the operation.

Comment. This case illustrates several important clinical points. This benign tumor in the region of the foramen magnum caused weakness to progress from the ipsilateral upper extremity to the ipsilateral leg and then to the contralateral leg, as often observed in fora-

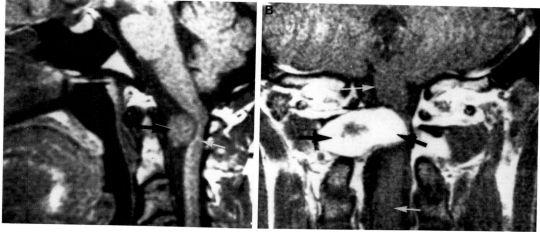

Figure 6–8. Spinal neurofibroma at C1–2 level. (A) This nonenhanced sagittal MRI demonstrates the neurofibroma (black arrow) anterior and compressing the spinal cord (white arrow). (B) This gadolinium-enhanced coronal MRI demonstrates the tumor (black arrows) lateral to the spinal cord (white arrows). (Courtesy of Dr. Joseph Piepmeier.)

men magnum mass lesions (see Chapter 2). The symptoms were slowly progressive, but the patient markedly deteriorated following incidental trauma, as is sometimes observed with spinal cord compression. Furthermore, despite severe spinal cord compression as observed on the MRI, the patient had a relative paucity of neurological signs consistent with the long evolution of spinal cord compression. Finally, the patient had an excellent outcome following surgical removal.

VASCULAR MALFORMATIONS AND VASCULAR TUMORS

The classification and nomenclature of vascular malformations and tumors have represented a great problem for the pathologist and clinician from the time these lesions were first described.[46,47] Several pathological classifications have been proposed (Table 6–1). Hemangioblastomas are neoplasms and arteriovenous malformations are not true neoplasms, but both are capable of growth and compression of neighboring tissue. They may be very difficult to differentiate clinically, because both may present as enlarging mass lesions, may hemorrhage, or may cause ischemic neurological symptoms. Finally, they may be difficult to separate clinically because in 48% of spinal hemangioblastomas,[48,49] an associated meningeal varicosity or arteriovenous malformation (AVM) is found.

The frequency of vascular malformations and neoplasms of the spine is diffi-

Table 6–1. **Classification of Spinal Vascular Malformations and Vascular Tumors**

Vascular Malformations	Vascular Tumors
Capillary Telangiectasia	Capillary Hemangioblastoma
Cavernous Angioma	Angiosarcoma
Arteriovenous Malformation	
Dural	
Intradural	
Venous Malformation	

cult to ascertain with certainty because the malformations may be clinically silent. Collectively, vascular malformations and neoplasms have been estimated to account for approximately 5% to 10% of primary "tumors" of the spine.[49,50] Vascular malformations are much more frequent than vascular tumors.[49]

Vascular Malformations

While in the past spinal arteriovenous malformations had been described pathologically, more recently they have been classified according to the location of the arteriovenous shunt.[47] With the development of spinal arteriography, these lesions are now distinguished on the basis of their location in relation to the dura and whether there are intervening abnormal vessels between the feeding artery and draining vein. Using arteriography, in 1977 Kendall and Logue[52] classified spinal arteriovenous malformations into two major types, dural and intradural. Dural AVMs are arteriovenous fistulas (here called dural AV fistulas or dural AVFs) and are defined as spinal vascular lesions in which the vascular nidus of the AV shunt is embedded in the dura, typically at the proximal nerve root sleeve.[53] Alternatively, intradural AVMs are defined as le-

sions in which the vascular nidus is located within the spinal cord or pia mater. Intradural AVMs are supplied by medullary arteries,[54] and may be further classified as intramedullary AVMs (juvenile and glomus types) and direct AV fistulas.

More recently, spinal vascular malformations have been classified into 4 types: type I—dural arteriovenous fistula (AVF); type II—spinal cord AVM; type III—juvenile AVM; and type IV—perimedullary AVF. Type I is dural and Types II–IV are intradural. Types I–III occur in decreasing frequency. Type IV, however, is more common than type III but less common than types I and II (Table 6–2).[55,56]

Type I vascular malformations, dural AVFs, are thought to be acquired lesions and are the most prevalent type of spinal AVM, accounting for over 80% of cases. They are most common in males in their fourth to sixth decade and are typically found in the lower thoracic region and conus medullaris. The feeding artery is usually a branch of an intercostal or lumbar artery. The branch enters the dura in the region of a root sleeve that makes a fistula within or beneath the dura and flows into medullary veins on the dorsal surface of the spinal cord (Fig. 6–9). McCutcheon et al.[53] have shown in a microangiographic study from en bloc resections of dural vascular abnormalities that these are direct

Table 6–2. **Comparison of Characteristics of Type I (Dural) and Type II, III, and IV (Intradural) Spinal AVMs***

Characteristic	Type I (Dural) AVM	Type II, III, and IV (Intradural) AVMs
Percentage of AVMs	85%–90%	10%–15%
Average age of patient at onset	40–50 year	10–25 year (older with type IV)
Etiology	Acquired	Congenital
Spinal location	Thoracolumbar > thoracic (cervical location rare)	Entire spinal axis
Acute symptom onset	Uncommon (10%–15%)	Common (50%–70%)
Chronic symptoms	Common (85%–95%)	Less common (30%–50%)
Subarachnoid hemorrhage	Rare	Common (50%–70%)
Symptom progression	Progressive worsening typical without significant clinical improvement	Spontaneous improvement to some degree common with recurrence of symptoms

*AVM = arteriovenous malformation.
From Hamilton, M, et al. 68, p. 2276, with permission.

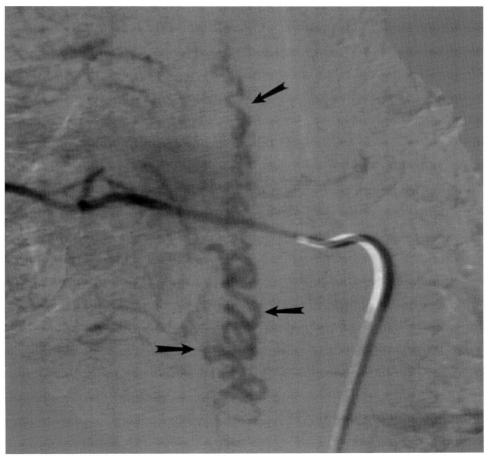

Figure 6–9. A middle-aged man presented with a rapidly progressive thoracic myelopathy. An MRI demonstrated venous congestion and a dorsal irregular vascular mass. As this angiogram demonstrates, there is an AV fistula (arrows) filling from T8 on the right. The feeding vessel was ligated surgically (extraspinally). The patient immediately improved to a functional ambulatory state.

AV fistulas that lack a glomerular nidus of capillaries of the sort classically seen in AVMs. Normally there is no vascular connection between the dural artery, feeding both the dural root sleeve and its adjacent spinal dura, and the medullary vein, which drains the spinal cord via the coronal venous plexus and radial arteries of the spinal cord. In the case of a spinal dural fistula, there is an abnormal shunt between the dural branch of an intercostal artery or lumbar artery and the intradural spinal veins. Since the AV fistula is drained by intradural medullary veins, the high arterial pressure from the AV fistula is transmitted to the intradural venous system and flow is reversed in the in-

tradural venous system. Accordingly, the coronal venous plexus and intraparenchymal radial veins of the spinal cord become engorged, causing venous hypertension within the spinal cord.[53] The resulting abnormal tangle of blood vessels on the surface of the cord represents the venous outflow system, which previously had been thought to represent an intradural AVM. Rather, these vessels represent the arterialized coronal venous plexus, which receives blood from the fistulous communication between the dural artery and medullary vein. In the microangiographic study of McCutcheon et al.[53] cited above, the most typical finding was that there were multiple feeding arteries and a single draining vein in the dural AVFs studied. In addition, some patients may have had more than one segmental feeding vessel supplying the arteriovenous fistula.[54,57]

Type II spinal cord AVMs are congenital high-flow, high-pressure, intramedullary lesions that have a true nidus of abnormal vessels within the parenchyma of the spinal cord. These lesions are often referred to as *glomus AVMs*. Type II AVMs are fed by branches of the anterior spinal artery and intadural arterial system. There may be a common arterial system feeding the AVM and spinal cord, which is critically important in treatment planning. Like intracranial AVMs, they often have multiple feeding arteries. Also like intracranial AVMs, symptoms frequently arise from hemorrhage or via the vascular steal phenomenon.

Type III vascular malformations, also called juvenile AVMs, are rare congenital high-flow, high-pressure lesions. They are usually very large, and they may be fed by arteries from multiple different spinal levels. Furthermore, they may extend beyond the spinal parenchyma per se into the extramedullary space or even extraspinal locations. They are very difficult to treat because of extraspinal, spinal column, and spinal cord involvement. Similarly, they usually present via hemorrhage or the steal phenomenon.

Type IV vascular malformations are intradural, extramedullary, or perimedullary arteriovenous fistulae. Originally described in 1977 by Djindjian and colleagues,[58] they were classified as type IV AVMs by Heros et al. in 1986.[59] Most are located anterior to the cord and are fed by the anterior spinal artery. They have been further subclassified into type, IVa, IVb, and IVc depending on their anatomic characteristics and size.[55,56] They often present with a progressive neurological defect due to venous hypertension. Less commonly, they present with hemorrhage.

The rostral–caudal location of spinal AVMs depends upon the type. Intradural AVMs have been found to be more uniformly distributed along the spinal axis than dural AVMs, which show a predilection for the low thoracic and lumbar areas.[54,60]

The etiology of AVMs is controversial. It has been suggested that dural AVMs may be acquired, and intramedullary AVMs are congenital in origin.[54]

PATHOGENESIS OF NEUROLOGIC MANIFESTATIONS

The pathogenic explanations for neurological dysfunction in spinal AVMs include venous hypertension, arterial steal, hemorrhage, venous thrombosis and, when present, compressive effects from dilated varices and aneurysms. The clinical presentation and pathogenesis of neurological manifestations are to a large extent determined by the type of AVM. As discussed above, in the case of dural AV fistulas, it is suggested that the valveless venous system allows high venous pressure from the AV fistula to be transmitted to the spinal veins, causing congestive myelopathy. (The characteristic angiographic feature of dural AV fistulas is the early filling of pial veins following injection of intercostal or lumbar arteries.) It is this direct communication between the arterial system and the pial veins which causes venous hypertension within the spinal cord. Furthermore, the caudal cord and conus medullaris are typically involved in cases of dural AV fistulas, a finding which has been recently explained on the basis of gravity and its effect on the congestive edema.[60]

Pathological examination of the cord in a recent report confirmed the concept that venous hypertension contributes to the pathophysiology of progressive myelopathy.[57] The histopathology demonstrated hyalinized blood vessels, arterialized veins, vascular calcification, and thrombosis along with necrosis of gray and white matter, gliosis, and lipid-laden macrophages. The histopathology described was identical to that seen in Foix-Alajouanine syndrome.[57] Arterial steal and hemorrhage are not likely explanations for the pathogenesis of neurological dysfunction in dural AVMs. However, with intradural AVMs, all pathogenic mechanisms noted above are considered possible explanations.[54]

CLINICAL FEATURES

Spinal vascular malformations occur more commonly in men than in women. Over two-thirds of patients in most series are men.[50,54,61] The clinical presentation is highly dependent upon whether the lesions are dural or intradural (Table 6–2). The average age of patients presenting with dural AVMs is greater than that of patients with intradural AVMs. In one series,[54] the average age of patients with dural AV fistulas was 49 years (range: 22–72); whereas the average age of those with intradural AVMs was 27 (range: 4–58), with 65% of patients under 25 years of age.

The symptoms caused by vascular malformations are similar to those of other space-occupying lesions of the spine—pain, motor deficit, sensory loss, and sphincter disturbance (Table 6–3). Pain may be local, funicular, and/or radicular in nature. When due to hematomyelia or subarachnoid hemorrhage, it can be meningeal, radicular, or funicular in origin. Precipitating factors found to play a role in the onset of spinal AVMs in occasional patients include physical exertion, trauma, and pregnancy.[50,54,61]

As shown in Table 6–3, paresis is the most common presenting symptom in patients with dural AVMs, whereas hemorrhage, common in conjunction with intradural AVMs, is not observed with dural fistulas. Weakness is usually manifested as spastic paraparesis; loss of pain and temperature is the most common sensory complaint. When a sensory level is present, it often corresponds to the level of the vascular nidus. Spinal bruits usually indicate high-flow intradural lesions. Some authors have found that intermittent neurogenic claudication may be the presenting complaint of spinal arteriovenous malformations.[62,63] Madsen and Heros[64] review the pathogenesis of neurogenic claudication and postulate that venous hypertension could be the mechanism that explains some of the neurological manifestations of spinal AVMs.

The temporal profile of clinical presentation of vascular malformations varies widely and, again, depends to a significant extent upon the type of AVM (see Table 6–2). Type 1 lesions typically present with a long history of progressive myeloradiculopathy, which may resemble the temporal profile of a spinal neoplasm.[57,65] The lower extremities are involved, typically

Table 6–3. Initial Symptoms and Symptoms at Diagnosis of Spinal AVM[*†]

Symptom	Initial Symptoms		Symptoms at Diagnosis[‡]	
	Dural AVMs	Intradural AVMs	Dural AVMs	Intra-dural AVMs
Back pain	2	8	11	10
Root pain	4	2	7	20
Paresis	12	16	21	50
Sensory change	5	5	18	40
Impotence	1	2	14	23
Hemorrhage	0	17	0	28
Bowel disturbance	1	1	17	24
Bladder dysfunction	2	3	22	40
Total cases	27	54	27	54

[*]From Rosenblum, B, et al.,[54] p. 798, with permission.
[†]AVM = arteriovenous malformation.
[‡]The values listed indicate the number of patients with those symptoms when the diagnosis of spinal AVM was established. Most patients had several of the symptoms.

with sparing of the arms. Apoplectiform loss of neurologic function is unusual given the fact that these lesions infrequently hemorrhage as compared to their intradural counterparts. Alternatively, type II and type III spinal AVMs are high-flow lesions, which like cerebral AVMs carry a significant risk of either intramedullary or subarachnoid hemorrhage. Furthermore, type II and type III lesions occur more evenly throughout the length of the spinal axis and are more evenly distributed between the sexes. Accordingly, the patient with a type II or III AVM more commonly presents at a younger age with an acute onset of neurologic dysfunction anywhere along the spinal axis. The clinical presentation of type IV lesions depends upon the size of the lesion and the rapidity of flow. Patients may present with either slow progressive manifestations or apoplectiform onsets. Both upper and lower extremities can be affected, and there is a relatively even distribution between the sexes. Presentation is typically between the third and sixth decades.

Spinal vascular malformations may be associated with AVMs elsewhere and with other physical findings. In the Klippel-Trénaunay-Weber syndrome, an accompanying cutaneous angioma is associated with a spinal vascular malformation. Other dysplasias associated with spinal angiomas have been reported.[49] Cerebral and spinal aneurysms may also be observed.[54] Furthermore, a vertebral angioma may be observed on radiological study of the spine.[50]

The Foix-Alajouanine syndrome[66,67] has been considered an example of progressive myelopathy secondary to a dural vascular malformation (type I, see above).[68] This syndrome is characterized by a subacute or chronic progressive course, leading over a period of months to paraplegia. Spasticity is said to occur early, but it evolves into a flaccid, areflexic paraplegia associated with sensory loss and impairment of sphincter function. Pathologically, in most cases there is evidence of venous hypertension and severe necrosis of gray and white matter, most marked in lumbosacral segments but extending upward in some cases to thoracic levels. Blood vessels show thickened, cellular, and fibrotic walls.[57,69–71]

LABORATORY AND DIAGNOSTIC IMAGING STUDIES

The CSF may show elevated protein and evidence of recent bleeding, but a normal CSF profile does not exclude a spinal angioma.[50,61] Myelography is reported to be abnormal in over 90% of cases of spinal vascular malformations and is specific for the diagnosis in nearly two-thirds.[61] It has been suggested that by demonstrating characteristic filling defects, myelography has been more sensitive than MRI in detecting enlarged intradural veins, especially those with low flow.[65,72] The rapid advances in MRI and MR angiography are expected to improve sensitivity of this modality (see below). Spinal angiography has also been found to be specific and critical for identifying the feeding vessels and draining veins, as well as the vascular nidus.[55,56,61,73] However, as demonstrated by the microangiographic study of McCutcheon et al.,[53] multiple collateral feeding arteries, which may not be visualized using spinal arteriography, are usually present. The CT is often abnormal but enhancement may be difficult to differentiate from neoplasms. Dynamic CT, in which CT images are obtained successively every few seconds, may help distinguish between a neoplasm and a vascular malformation.[39]

An MRI provides several advantages in evaluating spinal AVMs. There have been several studies reporting the results of MRI in cases of dural AVFs which are reviewed below. These include not only the demonstration of an abnormally enlarged and tortuous venous system in some cases but also the effects on the spinal cord itself. For example, cord edema, diffuse increase in cord diameter, abnormal cord enhancement, and myelomalacia have been reported.[55–57,74–76)] As noted previously, the caudal cord and conus medullaris are typically involved in cases of dural AV fistuals regardless of the level of the abnormal vascular nidus. Accordingly, MRI may show cord signal abnormality extending from the conus ros-trally.[57,60] In a study of 14 patients with spinal dural arteriovenous fistulas, all patients had regions of abnormal signal on T_2-weighted images, 93% had focal increased cord caliber, and 57% had prominent intradural vessels.[77] However, these findings were considered relatively non-specific. Other authors have reported that the findings on MRI may be difficult to distinguish from neoplasms.[57,78] An MRI may not reliably demonstrate the vascular fistula in types I and IV spinal AVMs.[68] It has been reported that when the MRI is nonspecific, myelography may improve diagnostic sensitivity.[79] In cases of type II and III spinal AVMs, MRI can often visualize the vacular nidus of the AVM.[68] With MR angiography, the arterial pedicles of spinal AVMs have been shown.[80]

Arteriography is the specific diagnostic test that permits visualization of the feeding arteries and draining veins. When there is a high index of suspicion that a spinal AVM exists, but confirmation via other imaging modalities has not been forthcoming, spinal angiography may be required to establish the diagnosis. Spinal angiography can be helpful (*1*) in confirming the diagnosis, (*2*) identifying the vascular anatomy of the lesion, and (*3*) classifying the AVM. This information is important in planning therapy in choosing between endovascular and surgical interventions.[81]

THERAPY

The management of spinal AVMs is controversial and difficult.[47,68] For the most part, it is dictated by the type of malformation, its site of origin, and its extent.[82] Barrow and Anson and Spetzler presented general recommendations based on these factors.[55,56] With the advent of microsurgical techniques and spinal angiography, treatment has improved. For example, type I (dural) AVMs have been obliterated by surgically ligating the feeding vessels to the AVM.[83] Using this technique, Spetzler and colleagues[68] reported that 18 (72%) of 25 patients with type I spinal AVMs clinically improved, 6 (24%) stablized, and 1 (4%) worsened. For patients with

intradural AVMs, endovascular embolization has become an alternative to surgery or has been performed preoperatively.[68,73,79] However, both surgery and embolization carry the significant risk of worsening the neurological deficit. Thus, in some cases no intervention is recommended. Patients should be managed by physicians with a large experience with these rare and often devastating lesions.[54,73,83]

Spinal Vascular Neoplasms

A review of spinal hemangioblastomas[2,48,51] reported that they represent approximately 2% of all spinal tumors, 3% of intramedullary neoplasms, 2% of extra-medullary–intradural tumors, and 4% of extradural tumors. It should be recognized that these surgical series tend to exclude metastatic neoplasms.

CLINICAL FEATURES OF SPINAL HEMANGIOBLASTOMAS

Some of the clinical features of spinal cord hemangioblastomas, which affect both sexes equally, are shown in Table 6–4.[48] The average age of patients with spinal hemangioblastomas is approximately 30 years. Of 85 hemangioblastomas, Browne et al. found the following levels of involvement: cervical, 38%; thoracic, 48%; and lumbar, 16% (Table 6–4).[48]

In the spinal cord, lesions are single in nearly 80% of cases. Lindau disease, characterized by hemangioblastomas occurring at multiple sites throughout the central nervous system, was found in nearly one-third of the patients in one review.[48] The associated hemangioblastomas were most common in the medulla, cerebellum, and retina. Of clinical importance is the observation that when cerebellar or retinal hemangioblastomas coexist with spinal lesions, the former usually become clinically symptomatic before those in the spine.

As most hemangioblastomas are situated in the dorsal aspect of the spinal cord, sensory loss and radicular pain are common early symptoms. As the other spinal tracts become involved, symptoms

Table 6–4. **Histologically Demonstrated Cases of Spinal Cord Hemangioblastoma***

	No. (%) of Patients	
Sex		
Male	42	(52.5)
Female	38	(47.5)
No. of Hemangioblastomas		
Single	59	(78.7)
Multiple	16	(21.3)
Position of Hemangioblastoma		
Intramedullary	45	(60.0)
Extramedullary–intradural	16	(21.3)
Intramedullary and	8	(10.7)
extramedullary		
Extradural	6	(8.0)
Level of Hemangioblastomas		
Cervical	30	(37.5)
Cervicothoracic	3	(3.7)
Thoracic	38	(47.5)
Lumbar	13	(16.2)
Lumbosacral	3	(3.7)
Sacral	2	(2.5)
Cauda equina	7	(8.7)
Syringomyelia		
Present	34	(43.0)
Absent	45	(57.0)
Meningeal Varices		
Present	34	(47.9)
Absent	37	(52.1)
Lindau disease	26	(32.5)
Coincident Hemangioblastomas		
Any location	26	(32.5)
Medulla	18	(22.5)
Cerebellum	15	(18.7)
Retina	14	(17.5)
Supratentorial area	3	(3.7)
Visceral Lesions of	18	(22.5)
Lindau Disease		
Family History of		
Hemangioblastoma		
Present	11	(23.9)
Absent	35	(76.1)

*From Browne, TR, et al.,[48] p. 439, with permission.

and signs extend to include motor findings. Spinal hemangioblastomas may remain clinically silent throughout life and be found incidentally at autopsy.[84,85]

The CSF in cases of spinal hemangioblastoma is often xanthochromic, and it has an elevated protein level.[86] Plain radiograph abnormalities were found in 37% of the cases shown in Table 6–4.[48] The most commonly encountered findings were widening of the interpedicular distance and the anteroposterior diameter of the vertebral canal. Several contiguous vertebrae are often found to have erosion of vertebral bodies and pedicles due to the expanding intraspinal mass.[87]

When performed, myelography is abnormal in over 90% of cases.[48] Depending upon the location of the tumor, both intramedullary and extramedullary masses may be found. When an associated syringomyelia has developed, the cord may be widened. This diagnosis should be considered dilated serpiginous vessels are encountered. Spinal angiography has been useful in the evaluation of these lesions.[88–90] A CT often reveals a soft-tissue mass with dramatic contrast enhancement,[39] and a cyst or syringomyelic cavity may be demonstrated. Several abnormalities may be observed using MRI, including diffuse enlargement of the spinal cord, cystic areas, and edema extending several segments beyond the limits of the tumor.[91] Following the administration of paramagnetic contrast agents, enhancement has been reported in spinal hemangioblastomas (Fig. 6–10).[26] The nidus of tumor may enhance, distinguishing it from an adjacent cyst.[28,92]

The definitive treatment of spinal hemangioblastomas is surgery (usually laminectomy).[48] Recent investigators have reported successful removal of spinal hemangioblastomas with improvement in neurological function postoperatively using microsurgical techniques.[93,94] In cases where larger lesions or strategically placed tumors may make complete removal impossible without unacceptable neurological injury, radiation therapy has been used following incomplete resection of the hemangioblastoma, or occasionally as primary therapy.[48] When the heman-

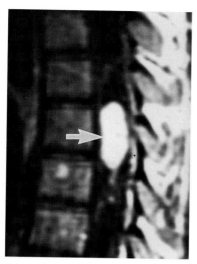

Figure 6–10. Thoracic spine MRI (sagittal image) reveals an enhancing intramedullary lesion (arrow) which was found at surgery to be a hemangioblastoma. (Courtesy of Dr. Richard Becker.)

gioblastoma nodule cannot be completely resected, it usually recurs. Infantile spinal hemangiomas may respond to steroid therapy.[45]

EPIDERMOID AND DERMOID CYSTS AND TERATOMAS

Epidermoid and dermoid cysts and teratomas comprise approximately 1% to 2% of primary spinal tumors. In the Mayo Clinic analysis of 1322 tumors of the spine, 18 (1.4%) were one of these histological types. Of this group, ten were intramedullary tumors; however, these neoplasms also may reside in the extramedullary–intradural space. Among children, these tumors account for nearly 5% of primary spinal tumors.[95]

The wall of an epidermoid cyst is composed of connective tissue lined by stratified squamous epithelium.[96–99] The central cavity of the cyst contains fat-laden keratinized debris produced by the epithelium.[100] The wall of a dermoid cyst has a similar composition, but it also contains such dermal appendages as hair follicles, sebaceous glands, and occasional sweat glands.[101] The central cavity may also contain hair and glandular secretions. When

either cyst is present in the subarachnoid space, it may be surrounded by signs of chronic inflammation. These cysts may release their contents, resulting in arachnoiditis.[102,103]

Epidermoid and dermoid cysts arise either as a result of an error in development in which cutaneous ectoderm is enclosed within the neural tube[104] or, possibly, as a result of the introduction of skin at the time of lumbar puncture.[105–107] Evidence suggests that epidermoid tumors may develop years after lumbar puncture is performed.[108] When the tumors occur in the setting of a developmental error, other anomalies may be found, such as spina bifida occulta, posterior dermal sinuses, syringomyelia, and diastematomyelia.[104,108] Dermal sinus tracts, beginning in the skin, may extend into the spinal canal and terminate intradurally in a dermoid cyst.[108–110]

Other related tumors and cysts may be more complex, exhibiting elements of mesodermal tissue and thus classified as teratomas.[111,112] Teratomas in the spinal canal are rare, with the majority appearing in childhood.[113] Other developmental abnormalities, such as spina bifida, are often found in association with such teratomas.[114]

Epidermoid and dermoid cysts are slow-growing mass lesions. They may occur at any level of the spinal axis,[114] but more often they are found in the lumbar region, causing symptoms referable to the cauda equina and conus medullaris. When they arise at a higher level in the spinal canal, symptoms and signs referable to these levels develop.

In cases associated with developmental anomalies, cutaneous stigmata consisting of hypertrichosis, pigmented skin, and cutaneous angiomas may be found. Repeated bouts of sterile meningitis due to rupture of the cysts may herald their presence. Examination of CSF under polarized light may demonstrate the presence of keratin released by an epidermoid cyst. In cases of developmental origin, vertebral defects may be noted on plain radiographs of the spine. Myelography and CT myelography[39] may demonstrate dermoids and epidermoids; MRI is expected to be useful in their evaluation.[26]

Surgery (usually laminectomy) is the treatment of choice. Gross total resection can usually be achieved.

LIPOMA

Spinal lipomas are rare primary tumors of the spinal canal composed of lobules of adult adipose tissue.[17,51,115] Many intraspinal lipomas are associated with other developmental defects of the vertebral arches, dura, and subcutaneous tissue. These lesions thus may be considered as part of a myelovertebral malformation rather than as an isolated spinal neoplasm. Such developmental lipomas are often transdural when observed in association with meningocele or myelomeningocele. A tethered conus medullaris may also be observed in such cases. The developmental lipomas associated with spinal dysraphism commonly occur in the caudal spinal canal and present in the early decades of life;[116–118] they are excluded from the present discussion.

Intradural spinal lipomas constitute approximately 1% of primary spinal tumors. In the Mayo Clinic series,[2] there were 6 (0.5%) lipomas among 1322 primary spinal neoplasms. Another study[118] found 6 (1.6%) intradural spinal lipomas among 378 primary spinal tumors. The tumors most frequently are located on the posterior surface of the spinal cord in the midline; this observation has led to the suggestion that they arise from embryologically misplaced cells.[46]

The lipoma is often covered on its dorsal surface by pia mater.[118] The neoplasm is usually adherent to the underlying spinal cord and may often extend into the substance of the cord itself. Lipomas are thus often both intramedullary and intradural–extramedullary in location. Any segmental level of the spinal axis may be the site of an intraspinal lipoma,[119] but the cervicothoracic region has been found to be a favored location.[118]

Although Giuffre[118] excluded spinal lipomatous malformations from his review, he still found that one-third of intradural lipomas were associated with other lesions, predominantly malforma-

tions, including spina bifida occulta, cranial osteomas, craniopharyngioma, subcutaneous lipoma at the same level, hydrocephalus, extradural lipoma, and intracranial lipoma. Thus, as with teratomas and epidermoid and dermoid cysts, the distinction between developmental anomalies and true neoplasms may be difficult.[112,114]

Intradural lipomas appear to show no predilection for either sex.[118] Although they may present at any age, approximately two-thirds of patients report that symptoms began before age 30.[118] Symptoms often are present for long periods of time prior to diagnosis. In the Mayo Clinic series,[2] the average duration of symptoms prior to surgery was 11 years, 8 months; the longest duration was 31 years. In the more recent review by Giuffre,[118] 56% of patients had symptoms exceeding 3 years; in 10%, the symptoms were present for over 20 years. The tumor may come to clinical attention after trauma, Valsalva maneuver (such as a sneeze), or pregnancy.[118,120]

Although pain was the first symptom in four of six patients in the Mayo Clinic series,[2] Giuffre[118] has commented on the infrequency of radicular pain in patients with intradural lipomas. In his review, numbness and ataxia were the most common presenting complaints. Despite the intramedullary location of some of these tumors, a suspended segmental sensory loss has been infrequently found.[118] As spinal cord compression or cauda equina compression ensues, the symptoms and signs are those of other space-occupying lesions of the spine. As with other spinal tumors, remissions and exacerbations have been reported in a minority of patients. The long duration of symptoms appears to be the most characteristic feature of intradural lipomas.

Plain radiographic abnormalities of the vertebral column are observed in approximately one-half of cases of intradural lipoma.[118] Widening of the spinal canal, abnormal curvature, and congenital abnormalities are the most frequently encountered characteristics. Myelography usually shows a mass lesion.[118] On CT, the tumor is usually observed as a noncontrast-enhancing, homogenous mass of low attenuation.[23,39,121] Magnetic resonance imaging is a sensitive technique for imaging lipomas. It plays a dominant role in their diagnosis and management.[26] When the intraspinal lipoma is associated with spinal dysraphism, many other abnormalities are observed.[22,122]

Surgery (usually laminectomy) is the treatment of choice for spinal cord compression with neurological deficit due to lipoma.[118] Recovery or improvement in function typically follows. If feasible, complete resection is preferred, but laminectomy alone may lead to a long period of clinical stabilization.[123] Complete resection may be difficult or dangerous due to an unclear demarcation between tumor and spinal cord.

INTRAMEDULLARY TUMORS

Gliomas are among the most common intramedullary spinal neoplasms: They are found in 0.01% to 0.06% of routine autopsies.[124] In the Mayo Clinic series of primary tumors of the spinal canal,[2] gliomas were the third most common tumor (after nerve sheath tumor and meningioma), accounting for 22% of all neoplasms encountered. Gliomas arise from neuroglia and may be classified in the spinal cord as ependymomas, astrocytomas, oligodendrogliomas, spongioblastomas, or subependymal gliomas.[2]

Over 60% of spinal gliomas are ependymomas; astrocytomas claim 25%, and glioblastoma and oligodendroglioma comprise 7.5% and 3%, respectively.[124] Among children alone, however, spinal astrocytoma is more common than ependymoma. Approximately 50% of all spinal gliomas are located in the caudal segments and filum terminale.[124] Oligodendrogliomas of the spinal cord are extremely rare; only 38 cases were reported prior to a review published in 1980.[125] Subependymal gliomas are similarly rare.[2] Spongioblastomas have been classified as astrocytomas.[17] Yagi and colleagues[126] have reported that intramedullary spinal cord tumors in patients with neurofibromatosis type 1 tend to be astrocytomas. Although

primary intramedullary spinal lymphoma[127] has been rarely reported, its frequency may increase as the incidence of primary CNS lymphoma rises.[128]

Ependymoma

Spinal ependymomas arise from ependymal cells and may occur as intramedullary growths throughout the length of the spinal cord or in the region of the cauda equina. Ependymal cells are those that line the central cavities of the central nervous system. In addition, ependymal cells have been found in abundance in the region of the filum terminale. Detailed histological studies of this structure found that the filum terminale is not merely a fibrous band; it contains multiple islands of ependymal cells.[129] These observations may explain the high frequency of ependymomas in the caudal spine.[130]

When ependymomas occur within the spinal parenchyma, they characteristically form a cylindrical mass surrounded by normal spinal tissue. The spinal cord may enlarge to cause a complete subarachnoid block. The tumor may extend from the intramedullary region of the spinal cord to breach the pia mater into the subarachnoid space.[2] When the tumor develops in the filum terminale, it forms a nodular or fusiform swelling in the caudal spinal canal. The tumor often grows between and invades the cauda equina.

Most ependymomas are histologically benign, although remote metastases may occur.[124] The presence of ependymal rosettes is a characteristic and, essentially, a diagnostic feature.[17] According to the histological classification used by Sloof, Kernohan, and MacCarty,[2] ependymomas may be graded from 1 to 4; grade 1 is the most benign form and grade 4 the most malignant. In their series of 169 cases, 108 were grade 1, 56 were grade 2, and 5 were grade 3 ependymomas; there were no grade 4 ependymomas. Furthermore, ependymomas may be classified as cellular, papillary, epithelial, myxopapillary, and mixed, according to their histological appearance. Although myxopapillary ependymomas are virtually restricted to the region of the conus medullaris and cauda equina, the other histological types also may occur in this region.[124]

Among primary spinal tumors, ependymomas were found in 13% [169] of the Mayo Clinic series of 1322 primary spinal tumors.[2] Ependymomas constitute the most common histological type of intramedullary glioma in the spinal cord including the filum terminale. In the large Mayo Clinic series, 62% of intramedullary and filum terminale gliomas were ependymomas.

LOCATION

Ependymomas may arise at any level of the central nervous system. In a clinical survey of 74 ependymomas cases,[131] 64% were intracranial and 36% were spinal.

Within the spinal canal, ependymomas are classified as intramedullary tumors when at the level of the spinal cord, or as neoplasms of the cauda equina. Of the 169 cases in the Mayo Clinic series,[2] 57% were at the level of the cauda equina and 43% were intramedullary. In other series of ependymomas,[2,131,132] 49% occurred at the level of the cauda equina and 50% were intramedullary (20% cervical and 31% thoracic).[133]

When ependymomas arise within the substance of the spinal cord, they often extend over multiple segments. In one surgical series of intramedullary spinal cord tumors,[134] the mean length of solid tumor was 4.7 segments. Occasionally spinal ependymomas may metastasize throughout the neuraxis.[135]

Among primary caudal tumors, ependymoma has been reported as the most frequent histological type.[136] In a series of 100 primary caudal tumors,[130] ependymoma accounted for 88% of cases. The second most common tumor in this series was astrocytoma, responsible for 8%.

CLINICAL FEATURES

Spinal ependymomas are more frequent in men than in women. Men accounted for 63%[131] and 59%[2] of cases in two series.

Spinal ependymomas may occur at any age from childhood to late life but, unlike

their intracranial counterparts, they appear to be rare in infancy and early childhood.[133] The youngest patient among 169 cases in one series[2] was 6 years old; the youngest in another was 14. The average age of patients with ependymomas of the filum terminale has been reported as 35 years, whereas the average age of those with intramedullary spinal cord ependymomas was 42 years.[2]

The interval of time between the onset of symptoms and diagnosis of spinal ependymoma ranges from days to years. In one series,[131] one patient presented after two days of leg weakness associated with coughing. At the other extreme, a patient with a caudal tumor had a 20-year history of coccygeal pain. Trauma often appears to precipitate symptoms; in the same series,[131] 33% of patients with spinal ependymomas attributed their symptoms to trauma.

In the detailed analysis of the Mayo Clinic series,[2] the average duration of symptoms was 56 months for grade 1 ependymomas and 33 months for grade 2. The average duration was similar for grade 1 lesions in the spinal cord as compared with the filum terminale (52 versus 58 months). For grade 2 tumors, however, the average preoperative duration was only 17 months for filum terminale lesions, compared with 49 months for intramedullary ones. Among the entire series for all sites, two thirds had symptoms for less than 4 years.[2]

The primary symptoms and signs in spinal ependymoma may be classified as pain, motor dysfunction, sensory disturbance, and sphincter disturbances. Pain, the most common initial symptom, may be due to vertebral compression (local), nerve root irritation (radicular), and/or ascending spinal tract involvement (funicular). Although these types of pain may occur separately, they more often occur in combination. As discussed in Chapter 2, the pain associated with intramedullary tumors is more often funicular than radicular.[137] Furthermore, funicular pain is usually bilateral, poorly localized, diffuse, and burning. Dysesthetic pain has been reported to be a common manifestation of cervical ependymomas, whereas motor dyfunction was found as the primary manifestaion in only five of 38 cases.[138] In the thoracic spine, scoliosis is a common clinical presentation.[139] Alternatively, pain due to cauda equina compression is usually radicular, although it may commonly be bilateral.

Among the 149 patients with spinal ependymomas, 117 experienced pain as the presenting symptom.[2] Back pain was the most common (60 patients), but back and limb pain (9 patients), lower extremity pain alone (16 patients), neck/upper extremity pain,[14] and truncal pain (6) also were reported. Coccygeal pain has also been observed as a presenting complaint.[131,133] In the series cited above,[2] three patients initially reported rectal discomfort.

In the same series,[2] the second most common presenting complaint was sensory disturbance. Twenty-one of 149 patients initially had sensory symptoms, generally in the form of numbness, coldness, and hypesthesia. The sensory disturbances could involve any region of the body. Motor disturbance was the third most common presenting symptom, reported in 15 patients. As with sensory complaints, motor disturbances more frequently involved the legs than the arms, but they could occur at any location. Sphincter disturbance or impotence was the presenting complaint in five patients.

LABORATORY AND DIAGNOSTIC IMAGING STUDIES

The cerebrospinal fluid usually demonstrates an elevated protein concentration, especially when the tumor causes a block of cerebrospinal pathways.[2,131] Occasionally a dry tap is encountered, especially with tumors of the filum terminale. A CSF pleocytosis is occasionally encountered; the average number of cells in the cerebrospinal fluid in the Mayo Clinic series[2] was 5 to 6 per cubic millimeter.

Plain radiographs of the spine have been reported as abnormal in a minority of patients with spinal ependymomas.[2] The abnormalities usually consist of widening of the interpedicular distance, erosion of the medial surface of the pedicle, and concavity of the posterior surface of the vertebral body. In one series,[131] these abnormalities were encountered in 38% of patients.

With myelography, intramedullary spinal tumors may show widening of the spinal cord. Alternatively, the width of the spinal cord may appear normal despite the presence of an intramedullary neoplasm. In the region of the filum terminale, an ependymoma may displace and compress the cauda equina. A CT is often complementary to myelography in cases of spinal ependymoma. A thin rim of intrathecal contrast may be observed on CT that is not evident with plain myelography, thus demonstrating the intramedullary location of the tumor. Nonenhanced CT of ependymomas frequently demonstrates a decreased attenuation or isodense tumor as compared with the cord.[39] Ependymomas may contrast-enhance following intravenous contrast administration.[24,39,140] Contrast enhancement of ependymomas may be prominent and has been found to be similar to that of intramedullary astrocytomas.[140]

Magnetic resonance imaging has been found useful in distinguishing syringomyelia from intramedullary tumors with or without associated tumor cavities.[26,74,141] With the use of paramagnetic contrast-enhanced MRI, spinal ependymomas may be readily observed (Fig. 6–11). Thus MRI is the initial imaging modality of choice in evaluating intramedullary spinal cord neoplasms.[141,142] T_1-weighted images may demonstrate cysts associated with the tumor and distinguish a cyst from solid tumor. Injection with contrast may reveal contrast enhancement that helps delineate the neoplasm from surrounding edema of the cord.[139] Patients with caudal spinal ependymomas should be evaluated for an intracranial ependymoma that is presenting with a drop metastasis.

THERAPY

While conservative surgery followed by radiotherapy had been recommended by some investigators,[143] the advent of improved surgical techniques has led to radi-

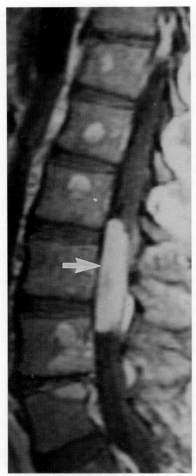

Figure 6–11. Ependymoma of the filum terminale. A 45-year-old woman presented with low back pain and sciatica. An MRI with contrast enhancement revealed a large enhancing mass (arrow) occupying most of the spinal canal. Surgical removal of the neoplasm revealed a myxopapillary ependymoma that was subtotally resected. She was treated with postoperative radiotherapy and did not have recurrence of her ependymoma for five years, at which time she died from acute leukemia. (Courtesy of Dr. Richard Becker.)

cal surgical resection of these lesions without routine adjuvant postoperative radiotherapy.[134,139] In a recent study of pediatric spinal cord ependymomas, 70% of tumors were totally removed.[144] In another series, clinical improvement or stabilization was reported in 21 of 29 patients (72%) undergoing radical resection of intramedullary tumors, usually via laminectomy (14 of the 29 patients had ependymomas).[134]

Ependymomas may be curable via aggressive surgery, particularly in cases in which a clear plane between tumor and spinal cord parenchyma exists. As with all intramedullary lesions, surgery entails a myelotomy, usually in midline, followed by suction and blunt dissection of the tumor and extirpation from its gliotic tumor bed within the parenchyma of the spinal cord.

The efficacy of postoperative radiotherapy following incomplete resection of spinal ependymomas is controversial. Withholding immediate postoperative radiotherapy following complete resection has been suggested,[139] but routine postoperative radiotherapy has been recommended in cases of incomplete resection.[45,143,145] Its value has been questioned by others.[139,146–148] In a recent retrospective study of 22 patients with spinal ependymal tumors treated between 1979 and 1993, it was concluded that radiotherapy is indicated after less than total resection of low-grade ependymal tumors, but not after total resection of ependymomas.[149] Other authors have suggested close follow-up of patients with low-grade ependymomas using serial MRI scans, reserving postoperative radiotherapy for those patients with rapid tumor growth or in cases where the ependymoma can not be removed radically.[139]

The prognosis for survival of patients with spinal ependymomas is relatively favorable. Of 51 patients with spinal ependymomas reported in one study,[146] 72% were alive at ten years. In a more recent study, the actuarial survival rate at five years was 96%.[149] In this latter series, there was no difference in survival between the group undergoing gross total resection versus those undergoing partial resection followed by radiotherapy. Patients with cauda equina tumors have a better prognosis than those with intramedullary neoplasms, and those with myxopapillary histology fare better than those with cellular pattern.[146]

Astrocytoma

Astrocytomas and ependymomas are the two most common intramedullary tumors of the spinal cord.[150] In the Mayo Clinic series,[2] 86 (7%) of the entire group of 1322 primary spinal tumors were astrocytomas. Although ependymomas (13%) were the most commonly encountered intramedullary tumor if the filum terminale is included in that designation, among tumors arising within the spinal cord per se, astrocytoma was the most common. Astrocytoma of the filum terminale is unusual, with only 7% of the cases of astrocytoma appearing in this region in the Mayo Clinic series.[2] In another surgical series of intramedullary tumors (excluding the filum terminale),[134] there were 14 ependymomas and ten astrocytomas. Among purely intramedullary spinal tumors in children, astrocytomas are approximately twice as frequent as ependymomas.[151,152]

As in the brain, spinal astrocytomas are often histologically classified from grade 1 to 4. The less malignant grades 1 and 2 are much more frequently encountered in the spinal cord than are the higher grade lesions.[153] Among the Mayo Clinic series, 76% were either grade 1 or 2.[2] A much higher incidence of more malignant astrocytomas is encountered in the brain.[2] Cysts or syringomyelia may be associated with spinal cord astrocytomas.[2,154]

LOCATION

The thoracic spine is the most frequent location for spinal cord astrocytomas.[2,134] In the Mayo Clinic series[2] 20% were in the cervical region, 13% in the cervicothoracic area, and 48% in the thoracic spine; only 5% were in the lumbar region alone. These observations correspond to the expected frequency of spinal cord tumors based on the relative length and mass of the spinal cord.[153] Using microsurgical techniques, Cooper and Epstein[134] found that the mean length of solid tumor in patients with astrocytoma was 5.3 segments.

CLINICAL FEATURES

Spinal cord astrocytomas are more frequently observed in men than in women.[153] Of 86 patients in the Mayo Clinic series,[2] 48 were males. These tumors may arise at any age, although the average patient is middle-aged. Patients with lower-grade tumors tend to be slightly older than those with more malignant lesions; in one series,[155] the average age of patients with astrocytoma grade 1 or 2 was 40 years, whereas that of patients with astrocytoma grade 3 or 4 was 34. The Mayo Clinic series[2] found the average age of patients with astrocytoma grade 1 or 2 was 37 years, whereas that of patients with glioblastoma was 23.

Although there is a considerable range, the mean duration of symptoms prior to diagnosis depends to some extent upon the grade of the astrocytoma. The average duration of symptoms in the Mayo Clinic series was reported to be 41 months for grade 1, 29 months for grade 2, 7 months for grade 3, and 4 months for grade 4.[2] The range of duration of symptoms was very broad, especially for lower-grade tumors; the interval ranged from 1 month to 12 years for grade 1 astrocytomas.

As in other spinal tumors, the most common presenting symptoms of patients with spinal astrocytomas are pain, motor disorders, sensory disturbances, and sphincter dysfunction. Pain is the most frequent presenting complaint,[2] and may be local, radicular, or funicular in nature; the site of referral depends on the location of the tumor. Motor disturbances are the second most frequent presenting complaint and include weakness, spasticity, or atrophy. When the lesion is in the cervical spine, upper extremity atrophy may be accompanied by lower extremity spasticity. Sensory and sphincter disturbances are less frequent presenting complaints. Sensory abnormalities often occur in a suspended distribution (see Chapter 2). At the time of diagnosis, most patients have more than one symptom, and they usually demonstrate multiple abnormalities on their neurological examination.[2]

LABORATORY AND DIAGNOSTIC IMAGING STUDIES

The cerebrospinal fluid usually shows signs of elevated protein, varying according to the degree of spinal block. Pleocytosis is occasionally found; the average number of white cells in the Mayo Clinic series[2] was 7 per cubic millimeter. On rare occasions, malignant astrocytomas may spread via the subarachnoid pathways and seed the leptomeninges throughout the neuraxis.[156] In such cases, the CSF may demonstrate malignant cells.

Plain radiographs of the spine are usually not helpful in evaluating patients with spinal astrocytomas. Among 74 patients undergoing such studies, only five demonstrated signs diagnostic of tumor.[2] Myelography is usually diagnostic of an intramedullary tumor but may occasionally be normal. A CT following the administration of intrathecal contrast is considered sensitive. A second series of CT scans obtained 12–24 hours following the intrathecal administration of contrast material may demonstrate the presence of an intramedullary cyst because the cystic cavities fill with dye.[23,134] An MRI may demonstrate the location and extent of these tumors, including the presence of an associated cyst or syringomyelia.[74,141] Following the administration of paramagnetic contrast material, MRI has been found to characterize and delineate of intramedullary astrocytomas.[26,92] Areas of contrast enhancement may identify regions of neoplastic tissue (Fig. 6–12).[92] The initial imaging procedure of choice for intramedullary spinal neoplasms is MRI.[139,141,142]

Somatosensory-evoked potentials (SSEP) have been used to evaluate intramedullary cord tumors and syringomyelia.[157] According to Restuccia and colleagues, the SSEP was frequently more sensitive than the clinical neurologic examination in defining the extent of involvement. This modality may offer an adjunct to the clinical examination and MRI scan in evaluating response to therapy, particularly in patients with subtle neurologic signs.

THERAPY

The therapy of intramedullary astrocytomas is controversial. While biopsy followed by radiotherapy has been recommended by many investigators,[143,149,158,159] recent advances in surgical techniques have led to reports of total or near-total resection of these tumors (via laminectomy as described for ependymomas) followed by improvement or stabilization of the clinical status in selected patients.[45,134,152,160,161] However, while a recent study reported that total resection could be achieved in 33% of pediatric patients with spinal astrocytomas, these authors concluded that the extent of resection did not significantly influence prognosis.[144] Postlaminectomy spinal deformities may be a significant postoperative complication, especially in children.[152] Although the benefits of adjuvant postoperative radiotherapy are controversial,[139,162] many authors recommend its use, especially in cases where there has been incomplete resection of the tumor.[45,149,152,158,159] In children, consideration needs to be given to the impact of radiotherapy on the developing nervous and osseous systems.[139]

Survival is related to the grade of the neoplasm.[158,159] In children and adolescents, grade 1 and 2 astrocytomas have a 5-year and 10-year survival rate of approximately 80% and 55%, respectively,[152] while patients with grade 3 or 4 lesions have a median survival of less than 1 year.[152,155,160] Alternatively, a Mayo Clinic report differentiated astrocytomas into pilocytic and diffuse fibrillary histologies.[159] Of 79 cases, 54% were pilocytic astrocytomas and 32% were diffuse fibrillary astrocytomas. (The remainder could not be classified further.) The 10-year survival rate for the pilocytic group was 81% and that for the diffuse fibrillary group was 15%. In the Mayo series,[159] the extent of surgical resection (i.e., biopsy, versus subtotal resection, versus gross total resection) did not significantly impact the survival of patients with pilocytic or nonpilocytic astrocytomas. Furthermore, patients undergoing postoperative radiotherapy (RT) had a longer survival than those not undergoing RT. The increased survival was more evident in the diffuse fibrillary histology type than the pilocytic type.

Chemotherapy has been used in selected cases of malignant astrocytoma of the spinal cord.[160] Using postoperative radiotherapy and the "8 drugs in 1 day" chemotherapy regimen in 13 children with high-grade gliomas of the spinal cord, Allen and colleagues [163] reported 5-year progression-free and total survival rates of 46 ± 14% and 54 ± 14%, respectively.

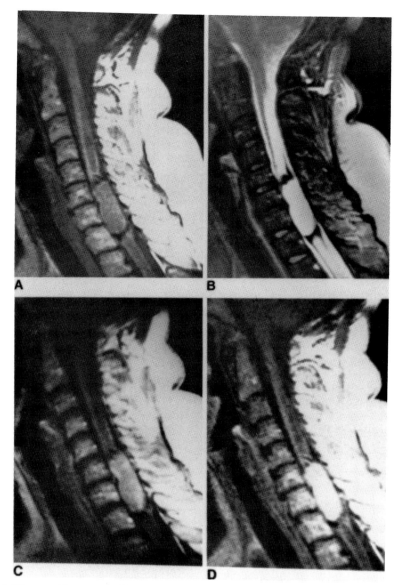

Figure 6–12. A 55-year-old woman with a spinal cord astrocytoma. (A) and (B) Noncontrast sagittal MRI demonstrates a central nidus with superior and inferior cysts. The markedly hypointense rim was shown pathologically to be hemosiderin deposition. (C) Gadolinium-enhanced MR sagittal image 30 minutes after administration of contrast material, disclosing peripheral enhancement of the central lesion. (D) One-hour-delayed gadolinium-enhanced sagittal scan showing enhancement of the central focus. Associated syrinxes are not surrounded by enhancing cord parenchyma, which suggests that they are probably benign reactive cysts (a finding confirmed at surgery) rather than tumor cysts. The necrotic nature of the tumor was shown pathologically and was probably responsible for delayed enhancement. (From Sze, G, et al.,[92] with permission.)

Intramedullary Metastasis

Intramedullary spinal cord metastases are rare and present difficult diagnostic and management problems. Approximately 100 cases had been reported as of a de-tailed review in 1985.[164] In an autopsy study 21 of 1066 patients with disseminated cancer, 200 had intraparenchymal central nervous system metastases. Of this group, an intramedullary spinal cord metastasis was found in ten. Thus in a detailed autopsy series, less than 1% of patients dying of malignancy were found to have intramedullary spinal cord metastasis. Using the same data, however, it may be concluded that the spinal cord is more susceptible to metastasis than is the brain.[165] Although the weight of the spinal cord is only 2% that of the brain, the autopsies found that 5% of intraparenchymal CNS metastases were to the spinal cord.[166] In another study of patients with small-cell lung cancer,[167] which has a high incidence of CNS metastases, 49% of patients had CNS metastases but only 6% had intraspinal involvement. Among the patients with intraspinal invasion, all had leptomeningeal metastases as well.

SITE OF PRIMARY TUMORS

Carcinoma of the lung appears to be the most common primary tumor causing intramedullary spinal cord metastasis. In a review of 55 cases of spinal cord metastases in the literature,[164] 49% were due to lung cancer; breast cancer accounted for 15%, followed by lymphoma (9%), colorectal (7%), head and neck (6%), renal cell (6%), and miscellaneous other neoplasms. In a review of 13 autopsied cases,[168] lung cancer accounted for 85% of cases, followed by breast cancer and melanoma, each responsible for 7.5%.

LOCATION AND PATHOLOGICAL FINDINGS

The spinal level of intramedullary spinal cord metastasis is roughly proportional to the length of spinal cord. Thus among 55 cases,[164] the cervical region had 31%; the thoracic cord, 42%; and the lumber region, 15%. The cervicothoracic and thoracolumbar areas accounted for the remaining cases.

In a gross pathological study, the spinal cord at the level of the tumor may or may not be enlarged.[168] Such absence of cord enlargement accounts for the lack of myelographic abnormalities in many cases. The metastasis may extend from one to several segments along the rostro-caudal axis.

The pathogenesis may be either direct metastasis to the cord, with occasional extension into the adjacent dorsal root or subarachnoid space, or, alternatively, leptomeningeal metastases with secondary extension into the spinal parenchyma. One pathological study[168] found 9 of 13 cases with direct metastasis to the spinal cord and 4 cases representing extension from the subarachnoid space to the spinal parenchyma.

A pathological study[169] concluded that most intramedullary metastases are the result of hematogenous dissemination to the cord directly rather than via transdural or perineural spread. It could not be determined whether the hematogenous spread occurred via venous or arterial routes or both. In a case report in which an intramedullary metastasis was associated with a spinal infarct[170] the authors suggested that the metastasis arose as a tumor embolus via the arterial system, which secondarily caused a spinal infarction.

CLINICAL FEATURES

As with epidural or leptomeningeal metastases from systemic cancer, intramedullary spinal cord metastases may herald the diagnosis of malignancy or develop years after the original diagnosis. In a review of 55 cases (Table 6–5),[164] the most frequent presenting complaints are pain and weakness. These symptoms usually occurred together in 33% of patients, but a similar proportion of patients presented with a single symptom. As presenting features, paresthesias and sphincter dysfunction were observed in 27% and 9%, respectively.

All 55 patients had weakness or paralysis on initial examination. Weakness was found in the following patterns: paraparesis (23 patients), monoparesis (15 patients), quadriparesis,[9] and hemiparesis.[8] An asymmetrical motor examination was found in 51% of cases. Atrophy was not common. Sensory deficits were observed in 64%; a sensory level was present in 49%. Despite a low incidence of bowel and bladder symptoms, signs of sphincter disturbance were observed in the majority (71%).

The time course between the onset of symptoms and the development of the full

Table 6–5. **Neurological Symptoms and Signs at the Time of Initial Evaluation of 55 Patients with Intramedullary Spinal Cord Metastasis***

Symptoms	No. of Patients (%)	
Pain	34	(62)
Nonradicular	16	(29)
Radicular	18	(33)
Motor Deficit	35	(64)
Paresthesias	15	(27)
Bowel/Bladder Dysfunction	5	(9)

Signs	No. of Patients (%)	
Motor Deficit	55	(100)
Sensory Level to Pin, etc.	27	(49)
Dermatomal Sensory Loss	7	(13)
Paresthesias	15	(27)
Atrophy of Musculature	3	(5)
Bowel/Bladder Dysfunction	39	(71)
Upgoing Toes	17	(31)
Tenderness Over Spine	4	(7)
Pain on Straight Leg Raising or Neck Flexion	6	(12)
Horner's Syndrome	2	(4)
Completed Neurological Deficit		
Flaccid paralysis	25	(45)
Spastic paresis/plegia	5	(9)
Brown-Séquard syndrome	6	(11)

*From Grem, JL, et al.,[164] p. 2310, with permission.

neurological deficit was less than 1 week in 22%, between 1 week and 1 month in 49%, and from 5 weeks to 6 months in 24%. In 5%, the neurological syndrome evolved for more than 6 months.[164]

LABORATORY AND DIAGNOSTIC IMAGING STUDIES

The cerebrospinal fluid in patients with intramedullary spinal cord metastasis is frequently abnormal, but the abnormalities are usually nonspecific. Protein levels are often elevated, and there may be pleocytosis. In cases of leptomeningeal metastases with secondary invasion of the spinal cord, there may be cytological evidence of malignant cells.

Radiological studies are usually necessary to confirm the clinical impression. Plain radiographs of the spine show evidence of vertebral metastases in 25% of cases;[164] the remainder are judged as normal.

Myelography was the most important diagnostic technique prior to the advent of MRI. On myelography, the characteristic appearance of an intramedullary spinal cord metastasis is widening of the cord in two perpendicular views.[164] A lobulated mass or prominent pial vessels may also be observed on the surface of the cord.[165] In one study,[164] 48% of myelograms demonstrated evidence of widening (fusiform swelling) of the spinal cord on two views. A partial or complete block, lobular filling defect, or abnormal dilated blood vessels were also observed. In the remaining 42% of cases, however, the myelogram was normal.

A CT of the spine following the intrathecal administration of contrast may be very sensitive to recognizing slight enlargement of the spinal cord. High-resolution CT of the spinal cord without intrathecal contrast may demonstrate the metastasis as an area of increased density in the spinal cord.[171]

The MRI is the diagnostic test of choice for identifying intramedullary metastases.[92,141,142] Contrast-enhanced studies typically show a well defined area of intramedullary enhancement, and when there is leptomeningeal disease, there may be enhancment of the meninges or nerve roots.[28,172]

CASE ILLUSTRATION

A 34-year-old woman was referred for increasing left upper extremity weakness and gait difficulty. She had a history of metastatic breast cancer to bone, lungs, liver, and brain. She had received whole brain irradiation five months earlier for a cerebellar metastasis. During the two weeks prior to referral, she noticed progressive left upper extremity weakness and occipital headache.

General physical examination demonstrated an enlarged liver and ascites. On neurological examination, she had normal higher integrative functions and cranial nerves. There was no nystagmus. Funduscopic examination was benign. There was weakness of the left arm

(4 - /5) and left leg (4/5) but no weakness of the right side. No sensory deficit was found, and there was no cerebellar disturbance. Gait was unsteady, with left lower extremity weakness. There were increased reflexes on the left and sustained left ankle clonus. Both toes were downgoing on plantar stimulation. The differential diagnosis was considered to be recurrent brain or cervical spine metastasis (possibly lep-tomeningeal cancer) or, less likely, radiation-induced CNS dysfunction.

A CT was performed to exclude recurrent cerebral metastases. It demonstrated no evidence of metastatic disease or hydrocephalus. A total spine MRI without and with gadolinium enhancement demonstrated an enhancing intramedullary metastasis in the cervical spine (Fig. 6–13)

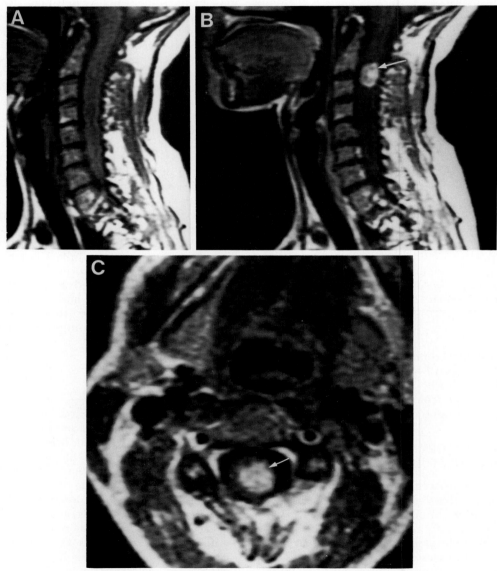

Figure 6–13. A cervical spine MRI is shown with an enhancing intramedullary metastasis from breast cancer. (A) Nonenhanced sagittal MRI shows a subtle spinal cord abnormality. (B) Enhancement of an intramedullary mass is observed following the administration of gadolinium. (C) Axial section showing enhancing metastasis within the spinal cord.

but no other evidence of metastases. The patient showed an excellent neurological response to corticosteroids and radiation therapy to the cervical spine.

DIFFERENTIAL DIAGNOSIS

Intramedullary spinal cord metastases cannot be clinically differentiated from epidural metastasis on the basis of symptoms or signs.[165] Pain, motor disturbances, sensory findings (dissociated or otherwise), and sphincter disturbances do not discriminate between these two locations.[165] In such cases, the clinician must resort to radiological procedures to discriminate between intramedullary and epidural metastasis. As discussed in Chapter 5, myelography and usually MRI will confidently demonstrate an epidural metastasis compressing the spinal cord.

When the cancer patient develops symptoms and signs of myelopathy and the radiological workup fails to reveal an epidural metastasis, the physician is confronted with a difficult diagnostic problem. The diagnostic possibilities may include metastatic disease (e.g., leptomeningeal metastases, intramedullary spinal cord metastasis); untoward effects of antineoplastic therapy (e.g., radiation myelopathy and myelopathy caused by intrathecal chemotherapy); remote effects of cancer (e.g., paraneo-

plastic necrotizing myelopathy); or causes unrelated to the cancer or its treatment, such as multiple sclerosis, subacute combined degeneration, spondylosis, or trauma. The clinical differentiation of intramedullary spinal cord metastasis from radiation myelopathy, paraneoplastic necrotizing myelopathy, and leptomeningeal metastases may present the clinician with a daunting task (Table 6–6).

The various clinical syndromes of radiation myelopathy are more fully discussed in Chapter 8. The most common syndrome is the early transient disorder consisting of Lhermitte's sign, which occurs within a few months of radiation therapy and is associated with a normal neurological examination. The second most common form of radiation myelopathy is the delayed chronic progressive myelopathy, which may more commonly be mistaken for intramedullary spinal cord metastasis. However, the two usually can be differentiated by their tempo of evolution. The onset of symptoms of intramedullary spinal cord metastasis is usually abrupt, with a rapidly progressive course over days or weeks; infrequently it may progress over months or, rarely, years.[165] Chronic progressive radiation myelopathy, however, generally evolves over several months or years and may arrest at a stage of incomplete myelopathy.

Table 6–6. Neurological Features of Differential Value in the Diagnosis of a Noncompressive Myelopathy in a Patient with Cancer*

Myelopathy	Pain	Progression of Spinal Disease			Size of Affected Spinal Segments as Seen on Myelogram			Tumor Cells in CSF
		Tempo		Ascending or Descending	Normal	Enlarged	Small	
		Subacute	Chronic					
Intramedullary spinal cord metastasis	+	+	−	+	+	+	−	−
Leptomeningeal metastases	+	+	−	NA	+	−	−	+
Radiation myelopathy	−	−	+	−	+	+	+	−
Necrotizing myelopathy	−	+	−	+/−	+	+	−	−

*From Winkelman, MD, et al.,[185] p. 529, with permission.
†CSF, cerebrospinal fluid; NA, not applicable; +, present; −, absent; and +/−, may be present or absent.

The amount of radiation received also is important in the diagnosis of chronic progressive radiation myelopathy. Not only the total dose but also the fractionation schedule and the length of the spinal cord irradiated are important parameters.[173] Factors such as hyperbaric oxygenation[174] and idiosyncratic sensitivity may allow radiation myelopathy to occur at levels otherwise considered safe.[173,175] The primary tumor most frequently associated with radiation myelopathy has been head and neck cancer (82% of cases according to one report).[176] In this case, the cervical spinal cord is included in the radiation port due to its proximity to the primary tumor. On the other hand, the most common tumors associated with intramedullary spinal cord metastasis are lung and breast cancer (68% of cases according to one report).[176] In the irradiation of these primary malignancies, the spine usually does not receive radiation at doses sufficient to cause chronic progressive radiation myelopathy.

Occasionally, intramedullary metastasis may be difficult to differentiate clinically from leptomeningeal metastases. Although leptomeningeal metastases usually cause symptoms and signs at multiple levels throughout the neuraxis, the cauda equina syndrome caused by metastases to this site alone may be identical to the clinical presentation of an intramedullary metastasis to the conus medullaris. As discussed in Chapter 2, it is not possible on clinical grounds alone to discriminate between the conus medullaris and cauda equina syndromes.[130,177]

In cases of leptomeningeal metastases, the CSF cytology and myelography, which may show thickening or nodularity of nerve roots and normal-size spinal cord, are helpful.[178,179] Furthermore, head CT scanning may show evidence of leptomeningeal seeding or communicating hydrocephalus.[180] Although plain MRI has had limitations in the evaluation of leptomeningeal spread from tumor,[181] contrast-enhanced MRI may be more sensitive.[29,92] It should be stressed that some patients develop intramedullary tumors secondary to leptomeningeal spread, so the two may coexist.[168] Finally, clinical follow-up of the patient should differentiate between the two because their clinical courses are different.

Necrotizing myelopathy, discussed in Chapter 8, is a very rare remote effect of cancer that is in the differential diagnosis of myelopathy in the cancer patient with negative radiological studies; it thus must be differentiated from intramedullary spinal cord metastasis.[182] Patients with necrotizing carcinomatous myelopathy do not complain of local or radicular pain.[34,183] Instead, they usually complain of vague, intermittent paresthesias in the lower extremities for weeks or months before an ascending transverse myelopathy develops. Necrotizing myelopathy usually begins in the thoracic spinal cord and then ascends and descends through the cord. Thus patients initially may have spastic paraplegia, followed by flaccid, areflexic paraplegia.[176] Radiological and CSF studies are nondiagnostic. As in cases of intramedullary metastasis, the course may be subacute. Because intramedullary metastases usually develop in the setting of widespread visceral and cerebral metastases, the law of parsimony would favor a diagnosis of intramedullary metastasis rather than a remote effect of cancer in such cases. Alternatively, visceral metastases occasionally may be found in patients with necrotizing carcinomatous myelopathy.

THERAPY

The management of intramedullary spinal metastasis is based on anecdotal reports because there are no large prospective series. Because many cases occur in the setting of widely disseminated disease, surgical therapy is infrequently undertaken. Furthermore, intramedullary metastases are often multiple or associated with intracerebral and/or leptomeningeal metastases; treatment therefore should consider the extent of CNS dissemination. Radiation therapy has been the primary treatment in most cases. The extent of the radiation port is determined by imaging studies, clinical involvement, and consideration of bone marrow tolerance. (Irradiation of the vertebral column may cause significant bone marrow suppression.)[176]

When leptomeningeal metastases are present, intrathecal chemotherapy may be used in addition to radiotherapy. The prognosis for patients with intramedullary spinal cord metastasis is poor; over 80% died within three months in one recent series.[164] Therefore, surgery (usually laminectomy) for intramedullary spinal metastases is usually relegated to diagnostic biopsy or resection in cases where life expectancy is greater than three months and ambulation is threatened.

SUMMARY

Tumors involving the spine may be classified according to either the epidural or intradural location. Intradural tumors may be further classified as intradural–extramedullary or intramedullary. Chapter 5 reviewed epidural tumors, and this chapter reviews intradural tumors, both intradural–extramedullary and intramedullary.

Intradural–extramedullary tumors include primary neoplasms such as meningioma and nerve sheath tumors (schwannoma and neurofibroma) as well as leptomeningeal metastases from systemic malignancies elsewhere. (Leptomeningeal metastases are discussed separately in Chapter 7 because they tend to have different diagnostic and therapeutic implications.) Intramedullary tumors may be primary neoplasms such as astrocytoma, ependymoma, and hemangioblastoma. Alternatively or they may metastasize from cancer elsewhere in the body.

Since meningiomas and nerve sheath tumors are histologically benign, patients may be restored to normal neurologic function and be cured if the diagnosis and treatment are undertaken before permanent neurologic sequelae develop. Intramedullary tumors such as ependymoma and astrocytoma present more difficult management problems. There have been reports of "cure" following gross total resection of ependymomas when there is a clear plane between the tumor and the spinal cord parenchyma. Astrocytomas are more inclined to be invasive and, accordingly, management more often includes

radiation therapy or chemotherapy. Less common tumors such as epidermoid cysts, teratomas, and lipomas are also briefly discussed,

Vascular malformations of the spine are presented in this chapter because although they may not be true neoplasms they may be difficult to differentiate from hemangioblastomas and other primary spinal neoplasms. With the recent development of MRI and spinal angiography, these lesions are more frequently recognized and present challenging diagnostic and management problems. These lesions are presented according to their current classification, which has been evolving. As these lesions are more frequently recognized, our understanding of their pathogenesis and management will increase.

REFERENCES

1. Alter M. Statistical aspects of spinal cord tumors. In Vinken PJ, Bruyn GW, editors. *Handbook of Clinical Neurology, Volume 19*. Amsterdam: North-Holland; 1975; pp. 1–22.
2. Coman DR, DeLong RP. The role of the vertebral venous system in the metastasis of cancer to the spinal column. *Cancer* 1951;4:610–8.
3. Gowers WR, Horsley V. Case of tumour of spinal cord: removal; recovery. *Med Chir Tr London* 1888;71:377–430.
4. Iraci G, Peserico L, Salar G. Intraspinal neurinomas and neurinomas. A clinical survey of 172 cases. *Int J Surg* 1971;56:289–303.
5. Nittner K. Spinal meningiomas, neurinomas and neurofibromas and hourglass tumors. In Vinken GW, Bruyn PJ, editors. *Handbook of Clinical Neurology, Volume 20*. Amsterdam: North-Holland; 1976; pp. 177–322.
6. Onofrio BM. Intradural extramedullary spinal cord tumors. *Clin Neurosurg* 1978;25:540–55.
7. Gonzalez-Vitale JC, Garcia-Bunuel R. Meningeal carcinomatosis. *Cancer* 1976;37:2906–11.
8. Patchell RA, Posner JB. Neurologic complications of systemic cancer. *Neurol Clin* 1985;3:729–50.
9. Bunn PA, Schein PS, Banks PM, DeVita VT. Central nervous system complications in patients with diffuse histiocytic and undifferentiated lymphoma: leukemia revisiteditor. *Blood* 1976;47:3–10.
10. Hermann G, Hermann P. Computerized tomography of the spine in metastatic disease. *Mt Sinai J Med* 1982;49:400–5.
11. Levitt LJ, Dawson DM, Rosenthal DS, et al. CNS involvement in non-Hodgkin's lymphomas. *Cancer* 1980;45:545–52.

12. Litam JP, Cabanillas F, Smith TL, et al. Central nervous system relapse in malignant lymphomas: risk factors and implications for prophylaxis. *Blood* 1979;54:1249–57.
13. Mead GM, Kennedy P, Smith JL, et al. Involvement of the central nervous system by non-Hodgkin's lymphoma in adults: a review of 36 cases. *Q J Med* 1986;60:699–714.
14. Perez-Soler R, Smith TL, Cabanillas F. Central nervous system prophylaxis with combined intravenous and intrathecal methotrexate in diffuse lymphoma of aggressive histologic type. *Cancer* 1986;57:971–7.
15. Oddsson B. *Spinal Meningioma*. Kopenhagen: H.P. Hansens; 1947.
16. Rand CW. Surgical experiences with spinal cord tumors. A survey over a forty-year period. *Bull Los Angeles Neurol Soc* 1963;28:260–8.
17. Rubinstein LJ. *Tumors of the Central Nervous System*. Washington, DC: AFIP; 1972.
18. Bull JWD. Spinal meningiomas amd neurofibromas. *Acta Radiol* 1953;40:283–300.
19. Levy WJ, Bay J, Dohn D. Spinal cord meningioma. *J Neurosurg* 1982;57:804–12.
20. Davis RA, Washburn PL. Spinal cord meningiomas. *Surg Gynecol Obstet* 1970;131:15–21.
21. McAlhany HJ, Netsky MG. Compression of the spinal cord by extramedullary neoplasms: a clinical and pathological study. *J Neuropathol Exp Neurol* 1955;14:276–87.
22. Banna M. *Clinical Radiology of the Spine and Spinal Cord*. Rockville, MD: Aspen Systems; 1985.
23. Kricun R, Kricun ME. Computed tomography. In Kricun ME, editor. *Imaging Modalities in Spinal Disorders*. Philadelphia: W.B. Saunders; 1988; pp. 376–467.
24. Grossman CB, Post MJD. The adult spine. In Gonzalez CF, Grossman CB, Masdeau JC, editors. *Head and Spine Imaging*. New York: John Wiley; 1985; pp. 781–858.
25. Kilgore DP. Thoracic spine. In Daniels DL, Haughton VM, Naidich TP, editors. *Cranial and Spinal Magnetic Resonance Imaging. An Atlas and Guide*. New York: Raven Press; 1987; pp. 263–84.
26. Masaryk TJ. Spine tumors. In Modic MT, Masaryk TJ, Ross JS, editors. *Magnetic Resonance Imaging of the Spine*. Chicago: Year Book Medical; 1988; pp. 183–213.
27. Graif M, Steiner RE. Contrast-enhanced magnetic resonance imaging of tumours of the central nervous system: a clinical review. *Br J Radiol* 1986;59:865–73.
28. Sze G. Gadolinium-DTPA in spinal disease. *Radiol Clin North Am* 1988;26:1009–24.
29. Sze G, Abramson A, Krol G, et al. Gadolinium-DTPA in the evaluation of intradural extramedullary spinal disease. *AJNR Am J Neuroradiol* 1988;9:153–63.
30. Gautier-Smith PC. Clinical aspects of spinal neurofibromas. *Brain* 1970;90:359–94.
31. Broager B. Spinal neurinoma. *Acta Psychiatr Scand Suppl* 1953;85:1–241.
32. Rasmussen TB, Kernohan JW, Adson AW. Pathologic classification, with surgical consider-

ation, of intraspinal tumors. *Ann Surg* 1940;111:513–30.
33. Elsberg CA. *Tumors of the Spinal Cord and Membranes*. New York: Paul A. Hoeber; 1925.
34. Handforth A, Nag S, Sharp D, et al. Paraneoplastic subacute necrotic myelopathy. *Can J Neurol Sci* 1983;10:204–7.
35. Hollis PH, Malis LI, Zappulla RA. Neurological deterioration after lumbar puncture below complete spinal subarachnoid block. *J Neurosurg* 1986;64:253–6.
36. Osborn RE, DeWitt JD. Giant cauda equina schwannoma: CT appearance. *AJNR am J Neuroradiol* 1985;6:835–6.
37. Coleman BG, Arger PH, Dalinka MK, et al. CT of sarcomatous degeneration in neurofibromatosis. *AJR Am J Roentgenol* 1983;140:383–7.
38. Cohen LM, Schwartz AM, Rockoff SD. Benign schwannomas: pathologic basis for CT inhomogeneities. *AJR Am J Roentgenol* 1986;147:141–3.
39. Haughton VM, Williams AL. *Computed Tomography of The Spine*. St. Louis: C.V. Mosby; 1982.
40. Tadmor R, Cacayorian ED, Kieffer SA. Advantages of supplementary CT in myelography of intraspinal masses. *AJNR Am J Neuroradiol* 1983;4:618–21.
41. Li M, Holtas S. MR imaging of spinal neurofibromatosis. *Acta Radiol* 1991;32:279–85.
42. Schroth G, Thron A, Guhl L, Voigt K, Niendorf H-P, Garces LR-N. Magnetic resonance imaging of spinal meningiomas and neurinomas. *J Neurosurg* 1987;66:695–700.
43. Levine E, Huntrakoon M, Wetzel L. Malignant nerve sheath neoplasms in neurofibromatosis: distinction from benign tumors using imaging techniques. *AJR Am J Roentgenol* 1987;149:1059–64.
44. Donner T, Voorhies R, Kline D. Neural sheath tumors of major nerves. *J Neurosurg* 1994;81:362–73.
45. Kornblith PL, Walker MD, Cassady JR. *Neurologic Oncology*. Philadelphia: J.B. Lippincott; 1987.
46. Burger PC, Vogel FS. *Surgical Pathology of the Nervous System and Its Coverings*. New York: John Wiley; 1976.
47. Awad I, Barrow D. *Spinal Vascular Malformations*. Park Ridge, IL: AANS; 1998.
48. Browne TR, Adams RD, Robertson GH. Hemangioblastoma of the spinal cord. *Arch Neurol* 1976;33:435–41.
49. Jellinger K. Pathology of spinal vascular malformations and vascular tumors. In Pia HW, Djindjian R, editors. *Spinal Angiomas: Advances in Diagnosis and Therapy*. New York: Springer-Verlag; 1978; p. 18.
50. Pia HW. Symptomatology of spinal angiomas. In Pia HW, Djindjian R, editors. *Spinal Angiomas: Advances in Diagnosis and Therapy*. New York: Springer-Verlag; 1978; pp. 48–74.
51. Elsberg CA. *Surgical Diseases of the Spinal Cord, Membranes and Nerve Root*. New York: Hoeber; 1941.
52. Kendall BE, Logue V. Spinal epidural angiomatous malformations draining into intrathecal veins. *Neuroradiology* 1977;13:181–9.

53. McCutcheon I, Doppman J, Oldfield E. Microvascular anatomy of dural arteriovenous abnormalities of the spine: a microangiographic study. *J Neurosurg* 1996;84:215–20.
54. Rosenblum B, Oldfield EH, Doppman JL, DiChiro G. Spinal arteriovenous malformations: a comparison of dural arteriovenous fistulas and intradural AVM's in 81 patients. *J Neurosurg* 1987;67:795–802.
55. Anson J, Spetzler R. Spinal dural arteriovenous malformations. In Awad I, Barrow D, editors. *Dural Arteriovenous Malformations.* Park Ridge IL: AANS; 1993; pp. 175–91.
56. Barrow D. Spinal vascular malformations. In Welch K, Reiss D, Caplan L, Siesjo B, editors. *Primer on Cerebrovascular Diseases.* New York: Academic Press; 1997.
57. Hurst R, Kenyon L, Lavi E, et al. Spinal dural arteriovenous fistula: the pathology of venous hypertensive myelopathy. *Neurology* 1995;45:1309–13.
58. Djindjian M, Djindjian R, Rey A, et al. Intradural extramedullary spinal arterio-venous malformations fed by the anterior spinal artery. *Surg Neurol* 1977;8:85–93.
59. Heros R, Debrun G, Ojemann R, et al. Direct spinal arteriovenous fistula: a new type of spinal AVM. Case report. *J Neurosurg* 1986;64:134–9.
60. Kohno M, Takahashi H, Yagashita A, et al. Preoperative and postoperative magnetic resonance imaging (MRI) findings of radiculomeningeal arteriovenous malformations: important role of gravity in the symptoms and MRI. *Surg Neurol* 1997;48:352–6.
61. Djindjian M. Clinical symptomatology and natural history of arteriovenous malformations of the spinal cord—a study of the clinical aspects and prognosis based on 150 cases. In Pia HW, Djindjian R, editors. *Spinal Angiomas: Advances in Diagnosis and Therapy.* New York: Springer-Verlag; 1978; pp. 75–83.
62. Jellinger K, Neumayer E. Claudication of the spinal cord and cauda equina. In Vinken PJ, Bruyn GW, editors. *Handbook of Clinical Neurology, Volume 12.* Amsterdam: North-Holland; 1972; pp. 507–47.
63. Verbiest H. Neurogenic intermittent claudication—lesions of the spinal canal and cauda equina, stenosis of the vertebral canal, narrowing of intervertebral foramina and entrapment of peripheral nerves. In Vinken PJ, Bruyn GW, editors. *Handbook of Clinical Neurology, Volume 20.* Amsterdam: North-Holland; 1976; pp. 611–804.
64. Madsen JR, Heros RC. Spinal arteriovenous malformations and neurogenic claudication. Report of two cases. *J Neurosurg* 1988;68:793–7.
65. Nacimiento W, Thron A. Spinal A-V. Fistula (letter). *Neurology* 1996;47:1108.
66. Foix C, Alajouanine T. La myelite necrotique subaigue. *Rev Neurol* 1926;2:1–42.
67. Greenfield JG, Turner JWA. Acute and subacute necrotic myelitis. *Brain* 1939;62:227–52.
68. Hamilton M, Anson J, Spetzler R. Spinal vascular malformations. In Tindall G, Cooper P, Barrow D, editors. *The Practice of Neurosurgery, Volume 2.* Baltimore: William and Wilkins; 1996.
69. Buchan AM, Barnett HJM. Infarction of the spinal cord. In Barnett HJM, Mohr JP, Stein BM, Yatsu FM, editors. *Stroke: Pathophysiology, Diagnosis and Management.* New York: Churchill Livingstone; 1986; pp. 707–19.
70. Rose FC, Brett EM, Burston J. Zoster encephalomyelitis. *Arch Neurol* 1964;11:155–72.
71. Mair WGP, Folkerts JF. Necrosis of the spinal cord due to thrombophlebitis (subacute necrotic myelitis). *Brain* 1953;76:563–75.
72. Koenig E, Thron A, Schrader V, Dichgans J. Spinal arteriovenous malformations and fistulae: clinical, neuroradiological, and neurophysiological findings. *J Neurol* 1989;236:260–6.
73. Choi IS, Berenstein A. Surgical neuroangiography of the spine and spinal cord. *Radiol Clin North Am* 1988;26:1131–41.
74. DiChiro G, Doppman JL, Dwyer AJ, et al. Tumors and arteriovenous malformations of the spinal cord: assessment using MR. *Radiology* 1985;156:689–97.
75. Masaryk TJ, Ross JS, Modic MT, Ruff RL, Selman WR, Ratcheson RA. Radiculomeningeal vascular malformations of the spine: MR imaging. *Radiology* 1987;164:845–9.
76. Hasuo K, Mizushima A, Mihara F, et al. Contrast-enhanced MRI in spinal arteriovenous malformations and fistulae before and after embolization therapy. *Neuroradiology* 1996;38:609–14.
77. Jones B, Ernst R, Tomsick T, Tew J. Spinal dural arteriovenous fistulas: recognizing the spectrum of magnetic resonance imaging findings. *J Spinal Cord Med* 1997;20:43–8.
78. Montine T, O'Keane J, Eskin T, et al. Vascular malformations presenting as spinal cord neoplasms: case report. *Neurosurgery* 1995;36:194–7.
79. Hodes J, Merland J, Casasco A, et al. Spinal vascular malformations: Endovascular therapy. *Neurosurg Clin North Am* 1994;5:497–509.
80. Masalchi M, Quilici N, Ferrito G, et al. Identification of the feeding arteries of spinal vascular lesions via phase-contrast MR angiography with three-dimensional acquisition and phase display. *AJNR Am J Neuroradiol* 1997;18:351–8.
81. Berenstein A, Lasjaunias P. *Spinal Neuroangiography: Endovascular Treatment of Spine and Spinal Cord Lesions, Volume 5.* New York: Springer-Verlag; 1992.
82. Martin N, Khanna R, Batzford U. Posterolateral cervical or thoracic approach with spinal cord rotation for vascular malformations or tumors of the ventrolateral spinal cord. *J Neurosurg* 1995;83:254–61.
83. Michelsen WJ. Arteriovenous malformation of the brain and spinal cord. In Johnson RT, editor. *Current Therapy in Neurologic Disease–2.* Toronto: B.C. Decker; 1987; pp. 170–3.
84. Kinney TD, Fitzgerald PJ. Lindau-von Hippel disease with hemangioblastoma of the spinal cord and syringomyelia. *Arch Pathol* 1947;43:439–55.

85. Rho YM. Von Hippel-Lindau's disease: a report of five cases. *Can Med Assoc J* 1969;101:135–42.

86. Guidetti B, Fortuna A. Surgical treatment of intramedullary hemangioblastoma of the spinal cord: report of six cases. *J Neurosurg* 1967;27:530–40.

87. Kendall B, Russell J. Hemangioblastoma of the spinal cord. *Br J Radiol* 1966;39:817–23.

88. Herdt JR, Shimkin PM, Ommaya AK, et al. Angiography of vascular intraspinal tumors. *J Roentgenol Radium Ther Nucl Med* 1972;115:165–70.

89. Kendall B. Application of angiography to tumors affecting the spinal cord. *Proc R Soc Med* 1970;63:185–7.

90. Yasargil MG, Fiedeler RW, Rankin TP. Operative Treatment of Spinal Angioblastomas. In Pia HW, Djindjian R, editors. *Spinal Angiomas: Advances in Diagnosis and Therapy*. Berlin: Springer-Verlag; 1978; pp. 171–88.

91. Solomon RA, Stein BM. Unusual spinal cord enlargement related to intramedullary hemangioblastoma. *J Neurosurg* 1988;68:550–3.

92. Sze G, Krol G, Zimmerman RD, Deck MDF. Intramedullary disease of the spine: diagnosis using gadolinium-DTPA-enhanced MR imaging. *AJNR Am J Neuroradiol* 1988;9:847–58.

93. Spetzger U, Bertalanffy H, Huffmann B, et al. Hemangioblastomas of the spinal cord and brainstem: diagnostic and therapeutic features. *Neurosurg Rev* 1996;19:147–51.

94. Xu Q, Bao W, Mao R. Magnetic resonance imaging and microsurgical treatment of intramedullary hemangioblastoma of the spinal cord. *Chin Med J* 1995;108:117–22.

95. Rand RW, Rand CW. *Intraspinal Tumors of Childhood*. Springfield, IL: Charles C. Thomas; 1960.

96. Alves AM, Norrell H. Intramedullary epidermoid tumors of the spinal cord. Report of a case and review of the literature. *Int Surg* 1970;54:239–43.

97. Craig RL. A case of epidermoid tumor of the spinal cord. Review of the literature of spinal epidermoids and dermoids. *Surgery* 1943;13:354–67.

98. Critchley M, Ferguson FR. The cerebrospinal epidermoids (cholesteatomata). *Brain* 1928;51:334–84.

99. Tytus JS, Pennybacker J. Pearly tumors in relation to the central nervous system. *J Neurol Neurosurg Psychiatry* 1956;19:241–59.

100. Manno NJ, Uihlein A, Kernohan JW. Intraspinal epidermoids. *J Neurosurg* 1962;19:754–65.

101. Boldrey EB, Elvidge AR. Dermoid cysts of the vertebral canal. *Ann Surg* 1939;110:273–84.

102. Cantu RC, Wright RL. Aseptic meningitic syndrome with cauda equina epidermoid tumor. *J Pediatr* 1968;73:114–6.

103. Decker RE, Gross SW. Intraspinal dermoid tumor presenting as chemical meningitis. Report of a case without dermal sinus. *J Neurosurg* 1967;27:60–2.

104. Black SPW, German WJ. Four congenital tumors found at operation within the vertebral canal. With observations on their incidence. *J Neurosurg* 1950;7 49–61.

105. Boyd HR. Iatrogenic intraspinal epidermoid. Report of a case. *J Neurosurg* 1966;24:105–7.

106. Choremis C, Oeconmos D, Papadatos C, Gargoulas A. Intraspinal epidermoid tumours (cholesteatomas) in patients treated for tuberculous meningitis. *Lancet* 1956;2:437–9.

107. Gibson T, Norris W. Skin fragments removed by injection needles. *Lancet* 1958;2:983–5.

108. Wilkins RH, Odom GL. Spinal intradural cysts. In Vinken PJ, Bruyn GW, editors. *Handbook of Clinical Neurology, Volume 20*. Amsterdam: North-Holland; 1976; pp. 55–101.

109. List CF. Intraspinal epidermoids,dermoids, and dermal sinuses. *Surg Gynecol Obstet* 1941;73:525–38.

110. Wright RL. Congenital dermal sinuses. *Prog Neurol Surg* 1971;4:175–91.

111. Furtado D, Marques V. Spinal teratoma. *J Neuropathol Exp Neurol* 1951;10:384–93.

112. Willis RA. *The Borderland of Embryology and Pathology*. London: Butterworth; 1962.

113. Ingraham FD, Bailey OT. Cystic teratomas and teratoid tumors of the central nervous system in infancy and childhood. *J Neurosurg* 1946;3:511–32.

114. Hughes JT. *Pathology of the Spinal Cord*. Philadelphia: W.B. Saunders; 1978.

115. Ehni G, Love JG. Intraspinal lipomas. Report of cases; review of the literature, and clinical and pathologic study. *Acta Neurol Psychiat* 1945;53:1–28.

116. Chapman PH. Congenital intraspinal lipomas: anatomical considerations and surgical treatment. *Child's Brain* 1982;9:37–47.

117. Emery JL, Lendon RG. Lipomas of the cauda equina and other fatty tumors related to neurospinal dysraphism. *Dev Med Child Neurol* 1969;2(Suppl 20):62–70.

118. Giuffre R. Spinal Lipomas. In Vinken PJ, Bruyn GW, editors. *Handbook of Clinical Neurology, Volume 20*. Amsterdam: North-Holland; 1976; pp. 389–414.

119. Drapkin AJ. High cervical intradural lipoma. *J Neurosurg* 1974;41:699–704.

120. Giuffre R. Intradural spinal lipomas. Review of the literature (99 cases) and report of an additional case. *Acta Neurochiur* 1966;14:69–95.

121. Dosseter RS, Kaiser M, Veiga-Pires JA. CT scanning in two cases of lipoma of the spinal cord. *Clin Radiol* 1979;30:227–31.

122. Fitz CR. The pediatric spine. In Gonzalez CF, Grossman CB, Masdeu JC, editors. *Head and Spine Imaging*. New York: John Wiley; 1985; pp. 759–80.

123. Thomas JE, Miller RH. Lipomatous tumors of the spinal canal. *Mayo Clin Proc* 1973;48:393–400.

124. Russell DS, Rubenstein LJ. *Pathology of Tumours of the Nervous System*. Baltimore: Williams & Wilkins; 1989.

125. Fortuna A, Celli P, Palma L. Oligodendrogliomas of the spinal cord. *Acta Neurochir* 1980;52:305–29.

126. Yagi T, Ohata K, Haque M, Hakuba A. Intra-medullary spinal cord tumour associated with neurofibromatosis type 1. *Acta Neurochir* 1997; 139:1055–60.

127. Hautzer NW, Aiyesmoju A, Robitaille Y. "Primary" spinal intramedullary lymphomas: A review. *Ann Neurol* 1983;14:62–6.

128. Hochberg FH, Miller DG. Primary central nervous system lymphoma. Review Article. *J Neurosurg* 1988;68:835–53.

129. Harmeier JW. Normal histology of intradural filum terminale. *Arch Neurol Psychiat* 1933;29: 308–16.

130. Norstrom CW, Kernohan JW, Love JG. One hundred primary caudal tumors. *JAMA* 1961; 178:1071–7.

131. Barone BM, Elvidge AR. Ependymomas: a clinical survey. *J Neurosurg* 1970;33:428–38.

132. Arseni C, Ionesco S. Les compressions medullaires dues a des tumeurs intra-rachidiennes. Etude clinico-statistique de 362 cas. *J Chir (Paris)* 1958;75:582–95.

133. Fischer G, Tommasi M. Spinal ependymomas. In Vinken GW, Bruyn PJ, editors. *Handbook of Clinical Neurology, Volume 20*. Amsterdam: North-Holland; 1976; pp. 353–87.

134. Cooper PR, Epstein F. Radical resection of intramedullary spinal cord tumors in adults: recent experience in 29 cases. *J Neurosurg* 1985; 63:492–9.

135. Davis C, Barnard RO. Malignant behavior of myxopapillary ependymoma: report of three cases. *J Neurosurg* 1985;62:925–9.

136. Ker NB, Jones CB. Tumours of the cauda equina: the problem of differential diagnosis. *J Bone Joint Surg* 1985;67B:358–61.

137. Shenkin HA, Alpers BJ. Clinical and pathological features of gliomas of the spinal cord. *Arch Neurol Psychiat* 1944;52:87–105.

138. Epstein F, Farmer J, Freed D. Adult intramedullary spinal cord ependymomas: the result of surgery in 38 patients. *J Neurosurg* 1993;79: 204–9.

139. Constantini S, Allen J, Epstein F. Pediatric and adult spinal cord tumors. In Black PM, Loeffler J, editors. *Cancer of the Nervous System* Cambridge, MA: Blackwell Science; 1997; pp. 637–52.

140. Lapointe JS, Graeb DA, Nugent RA, Robertson WD. Value of intravenous contrast enhancement in the CT evaluation of intraspinal tumors. *AJR Am J Roentgenol* 1986;146:103–7.

141. Council ScientificAffair. Magnetic resonance imaging of the central nervous system. *JAMA* 1988;259:1211–22.

142. Li M, Holtas S. MR imaging of spinal intramedullary tumors. *Acta Radiol* 1991;32:505–13.

143. Schwade JG, Wara WM, Sheline GE, et al. Management of primary spinal cord tumors. *Int J Radiat Oncol Biol Phys* 1978;4:389–93.

144. Innocenzi G, Raco A, Cantore G, Raimondi A. Intramedullary astrocytomas and ependymomas in the pediatric age group: a retrospective study. *Childs Nerv Syst* 1996;12:776–80.

145. Sonneland PRL, Scheithauer BW, Onofrio BM. Myxpapillary ependymoma: a clinicopathologic and immunocytochemical study of 77 cases. *Cancer* 1985;56:883–93.

146. Mork SJ, Loken AC. Ependymoma: a follow-up study of 101 cases. *Cancer* 1977;40:907–15.

147. Wen B, Hussey D, Hitchon P, et al. The role of radiation therapy in the management of ependymomas of the spinal cord. *Int J Radiat Oncol Biol Phys* 1991;20:781–6.

148. Whitaker S, Bessell E, Ashley S, et al. Postoperative radiotherapy in the management of spinal cord ependymoma. *J Neurosurg* 1991;74:720–8.

149. Shirato H, Kamada T, Hida K, et al. The role of radiotherapy in the management of spinal cord glioma. *Int J Radiat Oncol Biol Phys* 1995;33: 323–8.

150. Epstein F, Epstein N. Surgical treatment of spinal cord astrocytomas of childhood: a series of 19 patients. *J Neurosurg* 1982;57:685–9.

151. Epstein F, Epstein N. Intramedullary tumors of the spinal cord. In Shillito J, Matson DD, editors. *Pediatric Neurosurgery: Surgery of the Developing Nervous System*. New York: Grune and Stratton; 1982; pp. 529–39.

152. Reimer R, Onofrio BM. Astrocytomas of the spinal cord in children and adolescents. *J Neurosurg* 1985;63:669–75.

153. Arendt A. Spinal gliomas. In Vinken GW, Bruyn PJ, editors. *Handbook of Clinical Neurology, Volume 20*. Amsterdam: North-Holland; 1976; pp. 323–51.

154. Kan S, Fox AJ, Vinuela F, et al. Delayed CT metrizamide enhancement of syringomyelia secondary to tumor. *Radiology* 1983;146:409–14.

155. Kopelson G, Linggood RM. Intramedullary spinal cord astrocytoma versus glioblastoma: the prognostic importance of histologic grade. *J Neurosurg* 1982;50:732–5.

156. Johnson DL, Schwarz S. Intracranial metastases from malignant spinal-cord astrocytoma: case report. *J Neurosurg* 1987;66:621–5.

157. Restuccia D, Di Lazzaro V, Valeriano M, et al. Spinal responses to median and tibial nerve stimulation and magnetic resonance imaging in intramedullary cord lesions. *Neurology* 1996;46: 1706–14.

158. Jyothirmayi R, Madhaven J, Nair M, Rajan B. Conservative surgery and radiotherapy in the treatment of spinal cord astrocytoma. *J Neurooncol* 1997;33:205–11.

159. Minehan K, Shaw E, Scheithaueer B, et al. Spinal cord astrocytoma: pathological and treatment considerations. *J Neurosurg* 1995;83: 590–5.

160. Cohen AR, Wisoff JH, Allen JC, Epstein F. Malignant astrocytomas of the spinal cord. *J Neurosurg* 1989;70:50–4.

161. Guidetti B, Mercuri S, Vagnozzi R. Long-term results of the surgical treatment of 129 intramedullary spinal gliomas. *J Neurosurg* 1981;54: 323–30.

162. O'Sullivan C, Jenkin D, Doherty M, et al. Spinal cord tumors in children: Long term results of combined surgical and radiation treatment. *J Neurosurg* 1994;81:507–12.

163. Allen J, Aviner S, Yates A, et al. Treatment of high-grade spinal cord astrocytoma of childhood with "8-in-1" chemotherapy and radiotherapy: a pilot study of CCG-945. *J Neurosurg* 1998;88:215–20.

164. Grem JL, Burgess J, Trump DL. Clinical features and natural history of intramedullary spinal cord metastasis. *Cancer* 1985;56:2305–14.

165. Edelson RN, Deck MDF, Posner JB. Intramedullary spinal cord metastases: Clinical and radiological findings in 9 cases. *Neurology* 1972;22: 1222–31.

166. Chason JL, Walker FB, Landers JW. Metastatic carcinoma in the central nervous system and dorsal root ganglia. *Cancer* 1963;16:781–7.

167. Nugent JL, Bunn PA, Matthews MJ, et al. CNS metastases in small cell bronchogenic carcinoma—increasing frequency and changing patterns with lengthening survival. *Cancer* 1979; 44:1885–93.

168. Costigan DA, Winkelman MD. Intramedullary spinal cord metastasis: a clinicopathological study of 13 cases. *J Neurosurg* 1985;62:227–33.

169. Bechar M, Freud M, Kott E, et al. Hepatic cirrhosis with post-shunt myelopathy. *J Neurol Sci* 1970;11:101–7.

170. Hirose G, Shimazaki K, Takado M, et al. Intramedullary spinal cord metastasis of the spinal cord associated with pencil-shaped softening of the spinal cord. *J Neurosurg* 1980;52:718–21.

171. Reddy SC, Vijayamohan G, Gao GR. Delayed CT myelography in spinal intramedullary metastasis: case report. *J Comput Assist Tomogr* 1984; 8:1182–5.

172. Fredericks RK, Elster A, Walker FO. Gadolinium-enhanced MRI: a superior technique for the diagnosis of intraspinal metastases. *Neurology* 1989;39:734–6.

173. Kagan AR, Wollin M, Gilbert HA, et al. Comparison of the tolerance of the brain and spinal cord to injury by radiations. In Gilbert HA, Kagan AR, editors. *Radiation Damage to the Nervous System.* New York: Raven Press; 1980; pp. 183–90.

174. Brenk HASVd, Richter W, Hurley RH. Radiosensitivity of the human oxygenated cervical spinal cord based on analysis of 357 cases receiving 4 MeV X rays in hyperbaric oxygenation. *Br J Radiol* 1968;41:205–14.

175. Brown WJ, Kagan AR. Comparison of myelopathy associated with megavoltage irradiation and remote cancer. In Gilbert HJ, Kagan AR, editors. *Radiation Damage to the Nervous System.* New York: Raven Press; 1980; pp. 191–206.

176. Helms CA, Cann CE, Brunelle FO, et al. Detection of bone marrow metastases using quantitative computed tomography. *Radiology* 1981;140: 745–50.

177. Levitt P, Ransohoff J, Spielholz N. The differential diagnosis of tumors of the conus medullaris and cauda equina. In Vinken PJ, Bruyn GW, editors. *Handbook of Clinical Neurology, Volume 19.* Amsterdam: North-Holland; 1975; pp. 77–90.

178. Bleyer WA, Byrne TN. Leptomeningeal cancer in leukemia and solid tumors. *Curr Probl Cancer* 1988;12:185–238.

179. Grogan JP, Daniels DL, Williams AL, et al. The normal conus medullaris: CT criteria for recognition. *Radiology* 1984;151:661–4.

180. Jaeckle KA, Krol G, Posner JB. Evolution of computed tomographic abnormalities in leptomeningeal metastases. *Ann Neurol* 1985;17: 85–9.

181. Barloon TJ, Yuh WTC, Yang CJC, et al. Spinal subarachnoid tumor seeding from intracranial metastasis: MR findings. *J Comput Assist Tomogr* 1987;11:242–4.

182. Mancall EL, Remedios KR. Necrotizing myelopathy associated with visceral carcinoma. *Brain* 1964;87:639–55.

183. Ojeda VJ. Necrotising myelopathy associated with malignancy: a clinicopathological study of two cases and literature review. *Cancer* 1984;53: 1115–23.

184. Leeds NE, Elkin CM, Leon E, et al. Myelography. In Kricun ME, editor. *Imaging Modalities in Spinal Disorders* Philadelphia: W.B. Saunders; 1988; pp. 325–75.

185. Winkelman MD, Adelstein DJ, Karlins NL. Intramedullary spinal cord metastasis: Diagnostic and therapeutic considerations. *Arch Neurol* 1987;44:526–31.

Chapter 7

LEPTOMENINGEAL METASTASES

Metastases to the leptomeninges from systemic malignancies or primary central nervous system neoplasms are a frequent cause of symptoms and signs of spinal cord and cauda equina dysfunction. Thus leptomeningeal cancer must be considered in the differential diagnosis of patients with these complaints and findings. This is especially true among patients with known malignancy. Approximately 5% to 8% of patients dying of solid tumors develop leptomeningeal metastases.[1,2]

CLINICAL ANATOMY

The spinal cord and spinal roots are surrounded by three meninges: the dura mater, arachnoid, and pia mater. The arachnoid and pia mater are collectively called the leptomeninges (Fig. 7–1).

The outermost covering, the dura mater, consists of a tough fibrous tissue that forms a barrier to prevent the invasion of neoplastic cells into the central nervous system. Despite the frequency of vertebral metastases with epidural extension, epidural neoplasms rarely breach the dura mater and enter the CNS. In patients with epidural tumors, the region of the nervous system jeopardized is only that which is adjacent to or underlying the tumor and therefore subject to compression.

The leptomeninges are composed of trabeculated arachnoid and pia mater. While the outer arachnoid membrane is apposed to the dura mater, the pia mater closely follows the contours of the cerebral cortex and spinal cord.[3] Within the brain and spinal cord, the pia mater merges with glial elements to form the pia–glial membrane.

The subarachnoid space is located between the outer arachnoid and the pia mater. In addition to containing cerebrospinal fluid (CSF), the subarachnoid space also houses nerve roots, blood vessels, and connective tissue. As blood vessels penetrate the spinal cord, they are ensheathed by arachnoid and pia–glial tissues. The Virchow-Robin space, which is perivascular in nature, is formed between the blood vessel and this adventitial sheath. This space is clinically significant because it is continuous with the subarachnoid space and therefore allows invasion

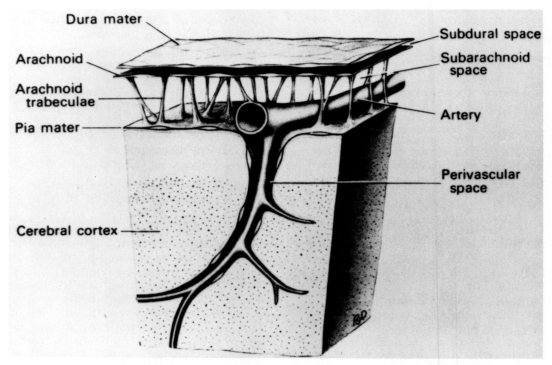

Figure 7–1. The anatomical relationship between the meninges and the brain parenchyma. (From Carpenter, MB,[3] with permission.)

of neoplastic cells deep into the substance of the spinal cord and brain.

Spinal roots are surrounded by sheaths of arachnoid and by extensions of the subarachnoid space that extend as far laterally as their exit from the vertebral canal. This has clinical importance because leptomeningeal invasion can extend out in a sheath-like fashion.

Within the subarachnoid space, CSF flows freely from the ventricular system through the spinal axis to the region over the convexities of the cerebral hemispheres, where it is reabsorbed by the arachnoid villi of the dural sinuses. This unobstructed flow provides a pathway for neoplastic cells that have seeded any region of the subarachnoid space to spread throughout the neuraxis. With this spread, disturbances of cerebral, cranial nerve, and/or spinal functions are often encountered. Thus the clinical hallmark of leptomeningeal metastases is multifocal neurological abnormalities at different levels of the neuraxis.

PATHOGENESIS

The basic concepts underlying the metastatic process are discussed in Chapter 5. However, the specific mechanisms whereby malignant cells spread to the leptomeninges are important to review here. Understanding them will aid the physician in diagnosing and managing of these patients.

Several mechanisms have been proposed to explain metastasis to the leptomeninges. The most frequent hypotheses suggest that metastases extend to the leptomeninges from a parameningeal site or via hematogenous routes. According to the first hypothesis, neoplastic cells would invade the leptomeninges from parameningeal foci such as brain or spinal cord parenchyma, the epidural space, choroid plexus, or bone marrow. In support of this explanation, it has been found that intraparenchymal CNS tumors such as malignant gliomas, ependymomas, medulloblastomas, and cerebral metastases may seed the leptomeninges.[4–7] Leptomeningeal invasion also has been shown to occur via nerve roots from paravertebral locations and along vascular channels from bone marrow involvement.[8,9] In lymphoma patients with bone marrow involvement, epidemiological studies have demonstrated an increased risk of leptomeningeal metastases.[9–11] Metastatic involvement of the choroid plexus provides additional access to the leptomeninges.[12]

Despite these reports, many patients with leptomeningeal metastases do not have a parameningeal tumor. In such cases, hematogenous dissemination is the most probable explanation.[13] There is strong experimental and clinicopathological support for this idea. In an experimental animal model, transvascular migration of leukemia cells has been shown to occur in the arachnoidal veins of guinea pigs.[14] One clinicopathological report provides a detailed histopathological study of the CNS of 126 children dying from leukemia.[15] Among the 70 cases with evidence of arachnoidal leukemia, the following pathogenesis was demonstrated: The arachnoidal veins bridging the subarachnoid space were the initial site of invasion by the leukemic cells. As the malignant cells invaded the supporting adventitia of the vessels, they extended into the CSF pathways of the subarachnoid space. Once in the CSF, the leukemic cells could follow the CSF pathways throughout the length of the neuraxis. Later, they were found to have invaded deep within the white and gray matter of the brain and spinal cord via the perivascular spaces. In the most advanced cases, the parenchyma of the brain and spinal cord was invaded, as also the pia–glial membrane was further disrupted by the invading leukemic cells.

Aside from providing a route for CNS dissemination, the fact that malignant cells invade blood vessels is significant in the pathogenesis of neurological symptoms and signs. Histopathological evidence of infarction and hemorrhage, considered secondary to blood vessel invasion by leukemic cells, has been reported.[15] A more recent report has shown that regional cerebral blood flow was diminished in nearly 90% of patients with leptomeningeal metastases.[16] Although the

cause of reduced cerebral blood flow may be multifactorial, compression of blood vessels is one probable determinant.

PATHOLOGICAL FINDINGS

The pathological findings of leptomeningeal metastases include diffuse and widespread multifocal infiltration of the leptomeninges. These findings are similar for cases caused by solid tumors,[17] leukemia,[15] and lymphoma.[8] We have detailed histopathological findings on the extent of nervous system involvement in cases of leptomeningeal invasion by lymphoma and solid tumors;[17] among 19 cases undergoing postmortem study, 15 demonstrated evidence of diffuse neoplastic involvement of the intracranial (supratentorial and infratentorial) and spinal leptomeninges. Intraparenchymal brain metastases were present in nearly half. Spinal leptomeninges alone were involved in two cases, a phenomenon that has been described by others.[18] In two other cases, only the basilar and spinal leptomeninges were involved.

Gross examination of the brain, spinal cord, and roots often shows tumor nodules studding these structures and the overlying leptomeninges (Fig. 7–2). Myelography and MRI with contrast can be helpful in identifying these nodules in the cauda equina. In occasional cases, however, the leptomeninges may not reveal thickening on gross examination.[17]

Communicating hydrocephalus frequently has been found pathologically and clinically in patients with leptomeningeal metastases.[17] It is explained by the predilection of such metastases for the basilar meninges. The association between hydrocephalus and leptomeningeal metastases has been found for all types of cancer, but its pathogenesis was studied most closely in a detailed report of patients (primarily children) with leukemia. Moore and colleagues[19] found that 75% of patients dying with leptomeningeal leukemia had communicating hydrocephalus at autopsy. The communicating hydrocephalus could not be explained by invasion of the pacchionian granulations in

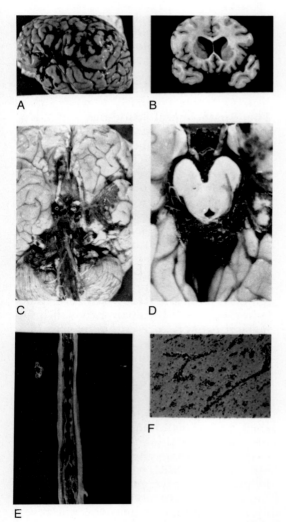

Figure 7–2. Leptomeningeal metastases due to melanoma. The pigmentation of the tumor identifies the regions where tumor is most heavily concentrated. (A) Lateral view of the cerebral hemispheres showing tumor concentrated in the sylvian fissure and sulci. (B) Coronal section through the anterior portion of the sylvian fissure demonstrates extension of leptomeningeal tumor into the brain parenchyma of both temporal cortices. The lateral ventricles are dilated secondary to communicating hydrocephalus. (C) The base of the brain is shown, with tumor involving several cranial nerves. (D) Transverse section through the midbrain showing tumor on the surface of the cord and tumor nodules along nerve roots. (F) Microscopic section from a different patient with melanoma demonstrating tumor extending into the perivascular space deep within the basal ganglia. (From Olson, ME, et al.,[17] with permission.)

the dural sinuses or the choroid plexus. Rather, it most closely correlated with the degree of arachnoidal and perivascular invasion of the basilar meninges, where neoplastic infiltration may have obstructed CSF flow.

Clinically, communicating hydrocephalus may cause gait difficulties and sphincter disturbances that must be differentiated from spinal cord and cauda equina dysfunction. Leptomeningeal metastases histopatholically consist of sheets of tumor cells that are surrounded by fibrosis and a small amount of inflammation.[17] Tumor cells tend to congregate around spinal nerve roots. Although the cerebral convexities generally show less tumor involvement, typically the basilar meninges are heavily involved, as are the spinal cord and its nerve roots.

A histopathological study of leptomeningeal invasion by solid tumors[17] demonstrated that tumor cells invade the brain and spinal cord parenchyma along the perivascular spaces, as in the case of leukemia.[15] Invasion of the spinal cord parenchyma secondary to cancer in the leptomeninges was found in four of 40 cases of leptomeningeal metastases.[20] Intraparenchymal spinal cord extension occurred either secondary to invasion of the pia mater or as a result of invasion along the perivascular spaces. Furthermore, along the spinal axis and basilar cisterns, tumor cells were again found to encase and invade spinal roots and cranial nerve structures. Thus the histopathological findings in cases of leptomeningeal invasion from solid tumors and lymphoma are similar to those previously described in leptomeningeal leukemia.[15,19]

PREVALENCE

In patients with systemic cancer, the overall prevalence of leptomeningeal metastases is approximately 5% to 8%.[2] The most common neoplasms that metastasize to the leptomeninges are breast and lung cancers, melanoma, non-Hodgkin's lymphoma, and leukemia.[2,9,13,17,19,21] However, the prevalence of leptomeningeal metastases from individual neoplasms is difficult to ascertain because the evolution of therapy for primary tumors has been associated with a change in the frequency of metastases to the CNS.[22] For example, because the CNS is a pharmacological sanctuary site,[13,23–26] the frequency of leptomeningeal leukemia dramatically increased as effective systemic treatments were developed for acute lymphoblastic leukemia.[21] Subsequently, with the advent of CNS prophylaxis for leptomeningeal leukemia, the frequency of this complication declined dramatically.[23,27]

Although these evolving patterns must be considered, some specific estimates of the risk for developing leptomeningeal metastases have emerged. Recent studies of patients with small-cell lung cancer have shown the risk to be approximately 9% to 18%.[25,28,29] Among patients receiving chemotherapy for breast cancer, approximately 5% develop leptomeningeal metastases.[26] In cases of non-Hodgkin's lymphoma, the frequency of leptomeningeal metastases is quite variable; it has been reported to range from 5% to 29%[10,11,23,30–33] Several other risk factors for involvement of the leptomeninges have been identified, including bone marrow and testicular involvement, extranodal disease, epidural invasion, diffuse histology, lymphoblastic lymphoma, and Burkitt's lymphoma.[9–11,32–34]

The interval of time between the diagnosis of malignancy and the development of leptomeningeal metastases also is quite variable. Although leptomeningeal metastases usually occur in conjunction with widespread systemic disease (as suggested by the risk factors identified above for non-Hodgkin's lymphoma), they may also be present at the time of diagnosis of the primary tumor or even herald the presence of malignancy.[9,13,25,35] Furthermore, because the CNS is a pharmacological sanctuary site, the leptomeninges may be the first site of recurrence in the absence of other metastases or may be affected while disease elsewhere is responding to chemotherapy.[9,25,29,35,36]

Leptomeningeal metastases may occur with or without coexisting intraparenchymal brain metastases or epidural spinal cord compression. The coexistence of these other metastases may make the clinical evaluation of these patients even more perplexing. For example, among a series of 90 patients with leptomeningeal metastases from solid tumors or lymphoma at Memorial Sloan-Kettering Cancer Center (MSKCC), one-third had coexisting intraparenchymal brain metastases or epidural spinal cord compression;[13] one patient had all three conditions. The presence of intraparenchymal brain metastases may help support the clinical impression of leptomeningeal metastases, or even an intramedullary spinal metastasis, if cytological and radiological confirmation is not forthcoming.[37,38]

CLINICAL MANIFESTATIONS

Spinal symptoms and/or signs are present on initial examination in approximately 70% of patients with leptomeningeal metastases.[39] The clinical hallmark of leptomeningeal metastases is multifocal involvement of the neuraxis at multiple levels. Since conventional neurological teaching emphasizes the identification of a single anatomical lesion to explain the patient's entire neurological deficit, this may be a diagnostically challenging problem. For example, a patient with known malignancy may present with chief complaints of back pain, gait difficulty, and burning dysesthesias of the lower extremities. Physical examination may reveal cognitive disturbances, facial asymmetry, asymmetric corneal responses, unilateral loss of biceps and knee reflexes, lax anal sphincter, apractic gait, and Babinski signs. In such a patient, although the history suggests spinal cord and/or cauda equina dysfunction alone, the physical examination may demonstrate evidence of dysfunction of the nervous system at multiple levels. Multiple levels of neurological disturbance, in which more abnormal neurological signs than symptoms are found, are characteristic of leptomeningeal metastases.[13]

The symptoms and signs of patients with suspected leptomeningeal metastases may be classified by abnormalities of spinal and radicular function, disturbances of cerebral function, or cranial nerve dysfunction.

Spinal/Radicular Symptoms and Signs

According to one detailed series from MSKCC, spinal and radicular symptoms and signs were present in 74 of 90 patients (82%) with leptomeningeal cancer (Table 7–1).[13] Lower extremity weakness was the most common symptom reported by patients. This weakness was of a lower motor neuron type and therefore was associated with depressed reflexes. The most common sign on physical examination (71%) was reflex asymmetry.

Pain is a common presenting manifestation, reported in approximately one-fourth of patients. The pain may be secondary to meningeal irritation or be due to spinal/radicular compression. When the pain is radicular, it may mimic that of epidural metastasis or degenerative disc disease. As with other forms of neuro-

pathic pain, it may be burning in character, or patients may describe the sensation as feeling as though the extremity(ies) were being wrapped.

Among all of the spinal roots, those of the cauda equina have the longest course in the subarachnoid space and are, therefore, most commonly affected. In the same series,[13] one-third of patients had signs of cauda equina dysfunction on initial examination; it was the presenting complaint in approximately 20% of patients. The symptoms and signs of cauda equina dysfunction usually include a combination of sphincter disturbance, lower extremity weakness of a lower motor neuron type (i.e., areflexic, hypotonic weakness), sensory loss in the lower extremities and in the sacral dermatomes over the buttocks, and pain in the back and lower extremities. Reflex abnormalities, weakness, and sensory loss are often asymmetric early in the course of the disease. It should be recalled that in a patient with cauda equina involvement, one would expect to find lower extremity weakness with depressed reflexes rather than hyperreflexia, which is typical of weakness due to upper motor neuron dysfunction. Alternatively, lower extremity weakness associated with asymmetric hyporeflexia may also be due to focal radiculopathies, lumbosacral plexus disease, or peripheral nerve disease. Furthermore, hyporeflexia in the cancer patient may be secondary to some chemotherapeutics such as vinca alkaloids. The peripheral neuropathy caused by these drugs, however, is usually symmetric rather than markedly asymmetric. Paresthesias, which are also frequent radicular complaints, may be vague and unfamiliar to the patient and thus be dismissed by the patient or the physician. Finally, rectal tone is frequently diminished when the cauda equina is invaded by leptomeningeal metastases.

Table 7–1. Leptomeningeal Metastases from Solid Tumors in 90 Patients: Spinal and Radicular Symptoms and Signs*

Symptoms	Number of Patients (%)	
Lower motor neuron weakness	34	(38)
Paresthesias	31	(34)
Radicular pain	19	(21)
Back/neck pain	23	(25)
Bowel/bladder dysfunction	12	(13)

Signs	Number of Patients (%)	
Reflex asymmetry	64	(71)
Weakness	54	(60)
Sensory loss	24	(27)
Straight-leg raising	11	(12)
Decreased rectal tone	10	(11)
Nuchal rigidity	7	(8)

*From Wasserstrom, WR, et al.,[13] p. 761, with permission.

Cerebral Symptoms and Signs

Cerebral symptoms and signs were found in 45 of 90 patients (50%) in the MSKCC study (Table 7–2).[13] Although they are not as common as spinal and root distur-

Table 7–2. **Leptomeningeal Metastases from Solid Tumors in 90 Patients: Cerebral Symptoms and Signs***

Symptoms	Number of Patients (%)
Headache	30 (33)
Mental change	15 (17)
Difficulty walking	12 (13)
Nausea/vomiting	10 (11)
Unconsciousness	2 (2)
Dysphasia	2 (2)
Dizziness	2 (2)

Signs	Number of Patients (%)
Mental change	28 (31)
Seizures	5 (6)
Generalized	3 (3)
Focal	2 (2)
Papilledema	5 (6)
Diabetes insipidus	2 (2)
Hemiparesis	1 (1)

*From Wasserstrom, WR, et al.,[13] p. 760, with permission.

bances, their recognition should suggest the possibility of leptomeningeal metastases rather than epidural spinal cord compression solely.

Headache, which may be secondary to raised intracranial pressure or irritation of innervated structures, is the most common cerebral complaint. Mental status change and gait difficulties also were very common. The latter is of interest since a spinal disorder must also be considered when patients offer this complaint. The most common cerebral abnormality found on neurological examination was mental status change (lethargy, memory loss, and confusion). In addition to these bicerebral disturbances, focal cerebral dysfunction was found in the form of dysphasia, seizures, hemiparesis, hemisensory disturbances, visual loss, and diabetes insipidus. Other reports of such cases have found similar examples of cerebral disturbances.[9,25,26,40] Finally, convulsive and nonconvulsive seizures may also be manifestations of cerebral involvement.[41]

Cranial Nerve Symptoms and Signs

Cranial nerve symptoms and signs were present in 50 of 90 patients (56%) with leptomeningeal metastases in the MSKCC series (Table 7–3).[13] While 38% of patients had cranial nerve symptoms as the presenting complaint, 56% had cranial nerve abnormalities at the time of diagnosis. Diplopia was overwhelmingly the most common of these symptoms; similarly, diplopia and dysconjugate gaze were the most common cranial nerve abnormalities among a group of patients with leptomeningeal lymphoma reported from Stanford.[9] Hearing loss and facial weakness are other common cranial neuropathies encountered.

Table 7–3. **Leptomeningeal Metastases from Solid Tumors in 90 Patients: Cranial Nerve Symptoms and Signs***

Symptoms	Number of Patients (%)
Diplopia	18 (20)
Hearing loss	7 (8)
Visual loss	5 (6)
Facial numbness	5 (6)
Decreased taste	3 (3)
Tinnitus	2 (2)
Hoarseness	2 (2)
Dysphagia	1 (1)
Vertigo	1 (1)

Signs	Number of Patients (%)
Ocular muscle paresis (III, IV, VI)	18 (20)
Facial weakness (VII)	15 (17)
Diminished hearing (VIII)	9 (10)
Optic neuropathy (II)	5 (6)
Trigeminal neuropathy (V)	5 (6)
Hypoglossal neuropathy (XII)	5 (6)
Blindness	3 (3)
Diminished gag (IX, X)	3 (3)

*From Wasserstrom, WR, et al.,[13] p. 761, with permission.

Comparison of the data presented in Tables 7–1 through 7–3 demonstrates that spinal/radicular symptoms and signs (present in 80%) are the most frequent initial complaints and findings on neurological examination of patients with leptomeningeal metastases.[13] Lower extremity weakness, the most common of these, is among the most vexing to evaluate because it may be due to cerebral dysfunction, spinal cord disease, cauda equina or lumbosacral plexus dysfunction, peripheral neuropathy, or nonneurological systemic causes. In evaluating gait difficulties in the oncology patient, one must especially consider the following etiologies: intraparenchymal brain metastases, epidural spinal cord compression, leptomeningeal metastases, peripheral neuropathy secondary to chemotherapy, cachexia, large tumor burden, and toxic–metabolic disturbances. More than one of these conditions may also coexist. Many cancer patients will have had multiple forms of chemotherapy and be suffering from advanced cancer. In this clinical setting, the history and physical examination may be helpful, but laboratory and diagnostic imaging studies usually are needed to confirm the clinical impression and exclude unexpected causes. To evaluate the spinal axis and exclude epidural spinal cord compression, which constitutes a medical emergency, MRI is most commonly used (see Chapter 5).[34,42–44]

LABORATORY AND DIAGNOSTIC IMAGING STUDIES

Cerebrospinal Fluid

Examination of the cerebrospinal fluid (CSF) is the single most useful laboratory test for the diagnosis of leptomeningeal metastases.[13,33,45] A lumbar puncture is routinely performed if there is no contraindication such as impending herniation from an intracranial mass or bleeding diathesis. The initial lumbar puncture CSF analysis usually reveals some abnormalities, possibly including an abnormally high opening pressure, elevated protein or white cell count, decreased CSF, glucose, or abnormal cytology. Although a CSF cytology that is positive for malignant cells is specific for leptomeningeal metastases, the other abnormalities are nonspecific. The CSF findings in two series of patients with leptomeningeal invasion from solid tumors and from lymphoma are shown in Tables 7–4 and 7–5.

In a study of 90 patients with leptomeningeal metastases from solid tumors (Table 7–4),[13] all but 3% showed at least one abnormality on initial routine CSF analysis. On repeated lumbar punctures, only one patient (1%) had persistently normal CSF analyses for all routine parameters. As in the case of lymphoma,[33] however, false-negative CSF cytologies are commonly encountered. The initial CSF yielded a positive cytology in only 54% of cases. When multiple CSF analyses were performed, a positive cytology for malignant cells was found in nearly 90% of cases; still, the diagnosis of leptomeningeal metastases from solid tumors could not be confirmed by CSF cytology in approximately 10% of patients. There were four cases in which the CSF cytology from the lumbar space was consistently negative, but the ventricular fluid (two cases) or the cisternal fluid (two cases) yielded malignant cells. Others have reported variations in the yield of CSF cytology and other routine parameters if CSF

Table 7–4. **Leptomeningeal Metastases From Solid Tumors in 90 Patients: CSF Findings**[*]

Parameter	Initial No. (%)		Total on All Punctures No. (%)	
Pressure > 160 mm CSF	45	(50)	64	(71)
Cells > 5/mm³	51	(57)	65	(70)
Protein > 50 mg/dl	73	(81)	80	(89)
Glucose < 40 mg/dl	28	(31)	37	(41)
Positive cytology	49	(54)	82	(91)
Normal	3	(3)	1	(1)

[*]From Wasserstrom, WR, et al.,[13] p. 762, with permission.

Table 7–5. **CSF Findings in 33 Patients with Leptomeningeal Lymphoma**[*]

Positive Findings	On First Lumbar Puncture No. (%)		Total on All Punctures No. (%)	
Pressure > 150 mm H_2O	17	(52)	22	(66)
White blood cells > 4/mm^3	22	(67)	24	(73)
Positive cytology	18	(54)	22	(67)
Protein > 50 mg/100 ml	23	(70)	29	(88)
Glucose < 50 mg/100 ml	11	(33)	19	(58)
No abnormalities	1	(3)	0	(0)

[*]From Young, RC, et al.,[33] p. 437, with permission.

is sampled at different levels of the neuraxis.[46]

In patients with leptomeningeal lymphoma (Table 7–5),[33] initial lumbar puncture was completely normal with regard to all routine parameters in only 3% of 33 patients. Although 97% of the patients showed some abnormality, the CSF cytology was diagnostic of lymphoma in only 54% of cases on initial lumbar puncture. Following repeated lumbar punctures, only 67% had a CSF cytology diagnostic of lymphoma; one-third of patients had persistently negative CSF cytology. Others also have found a high incidence of persistently false-negative CSF cytology in these patients despite involvement of the CNS from systemic lymphoma.[9]

The difficulties with regard to CSF cytological diagnosis of leptomeningeal leukemia are similar to those of lymphoma and other lymphoproliferative diseases; it is often difficult for the pathologist to distinguish reactive cells from leukemic cells.[15,47,48] Thus the brain, spinal cord, and nerve roots may be invaded by leukemic cells despite a negative CSF cytology in such cases.

The problem of false-negative CSF cytologies in patients with leptomeningeal metastases has been recognized since 1904.[49] Also, although most patients with malignant primary or metastatic intraparenchymal brain tumors have negative cytologies, occasionally the CSF of such patients reveals a positive cytology. Thus the clinical and pathological significance of a positive or negative CSF cytology under various circumstances needs to be defined.

Glass and colleagues[5] correlated CSF cytological examination during life with neuropathological findings at autopsy in an effort to determine the pathological significance and, therefore, the clinical implications of a positive CSF cytology. Among 66 cases at autopsy in whom only parenchymal or dural neoplasms were found, without pathological evidence of leptomeningeal involvement, a positive CSF cytology occurred in only one case. In this patient, the cytology reverted to negative while under treatment, suggesting that leptomeningeal disease may have been successfully eliminated prior to death. These findings suggest that a parenchymal primary or metastatic brain tumor will not yield a positive CSF cytology unless the leptomeninges have been seeded.

Another study,[50] however, reported that parenchymal tumors could cause a positive CSF cytology without leptomeningeal seeding. This study[5] also examined the rate of false-negative CSF cytologies in cases of leptomeningeal metastases. Of 51 patients with pathologically proven leptomeningeal involvement, the CSF cytology was positive in 59% during life.[5] Furthermore, the sensitivity of positive CSF cytology correlated with the extent of leptomeningeal invasion. For example, among patients found to have only focal leptomeningeal invasion, CSF cytologies were positive in only 38% of cases, but they were positive in 66% of those with diffuse leptomeningeal metastases. Of the 30 patients who had a positive CSF cytology, 25 (83%) had diffuse leptomeningeal metastases at autopsy. These results suggest, therefore, that when a CSF cytological examination is found to have malignant cells, it can be inferred that the patient has a high probability of diffuse and multifocal leptomeningeal metastases.

In addition, Glass and colleagues[5] found a false-negative cytology in 21 (41%) of 51 patients with documented leptomeningeal disease at autopsy; among them were 13 cases with disseminated leptomeningeal spread. They concluded that a negative CSF cytology does not exclude the presence of diffuse leptomeningeal spread, a finding which has been corroborated by several other clinical studies.[9,13,17,33,45,47]

On the issue of false-positive cytology, the same researchers[5] found two cases. Both patients had lymphoma and infection at the time of lumbar puncture; case one had sepsis and case two had herpes zoster. The reason for the false-positive cytologies was unknown, but it has been reported by other authors in the setting of lymphoma and CNS infections.[51–53]

The question is often asked, "How many lumbar punctures should be performed when evaluating the patient suspected of having leptomeningeal metastases if the initial CSF cytology is negative?" As noted above, in the setting of solid tumors, of 90 patients with proven leptomeningeal cancer, the initial lumbar puncture yielded a positive cytology in 49 (54%); an additional 27 (30%) positive cytologies were found on the second lumbar puncture, and subsequent lumbar punctures yielded a positive cytology in two additional cases. The rate of persistently false-negative CSF cytologies was near 10%.[13] In the case of lymphoma, the rate of false-negative cytology may be somewhat higher.[9,33] Therefore, when the diagnosis of leptomeningeal metastases is suspected, if the initial lumbar puncture is negative for malignant cells, it is generally recommended (if not contraindicated) that patients undergo a minimum of three lumbar punctures, if necessary, and that these samples for cytologic analysis be at least 5 to 10 cc each.[9,27]

The frequent finding of a false-negative CSF cytology for malignant cells in the setting of leptomeningeal lymphoma or leukemia is a significant clinical problem. Monoclonal antibodies may be helpful in differentiating normal from malignant cells in the cerebrospinal fluid,[54,55] identifying inflammatory mononuclear cells as T cells.[48] Thus B-cell lymphoproliferative neoplasms involving the leptomeninges may be differentiated from reactive pleocytosis.[47] This technique may improve the ability to confirm leptomeningeal invasion in cases of lymphoproliferative disease. Flow cytometry is another method used to examine CSF for malignant cells.[56,57] Aneuploid and hyperdiploid cells may be found in some cases of leptomeningeal metastases.

Biochemical Markers

There are several biochemical substances produced by neoplasms that could potentially be useful in early detection of malignancy.[58–61] In the serum, perhaps the most commonly assayed substance is carcinoembryonic antigen (CEA), which has emerged as a useful marker to screen patients for recurrence of a variety of different neoplasms.[62] Several studies have attempted to determine if measuring CEA and other biochemical markers in the CSF is useful in evaluating and managing patients with suspected leptomeningeal invasion.[61,63–68]

Carcinoembryonic antigen is a glycoprotein produced by both normal and malignant cells.[62] Originally thought to be a specific marker for gastrointestinal malignancies,[69] it has more recently been recognized to be elevated in a variety of malignant and nonmalignant conditions.[62] It is usually detectable in the serum of normal individuals at low concentrations. In the CSF of normal individuals, it is either undetectable or found in only trace concentrations.[66,70,71] Despite earlier reports to the contrary,[72,73] CEA has been found in the CSF of patients with serum CEA concentrations greater than 100 ng/ml; therefore, simultaneous measurement of plasma and cerebrospinal fluid CEA is recommended. At plasma levels greater than 100 ng/ml, CEA has been found to enter the CNS through an intact blood–brain barrier in the absence of CNS disease.[66] Other biochemical markers which, when found in the CSF strongly suggest leptomeningeal malignancy, include alpha fetoprotein (AFP), beta-HCG, and melanin (in cases of melanoma), except in cases where there is a very high serum concentration of the marker.[39]

Several nonspecific markers have been reported to be elevated in cases of leptomeningeal malignancy. Among others, these include beta-glucuronidase,[67] myelin basic protein,[74] isozyme V of lactic dehydrogenase,[75] and beta$_2$-microglobulin,[59] which may all be elevated in inflammatory or other diseases of the nervous system. Beta-glucuronidase is an intracellular enzyme that is normally present in both the gray and white matter of the brain, and it is found in relatively high concentrations within the pia–arachnoid and choroid plexus.[66] It is not unexpected, therefore, for it to be found under normal conditions in the CSF.[76] In the presence of malignancy in the CNS, however, the level of beta-glucuronidase has been found to rise.[76] Further studies have shown that the level of CSF beta-glucuronidase is often elevated in the setting of leptomeningeal metastases, but this elevation is not specific for this disease because elevated levels have also been found in cases of acute and chronic CNS infection.[66,67]

Both CEA and beta-glucuronidase have been studied in the CSF of patients suspected of having CNS metastases from adenocarcinoma, leukemia, lymphoma, or other malignancies.[66–68] Serial measurements of CEA may be useful in identifying patients with leptomeningeal relapse of breast cancer before other evidence of relapse.[68] Unlike beta-glucuronidase, CEA appears not to be consistently elevated in cases of chronic infectious meningitis.[66] Cerebrospinal fluid CEA and beta-glucuronidase are both useful tumor markers for the detection of leptomeningeal metastases, but not for intraparenchymal brain metastases or epidural tumor.[66] Cerebrospinal fluid levels of CEA were more accurate in detecting leptomeningeal metastases from lung carcinomas than those from breast cancer and melanoma. Neither CSF CEA nor beta-glucuronidase has been found to be very sensitive in the diagnosis of leptomeningeal lymphoma, however.[66]

An abnormal lactic dehydrogenase (LDH) isoenzyme pattern was found in some individuals with leptomeningeal metastases.[13] The CSF LDH-5/LDH-1 ratio was abnormal in 15 of 20 patients with leptomeningeal cancer in whom it was assayed. An elevated CSF lactic acid also was found in many patients with leptomeningeal cancer, as compared with controls.

Cerebrospinal fluid and serum immunoglobulins as well as beta$_2$-microglobulin have been assayed in patients with neoplastic diseases involving the CNS. In patients with lymphoproliferative diseases, and occasionally patients with nonlymphoid neoplasms, several abnormalities including presence of CSF and serum oligoclonal bands have been observed.[63] The results, however, were not sufficiently sensitive or specific to establish a diagnosis of CNS neoplastic involvement with certainty. Increased levels of beta$_2$-microglobulin have also been found in many cases of neoplastic involvement of the CNS.[63] However, this assay was associated with both false-positive and false-negative results. Furthermore, the study found that the CSF beta$_2$-microglobulin level increased during intrathecal treatment and/or CNS irradiation. Finally, CSF levels of beta$_2$-microglobulin, the IgG index, and the IgM index all increased when infectious complications in the CNS were found.

The cerebrospinal levels of vasopressin (ADH) and adrenocorticotrophic hormone (ACTH) have been assayed in patients suspected of harboring CNS metastatic disease from small-cell lung cancer.[64,65] As with the other biochemical markers described, the utility of these assays has been questioned due to their lack of specificity and sensitivity in accurately diagnosing leptomeningeal metastases. Attempting to explain this shortcoming, Pedersen and colleagues[65] cited evidence suggesting that with regard to production of biochemical markers, many tumors may be polyclonal; different metastatic clones might produce varying quantities of biochemical markers, creating an inherent difficulty in reliably measuring marker. Given the lack of specificity and sensitivity of the biochemical tumor markers in the evaluation of patients with suspected leptomeningeal metastases, they must be interpreted in the context of the other clinical and laboratory findings.

Diagnostic Imaging Studies

The modalities most frequently used for imaging the central nervous system are CT and MRI. Prior to MRI, myelography was frequently utilized to visualize leptomeningeal metastases.[9,13,17] Characteristic findings on myelography include a thickening of nerve roots and presence of nodules along the cauda equina due to metastases (Fig. 7–3.) Myelography was diagnostic in 13 of 49 patients in the MSKCC series.[13]

Contrast-enhanced CT of the brain has been used to identify leptomeningeal metastases.[77–80] The leptomeninges, cranial nerves, and superficial brain metastases commonly are abnormally enhanced because of breakdown of the blood–brain barrier. Communicating hydocephalus is also seen, due to obstruction of the basilar meninges.[81] Normal head CT scans are also often encountered in the presence of leptomeningeal metastases. One study[77] reported that a contrast-enhanced cranial CT was normal in 44% of patients with leptomeningeal cancer.

Spinal CT scanning following the introduction of intrathecal water-soluble contrast material may be more sensitive than myelography, however, in demonstrating the presence of nodules and thickening along nerve roots and the cauda equina.

Contrast-enhanced MRI can be helpful in the diagnosis and management of patients with leptomeningeal metastases.[81–83] On the other hand, noncontrast-enhanced MRI has been found to be insensitive to diagnosing leptomeningeal metastases. In one study,[84] noncontrast MRI of the brain was compared to contrast-enhanced cra-

nial CT. Many abnormalities seen on CT, such as sulcal and cisternal enhancement, or ependymal or subependymal metastases, were not as readily recognized on the noncontrast MRI or could not be differentiated from radiation effects or ventriculomegaly alone. In the study cited above,[77] Krol et al. also compared cranial CT with nonenhanced cranial MRI in the evaluation of leptomeningeal cancer. Nonenhanced MRI of the brain was normal in 65% of cases.

Similarly in the spine, noncontrast MRI was found to be relatively insensitive in detecting leptomeningeal metastases.[77,85] Alternatively, with the use of contrast-enhanced MRI, leptomeningeal metastases are frequently visualized (Fig. 7–4).[85–90] The sensitivity of gadolinium-enhanced MRI scans for leptomeningeal metastases appears to match that of myelography and postmyelography CT.[87] However, as in the case of myelography, the gadolinium-enhanced MRI may be normal in the setting of leptomeningeal metastases; thus, CSF cytology continues to be helpful in the evaluation of these patients.[87]

Although not specific, electrophysiological studies may occasionally help in evaluating patients with leptomeningeal metastases. The electroencephalogram may be diffusely or focally slow, and seizure activity may be seen.[17] Electrophysiological studies of the peripheral nervous system (i.e., spinal roots) may identify subclinical abnormalities in these patients.

The following case illustrates the protean manifestations of leptomeningeal cancer and the difficulties sometimes encountered in confirming a diagnosis with laboratory methods.

CASE ILLUSTRATION

A 24-year-old man with a history of diffuse histiocytic lymphoma was referred for evaluation of low back pain and gait difficulty. The patient reported that he had had intermittent but progressive low back pain for three to four weeks; during the past week he had developed left leg pain; and most recently he had developed neck and right arm pain. His gait difficulty began one to two weeks previously. Initially he noted

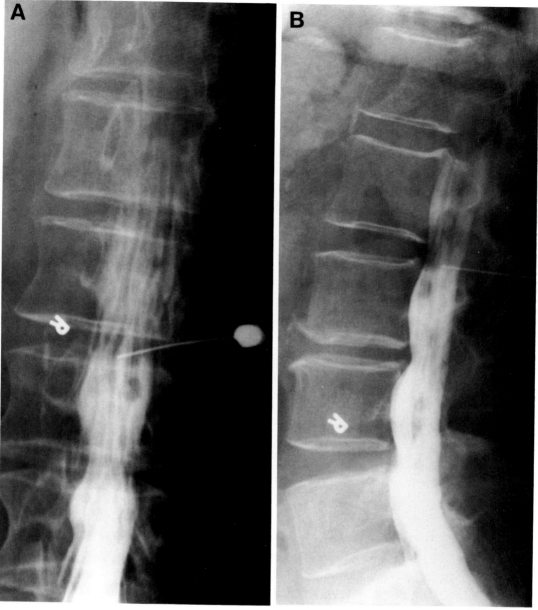

Figure 7–3. Myelogram showing leptomeningeal metastases from breast cancer. The patient had cauda equina symptoms and signs, and the myelogram reveals metastatic nodules involving the cauda equina. (A) Anteroposterior view. The largest filling defect is seen just above the spinal needle. (B) Lateral view.

left leg numbness and weakness, but more recently his right leg and right hand seemed to be getting weaker. During the past two weeks, he had also noted increasing difficulty sustaining an erection. He denied headache, diplopia, dysarthria, change in cognitive function, bowel

or bladder difficulties, fever, chills, or other symptoms of infection.

His past medical history was significant only for lymphoma, which had been diagnosed 18 months earlier. He had received several cycles of chemotherapy, some of which had included

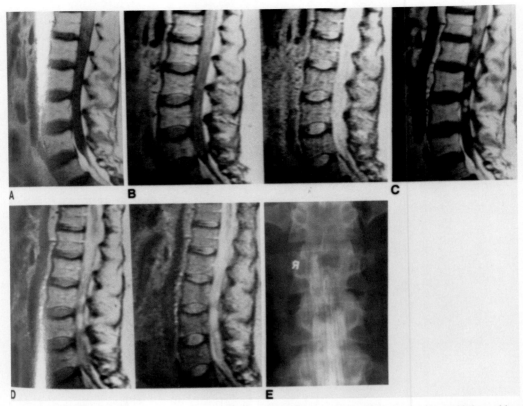

Figure 7–4. A 28-year-old man with known cerebral glioblastoma presenting with back pain and bilateral lower extremity weakness. The clinical history, examination, myelogram, and positive CSF cytology were all consistent with leptomeningeal metastases. Sagittal lumbar MR images are shown in A through D. (A) T_1-weighted noncontrast image was considered negative except for poor definition of the conus and proximal nerve roots. In retrospect, vague nodules may be present in the subarachnoid space. (B) Proton-density (left panel) and T_2-weighted (right panel) images were also considered equivocal; there was a suggestion of high intensity near the conus. (C) T_1-weighted image after contrast administration shows enhancing subarachnoid tumor encasing the nonenhancing distal spinal cord. Multiple metastases are seen. (D) Proton-density (left panel) and T_2-weighted (right panel) scans after contrast administration show that the lesions enhance (white nodular areas in the spinal canal). (E) Myelogram confirms the presence of multiple nodules, and block at the level of the conus. (From Sze, G, et al.,[85] with permission.)

vinca alkaloids. A recent extent-of-disease evaluation showed bone marrow involvement by lymphoma and enlarging retroperitoneal adenopathy.

Physical examination revealed a chronically ill young man with normal vital signs. He had palpable cervical and axillary adenopathy and an enlarged spleen. The remainder of the general physical examination was unremarkable. The neurological examination revealed a normal mental status, normal funduscopic examination, and normal cranial nerve function. The neck was supple and deep tendon reflexes were asymmetric: The biceps and triceps reflexes were absent on the right side but present on the left. Both brachioradialis reflexes were absent. The patellar reflex was absent on the left but intact on the right. Both ankle jerks were depressed. No Babinski signs were elicited, and the superficial abdominal reflexes were present and symmetric. The right upper extremity strength was 4/5 proximally and 4-/5 distally. The left leg strength was 4-/5 throughout and the right leg strength was 4/5. No fasciculations were seen, and there was no atrophy. Sensory examination showed a stocking-glove sensory loss to pin, vibration, and temperature. There was also decreased pin sensation in the right proximal upper extremity and markedly decreased sensation over the sacral dermatomes of the buttocks. The anal sphincter was lax.

The clinical impression was that the patient had leptomeningeal metastases from lymphoma. Routine laboratory studies were unremarkable. Total spine films did not demonstrate a compression fracture or paravertebral mass. Because epidural spinal cord compression could not be excluded on the basis of the examination alone, the patient was treated with corticosteroids. A total spinal myelogram with metrizamide was followed by CT scanning. There was no evidence of epidural tumor or leptomeningeal seeding on the radiological studies. The CSF studies revealed a protein of 84 mg per dl, glucose 51 mg per dl, 25 nucleated cells (1% polymorphonuclear cells, 90% lymphocytes, 9% monocytes). Cytology was negative for malignant cells, and infectious disease studies (routine, AFB, fungal studies, and cryptococcal antigen) were all negative.

In the absence of laboratory confirmation of leptomeningeal metastases, the patient underwent two more lumbar punctures during the following week. In each case, there was persistent CSF pleocytosis, elevated protein, and negative cytology for malignant cells. The infectious disease workup was repeated (including serum Lyme titer and FTA-ABS) and again found to be negative. During this period of time, the patient developed progressive bilateral upper extremity weakness and lower extremity weakness. The deep tendon reflexes that had been present initially were lost. He developed memory difficulties. He began to complain of diplopia and was found to have a partial left third-nerve palsy with inability to adduct and elevate the eye. A questionable left facial paresis was also seen. A contrast-enhanced head CT scan was performed and was normal.

After one week of hospitalization, despite the lack of definitive laboratory confirmation, leptomeningeal lymphoma was considered the most likely diagnosis and treatment was initiated. Despite whole neuraxis radiation therapy and intrathecal chemotherapy (his CSF cytologies remained negative for malignant cells), his neurological condition deteriorated and he died two weeks later of respiratory failure.

At postmortem examination, this patient's leptomeninges were studded with lymphoma; the heaviest concentration was in the spinal axis. The cranial nerves were involved, and lymphoma was found to cuff leptomeningeal blood vessels. Areas of cerebral infarction were seen on histopathological examination.

Comment. This case illustrates the difficulties often encountered in the evaluation of patients with leptomeningeal metastases. Initially, only radicular abnormalities were found, but during further observation cranial nerve and cerebral symptoms and signs developed, which helped to confirm the clinical impression. The laboratory workup showed no definite signs of leptomeningeal lymphoma, but the CSF was persistently abnormal in terms of cell count, protein, and glucose determinations. When the other causes of chronic meningitis were confidently excluded, and the clinical examination confirmed the presence of multiple levels of neuraxis involvement, the patient was treated for leptomeningeal metastases. It should be noted that the clinical diagnosis also was supported by the histological type of lymphoma which showed bone marrow involvement (diffuse histiocytic lymphoma), a risk factor for leptomeningeal invasion.

APPROACH TO THE PATIENT SUSPECTED OF HAVING LEPTOMENINGEAL METASTASES

As has been emphasized throughout this chapter, the clinical manifestations of leptomeningeal metastases are typically by the very nature of the disease multifocal and therefore protean. Occasionally, cancer patients with no neurological complaints undergo lumbar punctures for unrelated reasons, and malignant cells are found. Patients also may have solitary symptoms or signs as the initial manifestation of leptomeningeal involvement. In cancer patients with multifocal involvement of the nervous system, there may be a high index of suspicion that the patient has leptomeningeal metastases, but the CSF may fail to reveal malignant cells to confirm the clinical impression. Thus no single approach can be recommended. In the absence of definitive laboratory confirmation, only guidelines can be offered. Decision-making and management should be modified on the basis of the patient's individual circumstances.

The diagnosis of leptomeningeal cancer is usually suspected in the cancer patient with the appropriate clinical history and examination. In addition to the clinical data, the clinician should consider the primary tumor type, the extent of disease elsewhere, and the risk factors for the development of leptomeningeal metastases. All of these factors may provide clinical evidence for or against the diagnosis. Laboratory data such as CSF cytology will usually confirm the clinical impression, but as seen above, CSF cytology may continue to be negative.

In the patient presenting with spinal symptoms and signs, leptomeningeal metastases may be considered if the patient has symptoms or signs of intracranial disease or other signs of multifocal involvement that cannot be explained on the basis of epidural spinal cord compression alone. In the setting of coexisting cerebral or cranial nerve disturbances, a head CT scan or MRI will identify a mass lesion or hydrocephalus. However, as cited above, contrast-enhanced studies are needed to demonstrate leptomeningeal metastases apart from the nonspecific finding of communicating hydrocephalus.[81]

If the clinical presentation suggests the possibility of epidural spinal cord compression, then MRI (or myelography) will identify an epidural mass. If myelography is performed, CSF may be obtained at the time of myelography. While nonenhanced MRI is usually sufficient for identifying metastatic epidural spine compression, contrast-enhanced MRI of the spine should be performed to evaluate for leptomeningeal disease. If no epidural compression is seen that could explain the patient's clinical findings, then (if there is no contraindication) a lumbar puncture with CSF studies sent for cell count, protein, glucose, cytology, and infectious disease studies (including bacterial, AFB, fungal studies, cryptococcal antigen, and VDRL) may confirm the clinical impression of leptomeningeal metastases. If the initial cytology is negative, two or three repeat CSF analyses may be performed. If the CSF cytologies are persistently negative for ma-

lignant cells and the imaging findings are not diagnostic, other less common infectious etiologies (including Lyme disease and syphilis) and noninfectious causes of chronic meningitis[91] should be considered.[83] If the diagnosis cannot be confirmed by laboratory studies, repeat CSF analyses and repeat contrast-enhanced head MRI scans may be helpful. If the patient has leptomeningeal metastases, some laboratory evidence supporting this diagnosis, such as a markedly depressed CSF glucose or persistent CSF pleocytosis, is usually seen in the absence of infectious or other nonneoplastic etiology.

If the clinical evidence for leptomeningeal cancer is not strong, relatively specific laboratory findings such as positive CSF cytology, enhancing metastases on MRI, or metastatic neoplasms on nerve roots should be demonstrated before a diagnosis is made.[13,39,81] Given the difficult diagnostic and management issues in cases where a definitive clinical and laboratory diagnosis is not forthcoming, consultation with an experienced neurological clinician and other specialists, as the circumstances indicate, is recommended.

THERAPY

Treatment of leptomeningeal metastases must be directed to both the intracranial compartment and spinal axis because malignant cells circulate throughout the entire subarachnoid space. Radiotherapy, intrathecal chemotherapy, and systemic chemotherapy have each been used alone and in combination.[92,93] For example, systemic high-dose methotrexate with leukovorin rescue[94] and high-dose cytosine arabinoside[95] have been used in patients with leptomeningeal leukemia. Although radiotherapy is generally effective in treating leptomeningeal cancer, it usually cannot be delivered to the entire neuraxis without significant bone marrow suppression. Thus radiotherapy directed to symptomatic sites—in combination with intrathecal chemotherapy consisting of methotrexate, cytosine arabinoside (ARA-C), or thiotepa—is often used.[39,96,97] Investigational approaches include immuno-toxin therapy and the use of radiolabeled monoclonal antibodies.[98–102]

Intraventricular administration of chemotherapy provides better distribution of the drug throughout the neuraxis than does intralumbar administration.[103–105] Two independent studies have shown the clinical advantage of intraventricular chemotherapy in overt leptomeningeal leukemia.[106,107] In both studies, patients served as their own controls: In the first, the median duration of remission was increased from 9.5 months in the intralumbar-treated period to 16 months in the intraventricular-treated period ($p < 0.05$).[106] In the other study, the monthly incidence of CNS relapses in the intraventricular-treated period was one fourth that of the intralumbar-treated period ($p < 0.05$).[107]

Toxicities from treatment include neurotoxicity, mucositis, and bone marrow suppression from radiotherapy and intrathecal chemotherapy. Systemic toxicities from intrathecal methotrexate may be reduced by administering oral or parenteral leukovorin. Complications from the placement of the Ommaya reservoir are infrequent. Posner has reported that hemorrhage into the brain at the time of placement occurs in less than 1% of patients, and infectious complications occur in about 5%.[39,108] If the catheter is not placed properly in the ventricle, instillation of chemotherapy directly into the brain can cause leukoencephalopathy surrounding the catheter.

The treatment of leptomeningeal metastases and of toxicities associated with various forms of therapy (e.g., leukoencephalopathy) has been reviewed.[27,39] In general, leukemic and lymphomatous meningitis respond best to aggressive therapy. Leptomeningeal disease from breast cancer has shown variable responses, including 25% one-year survival with intensive intraventricular methotrexate treatment reported by Ongerboer de Visser et al.[109] On the other hand, other groups have found less favorable responses to therapy.[110,111] The outcome from therapy of non-small-cell lung cancer and other adenocarcinomas involving the leptomeningeas is usually poor.[39,112] The median survival of patients with leptomeningeal metastases from solid tumors has been reported to be four to six months.[13,27]

SUMMARY

Neoplastic cells which enter the cerebrospinal fluid are called leptomeningeal metastases. Such metastases may arise from systemic malignancies or primary CNS cancer. Leptomeningeal metastases were first recognized as a significant clinical problem in neuro-oncology when children with acute lymphoblastic leukemia were successfully treated with chemotherapy. Because the CNS is a "pharmacologic sanctuary site," children who were successfully placed in systemic remission by chemotherapeutic agents were found to relapse in the leptomeninges. (This experience recalled a similar phenomenon in the treatment of tuberculosis with streptomycin.) With the advent of more successful chemotherapeutic agents for other malignancies (e.g., breast cancer), leptomeningeal metastases have become an increasingly frequent problem for patients with malignancies.

Since neoplastic cells circulate throughout the CNS, they frequently cause perplexing clinical manifestations. Accordingly, patients may present alone or with any combination of (1) cerebral disturbance, (2) cranial neuropathy, and/or (3) spinal dysfunction. This presents a difficult diagnostic problem because we are often taught to think of a single lesion which causes the patient's neurologic disorder. Furthermore, imaging and laboratory diagnosis are fraught with pitfalls. For example, while nonenhanced MRI scanning is very sensitive in diagnosing epidural spinal metastases, contrast enhancement is needed to reveal most cases of leptomeningeal metastases. Furthermore, CSF analysis may not yield malignant cells on the first tap and may require multiple analyses. In cases of lymphoma or leukemia, where the neoplastic cells resemble normal lymphocytes, the laboratory diagnosis may be particularly vexing.

Once a diagnosis is established the entire neuraxis requires therapy in order to clear the leptomeninges of neoplastic cells. Radiation therapy is frequently administered, but because radiation to the entire neuraxis includes an extensive region of bone marrow, it must often be limited to the symptomatic sites and supplemented with chemotherapy to treat subclinical disease elsewhere. Chemotherapy may be administered either directly into the CSF (e.g., via Ommaya reservoir) or systemically in doses and by agents which penetrate the CNS. This chapter reviews the clinical manifestations and imaging and laboratory features of leptomeningeal metastases and briefly comments upon principles of therapy. The interested reader is referred to oncologic texts and articles for specific recommendations regarding current therapies.

REFERENCES

1. Gonzalez-Vitale JC, Garcia-Bunuel R. Meningeal carcinomatosis. *Cancer* 1976;37: 2906–11.
2. Patchell RA, Posner JB. Neurologic complications of systemic cancer. *Neurol Clin* 1985;3: 729–50.
3. Carpenter MB. Meninges and Cerebrospinal Fluid. *Human Neuroanatomy*. Baltimore: William & Wilkins; 1976; pp. 1–19.
4. Edwards MS, Levin VA, Seager ML, Wilson CB. Intrathecal chemotherapy for leptomeningeal dissemination of medulloblastoma. *Child's Brain* 1981;8:444–51.
5. Glass JP, Melamed M, Chernik NL, Posner JB. Malignant cells in cerebrospinal fluid (CSF): the meaning of a positive CSF cytology. *Ann Neurol* 1979;29:1369–75.
6. Johnson DL, Schwarz S. Intracranial metastases from malignant spinal-cord astrocytoma: case report. *J Neurosurg* 1987;66:621–5.
7. Yung W-K, Horten BC, Shapiro WR. Meningeal gliomatosis: a review of 12 cases. *Ann Neurol* 1980;8:605–8.
8. Griffin JW, Thompson RW, Mitchinson MJ. Lymphomatous leptomeningitis. *Am J Med* 1971;51:200–8.
9. Mackintosh FR, Colby TV, Podolsky WJ, et al. Central nervous system involvement in non-Hodgkin's lymphoma: an analysis of 105 cases. *Cancer* 1982;49:586–95.
10. Herman TS, Hammond N, Jones SE, et al. Involvement of the central nervous system by non-Hodgkin's lymphoma: the southwest oncology group experience. *Cancer* 1979;43: 390–7.
11. Levitt LJ, Dawson DM, Rosenthal DS, et al. CNS involvement in non-Hodgkin's lymphomas. *Cancer* 1980;45:545–52.
12. Grain GO, Karr JP. Diffuse leptomeningeal carcinomatosis. Clinical and pathologic characteristics. *Neurology* 1955;5:706–22.
13. Wasserstrom WR, Glass JP, Posner JB. Diagnosis and treatment of leptomeningeal metastases from solid tumors: Experience with 90 patients. *Cancer* 1982;49:759–72.
14. Azzarelli B, Mirkin LD, Goheen M, Muller J, Crockett C. The leptoemeningeal vein: a site of re-entry of leukemic cells into the systemic circulation. *Cancer* 1984;54:1333–43.
15. Price RA, Johnson WW. The central nervous system in childhood leukemia: I. The arachnoid. *Cancer* 1973;31:520–33.
16. Siegal T, Mildworf B, Stein D, Melamed E. Leptomenigeal metastases: reduction in regional cerebral blood flow and cognitive impairment. *Ann Neurol* 1985;17:100–2.
17. Olson ME, Chernik NL, Posner JB. Infiltration of the leptomeninges by systemic cancer; a clinical and pathologic study. *Arch Neurol* 1974;30: 122–37.
18. Parsons M. The spinal form of carcinomatous meningitis. *Q J Med* 1972;41:509–18.
19. Moore EW, Freireich EJ, Shaw RK, Thomas LB. The central nervous system in acute leukemia. *Arch Int Med* 1960;105:451–67.
20. Costigan DA, Winkelman MD. Intramedullary spinal cord metastasis: a clinicopathological study of 13 cases. *J Neurosurg* 1985;62:227–33.
21. Yuill GM. Leukemia: neurological involvement. In Vinken PJ, Bruyn GW, editors. *Handbook of Clinical Neurology, Volume 39*. Amsterdam: North-Holland; 1980; pp. 1–25.
22. Posner JB. Neurologic complications of systemic cancer. *Dis Mon* 1978;25:1–60.
23. Bunn PA, Schein PS, Banks PM, DeVita VT. Central nervous system complications in patients with diffuse histiocytic and undifferentiated lymphoma: leukemia revisited. *Blood* 1976; 47:3–10.
24. Nugent JL, Bunn PA, Matthews MJ, et al. CNS metastases in small cell bronchogenic carcinoma–increasing frequency and changing patterns with lengthening survival. *Cancer* 1979; 44:1885–93.
25. Rosen ST, Aisner J, Makuch RW, et al. Carcinomatous leptomeningitis in small cell lung cancer: a clinicopathologic review of the National Cancer Institute experience. *Medicine* 1982;61: 45–53.
26. Yap H-Y, Seng B-S, Tashima CK, DiStefano A, Blumenschein GR. Meningeal carcinomatosis in breast cancer. *Cancer* 1978;42:283–6.
27. Bleyer WA, Byrne TN. Leptomeningeal cancer in leukemia and solid tumors. *Curr Prob Cancer* 1988;12:185–238.
28. Aroney RS, Dalley DN, Chan WK, Bell DR, Levi JA. Meningeal carcinomatosis in small cell carcinoma of the lung. *Am J Med* 1981;71: 26–32.
29. Balducci L, Little DD, Khansur T, Steinberg MH. Carcinomatous meningitis in small cell lung cancer. *Am J Med Sci* 1984;287:31–3.
30. Litam JP, Cabanillas F, Smith TL, et al. Central nervous system relapse in malignant lym-

phomas: risk factors and implications for prophylaxis. *Blood* 1979;54:1249–57.

31. Mead GM, Kennedy P, Smith JL, et al. Involvement of the central nervous system by non-Hodgkin's lymphoma in adults: a review of 36 cases. *Q J Med* 1986;60:699–714.

32. Perez-Soler R, Smith TL, Cabanillas F. Central nervous system prophylaxis with combined intravenous and intrathecal methotrexate in diffuse lymphoma of aggressive histologic type. *Cancer* 1986;57:971–7.

33. Young RC, Howser DM, Anderson T, et al. Central nervous system complications of non-Hodgkin's lymphoma. *Am J Med* 1979;66:435–43.

34. Smoker WRK, Godersky JC, Knutzon RK, Keyes WD, Norman D, Bergman W. The role of MR imaging in evaluating metastatic spinal disease. *AJR Am J Roentgenol* 1987;149:1241–8.

35. Sorensen SC, Eagen RT, Scott M. Meningeal carcinomatosis in patients with primary breast or lung cancer. *Mayo Clin Proc* 1984;59:91–4.

36. Cairncross JG, Posner JB. Neurological complications of malignant lymphoma. In Vinken PJ, Bruyn GW, editors. *Handbook of Clinical Neurology, Volume 39*. Amsterdam: North-Holland; 1980; pp. 27–62.

37. Grem JL, Burgess J, Trump DL. Clinical features and natural history of intramedullary spinal cord metastasis. *Cancer* 1985;56:2305–14.

38. Winkelman MD, Adelstein DJ, Karlins NL. Intramedullary spinal cord metastasis: diagnostic and therapeutic considerations. *Arch Neurol* 1987;44:526–31.

39. Posner J. *Neurologic Complications of Cancer.* Philadelphia: FA Davis; 1995; Contemporary Neurology Series.

40. Yap H, Tashima CK, Blumerschein GR, Eckles N. Diabetes insipidus in breast cancer. *Arch Int Med* 1979;139:1009–11.

41. Broderick JP, Cascino TL. Nonconvulsive status epilepticus in a patient with leptomeningeal cancer. *Mayo Clin Proc* 1987;62:835–7.

42. Daffner RH, Lupetin AR, Dash N, Deeb ZL, Sefczek RJ, Schapiro RL. MRI in detection of malignant infiltration of bone marrow. *AJR Am J Roentgenol* 1986;146:353–8.

43. Sze G, Krol G, Zimmerman RD, Deck MDF. Gadolinium-DTPA: malignant extradural spinal tumors. *Radiology* 1988;167:217–23.

44. Zimmer WD, Bergquist TH, McLeod RA, et al. Bone tumors: magnetic resonance imaging versus computed tomography. *Radiology* 1985;155:709–18.

45. Theodore WH, Gendelman S. Meningeal carcinomatosis. *Arch Neurol* 1981;38:696–9.

46. Murray JJ, Greco FA, Wolff SN, Hainsworth JD. Neoplastic meningitis: marked variations of cerebrospinal fluid composition in the absence of extradural block. *Am J Med* 1983;75:289–94.

47. Ernerudh J, Olsson T, Berlin G, Gustafsson B, Karlsson H. Cell surface markers for diagnosis of central nervous system involvement in lymphoproliferative diseases. *Ann Neurol* 1986;20:610–5.

48. Moench TR, Griffin DE. Immunocytochemical identification and quantitation of the mononuclear cells in cerebrospinal fluid, meninges, and brain during acute viral meningoencephalitis. *J Exp Med* 1984;159:77–88.

49. Dufour MH. Meningite sarcomateuse diffuse avec encaissement de la moelle et des racines: cytologie positive et special du liquide cephalo-radichien. *Rev Neurol (Paris)* 1904;12:104–6.

50. Choi HH, Anderson PJ. Diagnostic cytology of cerebrospinal fluid by the cytocentrifuge method. *Am J Clin Pathol* 1979;72:931–43.

51. Davies SF, Gormus BJ, Yarchoan R, et al. Cryptococcal meningitis with false-positive cytology in the CSF: use of T-cell rosetting to exclude meningeal lymphoma. *JAMA* 1978;239:2369–70.

52. Naylor B. The cytologic diagnosis of cerebrospinal fluid. *Acta Cytol* 1964;8:141–9.

53. Rawlinson DG, Billingham ME, Berry PF, et al. Cytology of the cerebrospinal fluid in patients with Hodgkin's disease or malignant lymphoma. *Acta Neuropathol (Berlin) (Suppl)* 1975;VI:187–91.

54. Coakham HB, Brownell B, Harper EI, et al. Use of monoclonal antibody panel to identify malignant cells in cerebrospinal fluid. *Lancet* 1984;1:1095–7.

55. Coakham HB, Harper EI, Garson JA, Brownell B, Lane EB. Carcinomatous meningitis diagnosed with monoclonal antibodies. *Br J Med* 1984;288:1272.

56. Dux R, Kindler-Rohrborn A, Annas M, et al. A standardized protocol for flow cytometric analysis of cells isolated from cerebrospinal fluid. *J Neurol Sci* 1994;121:74–8.

57. ESCibas, Malkin M, Posner J. Detection of DNA abnormalities by flow cytometry in cells from cerebrospinal fluid. *Am J Clin Pathol* 1987;88:570–7.

58. Nakagawa H, Kubo S, Murasawa A, et al. Measurements of CSF biochemical tumor markers in patients with meningeal carcinomatosis and brain tumors. *J Neurooncol* 1992;12:111–20.

59. Hansen P, Kjeldsen L, Dalhoff L, et al. Cerebrospinal fluid beta-2-microglobulin in adult patients with acute leukemia or lymphoma: a useful marker in early diagnosis and monitoring of CNS-involvment. *Acta Neurol Scand* 1992;85:224–7.

60. Musto P, Modini S, Ladogana S, et al. Increased risk of neurological relapse in acute lymphblastic leukemias with high levels of cerebrospinal fluid thymideine kinase at diagnosis. *Leuk Lymphoma* 1993;9:121–4.

61. Zanten AV, Twiijnstra A, Visser BOd, et al. Cerebrospinal fluid tumour markers in patients treated for meningeal malignancy. *J Neurol Neurosurg Psychiatry* 1991;54:119–23.

62. McIntire KR. Tumor markers. In DeVita Jr. VT, Hellman S, Rosenberg SA, editors. *Cancer: Principles and Practice of Oncology*. Philadelphia: J.B. Lippincott; 1985; pp. 375–88.

63. Ernerudh J, Olsson T, Berlin G, Schenck Hv. Cerebrospinal fluid immunoglobulins and beta 2-microglobulin in lymphoproliferative and

other neoplastic diseases of the central nervous system. *Arch Neurol* 1987;44:915–20.

64. Pedersen AG, Hammer M, Hansen M, Sorensen PS. Cerebrospinal fluid vasopressin as a marker of central nervous system metastases from small-cell bronchogenic cancer. *J Clin Oncol* 1985;3:48–53.

65. Pedersen AG, HAnsen M, Hummer L, Rogowski P. Cerebrospinal fluid ACTH as a marker of central nervous system metastases from small cell carcinoma of the lung. *Cancer* 1985;56:2476–80.

66. Schold SC, Wasserstrom WR, Fleisher M, Schwartz MK, Posner JB. Cerebrospinal fluid biochemical markers of central nervous system metastases. *Ann Neurol* 1980;8:597–604.

67. Tallman RD, Kimbrough SM, O'Brien JF, Goellner JR, Yanagihara T. Assay for beta-glucuronidase in cerebrospinal fluid: usefulness for the detection of neoplastic meningitis. *Mayo Clin Proc* 1985;60:293–8.

68. Yap B-S, Yap H-Y, Fritsche HA, Blumenschein G, Bodey GP. CSF carcinoembryonic antigen in meningeal carcinomatosis from breast cancer. *JAMA* 1980;244:1601–3.

69. Gold P, Freeman SO. Demonstration of tumor-specific antigens in human colonic carcinomata by immunologic tolerance and absorption techniques. *J Exp Med* 1965;121:439–66.

70. Kido D, Dyce B, Haverback BJ, Rumbaugh C. Carcinoembryonic antigen in patients with untreated central nervous system tumors. *Bull Los Angeles Neurol Soc* 1976;41:47–54.

71. Snitzer LS, McKinney E. Carcinoembryonic antigen in cerebrospinal fluid (abstract). *Proc Am Soc Clin Oncol* 1976;17:249.

72. Snitzer LS, McKinney EG, Tejada F, Seigel M, Rosomoff H, Zubrod G. Cerebral metastases and carcinoembryonic antigen in CSF (letter). *N Engl J Med* 1975;293:1101.

73. Yap BS, Yap HY, Benjamin RS, Bodey GP, Freireich EJ. Cerebrospinal fluid carcinoembryonic antigen in breast cancer patients with meningeal carcinomatosis (abstract). *Proc Am Soc Clin Oncol* 1978;19:98.

74. Nakagawa H, Yamada M, Kanayama T, et al. Myelin basic protein in the cerberospinal fluid of patients with brain tumors. *Neurosurgery* 1994;34:825–33.

75. Wasserstrom W, Schwartz M, Fleisher M, et al. Cerebrospinal fluid biochemical markers in central nervous system tumors: a review. *Ann Clin Lab Sci* 1981;11:239–51.

76. Allen N, Reagan E. Beta-glucuronidase activities in cerebrospinal fluid. *Arch Neurol* 1964; 11:144–54.

77. Krol G, Sze G, Malkin M, Walker R. MR of cranial and spinal meningeal carcinomatosis: comparison with CT and myelography. *AJR Am J Roentgenol* 1988;151:583–8.

78. Jaeckle KA, Krol G, Posner JB. Evolution of computed tomographic abnormalities in leptomeningeal metastases. *Ann Neurol* 1985;17:85–9.

79. Lee YY, Glass JP, Geoffray A, Wallace S. Cranial computed tomographic abnormalities in lep-

tomenigeal metastases. *AJNR Am J Neuroradiol* 1984;5:559–63.

80. Enzmann DR, Krikorian J, Yorke C, Hayward R. Computed tomography in leptomeningeal spread of tumor. *J Comput Assist Tomogr* 1978; 2:448–55.

81. Freilich R, Krol G, DeAngelis L. Neuroimaging and cerebrospinal fluid cytology in the diagnosis of leptomeningeal metastasis. *Ann Neurol* 1995;38:51–7.

82. Yousem D, Patrone P, Grossman R. Leptomeningeal metastases: MR evaluation. *J Comput Tomogr* 1990;14:255–61.

83. Chamberlain M. Comparative spine imaging in leptomeningeal metastases. *J Neurooncol* 1995; 23:233–38.

84. Davis PC, Friedman NC, Fry SM, Malko JA, Hoffman JC, Braun IF. Leptomenigeal metastasis: MR imaging. *Radiology* 1987;163:449–54.

85. Sze G, Abramson A, Krol G, et al. Gadolinium-DTPA in the evaluation of intradural extramedullary spinal disease. *AJNR Am J Neuroradiol* 1988;9:153–63.

86. Barloon TJ, Yuh WTC, Yang CJC, Schultz DH. Spinal subarachnoid tumor seeding from intracranial metastasis: MR findings. *J Comput Assist Tomogr* 1987;11:242–4.

87. Sze G. Gadolinium-DTPA in spinal disease. *Radiol Clin North Am* 1988;26:1009–24.

88. Kramer E, Rafto S, Packer R, et al. Comparison of myelography with CT follow-up versus gadolinium MRI for subarachnoid metastatic disease in children. *Neurology* 1991;41:46–50.

89. Lim V, Sobel D, Zyroff J. Spinal cord pial metastases: MR imaging with gadopentetate dimeglumine. *AJNR Am J Neuroradiol* 1990;11:975–82.

90. Schukneckt B, Huber P, Buller B, et al. Spinal leptomeningeal neoplastic disease. Evaluation by MR, myelography and CT myelography. *Eur Neurol* 1992;32:11–6.

91. Wilhelm C, Ellner JJ. Chronic meningitis. *Neurol Clin* 1986;4:115–41.

92. Blaney S, Balis F, Poplack D. Pharmacological approaches to the treatment of meningeal malignancy. *Oncology* 1991;5:107–16.

93. Halperin E. Concerning the inferior portion of the spinal radiotherapy field for malignancies that disseminate via the cerebrospinal fluid. *Int J Radiat Oncol Biol Phys* 1992;26:357–62.

94. Balis FM, Savitch J, Reaman G, et al. Remission induction of meningeal leukemia with high-dose intravenous methotrexate. *J Clin Oncol* 1985;3:485–9.

95. Frick J, Ritch PS, Hansen RM, et al. Successful treatment of meningeal leukemia using systemic high-dose cytosine arabinoside. *J Clin Oncol* 1984;2:365–8.

96. Chamberlain M. A review of leptomeningeal metastases in pediatrics. *J Child Neurol* 1995;10: 191–9.

97. Fizazi K, Asselain B, Vincent-Salomon A, et al. Meningeal carcinomatosis in patients with breast carcinoma. Clinical features, prognostic factors, and results of a high-dose intrathecal methotrexate regimen. *Cancer* 1996;77:1315–23.

98. Myklebust A, Godal A, Fostad O. Targeted therapy with immunotoxins in a nude rat model for leptomeningeal growth of human small cell lung cancer. *Cancer Res* 1994;54:2146–50.

99. Walbridge S, Rybak S. Immunotoxin therapy of leptomeningeal neoplasia. *J Neurooncol* 1994; 20:59–65.

100. Zalutsky M, McLendon R, Garg P, et al. Radioimmunotherapy of neoplastic meningitis in rats using an alpha-particle-emitting immunoconjugate. *Cancer Res* 1994;54:4719–25.

101. Moseley R, Davies A, Richardson R, et al. Intrathecal administration of ^{131}I radiolabelled monoclonal antibody as a treatment for neoplastic meningitis. *BR J Cancer* 1990;62: 637–42.

102. Samlowski W, Park K, Galinsky R, et al. Intrathecal administration of interleukin-2 for meningeal carcinomatosis due to malignant melanoma: sequential evaluation of intracranial pressure, cerebrospinal fluid cytology and cytokine analysis. *J Immunother* 1993;13:49–54.

103. Shapiro WR, Young DF, Mehta BM. Methotrexate: distribution in cerebrospinal fluid after intravenous, ventricular and lumbar injections. *N Engl J Med* 1975;293:161–6.

104. Larson S, Schall G, DiChiro G. The influence of previous lumbar puncture and pneumoencephalography on the incidence of unsuccessful radioisotope cisternography. *J Nucl Med* 1971; 12:555–7.

105. Bleyer WA, Poplack DG. Intraventicular versus intralumbar methotrexate for central nervous system leukemia. *Med Pediatr Oncol* 1979;6: 207–13.

106. Bleyer WA, Poplack DG, Simon RM. "Concentration × Time" methotrexate via a subcutaneous reservoir: a less toxic regimen for intraventricular chemotherapy of central nervous system neoplasms. *Blood* 1978;51:835–42.

107. Shapiro WR, Posner JB, Ushio Y, et al. Treatment of meningeal neoplasms. *Cancer Treat Rep* 1977;61:733–43.

108. Obbens E, Leavens M, Beal J, et al. Ommaya reservoirs in 387 cancer patients: a 15 year experience. *Neurology* 1985;35:1274–8.

109. OngerboerdeVisser B, Somers R, Nooyen W, et al. Intraventricular methotrexate therapy of leptomeningeal metastases from breast cancer. *Neurology* 1983;33:1565–72.

110. Grossman D, Finkelstein D, Ruckdeschel J, et al. Randomized prospective comparison of intraventricular methotrexate and thiotepa in patients with previously untreated neoplastic meningitis. ECOG. *J Clin Oncol* 1993;11:561–9.

111. Boogerd W, Hart A, vanderSande J, et al. Meningeal carcinomatosis in breast cancer. Prognostic factors and influence of treatment. *Cancer* 1991;67:1685–95.

112. Grant R, Naylor B, Greenberg H, et al. Clinical outcome in aggressively treated meningeal carcinomatosis. *Arch Neurol* 1994;51:457–63

Chapter 8

NONCOMPRESSIVE MYELOPATHIES

Intrinsic or medullary diseases cause several disorders of the spinal cord that disrupt its structure and function. A broad range of pathological processes are affected by these diseases (Table 8–1):

1. Noninfectious diseases such as transverse myelitis, which occur following infection or vaccination or which may be idiopathic, and the demyelinating disease multiple sclerosis
2. Infectious diseases
3. Toxic diseases, such as those caused by irradiation
4. Metabolic disorders and vitamin deficiencies, such as the combined degeneration caused by vitamin B_{12}
5. Vascular diseases, including ischemia, hemorrhage, and vascular malformations
6. Neoplastic diseases

Most of these diseases clinically present with an acute or subacute myelopathy. Since biopsy of the cord is rarely performed and most of the diseases are inflammatory in nature, diagnosis and management rely mostly on the patient's history, examination, imaging findings, and exclusion of infectious diseases. Furthermore, since there is evidence that patients with acute noninfectious myelitis appear to respond to high-dose corticosteroids when given early in the course of the disease, it is

Table 8–1. **Noncompressive Causes of Myelitis and Myelopathy***

Postinfectious or Parainfectious Myelitis	*Toxic Myelopathy*
Postvaccinal	Ortho-cresyl phosphate
"Influenzal" and subsequent to viral infection	Following aortography
Spontaneous acute myelitis (acute dissemi-nated encephalomyelitis of unknown cause)	Arsenic
	Lathyrism
	Organic iodide contrast media
Demyelinating Myelitis of Unknown Etiology	Penicillin
Multiple sclerosis	Spinal anesthetics and arachnoiditis
Neuromyelitis optica	
Acute necrotizing myelitis	*Myelopathy Owing to Physical Agents*
	Irradiation
Primary Infectious Myelitis	Electrical injury to the central nervous system
Viral Myelitides	*Metabolic and Nutritional Myelopathy*
Poliomyelitis	Diabetes mellitus
Postpoliomyelitis syndrome	Cyanocobalamin deficiency
Myelitis with acute viral encephalomyelitis	Pellagra
Herpes zoster	Complex deficiencies without single identified nutrient
Rabies	
Subacute myoclonic spinal neuronitis	Myelopathy of chronic liver disease
HTLV-1[†]	
AIDS myelopathy	*Myelopathy Owing to Diseases of the Blood Vessels*
Bacterial and Spirochetal Myelitides	Arteriosclerosis
Acute suppurative myelitis with spinal abscess	Dissecting aortic aneurysm
Tuberculoma of spinal cord	Coarctation of the aorta
Syphilitic myelitis	Periarteritis nodosa
Lyme disease	Systemic lupus erythematosus
Rickettsial, fungous, and parasitic myelitides	Sjogren's syndrome
Typhus and spotted fever	Vascular malformations of the spinal cord
Actinomycosis, coccidioidomycosis, aspergillosis, torulosis	
Trichinosis, falciparum malaria, schistosomiasis	*Paraneoplastic myelopathy*
Myelopathy Secondary to Acute Intraspinal Infection	
Acute bacterial meningitis	
Tuberculous meningitis	

*Adapted from Plum, F and Olson, ME.[78]
[†]Human T-cell leukemia/lymphoma virus.

important to expeditiously evaluate and manage these patients.[1,2]

In the pre-MRI era, most patients presenting with a myelopathy that evolved over hours to days or weeks, and whose myelogram revealed no cord compression were diagnosed with acute or subacute transverse myelopathy. As defined by Ropper and Poskanzer in their classic paper, "transverse myelopathy is an acute intramedullary dysfunction of the spinal cord, either ascending or static, involving both halves of the cord, often over considerable length, and appearing without history of previous neurological disease."[3] These authors acknowledged that the term transverse myelopathy included several different neuropathological processes. Now MRI permits a more rapid diagnosis. In some cases it has permitted a refined approach to the differential diagnosis of patients with transverse myelopathy. The AIDS epidemic has also broadened the differential diagnosis to include several infectious disorders, such as HIV-1, cytomegalovirus, herpes zoster, toxoplasmosis, and other infections prevalent in the immunocompromised host. Accordingly, the diagnosis and management of transverse myelopathy has become more complex, especially in the immunocompomised patient. It is thus important to determine the HIV status of patients with transverse myelopathy.

In this chapter, we will review the common disorders that present as transverse myelopathy. The spectrum of diseases in immunocompromised hosts is rapidly evolving, and this text is not intended to cover the entire spectrum. Other sources should be consulted when evaluating patients with infectious diseases.

POSTINFECTIOUS, POSTVACCINATION, AND IDIOPATHIC MYELITIS

Acute and subacute transverse myelitides presumed to be secondary to an underlying autoimmune condition have been recognized for decades. They present a vexing clinical problem. These patients typically present with a rapidly evolving myelopathy and no specific etiology. Diagnosis is made on the basis of the clinical presentation, MRI findings, CSF analysis, and exclusion of etiologies requiring specific therapy, such as infections. Since some patients respond to corticosteroids, rapid evaluation is necessary.

In this section, we first consider the monophasic disease acute transverse myelitis, which may be postinfectious, postvaccination, or idiopathic; later, we will discuss multiple sclerosis and acute and subacute necrotizing myelitis. Collectively, these diseases of unknown etiology are the most common causes of acute transverse myelitis.[4] Although each may have a different antecedent, these diseases share a similar pathology and are thought to have an inflammatory pathogenesis. Unlike the viral myelitides, which show a predilection for the gray matter, this group of diseases usually involves white matter tracts, or both white and gray mat-

ter (thus earning the term transverse myelopathy).[4,5]

Acute Transverse Myelitis

Although the antecedent conditions are separable, postinfectious (sometimes termed parainfectious) myelitis shares a very similar clinical course and pathology with postvaccination myelitis.[6,7] Some of the exanthematous infections and vaccinations that are antecedent to myelitis are shown in Table 8–2. Although the most common antecedent infections are viral illnesses, bacterial mycoplasma[8] and other infections may also trigger myelitis.[6,9] In many cases, a myelopathy clinically and pathologically indistinguishable from postinfectious myelitis occurs without an apparent infection or vaccination.[4]

PATHOGENESIS

It is now recognized that postinfectious and postvaccination myelitis are not due to viral invasion of the central nervous system. On the contrary, immunological mechanisms play an important role in their pathogenesis.[10,11] Although the precise mechanisms of CNS injury are unknown, the histopathological similarity between postinfectious and postvaccination myelitis and experimental allergic en-

Table 8–2. **Some Antecedents of Parainfectious Myelitis**

Viral Disease
Rubeola (measles)
Rubella (German measles)
Mumps
Influenza
Mycoplasma pneumonia
Infectious mononucleosis
Varicella

Vaccinations
Tetanus
Poliomyelitis
Rabies
Smallpox

cephalomyelitis has suggested to many investigators that an autoimmune response to a CNS antigen such as myelin basic protein may be responsible.[12] Alternatively, it has been suggested that circulating immune complexes may play a role in the pathogenesis of these disorders by inducing a vascular injury.[13] The time interval between exposure to an infection or vaccination and development of the neurological disorder varies but is commonly seven to ten days.

PATHOLOGY

The clinical manifestations of postinfectious and postvaccination myelitis may include symptoms, signs, and/or MRI evidence of brain involvement. However, in occasional cases the spinal cord is the predominant (or only) site of involvement.

As noted above, the pathological findings of postinfectious and postvaccination myelitis are the same.[14] On gross examination, the spinal cord may be normal or swollen. On histopathological inspection of the gray and white matter, the most prominent findings are found in the blood vessels and the perivascular regions.[15] Hyperemia, perivascular cellular exudate and edema, and hemorrhage usually are found around arterioles, venules, and capillaries.[6] The perivenous areas infiltrated by inflammatory cells typically show regions of demyelination that may coalesce with other areas, so the perivascular localization is not apparent. In regions of severe inflammation, necrosis may be seen.[11,15]

CLINICAL FEATURES

The clinical features of acute transverse myelitis are highly variable. An antecedent history of viral illness or vaccination may be elicited in a third to a half of all patients. Systemic symptoms, which may appear first, include fever, malaise, nausea, vomiting, and muscular aching, suggesting an infectious etiology. When the spinal cord is the major clinical site of neurological involvement, paresthesias may be reported in the lower extremities. Although back pain and/or radicular pain may her-

ald the illness, the myelopathy can also develop without pain.

Any level of the spinal cord may be involved, but the thoracic region is the most frequent. Myelopathy may be accompanied or occasionally preceded by a polyradiculopathy and/or cerebral manifestations, in which case it may be designated encephalomyeloradiculitis rather than acute transverse myelitis. Symptoms and signs of cord involvement usually evolve acutely; the majority of patients develop maximal neurological deficit within several days to several weeks. Those with abrupt onset appear to have a worse prognosis.[3] Specific signs (weakness, sensory loss, and sphincter dysfunction) depend on the tracts involved and on whether the involvement is transverse, ascending, or multifocal.

Routine laboratory studies are usually normal or nonspecific. The CSF may be normal, but it typically shows a moderate lymphocytic pleocytosis. Other signs of CNS inflammation may include a slightly elevated protein (usually less than 120 mg/dl) level, elevated IgG, and the presence of oligoclonal bands. If polyradiculitis is part of the clinical presentation, or if there is a subarachnoid block secondary to cord swelling, then the protein may be further elevated. CSF glucose concentration is typically normal.[3]

The advent of MRI has revolutionized diagnostic imaging ability where transverse myelopathy is concerned, and it may shed light on the pathogenesis in some cases. Choi and colleagues[16] evaluated MR characteristics of 17 patients with idiopathic transverse myelitis. Common MR abnormalities included a central hyperintensity occupying more than two-thirds of the cross-sectional area of the cord in 88% of cases; a rostrocaudal length of three to four vertebral bodies (53%); cord expansion (47%); focal peripheral cord enhancement (53%); and a slow regression of T_2 hyperintensity with an enhancing nodule. Tartaglino and others[17] studied MR findings in 19 patients with idiopathic acute transverse myelitis (53% had experienced recent upper respiratory infections or vaccination). On T_2-weighted axial images, 13 of 18 lesions showed holocord signal abnormalities, 39% had gray matter abnormalities, as often seen in ischemic lesions of the cord, and 16% had isolated white matter lesions. Enhancement patterns were variable, and in 17% of cases enhancement of the cauda equina occurred in a pattern similar to that of Guillain-Barré syndrome. These authors concluded that a small-vessel vasculopathy may be the basis for some cases of transverse myelitis.

In patients with lupus, Provenzale et al.[18] reported MR findings in four patients with eight episodes of transverse myelitis. There was prolongation of T_1 or T_2 signal (or both) in all eight episodes. Spinal cord enlargement was seen in six episodes (75%), and spinal cord enhancement was seen in three of six episodes. During periods of remission, the spinal cord diameter returned to normal and enhancement resolved, although abnormal cord signal could also persist. Improvement in MR findings correlated with clinical improvement.

THERAPY

Although there are no randomized controlled trials that show corticosteroids are effective in treating transverse myelitis, the suspected autoimmune basis for this disorder has led to the use of these drugs.[18a,b] Retrospective studies showing their benefit have begun to emerge. In a series of five children with acute transverse myelopathy, Sebire and colleagues[1] treated them with high-dose intravenous methylprednisolone and compared their outcomes with historical controls. These authors found that the median time to walking independently was significantly reduced (23 versus 97 days), and the proportion with full recovery within 12 months was dramatically higher (80% versus 10%). No significant adverse effects from the corticosteroids were reported.

Harisdangkul and colleagues[2] reported the outcome of seven patients with transverse myelopathy associated with systemic lupus erythematosus (four of whom had no prior history of lupus). Only two patients, who received high-dose IV pulse steroid within one week of onset of transverse myelopathy, had a good outcome. These authors concluded that early diagnosis and early treatment with high-dose steroids reduced mortality and improved functional outcome.

Urinary retention may require intermittent catheterization or an indwelling catheter, and careful attention is needed to prevent development of a urinary tract infection. If bladder dysfunction persists, urodynamic studies usually are undertaken to determine the specific mechanism of impairment. Constipation is also a common problem and may be due to ileus. When ileus has resolved and oral feedings have resumed, a stool softener or enemas may be needed. Attention also must be given to preventing skin breakdown, as in other patients with spinal cord injury.

Patients with acute transverse myelitis present two questions: (*1*) What is the immediate prognosis for recovery of spinal cord function? and (*2*) What is the risk of developing multiple sclerosis? Patients with abrupt onset tend to have a worse prognosis that those whose myelopathy develops over several days or weeks. Furthermore, Scott and colleagues,[19,19a] report that spinal cord swelling present on MRI scanning predicts a poor outcome, whereas normal spine and brain MRI indicate a good prognosis. In the study by Scott et al[19a] there were 20 patients with transverse myelitis. Of 11 with normal MRI scans of the cord, all 11 had a complete or near-complete neurologic recovery. Of nine patients with abnormal MRI scans of the spinal cord, seven had minimal or no neurologic recovery. In regard to the risk of later development of multiple sclerosis, several studies have shown risks ranging from 3% to 72%.[3,20–22] It appears that in patients with symmetric transverse myelopathy risk for multiple sclerosis is low. In patients with incomplete spinal cord syndromes, the risk appears to be much higher.[19a,22a] In a study by Scott et al.[19a] 20 patients with transverse myelitis (TM) were compared to 16 patients presenting with acute myelopathic multiple sclerosis (MMS). Motor dysfunction was the presenting manifestation in all 20 TM patients and in 15 of the 16 MMS patients. The MMS patients had asymmetric motor or sensory findings in 15 of 16 cases, whereas among the TM patients 19 of 20 patients had symmetric motor and sensory findings. These authors concluded that TM can be distinguished from MMS on the basis of symmetry of motor and sensory findings in TM, and on the basis of asymmetry of motor and sensory findings in MMS. In an average follow-up of 4.5 years, none of the TM patients developed MS. In the extensive experience of Paty et al.[23] only 0.7% of their 3500 patients with multiple sclerosis presented with acute complete transverse myelitis. Relapse of transverse myelitis has been reported to occur at the same level.[23a]

MULTIPLE SCLEROSIS

The clinical manifestations of multiple sclerosis are protean. Although the history, findings on neurological examination, or laboratory studies (MRI or evoked responses) often demonstrate a multifocal distribution of lesions, the spinal cord is a common site of initial clinical involvement. In one series,[24] for example, limb sensory symptoms (30.7%) were the most common presenting complaint (Table 8–3). Other spinal symptoms, such as Lhermitte's sign, gait difficulties, extremity weakness, and sphincter disturbances, also were very common, so the spinal cord was considered the site of initial involvement in over one-half of patients presenting with multiple sclerosis.[25]

Pathology

In a classic study, Lumsden[26] drew attention to the presence of demyelinated plaques (on postmortem examination) in the spinal cords of most multiple sclerosis patients. Lumsden also commented on the relative symmetry of demyelination in cases of multiple sclerosis, with similar lesions on both sides of the midline in many cases (Fig. 8–1).

Fog[27] noted that fan-shaped plaques in the lateral columns are especially common, suggesting that demyelination is

Table 8–3. Initial Symptoms in 1721 Patients With Clinically Defined Multiple Sclerosis From the University of British Columbia Multiple Sclerosis Clinic*

Sensory in limbs	30.7%
Visual loss	15.9%
Motor, slowly developing	8.9%
Diplopia	6.8%
Gait disturbance	4.8%
Motor, acute onset	4.3%
Sensory in face	2.8%
Balance problem	2.9%
Vertigo	1.7%
Lhermitte's symptom	1.8%
Bladder symptom	1%
Acute transverse myelopathy	0.7%
Limb ataxia	1%
Pain	0.5%
Other	2.5%
Polysymptomatic onset	13.7%

*From Paty, DW and Ebers, GC,[24] p. 56, with permission.

most likely to occur in the vicinity of veins within the spinal cord. More recently, Oppenheimer[28] observed that plaques in the cervical cord are about twice as common as those at lower levels. On the basis of the distribution of lesions in the transverse plane, he suggested that mechanical stresses, transmitted to the cord via the denticulate ligaments, might play a role in determining the site of multiple sclerotic lesions in the spinal cord. This suggestion remains controversial. It is now clear that in addition to demyelination at least some degree of axonal degeneration occurs in multiple sclerosis.[29–31]

Clinical and Laboratory Features

Clinical features of the spinal form of multiple sclerosis (cases characterized by solely spinal symptomatology) have been described. A study[32] found that 109 out of a pool of 1271 multiple sclerosis patients had cases of spinal MS (9%). This figure is somewhat lower than the 25% reported by

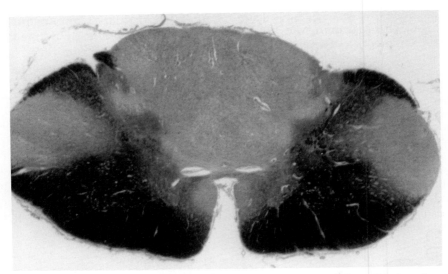

Figure 8–1. Multiple sclerosis involving the spinal cord. Note the nearly total demyelination of posterior and lateral columns. (Courtesy of Dr. Lysia Forno.)

others,[33] whose patients were characterized by current symptoms only, not excluding patients with a history of extraspinal symptoms. There was a slight preponderance of females among the 109 cases.[32] Both studies note a higher age at onset of spinal MS compared with other forms and a higher percentage of cases with a progressive course.[32,33] Signs and symptoms of pyramidal tract and posterior column dysfunction are especially prominent, although sensory ataxia, impairment of sensibility for light touch and temperature, and sphincter/sexual impairment also occur. Many patients with spinal forms of multiple sclerosis harbor subclinical demyelinated plaques in other regions of the CNS. Why these lesions remain asymptomatic remains conjectural.[34]

How frequently will multiple sclerosis develop in patients who present with isolated spinal cord syndromes? Some authors have suggested that in patients without evidence of cord compression, clinically definite multiple sclerosis will develop in a higher proportion of patients with chronic progressive myelopathies than in patients with acute myelopathies. In an autopsy series,[35] multiple sclerosis was found in 34% of patients with undiagnosed, chronic progressive myelopathies. Other researchers[36] have observed oligo-

clonal bands and/or abnormal visual evoked potentials in 44% of patients with chronic progressive myelopathy.

Hume and Waxman[37] examined visual somatosensory, and brain-stem auditory evoked potentials in 222 patients referred to Yale–New Haven Hospital for suspected multiple sclerosis. Thirty-two had a history and signs of isolated spinal cord disease. Of these, four developed clinically definite multiple sclerosis (McAlpine criteria) on 2 1/2-year follow-up; all four of these patients had positive visual or brain-stem-evoked potentials, demonstrating slowed conduction outside the spinal cord at the time of presentation. Three of the other 28 recovered and showed no further symptoms; none of the other patients had positive evoked potentials. Notably, three of these other patients referred for suspected multiple sclerosis harbored structural lesions causing cord compression (cervical disc disease, cervical cord tumor, foramen magnum meningioma); in each of these cases, the visual and brain-stem-evoked potentials were normal. These patients illustrate the danger in making a premature diagnosis of spinal multiple sclerosis.[37]

A study of patients with acute myelopathies[38] found abnormal visual evoked responses in only 10%. A follow-up study[3] on patients presenting with acute myelitis and subacute transverse myelopathy found multiple sclerosis in only about 10% of cases; a subsequent study[39] observed normal visual, brain-stem auditory, and median somatosensory-evoked potentials in 12 patients with complete, acute transverse myelitis, which suggests that acute transverse myelitis usually is a monophasic illness distinct from multiple sclerosis.

In a series of 121 patients with isolated noncompressive spinal cord syndromes,[40] brain and spinal MRI showed lesions in the appropriate spinal cord region in 64% of patients with a cervical syndrome and 28% of patients with a thoracic or lumbar syndrome. In patients with chronic progressive spinal cord syndromes, MRI revealed cerebral lesions in 72%; most lesions were similar to those characteristic of multiple sclerosis. An MRI revealed lesions in the white matter of the cerebral hemispheres in 79% of patients with chronic relapsing spinal cord syndromes. In patients with acute spinal cord syndromes (defined as a single clinical episode, fully developed within 14 days of onset), MRI of the brain was abnormal in 56%, often showing lesions indistinguishable from those seen in multiple sclerosis. The authors point out that the finding of multiple lesions at presentation cannot be used to make a diagnosis of clinically definite multiple sclerosis because the criteria of time and number are not met; either serial MRI scanning showing dissemination of lesions or a second clinical bout is required.[41,42] Other investigators also have found cranial MRI helpful in the evaluation of patients with myelopathy of undetermined etiology when demyelinating disease is the cause.[43]

Unexpected spinal cord compression occasionally is seen in patients with remitting and/or mild symptoms of spinal cord dysfunction. As noted above, three patients with spinal cord compression were among 32 patients referred to a teaching hospital because of suspected spinal multiple sclerosis. In a series[40] of 130 patients referred to a neurological hospital for evaluation of a spinal cord syndrome in which a compressive cause was considered

unlikely, nine (two of whom had negative myelograms, 1 and 3 months earlier) had compressive lesions demonstrated by MRI. Several of these patients had a remitting spastic paraparesis that had been previously diagnosed as multiple sclerosis. None of these patients had symptoms or signs referable to levels of the neuraxis above the foramen magnum. This demonstration of unexpected compressive lesions in patients with remitting myelopathies emphasizes the importance of carefully considering cord compression in patients with undiagnosed spinal cord syndromes and of rethinking the diagnosis if there is progression of signs.

Although the clinical presentation of spinal multiple sclerosis may resemble postinfectious myelitis, the evolution of myelopathy in multiple sclerosis frequently occurs over a few weeks rather than hours or days. The CSF sometimes shows signs of inflammation with pleocytosis, and elevations of protein (usually to levels less than 100 mg per deciliter). The IgG is also usually elevated, and oligoclonal bands are often present. Imaging of the spine by MRI may demonstrate evidence of demyelination (Fig. 8–2).

Pain syndromes and paroxysmal symptoms and signs are common manifestations of myelopathy in patients with multiple sclerosis. Paroxysmal symptoms are brief episodes of neurologic dysfunction which may take the form of tingling, numbness, weakness, painful tonic spasms of muscle, tonic seizures, or pain. They usually have an abrupt onset and spontaneously remit, and they may occur several times per day. The pathogenesis is not known, but it has been attributed to ephaptic transmission at sites of demyelination.[44] These paroxysmal events may (1) occur spontaneously at a site of previous demyelination, (2) herald a new demyelinating event, or (3) be induced by an intercurrent illness such as urinary tract infection or fever at a site of prevous demyelination (pseudorelapse). Paroxysmal symptoms in patients with multiple sclerosis commonly respond to anticonvulsants such as carbamazepine or phenytoin.

Neurogenic pain is a common finding in patients with multiple sclerosis. The pain

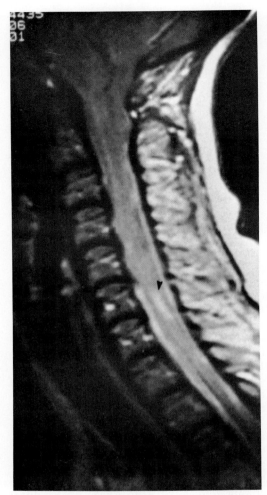

Figure 8–2. An MRI of spinal cord in a patient with multiple sclerosis. Note the demyelinating plaque (white) in the lower cervical spine. (From Sze, G,[239] with permission.)

is wise to consider other causes such as neural compression or herniated discs. Treatment of these neuropathic pain syndromes can be challenging, but use of anticonvulsants or tricyclics has been helpful in some patients.

Therapy

Although multiple sclerosis remains incurable, therapies that can significantly alter the disease course in the relapsing form of multiple sclerosis have become available over the past several years. With the introduction of interferon beta-1b, interferon beta-1a, and glatiramer acetate the clinical deterioration and MRI progression of the disease may be slowed.

Interferon beta-1b has been shown to reduce the incidence of relapse by 34%, increase the percent of relapse-free patients, decrease the number of days of hospitalization in the treated group, and showed a trend in favor of delayed progression in the treated population.[49,50] Interferon beta-1b's effect on disease activity was remarkable as exhibited by MRI. A 90% decrease in disease activity was measured by detecting new lesions and expanding old lesions with T_2-weighted cranial MRIs.[51] Another study using interferon beta-1a was reported in 1995.[52] In addition to a significant effect on the relapse rate, this study demonstrated a statistically significant slowing in the progression of disease as measured by the expanded disability status scale (EDSS). Although a different MRI analysis strategy was pursued in this study, again a substantial effect on brain MRI disease activity was seen.[52,53]

Significant flu-like symptoms (fever, myalgia, and fatigue) may accompany initial treatment with these agents. Clinical experience has shown that tolerability of these agents in the first three months can be substantially enhanced by starting at a fraction of the usual dose and slowly escalating the dose over six to eight weeks. In addition, the generous use of antipyretics, such as acetaminophen or ibuprofen, has also been found to significantly increase the tolerability of interferon beta thera-

may be paroxysmal as described above or it may be chronic and persistent. In studies of patients with multiple sclerosis, pain has been reported to occur in approximately one-third to two-thirds of cases.[45,46] In a study of pain syndromes in multiple sclerosis patients, Moulin and colleagues[47] reported painful tonic spasms in 15% of cases and persistent extremity pain in 29%. In a similar study by Vermote et al.[48] paroxysmal tonic spasms were seen in 10%, radicular pain in 4%, and persistent extremity pain in 14%. When evaluating a patient with multiple sclerosis and pain, it pies. Treatment with interferon beta-1b is occasionally complicated by local skin reactions, including rare skin necrosis.[49–51]

Recently the FDA approved the use of glatiramer acetate, previously known as copolymer-1, for treatment of multiple sclerosis.[54] This is a synthetic polypeptide made up of four amino acids originally synthesized as an analogue of myelin basic protein. It has been shown to suppress the development of experimental allergic encephalomyelitis (EAE) in rodent and primate species regardless of whether the disease was induced by myelin basic protein (MBP), proteolipid protein (PLP), myelin-oligodendrocyte associated glycoprotein (MOG), or spinal cord homogenate. A small study performed by Bornstein et al. revealed a 75% decrease in relapse rate in patients with relapsing-remitting multiple sclerosis as a result of treatment with glatiramer acetate.[55] A subsequent small study on progressive forms of MS showed a trend in favor of treatment, but it was statistically insignificant.[56] More recently, a multicenter clinical trial has shown a significant effect of glatiramer acetate on relapse rate (29%) and on disease progression as measured by the EDSS.[57] This latter effect is comparable to that seen in the interferon beta-1a studies, and it is particularly notable in the three year extension study.[57] An adequately powered MRI study of the effects glatiramer acetate in MS patients has yet to be reported.

Skin reactions, particularly acute hypersensitivity and delayed-type hypersensitivity reactions, are common with this medication but are rarely of clinical significance. In the clinical study, 15% of treated patients reported at least one of a constellation of symptoms often referred to as postinjection reaction. Symptoms include chest tightness, shortness of breath, palpitations, lightheadedness, and erythroderma immediately after injection of the medication. The symptoms usually last 2 to 15 minutes and have not been associated with significant medical complications to date. The mechanism responsible for this reaction is not well understood, but it may be due to accidental intravascular injection of the medication, leading to the sudden degranulation of mast cells and basophils. This is only speculation.[54,57]

Acute relapses of multiple sclerosis respond to high-dose intravenous methylprednisolone treatment. More recent studies have suggested that similar doses of oral methylprednisolone are as effective as the intravenous formulations.[58]

Intravenous gamma globulin has been reported to effectively decrease the number of relapses and possibly alter the short-term course of a relapse in patients with multiple sclerosis.[59–61] Relatively low doses (200mg/kg) were used. The continually sparse supply of this agent has limited its usefulness in the management of multiple sclerosis.

Devic's Disease (Neuromyelitis Optica)

Devic's disease (neuromyelitis optica) has been considered by different authors to be a variant of multiple sclerosis, a form of acute disseminated encephalomyelitis, or a distinct disorder. It is characterized by involvement of the spinal cord (usually, although not invariably, in the thoracic region) and the optic nerve(s) or chiasm.[62,63] Devic's disease is characterized pathologically by a greater degree of axonal degeneration than is usual in multiple sclerosis. The spinal cord can present a frankly necrotic picture, in some cases leading to cavitation, which is also atypical for MS.

Spinal cord and optic nerve/chiasm involvement occur almost simultaneously. While optic neuritis and spinal cord involvement can occur together in cases of multiple sclerosis, Devic's disease presents a distinct constellation characterized by presentation at the extremes of age (before 10 and after 50 years of age). The CSF is characterized by a pleocytosis, which is often associated with an increase of protein of up to 200 mg per deciliter.

Clinical presentation reflects the sites of pathology. Thus, unilateral or bilateral visual impairment is followed within days or weeks by a transverse or ascending myelitis. Visual impairment often progresses rapidly, over the course of several hours. Paraparesis or paraplegia, together with a sensory level, develop with a similar rapid time course. In some cases, temporary remissions are followed by worsening. As would be expected from the necrotizing character of the lesions, remission is less likely than in typical cases of multiple sclerosis. Nevertheless, in several cases there have been claims of nearly total recovery.

ACUTE NECROTIZING MYELITIS

This rare disorder clinically presents as an acute or subacute transverse myelopathy.[3,64] Thus motor, sensory, and sphincter paralysis evolve over a matter of hours or days. Occasionally, the optic nerves may be involved.[5] Sensory disturbances tend to be more prominent early symptoms than are motor complaints.[15] Motor weakness rapidly evolves into an areflexic, flaccid paralysis. Some patients report a prior infectious illness, usually an upper respiratory infection.[15]

Acute necrotizing myelitis is distinguished from the other forms of myelitis above by its distinctive pathological findings.[15] The CSF demonstrates evidence of inflammation. Pathological characteristics include perivenous demyelination and diffuse necrosis of all spinal cord elements.[15] The appearance of the acute lesion of necrotizing hemorrhagic myelitis resembles necrotizing hemorrhagic leukoencephalitis.[5] The rostrocaudal extent of the lesions may involve several segments. Acutely, the spinal cord may be swollen, but eventually atrophy supervenes. Potentially, these gross pathological findings may be seen with imaging studies such as MRI.

VIRAL MYELITIS

Most viruses that invade the spinal cord demonstrate a predilection for gray matter with relative sparing of white matter. Viral myelitis may be distinguished by the location of spinal cord damage. For example, anterior horn cell damage is due to the poliomyelitis virus,[65] and posterior horn cell disease occurs as a result of infection by herpes zoster.

With the notable exceptions of human T-cell leukemia/lymphoma virus (HTLV)-1 myelopathy and AIDS myelopathy, the white matter tracts are characteristically spared in comparison with the major clinical and pathological involvement of the gray matter. This observation is important in distinguishing viral myelitis from other causes of myelopathy. For example, in cases of neoplastic or nonneoplastic spinal cord compression, white matter dysfunction is often a predominant finding. Furthermore, in cases of inflammation of the spinal cord where white matter tracts bear the brunt of involvement, one should initially consider causes other than viral myelitides (such as parainfectious and postvaccination myelitides, multiple sclerosis, and paraneoplastic myelopathy). In addition, involvement of multiple roots, as may occur with sacral radiculitis due to herpes simplex type 2, may be difficult to differentiate from myelopathy or conus medullaris involvement. The major clinical features of viral myelitis that are important in the differential diagnosis of spinal cord compression are discussed below.

Acute Anterior Poliomyelitis

Acute anterior poliomyelitis is a febrile illness associated with flaccid motor weakness or paralysis and signs of meningeal inflammation.[66] Before there was polio vaccine, epidemic paralytic poliomyelitis was caused by one of three antigenic types of poliovirus. (In areas where there has not been widespread vaccination or where it has lapsed, epidemic polio is, of course, still a major threat.) Even where the vaccination program has been successful, sporadic cases still occur.[67–70] For example, in the United States between 1969 and 1982, 208 cases of paralytic poliomyelitis were reported.[66,68,71] Although rare, the poliomyelitis virus has not been eradicated, and one can expect occasionally to encounter the clinical syndrome of acute anterior poliomyelitis. Similar clinical syndromes, usually milder, may be caused by other enteroviruses, echoviruses, and Coxsackie virus groups A and B.[72-77] Only the most common spinal manifestations of paralytic poliomyelitis will be reviewed here. For a more complete account, the reader is referred elsewhere.[67-71,78]

CLINICAL AND LABORATORY FEATURES

Most individuals with poliovirus infection have no symptoms or mild gastrointestinal or flu-like symptoms during the viremic phase of the disease. If an effective immune response is not mounted, aseptic meningitis and/or paralytic poliomyelitis may occur. The early spinal manifestations of the disease are characterized by fever, tenderness and spasm of the muscles, headache, neck and back pain, and other signs of meningeal irritation. Diffuse fasciculations of muscles may be present. Motor paralysis may occur abruptly, evolving over hours to tetraplegia, or may show a more indolent course over several days. The pattern of weakness is usually asymmetric and may, of course, involve bulbar muscles as well as those innervated by spinal motor neurons. Although hyperreflexia initially may be present, areflexia usually develops as flaccid paralysis ensues. Sensory loss is rarely found, although sensory complaints in the form of dysesthesias and paresthesias may be present. Transient urinary retention is seen in 50% of adults.[66] Transient papilledema lasting two to ten weeks is seen in 5% of seriously paralyzed cases.[78]

Although initially the CSF may be normal in 10% of cases, it typically shows signs of inflammation: pleocytosis, elevated protein, normal sugar levels, and normal pressure. The CSF white cell counts may exceed 2500; initially, the spinal fluid mostly contains polymorphonuclear cells, but later it evolves to contain primarily lymphocytes. The spinal fluid protein does not usually rise above 150 mg per deciliter. However, in cases associated with papilledema, the protein may be much higher and persist for several months.[78]

DIFFERENTIAL DIAGNOSIS

The syndrome of acute poliomyelitis from poliovirus must be distinguished from a variety of other paralytic diseases. Acute polyneuritis (Guillain-Barré syndrome) usually presents with symmetric areflexic weakness and no meningeal signs, fever, or signs of systemic illness; sensory changes are often present. Furthermore, the CSF in Guillain-Barré syndrome exhibits increased protein but rarely shows significant pleocytosis.

Epidemic neuromyasthenia (Iceland disease, benign myalgic encephalomyelitis) is an obscure illness with a clinical syndrome similar to that of poliomyelitis. It usually occurs in outbreaks in residential communities or in hospitals during the summer months.[66] It is characterized by fever, headache, and aching muscles. Muscle paresis develops in 10% to 80% of cases but, unlike the weakness seen in poliomyelitis, there is no muscle atrophy, and preserved reflexes or hyperreflexia rather than hyporeflexia is the rule.[66] Sensory complaints are often reported. Brainstem signs, emotional instability, and urinary retention also may be found.[66,78] The CSF is usually entirely normal. The causative agent of neuromyasthenia is unknown.[66]

Although usually less severe, the clinical syndrome of anterior poliomyelitis caused by the enteroviruses, echoviruses, and Coxsackie viruses is clinically indistinguishable from that caused by the poliomyelitis virus.[78] In areas where polio vaccination programs have all but eradicated this disease, these enteroviruses are responsible for the majority of cases of paralytic poliomyelitis syndrome.[66] Because the clinical and spinal fluid findings are similar, differentiation must be made on the basis of virus isolation or serological studies. With rare exception (e.g., Coxsackie A7 and some other enteroviruses), most cases of nonpolio enteroviral poliomyelitis do not occur as epidemics.[66,77] A polio-like syndrome also has been reported secondary to mumps virus,[79] infectious mononucleosis,[80] and rabies virus.[81,82]

POSTPOLIOMYELITIS SYNDROME

Many years following an attack of acute paralytic poliomyelitis, a slowly progressive syndrome of muscle weakness that has been termed the postpoliomyelitis syndrome may develop.[83–86] Because it has been estimated that 25% of patients with antecedent paralytic poliomyelitis will develop this late sequela,[87] nearly 60,000 individuals in the United States are at risk to develop this syndrome. The weakness, which is of a lower motor neuron type, is often most prominent in the areas of original paralysis. It is associated with fatigue and pain. The lack of upper motor neuron signs distinguishes this disease from amyotrophic lateral sclerosis.[66]

Recent pathological studies of spinal cords from patients with prior poliomyelitis (mean 20 years prior to autopsy) have been performed.[88] The histopathological findings in those suffering from the postpoliomyelitis syndrome did not differ from those without the syndrome. In both settings, there was evidence of atrophy of motor neurons, severe gliosis, and mild to moderate perivascular and parenchymal inflammation. The pathogenesis of the disorder is uncertain,[66,88] although it is suggested that late denervation of muscles previously reinnervated during the recovery phase from paralytic poliomyelitis is involved in its causation.[89]

Herpes Viruses

Herpes zoster, an acute viral infection involving the dorsal root ganglia, may extend into the spinal cord to cause a posterior horn myelitis at one or several cord segmental levels. In addition, segmental (radicular) weakness at the level(s) of sensory involvement as a result of anterior horn inflammation is a relatively frequent finding.[90,91] More rarely, a zoster-associated myelitis involving ascending and descending white matter tracts may occur.[92] Among 1210 cases of herpes zoster seen at the Mayo Clinic over a nine-year period, only one case of zoster-associated myelitis was reported.[93]

The pathogenesis of zoster-associated myelitis is uncertain.[92] The mechanisms suggested include direct viral invasion of the cord,[94] an associated vasculitis and thrombosis[15,95] or an immunologic parainfectious cause.[96] Recently, de Silva and colleagues[97] reported two immunocompromised patients with zoster myelitis in whom antiviral agents caused clinical improvement, leading these authors to conclude that, at least in immunocompromised patients, myelitis reflects viral invasion of the spinal cord. The development of zoster-associated myelitis may immediately follow cutaneous vesicular eruption or may be delayed by several weeks to months.[92] There have also been reports of cases with zoster radiculitis and no vesicular eruption (zoster sine herpete).[98,99] The neurological abnormalities found on examination depend upon the specific tracts involved. There may be progressive, relentless cord destruction with an ascending myelopathy.[94,95] The CSF generally shows pleocytosis, elevated protein, and a normal glucose level. Virus may sometimes be cultured from the CSF, but this test is not invariably positive.[97] Antibodies to VZV in the CSF may help verify the diagnosis. Recently, amplification of varicella zoster virus DNA in CSF has been reported as a diagnostic tool.[97,100] The MRI findings may be unremarkable or may reveal abnormal root and/or cord intensity with enhancement.[91,97,101]

It is important to note that secondary or symptomatic zoster[15] may develop at a segmental level of underlying spinal disease. Occasionally, patients with neoplastic epidural spinal cord compression may present with herpes zoster at the level of metastasis.[102] Thus, in diagnosing zoster-associated myelopathy, one should consider the possibility that another underlying disease process is responsible for the neurological deficit.

The optimal treatment for zoster-associated myelitis is evolving. Because virus has been isolated from the CSF and spinal cords of some patients, the administration of antiviral agents has been advocated.[97] Both acyclovir and famcyclovir have been associated with neurological improvement.[91,97]

HTLV-1-Associated Myelopathy and Tropical Spastic Paraparesis

Human T-cell lymphotropic virus type I (HTLV-1), a retrovirus, has recently been implicated as the causative agent of a slowly progressive myelopathy characterized by symmetric upper motor neuron paresis, sphincter disturbances, and mild sensory signs.[103] In Japan, this myelopathy was found to be associated with leukemia-like cells in the blood and CSF. It has been identified as HTLV-1-associated myelopathy (HAM).[104–107] In the tropics, a progressive myelopathy with similar clinical features has been recognized for many years. It is called tropical spastic paraparesis (TSP).[107–109]

In 1985, Gessain and colleagues[105] first demonstrated antibodies to HTLV-1 in 10 of 17 Caribbean patients clinically diagnosed with TSP. In Martinique, 78% of patients with TSP are seropositive for HTLV-1 (4% of the general population is seropositive).[107] The link between HTLV-1 infection and TSP was further confirmed when the virus was isolated,[110] and viral DNA was amplified from neural tissues of patients with TSP.[111,112] Patients with myelopathy found to be seropositive for HTLV-1 usually have antibodies in both the serum and CSF.[103,107,111] The retrovirus HTLV-1 also has been found to be associated with acute T-cell leukemia.[106,113,114] HTLV-I infection can be transmitted by sexual intercourse, intravenous drug use, breast feeding, or transfusion.[115]

The neuropathology of HAM/TSP reveals demyelination in the lateral and dorsal tracts, some axonal loss, and variable amounts of vacuolization and inflammation where the proviral DNA may be amplified.[116–118] The lateral columns are most severely affected.[119] Although myelopathy has been estimated to occur in less than 1% of infected individuals,[115,120] a recent study[121] of HTLV-1-infected blood donors revealed clinical signs of HAM in four of 166 HTLV-1 subjects (2.4%). The incubation period before developing myelopathy is variable but has been reported as early as 18 weeks after infection.[122] Alternatively, years may elapse between infection and the development of myelopathy.[120] Occasional patients may develop both adult T-cell leukemia and HAM/TSP.[109,115]

The pathogenesis of HTLV-1/TSP myelopathy is obscure but has been suggested to be immunologically mediated.[123] Various mechanisms of neurological injury have been recently discussed.[120] These include (1) a cytotoxic hypothesis, which predicts that infected CD4 T cells migrate into the CNS and infect cells, paving the way for cellularly mediated cytotoxic demyelination; (2) an autoimmune hypothesis, in which the target is an antigen in the CNS, such as occurs in experimental autoimmune encephalomyelitis; and (3) the bystander hypothesis, in which there is not a specific CNS antigen but rather an interaction between interferon-gamma-secreting HTLV-1-infected CD4 T cells and virally specific CD8 T cells, which induces cytokine release. Cytokines such as tumor necrosis factor (TNF)-alpha are toxic to myelin. Tumor necrosis factor receptor has been demonstrated in the CSF of afflicted patients, suggesting immune activation is necessary for disease pathogenesis.[124] With the increase in frequency of individuals seropositive for HTLV-1, HTLV-1-associated myelopathy may be encountered more frequently in the United States.[125] Some patients have been reported to be dually infected with the AIDS virus (HIV-1) and HTLV-1.[126] Since HIV-1 can also cause a myelopathy, clinical distinction may be difficult.

Another human retrovirus, HTLV-2, has been discovered, although the spectrum of disease is not fully understood. Lehky and colleagues[127] recently reported the findings of four patients infected with HTLV-2. These investigators found that the clinical and immunologic features resemble those found in HTLV-1-associated myelopathy patients. In a study[121] of 404 HTLV-2-infected blood donors, one (0.25%) demonstrated clinical signs of HAM (See Table 8–1).

CLINICAL FEATURES

The clinical presentation of HAM is usually progressive lower extremity weakness, often associated with lumbar or thoracic pain with or without lower extremity discomfort. Paresthesias are common, but prominent sensory disturbances are unusual. Bladder dysfunction is common. Signs and symptoms are usually bilateral and symmetric, but may also be asymmetric. Although weakness usually involves the legs more prominently than the arms, spasticity is typically found in all extremities. The course evolves over several months in most patients, but may occasionally be less than one month.[107] Most patients in recent series are women.[103,107,109] The CSF usually shows an inflammatory profile, with elevated protein, oligoclonal bands, pleocytosis, and HTLV-1 antibody.[128] Table 8–4 [121] demonstrates the epidemiologic, clinical, and laboratory data on four HTLV-1 cases and one HTLV-2 case identified at the time of blood donation. The clinical and epidemiologic features have been reviewed.[115]

Since the neuropathological features of HAM involve the white matter, it is not surprising that the MRI findings for HAM and multiple sclerosis are similar.[119,129] Godoy and colleagues[129] found a similar MRI appearance of brain lesions in patients with HAM/TSP and remitting relapsing multiple sclerosis, which suggested to these authors that demyelination is operative in the pathogenesis of HAM/TSP. An alternative comparison of MRI findings in the brains of patients with HAM and patients with multiple sclerosis has been reported by Kuroda and colleagues.[130] These authors found white matter lesions in the brains in 30 of 36 (84%) HAM patients; however, they felt these lesions were different from those seen in MS patients as defined by the criteria of Paty.[24] None of the patients with HAM had intracranial lesions below the tentorium. There have been few studies of the MRI spinal cord appearance of patients with HAM. Those that have been done reveal normal cord. Sometimes atrophy of the cord may be found.[115,119,121,130]

Lower limb somatosensory-evoked potentials have been studied in patients with HAM/TSP.[131] Among 96 such patients in one series, the central sensory conduction time (CSCT) was abnormal in 42 patients. Furthermore, there was a high correlation between the CSCT results and disability score. In some patients with normal sensory function, a delayed CSCT was found, suggesting that subclinical lesions of the spinal cord can be identified. This technique has the potential to provide a quantitative measure of disease progression or response to therapy.

THERAPY

Therapy of HAM/TSP remains unsatisfactory. Most of the therapeutic approaches have been based on the premise that anti-inflammatory agents might prevent the progression of the disease. Accordingly, corticosteroid therapy has been tried, and it may be temporarily effective in some patients. In patients treated with corticosteroids, the HTLV-1 antibody titers and IgG fall both in the serum and CSF, suggesting that HTLV-1 antibody may be important in the pathogenesis of the disorder. Alternatively, plasmapheresis, which may also be a temporarily effective treatment, does not lower the HTLV-1 antibody titer in the CSF. These findings and the observation that serum and CSF HTLV-1 antibody titers do not correlate with disease severity have cast doubt on the role of HTLV-1 antibody in the pathogenesis of HAM.[370] In one large scale study of 200 patients with HAM/TSP treated between 1986 and 1993, a variety of immunomodulating agents were used such as prednisolone, plasmapharesis and lymphocytapharesis, and interferon alpha.[132] The results of this open-label study suggested that immunomodulatory therapies have some, albeit limited, beneficial results. Whether the advent of specific antiretroviral therapy will impact the disease is not known at this time.

AIDS-Related Myelopathies

Patients with acquired immunodeficiency syndrome (AIDS) may develop myelopathies secondary to compression from infection

Table 8–4. **Epidemiologic, Clinical, and Laboratory Data on HAM Cases**[*]

	HTLV-I Cases				HTLV-II Case
Variable	**Case 1**	**Case 2**	**Case 3**	**Case 4**	**Case 5**
History					
Age/sex at onset	46F	58M	39F	30F	42F
Probable risk factor(s)	Sex with Caribbean person, blood transfusion	Sex with Japanese person	Unknown	Breastfed by Japanese person	Drug injection with shared needle, with sex IVDU
Estimated duration of infection	9–13 years	38 years	Unknown	30 years	0–14 years
Duration of symptoms	5 years	2 years	5 years	2 years	1 year
Neurologic Examination					
Patellar reflex	↑	↑	Normal	↑	↑
Plantar response	Extensor	Extensor	Extensor	Extensor	Unreactive
MRI	Thin cervical cord	Normal	Normal	Normal	Normal
Urologic diagnosis	Spastic bladder	Spastic bladder	Spastic bladder	Spastic bladder	Spastic bladder
Laboratory Evaluation					
Cerebrospinal fluid					
WBC cells/mm^3	7	3	2	N.A.[†]	1
Protein (mg/dl)	39	41	31	N.A.[†]	28
HTLV-antibody titer: serum/CSF	1:16,384/1:16	1:65,536/1:256	1:1,024/1:64	N.A.	1:320/1:20
HTLV: albumin index[‡]	0.55	0.78	15.97	N.A.	17.45
HTLV PCR (PBMC/CSF)	HTLV-1/HTLV-1	HTLV-1/HTLV-1	HTLV-1/HTLV-1	HTLV-1/N.A.	HTLV-2/Neg

[*]From Murphy, EL, et al.,[121] with permission.
[†]Not available since lumbar puncture was not performed.
[‡]Ratio of the CSF/serum antibody titer divided by the ratio of the CSF/serum albumin concentration. Values greater than 2.0 were deemed to represent intrathecal synthesis of HTLV antibodies.

or neoplasm, or induced by infection with the human immunodeficiency virus or other infectious diseases.[133–135/136] Whereas in adults with AIDS, vacuolar myelopathy may lead to a progressive myelopathy, in pediatric patients bilateral corticospinal tract degeneration may occur with a distinct histopathology.[61] Such children may develop progressive quadriparesis.

Vacuolar myelopathy[137,146] may occur in patients with AIDS and is often seen in patients with AIDS-related dementia[135/136] (Figs. 8–3 and 8–4). The lateral and posterior columns of the thoracic spinal cord appear to be predominantly affected.[146] Histopathological features are similar to those of subacute combined degeneration of the spinal cord secondary to vitamin B_{12} deficiency. Tan et al.[138] have suggested that a cellular deficiency in B_{12} might be pathogenetic as a result of increased demand for the vitamin. Furthermore, while earlier studies suggested that direct viral invasion is involved in the pathogenesis of this disorder,[135/136,139,140] more recent investigations using immunohistochemistry and in situ hybridization found that vacuolar myelopathy occurred independent of productive HIV-1 infection in the spinal cord.[134,141] Kamin and Petito[142] have shown that the pathological features of vacuolar myelopathy may occur in patients with other immunodeficiency states. Macrophages and microglia found within vacuoles may play a role in pathogenesis by releasing cytokines which are toxic to myelin.[143–145] HIV-1 may play a role in activating the inflammatory cells.

The most common clinical manifestations of vacuolar myelopathy are progressive spastic paraparesis, incontinence, and ataxia.[146] When peripheral neuropathy is also present, the deep tendon reflexes may be absent and there may be distal sensory loss and/or paresthesias. Of the 20 patients in one study,[146] dementia was present in 14 (70%). Other HIV-1-associated myelopathies that have been reported include acute myelopathy occurring at the time of initial infection,[146,147] spinal myoclonus,[148] and a remitting-relapsing myelopathy.[149] Because compressive myelopathies may clinically resemble vacuolar myelopathies, MRI and/or myelography is

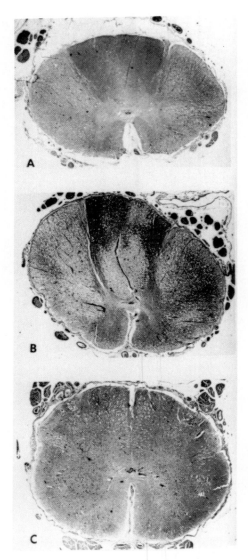

Figure 8–3. Vacuolar myelopathy shown in a patient with AIDS. The lower thoracic spinal cord (B) is most severely affected, with marked, confluent vacuolation of the posterior and lateral columns. The upper thoracic (A) and lumbar (C) spinal cord areas are less severely involved. Hematoxylin-eosin stain, × 7.92. (From Petito, CK, et al.,[146] p. 876, with permission.)

usually performed in such patients before a diagnosis is made.[140] In a postmortem MR study of spinal cords affected by vacuolar myelopathy, Santosh et al.[150] reported that with proton-density and T_2-weighted images, increased signal from the affected white matter tracts, usually with a symmetric pattern, was found.

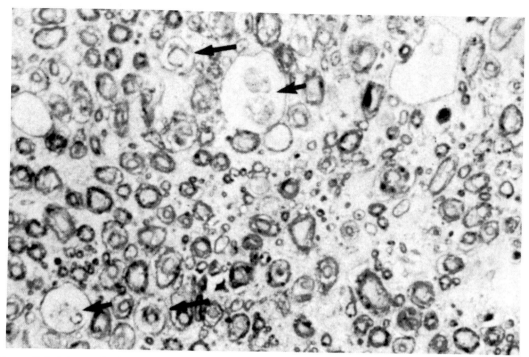

Figure 8–4. A 1-μm plastic-embedded section of the lateral column of a patient with moderately severe AIDS-related vacuolar myelopathy. Vacuoles surrounded by thin myelin sheaths are shown. Two vacuoles contain lipid-laden macrophages (short arrows). A few myelin sheaths show intramyelin swelling (long arrows). Toluidine blue stain, × 1085. (From Petito, CK, et al.,[146] p. 877, with permission.)

In addition to vacuolar myelopathy, patients with AIDS are at risk to develop a variety of infections that damage the spinal cord.[135/136,151] Herpes simplex types I and II and varicella-zoster virus have been found to cause myeloradiculopathies in patients with AIDS.[135/136,152,153] Cytomegalovirus (CMV) also has been reported to cause an ascending myelitis and radiculomyelitis.[134,154,155]

Clinically, CMV radiculomyelitis often presents with cauda equina dysfunction manifested as back and radicular pain, sphincter disturbance, and areflexic leg weakness. An ascending myelitis may occur, and the brain may ultimately be involved. The CSF characteristically shows an inflammatory profile with polymorphonuclear pleocytosis, low sugar, and high protein.[156] A CSF virologic culture may reveal the organism.[157,158] Imaging of the spine may reveal abnormal enhancement[101] or thickened nerve roots, or be normal.[159] Some reports suggest that

patients with neurologic CMV infection may respond to the antiviral agent ganciclovir;[156,157,160] however, this has been questioned.[161] Mycobacterial meningomyelitis and spinal toxoplasmoses are other identifiable CNS infectious complications of AIDS. [162,163] Intramedullary tuberculoma has also been reported in one patient.[164] Herpes simplex myelitis has been reported.[152] Toxoplasmosis, which is commonly present in the brains of patients dying of AIDS, can occasionally affect the cord.[165,166] Syphilis may also affect the central nervous system in patients with AIDS.[167]

Herpes zoster radiculitis is common in patients with AIDS, but zoster-associated myelitis has also been reported occasionally. Devinsky and colleagues[168] described a patient who developed flaccid paraplegia several days after rash. Chetrien et al.[169] described a fatal case of ascending necrotizing meningomyeloradiculitis without rash. Imaging may show a swollen cord. Antiviral agents have been reported to be beneficial in some cases.[97]

In addition to direct viral invasion of the spinal cord by opportunistic infections, patients with AIDS suffer from poor nutrition and toxic and metabolic derangements that may be responsible for some cases of myelopathy.[134,135/136] Finally, these patients also have an increased risk of primary CNS lymphoma and other systemic neoplasms that may cause spinal cord compression.[137,170,171]

SPIROCHETAL DISEASE OF THE SPINAL CORD

Syphilis

Syphilis has been a major public health problem that again appears to be increasing in incidence with the development of AIDS.[172] In a recent study of HIV-infected and HIV-noninfected patients, *Treponema pallidum*, the cause of syphilis, was found in the CSF of 30% of patients with primary or secondary syphilis.[173] The importance of syphilis in the evaluation of spinal cord disease was best expressed by Merritt et al.[174] (page 144), who wrote, "In summary, it should be said that with the combination of chronic meningitis, arterial disease, and granuloma formation, it is not surprising that almost every conceivable cord disease may be simulated clinically by spinal syphilis."

CLINICAL AND LABORATORY FEATURES

The spirochete *Treponema pallidum* usually invades the CNS, resulting in an acute syphilitic meningitis during the secondary stage of the disease.[15,174] Following a latent period of variable duration, the tertiary stage, characterized first by meningovascular syphilis and then parenchymal syphilis, may occur. Pathologically, the meningovascular form is an arteritis, the location of which determines the clinical neurological manifestations.[174] Clinical syndromes of spinal cord involvement from the meningovascular disease may be classified as syphilitic meningomyelitis,

syphilitic pachymeningitis, syphilitic spastic paraplegia (Erb's spastic paraplegia), and syphilitic amyotrophy.[15] Among these meningovascular forms, syphilitic meningomyelitis is the most common.[15] It is characterized pathologically by a granulomatous involvement of blood vessels called, Heubner's arteritis. As mentioned, the clinical syndromes are secondary to the areas of the spinal cord that are infarcted. Thus, patients may present with a Brown-Séquard syndrome or an anterior spinal artery syndrome. Alternatively, scattered smaller infarctions may cause a variety of other spinal presentations. In cases of syphilitic pachymeningitis, the pachymeninges and leptomeninges are the site of granulomatous inflammation. Some patients have only progressive spastic paraparesis with preservation of sensory function, which was formerly called Erb's spastic paraplegia; this must be differentiated from motor neuron disease and familial spastic paraplegia. Syphilitic meningovascular involvement also may give rise to a syndrome of amyotrophy as a result of nerve root involvement. This may or may not be associated with spastic paraplegia. Some authors question the relationship between syphilitic pachymeningitis and syphilitic amyotrophy.[175]

The parenchymal form of neurosyphilis involving the spinal cord is tabes dorsalis. More common than meningovascular forms of spinal syphilis,[175] tabes dorsalis is a parenchymal disease of the nervous system secondary to invasion by *Treponema pallidum*. Pathologically, changes in the posterior roots, thickening of the leptomeninges, and gliosis of the posterior columns are typically seen[15] (Fig. 8–5). Dominant symptoms and signs are lightning pains, ataxia, urinary incontinence, absent lower extremity deep tendon reflexes, and impaired vibratory and position sensibilities in the lower extremities. The ataxia is secondary to sensory disturbance. Argyll-Robertson pupils, constricting in accommodation but not to light, also are typically present. Some patients experience severe abdominal pain and diarrhea.

Although the CSF is usually abnormal in patients with neurosyphilis, some authorities report that it may be entirely nor-

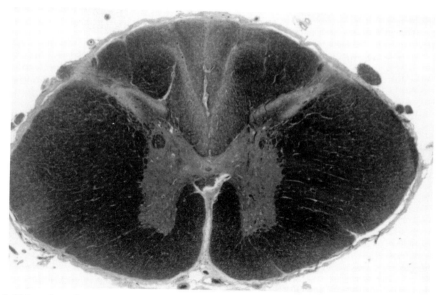

Figure 8–5. Tabes dorsalis. Note the symmetric loss of myelin in posterior columns. (Courtesy of Dr. Lysia Forno.)

mal by conventional testing in a significant number of patients.[176] Specific laboratory findings and the clinical constellation of neurosyphilis are discussed elsewhere in detail.[172,173,177–179]

The following is a case illustration of a syphilitic meningitis.

CASE ILLUSTRATION

A 34-year-old woman presented with a four-week history of back and leg pain, followed by headache and gait difficulty. There was also a history of maculopapular rash during this period, and night sweats. On physical examination, she had no adenopathy or splenomegaly but did have maculopapular rash. Neurological examination revealed papilledema on funduscopic examination and hypotonic lower extremity weakness (4/5) with depressed-to-absent lower extremity reflexes. She had a waddling gait due to proximal lower extremity weakness and could not stand on her toes or heels. There was slight sensory disturbance to touch and pin over the right distal lower extremity.

An MR scan of the entire spine with gadolinium showed enhancement of the cauda equina and clumping or nodularity of the nerve roots. A lumbar puncture demonstrated an opening pressure of 340 mm, with a CSF pleocytosis, protein 85 mg per deciliter, glucose 50 mg per

deciliter, and positive VDRL. The serum VDRL was positive, as was the serum FTA-ABS. The CSF IgG was 38 mg per deciliter (normal <5 mg per deciliter) and oligoclonal bands were present. The skin lesions were biopsied and showed perivascular plasma cells highly suggestive of spirochetal infection. A diagnosis of secondary syphilis with syphilitic meningitis was made, and the patient showed neurological recovery following high-dose intravenous penicillin.

Comment. This case illustrates a rare neurological manifestation of syphilitic meningitis. This patient had evidence of increased intracranial pressure and a cauda equina syndrome caused by syphilis. The MRI was done without and with gadolinium to look for leptomeningeal enhancement because the papilledema and cauda equina syndrome were considered suspicious for meningeal involvement. Although this clinical constellation of multifocal involvement of the CNS is often found in leptomeningeal cancer,[180] it is clear that other forms of chronic meningitis may cause a similar clinical picture.

THERAPY

Specific recommendations regarding the treatment of neurosyphilis are controversial and beyond the scope of this book. Accordingly, only general principles will be mentioned. Although there is general agreement that penicillin is the drug of choice for neurosyphilis, there is considerable controversy over the form and dosage.[173,176] Both intravenous aqueous crystalline penicillin G and intramuscular procaine penicillin plus probenecid have been recommended.[181,182] Despite these recommendations, subtreponemicidal levels of penicillin are found in the CSF of patients treated with benzathine penicillin,[179] and the adequacy of benzathine and procaine penicillin regimens has been questioned.[172] Furthermore, patients with coexistent HIV infection appear to be at increased risk for treatment failure[182] Careful neurological follow-up is important to determine the efficacy of therapy. Repeated CSF examinations following treatment are recommended to verify improvement of the CSF parameters.[175,179]

Lyme Disease

Lyme disease is caused by the spirochete *Borrelia burgdorferi*, which is transmitted by ticks and other arthropod vectors.[183–185] Lyme disease recently has been recognized to lead to a wide variety of neurological complications.[185–187] Although the disease's clinical manifestations have been classified in three stages, many patients do not demonstrate symptoms or signs of all three.[178]

The first stage of the disease often begins soon after infection and consists of a flu-like illness associated with erythema chronicum migrans, the characteristic skin lesion. The second stage usually begins within a few weeks to months of infection and may include neurological and/or cardiac involvement. As in the case of syphilis, it is during this secondary stage that the central nervous system may be seeded. In a study of patients with an acute disseminated infection of *B. burgdorferi,* invasion of the central nervous system was found in 8 of 12 cases by CSF analysis.[188] When neurological involvement occurs during the secondary stage, there is often evidence of meningitis, cranial neu-

ritis, radiculitis, and/or peripheral neuropathy.[178] The third stage, which may commence within several months to years after the initial infection, is often manifested as arthritis. However, neurological involvement may dominate this stage and the spinal cord may be the primary or sole site of clinical involvement.[189]

A demyelinating disease resembling multiple sclerosis and a variety of neuropsychiatric syndromes have been reported during the third stage,[178,187,190] of Lyme disease. However, recent studies have challenged the etiologic role of *B. burgdorferi* in the development of symptoms resembling multiple sclerosis.[191–193] Rarely, transverse myelitis also has been reported to dominate the neurological picture in late Lyme disease.[178] Acute transverse myelitis occasionally may occur as a presenting neurological manifestation of Lyme disease during the secondary phase of the disease and in association with meningitis.[194–196]

In many geographical areas, Lyme disease is very common and serum immunoreactivity against *B. burgdorferi* is widespread. Thus, it may be difficult to determine confidently whether a specific neurological disorder is due to Lyme disease. In an attempt to identify CNS disorders due to Lyme disease, researchers have reported that intrathecal production of specific antibodies appears to be a marker for active CNS involvement.[192,197,198] Because intrathecal antibody to *B. burgdorferi* has been found in only approximately 40%–50% of North American patients with late central nervous system involvement,[193,197] other laboratory techniques have been sought. Detection by PCR of *B. burgdorferi* in the central nervous system of patients with CNS involvement has yielded conflicting results. In one recent study, *B. burgdorferi* DNA was detected in the CSF in 6 (38%) of 16 patients with acute neuroborreliosis and in 11 (25%) of 44 with chronic neuroborreliosis.[199] An MRI of the spine may show intramedullary abnormalities and abnormal contrast enhancement of the cord and/or roots.[101]

As in the case of syphilis, patients with CNS involvement may respond to antibiotic therapy.[178,190,194] Ceftriaxone and penicillin have been used.[192,200]

TOXIC MYELOPATHIES

Myelopathies may occur secondary to toxic exposures. In many cases, the symptoms and signs of myelopathy are overshadowed by those of other organs affected. For example, although lead may cause a myelopathy, its toxic effect on the brain in children, and on peripheral nerves in adults, may be far more prominent findings. This section lists some of the more commonly encountered causes of toxic myelopathies. As further experience is gained with other substances, this list is expected to lengthen.

Orthocresyl Phosphate

Orthocresyl phosphates, which are used as industrial solvents, are highly toxic to the central and peripheral nervous system when ingested.[201] During the era of Prohibition, jake paralysis, an acute peripheral neuropathy secondary to the ingestion of ginger jake adulterated with triorthocresyl phosphate, was seen.[78] More recently, outbreaks have occurred when olive oil was contaminated with lubricating oil containing triorthocresyl phosphate.[202] The clinical picture is usually that of an acute peripheral neuropathy developing over a period of weeks, accompanied or followed by myelopathy. On pathological inspection, Wallerian degeneration is seen of both peripheral and central nervous system fibers.[15,203]

Myelopathy Following Aortography

On rare occasions, aortography contrast injection of the aorta has been followed by myelopathy.[204,205] The mechanism of pathogenesis is uncertain and in some cases it could be secondary to embolic infarction or vasospasm of the spinal cord; in other instances, the contrast material was considered toxic to the spinal cord.[15,78] This type of myelopathy may present immediately as spasms in the lower extremities during the injection of contrast material.[206] The patient may have a sensory level and loss of bowel and bladder function, as well as a flaccid paraplegia.[78] When due to anterior spinal artery infarction, posterior column function (position and vibration) may be spared.

Lathyrism

Lathyrism, a disease most often encountered in India and North Africa, is a relatively acute neurological syndrome of pain, sensory complaints, and weakness of the lower extremities that evolves into an ataxic, spastic paraplegia. (Lathyrism has been considered a cause of tropical spastic paraparesis.[207]) On pathological inspection, the anterior and lateral columns reveal degeneration.[208,209] Its specific etiology and pathogenesis have not been elucidated, but it is considered secondary to consumption of vetches such as *Lathyrus sativas*.[15]

Myelopathy Due to Intrathecal Agents

Myelopathy may follow the injection of a variety of agents into the subarachnoid space. Penicillin, which was frequently administered intrathecally in the past, may cause radiculitis, arachnoiditis, and transverse myelitis.[78,210–212] In the past, methylene blue was injected into the subarachnoid space to detect sites of CSF leak.[78] This compound was found to cause a myelitis and radiculitis, apparently without arachnoiditis.[213,214]

SPINAL ANESTHETICS

Although the frequency of this complication varies widely, both acute and delayed myelopathies have been reported to occur following the administration of spinal anesthetics.[215–218] Pathogenesis is unknown and has been considered secondary to the anesthetic[219] to contaminants such as phenol or detergents within the anesthetics.[217,220] In patients with acute myelopathy, paralysis may occur immediately following spinal anesthesia. On pathological examination, the spinal cord has been reported to show softening, petechial hemorrhages, and inflammatory cells.[217,221,222]

INTRATHECAL CHEMOTHERAPY

Both acute and delayed myelopathy have been reported following the intrathecal administration of methotrexate, cytosine arabinoside, and thiotepa.[223–227] Myelopathy may occur between 30 minutes and 48 hours (or, occasionally, up to 1 to 2 weeks) following administration.[228] Clinical presentation often is associated with leg pain, paraplegia, sensory level, and neurogenic bladder.[224,228,229] Improvement of the myelopathy, which can be partial or complete, may occur within days to months following its onset, or it may be permanent.[228]

Myelopathy may occur due to either intrathecal chemotherapy for the treatment of malignant leptomeningeal disease or prophylactic therapy. It appears to be unrelated to the administration of other systemic drugs or CNS irradiation.[80] Its pathogenesis is unknown but may be secondary to demyelination or another toxic phenomenon.[225]

Spinal Arachnoiditis

Spinal arachnoiditis is an uncommon disorder in which a nonspecific inflammatory reaction of the leptomeninges and fibrosis cause both root and spinal cord symptoms and signs. Although the etiology of the inflammatory reaction often is never uncovered, spinal arachnoiditis may occur secondary to intrathecal administration of contrast material (especially oil-soluble contrast media), antibiotics, and other agents, as well as trauma and spinal surgery.[230–232]

On pathological examination of the spinal cord and meninges, fibrosis may be widespread along the neuraxis, or it may be more circumscribed.[15] The spinal subarachnoid space may be obliterated from the process.[233] There may be a predilection for the thoracic spine. In addition, there may be loculated cystic areas that cause spinal cord and root compression. Although the pathogenesis of neurological dysfunction may be secondary to compression in some cases, vascular disturbances secondary to arachnoiditis also may occur,[15] and syringomyelia may result.[233a]

The clinical presentation of spinal arachnoiditis is most commonly that of multifocal spinal disease manifested by a combination of radicular and/or spinal cord symptoms and signs. Neuropathic pain, which may be burning and distributed in one or several spinal roots, is a common presenting symptom. Weakness of a lower motor neuron type may be seen, especially in cases with cauda equina involvement.[5] In patients with lumbosacral arachnoiditis, the straight-leg-raising sign is frequently positive, and neck flexion may cause pain in the lower extremities. If the spinal cord becomes involved, a progressive myelopathy with features of spasticity and ataxia may ensue.

The CSF is nearly always abnormal, and elevation of protein and pleocytosis are common. It may show oligoclonal bands.[24,234] Myelography with or without follow-up CT scanning usually reveals a characteristic appearance.[235,236] Patients with arachnoiditis may be sensitive to the administration of intrathecal contrast material, which may cause further irritation.[78,235] Tethered and clumped nerve roots and distortion of the thecal sac may be seen on noncontrast MRI studies.[237,238] Using gadolinium-DTPA, enhancement has recently been seen in some cases.[239] Several studies have shown the value of contrast-enhanced MRI in evaluating arachnoiditis.[239a–d]

The management of spinal arachnoiditis is difficult. While corticosteroids and surgery have been used, they remain controversial.[5,240,241]

Radiation Myelopathy

Radiation myelopathy may occur following radiation therapy in which the spinal cord is included within the radiation port. Despite advances in knowledge concerning the effects of radiation on the spinal cord, severe forms of radiation myelopathy are still occasionally encountered. For example, it has been found that some patients will develop chronic progressive radiation myelopathy despite the fact that they have received a dose of spinal irradiation considered safe for most individuals.[242,243] Furthermore, some agents, such as hyperbaric oxygenation, may increase the risk of radiation myelopathy.[244] Based upon its clinical manifestations, radiation myelopathy has been classified into four distinct syndromes (Table 8–5).[245]

EARLY-DELAYED RADIATION MYELOPATHY (TRANSIENT RADIATION MYELOPATHY)

Transient radiation myelopathy is characterized by the subjective complaints of paresthesias and electric-like shock sensations on neck flexion (Lhermitte's sign).[246,247] This form of myelopathy is a frequent sequela of standard doses of radiation to the spinal cord when neoplasms of the neck and upper thoracic region are irradiated. It has been estimated to occur in 15% of individuals undergoing standard mantle irradiation; higher doses of irradiation cause even more frequent transient radiation myelopathy.[247] Typically, symptoms begin 2 to 37 weeks (average, 16 weeks) following radiation therapy and spontaneously resolve after a period usually lasting 2 to 36 weeks (average 16 weeks).[248,249] Although Lhermitte's sign does not typically portend the later development of progressive spinal cord dysfunction, it may be an early manifestation of chronic progressive radiation myelopathy.[248]

Clinical features consist of painful electric-like shock sensations, elicited by neck

Table 8–5. **Classification of Radiation Myelopathy**

Transient myelopathy (Lhermitte's sign)
Lower motor neuron dysfunction
Acute transverse myelopathy
Chronic progressive radiation myelopathy

flexion or extension, which involve the body below the neck. Although the regions of the body involved are quite variable, the trunk, anterior or posterior lower extremities, and upper extremities, are typically affected individually or in combination (Fig. 8–6). Sensations usually are bilateral.

On neurological examination, no abnormalities are found. The differential diagnosis for the cause of Lhermitte's sign includes spinal metastasis and unrelated disorders such as cervical spondylosis and disc herniation,[250] subacute combined degeneration,[251,252,253] posttraumatic syndrome,[254] multiple sclerosis,[34,255] and complications from cisplatin chemotherapy.[256] The pathogenesis of the disorder is thought to be reversible damage to myelin in the ascending sensory tracts of the spinal cord, allowing axons to be abnormally sensitive to mechanical deformation, although there is no histologic proof of this.[248,257] Somatosensory-evoked potentials have been reported to be abnormally prolonged in some patients, supporting the impression that the pathology resides in the posterior columns and is demyelinating in nature.[258] Furthermore, in experimental animals, CSF myelin basic protein has been reported to be transiently elevated soon after irradiation.[259,260]

LATE-DELAYED RADIATION MYELOPATHY

Chronic Progressive Radiation Myelopathy

Chronic progressive radiation myelopathy is the most common form of severe irradiation-induced spinal cord injury.[261–265] The clinical syndrome is variable but commonly develops with spinal cord symptoms and signs beginning several months to many years following therapy.[245] Sensory symptoms beginning in the lower extremities, described as burning paresthesias and alterations in pain and temperature sensation, are often reported. As noted above, Lhermitte's sign may herald the development of chronic progressive myelopathy, but in this case it generally arises after a higher dose of radiation

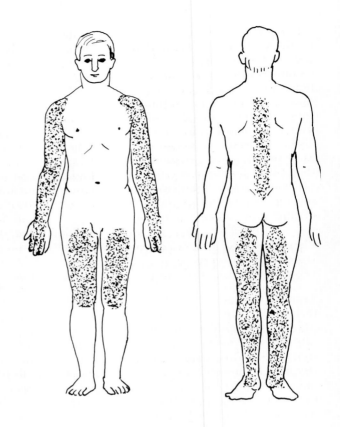

Figure 8–6. Anatomical areas commonly involved in electrical paresthesias (Lhermitte's symptom) in cases of transient radiation myelopathy.

therapy and after a more prolonged latent period (usually more than one year) than that seen in the transient form of radiation myelopathy.[248]

The neurological examination usually reveals spastic lower extremity weakness. Sphincter disturbance also develops. A Brown-Séquard syndrome is sometimes seen, or other forms of transverse myelopathy (incomplete) may predominate. An ascending sensory level may evolve over several weeks or months. Symptoms and signs usually are slowly progressive over several months but may ultimately stabilize. Spontaneous improvement rarely occurs.

The diagnosis of chronic radiation myelopathy requires the exclusion of compressive lesions of the cord, which are much more common, and treatable, in the cancer patient.[266] Scanning with MRI is usually effective in ruling out a compressive lesion and may show intramedullary cord abnormalities characteristic of chronic progressive myelopathy. In the acute phase, the cord may be swollen and enhance with intravenous contrast material, indicating a loss of normal blood–spinal cord barrier.[267,268] Investigational studies have shown that the blood–spinal cord barrier is disrupted early in the pathogenesis of radiation-induced myelopathy.[269] Later in the course, the cord may be atrophic on MRI. The CSF may show an elevated protein and other nonspecific findings. Cerebrospinal fluid cytology is negative for malignant cells.[245]

The main pathological finding consists of demyelination, which may begin in the posterior columns and extend into the lateral columns, causing necrosis and leukomalacia. The gray matter generally shows evidence of coagulative necrosis at the level of irradiation. Secondary ascending and descending tract degeneration (Wallerian degeneration) is seen. Vascular changes described include hyalinization of arterial walls, subendothelial intimal swelling, and luminal narrowing and thrombosis.[249,270–272]

The primary insult that causes this type of myelopathy has been debated; some authors favor a radiation-induced vascular etiology[273] while others suggest a direct radiation-induced glial injury.[270,274] Plasminogen activator inhibitor-1 has also been suggested to play a role in the pathogenesis of the disorder.[275]

The therapy of chronic radiation-induced myelopathy is unsatisfactory. In an experimental model of radiation myelopathy, high-dose corticosteroids produced some benefit in the neurological function of animals.[276] Occasional clinical reports suggest that corticosteroids may have a role in the management of this disorder.[273] A recent study suggests that anticoagulation with heparin and warfarin may benefit some patients.[277]

Lower Motor Neuron Dysfunction

The third form of radiation myelopathy, which appears to be very rare, presents as signs of lower motor neuron dysfunction.[245] In the patients described, painless amyotrophy and weakness, usually of the lower extremities, develops subacutely several years following high-dose radiation therapy to the spinal cord.[278–280] It has most frequently been reported in long-term survivors of pelvic tumors (such as testicular cancer), where the distal cord and cauda equina have been included in the radiotherapy port. It may be bilateral or unilateral.[281] Sensory abnormalities are not found, and sphincters remain intact. The differential diagnosis includes paraneoplastic motor neuronopathy and other pure motor neuropathies.

An MRI report of the cervical spine in an affected patient with brachial weakness revealed a cystic hypodensity from C4 to C6.[282] Electrodiagnostic studies demonstrate normal motor conduction velocities and denervation on electromyogram. The CSF protein may be elevated.[249] Pathogenesis is unknown, but the clinical constellation resembles the subacute motor neuronopathy that occurs secondary to ionizing radiation and/or activation of a latent virus.[283] Pathological examination has been rare and has not yielded an understanding of the pathogenesis.[284] The course is usually subacutely progressive but usually stabilizes.

Acute Transverse Myelopathy

The fourth form of radiation myelopathy is acutely developing paraplegia or quadriplegia, presumably secondary to infarction or hemorrhage into the spinal cord. It may be secondary to radiation-induced vascular pathology.[245] It is exceedingly rare and only a few cases have been reported.

In 1991, Allen and colleagues[285] described vascular changes in the brains and spinal cords of long-term survivors of radiotherapy. Vascular malformations resembling telangiectases may in some instances develop and hemorrhage. Accordingly, patients may develop the acute onset of pain and neurologic dysfunction below the level of the affected cord region. Posner has described a case of intramedullary cord hemorrhage that occurred many years after mantle irradiation for Hodgkin's disease in a patient taking nonsteroidal antiinflammatory medications.[286] He recommends that affected patients avoid aspirin and nonsteroidals, which may lead to subsequent hemorrhage.

Electrical Injuries

Spinal cord damage secondary to electrical injuries may be either acute or delayed. The cervical spinal cord is frequently the site of injury because electrical current often passes from hand to hand.[287] Acute injuries may be secondary to heating of tissue or ischemia. Both gray matter and white matter tracts may be damaged, so sensory, motor, and sphincter disturbances may occur. The motor weakness may be secondary to anterior horn cell damage resulting in amyotrophy. Such findings may be self-limited or may regress.[78]

Occasionally, a delayed progressive spinal cord syndrome develops following electrical injury; this syndrome may be difficult to differentiate clinically from spinal muscular atrophy or amyotrophic lateral sclerosis.[287–289] The pathogenesis of this delayed progressive myelopathy is not well understood; it may be secondary to vascular occlusive changes, as seen in some patients with delayed myelopathy following radiation therapy.[5]

METABOLIC AND NUTRITIONAL MYELOPATHIES

Metabolic and nutritional myelopathies may occur due to vitamin deficiencies or liver disease. Subacute combined degeneration due to vitamin B_{12} deficiency is discussed separately from other nutritional deficiencies.

Subacute Combined Degeneration of the Cord

This treatable disease was first described in detail at the turn of this century and usually presents with the insidious progression of paresthesias of the extremities.[290] Since the peripheral nervous system and the cerebrum are also affected, the clinical presentation can be protean.[291] Unlike some other deficiency myelopathies in which either the posterior or lateral columns may be involved alone, the designation "combined degeneration" refers to the fact that both the lateral and posterior columns are usually involved pathologically and clinically.[292] The disease results from vitamin B_{12} (cobalamin) deficiency and is often, but not invariably, associated with megaloblastic anemia.[293]

Degenerative and demyelinative changes occur in the white matter of the posterior and lateral columns of the spinal cord (Fig. 8–7). The white matter of the brain may show similar changes. The peripheral nerves also may show signs of demyelination and axonal degeneration.[294]

Initial neurological manifestations are generally sensory complaints, including paresthesias involving the distal extremities.[295] Many patients first note pins-and-needles tingling or numbness in the feet, followed by the hands. These symptoms, which may be due to sensory peripheral neuropathy and/or damage to ascending white matter tracts, are usually progressive and ascend the extremities. Vibration and position sensation are disturbed, and the Romberg usually becomes positive. The motor symptoms generally are weakness and stiffness in the lower extremities. The degree of spasticity and ataxia depends upon the relative degree of involvement of the descending and ascending

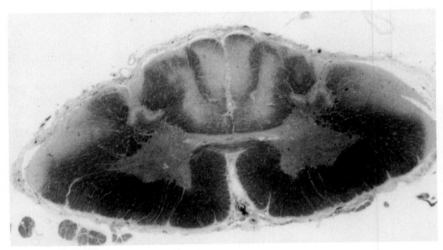

Figure 8–7. Subacute combined degeneration affecting the spinal cord. Note lateral and posterior column involvement. (Courtesy of Dr. Lysia Forno.)

tracts, respectively. Thus the patient may have primarily a spastic gait, an ataxic gait, or a combined spastic, ataxic gait. Involvement of the deep tendon reflexes depends upon the relative degree of central and peripheral nervous system involvement. Babinski signs eventually develop if the disease is not recognized and treated. Sphincter disturbances are atypical.[295] When the brain is involved, a variety of neuropsychiatric findings may occur, along with visual and other cerebral manifestations.[293]

A laboratory diagnosis is based on an understanding of cobalamin physiology.[291,296,297] Cobalamin is transported in the serum by at least three transport proteins (transcobalamin I, II, and III). The serum assay of cobalamin measures total cobalamin; however, it is believed that the metabolically active form is that bound to transcobalamin II. Accordingly, it is possible to have a normal serum cobalamin level and still be deficient.[298] Since cobalamin is needed as a cofactor for the metabolic conversion of both methylmalonic acid and homocysteine, elevated levels of either or both of these compounds have been used as a diagnostic tool to assess cobalamin deficiency. For example, using serum cobalamin levels of less than 200 pg/ml as an indicator of deficiency, there have been a number of studies that find a prevalence of cobalamin deficiency of 7% to 16% in the elderly population.[298] Alternatively, using a cobalamin level of less than 300 pg/ml as an indicator of deficiency, or elevation of the metabolites methylmalonic acid and homocysteine, Pennypacker et al.[297] and Yao et al.[299] reported a prevalence of deficiency at 14.5% and 21%, respectively. The clinical significance of these studies is not yet clear, since some of these patients may not be clinically deficient and there are other causes of elevated homocysteine and methylmalonic acid levels.[298] However, these studies underscore the importance of careful laboratory testing for cobalamin deficiency in the patient with an appropriate clinical syndrome. An algorithm for evaluating and treating cobalamin deficency has been published.[298]

Nutritional Myelopathy

Unlike subacute combined systems disease, myelopathy from nutritional deprivation may be due to a variety of (and possibly multiple) deficiencies.[207,300–303] Erbsloh and Abel[304] have classified the nutritional myelopathies as: (1) posterolateral myelopathy manifesting itself as mainly an ataxic syndrome, (2) anterolateral myelopathy presenting with a spastic syndrome, and (3) combined ataxic and spastic syndromes. Nutritional and vitamin deficiencies also are responsible for some of the reported cases of tropical spastic paraparesis and tropical ataxic neuropathy.[207]

Although clinical manifestations vary, Hughes[15] has summarized the most commonly encountered syndromes. Some patients present with a progressive spastic paraparesis that may evolve to quadriparesis. Bowel and bladder function are involved in advanced cases, as are mental changes. Sensory findings are less frequent. Pathological studies[302] have revealed bilateral corticospinal tract degeneration, and posterior column degeneration may also be seen.

Clinical and pathological findings similar to those of nutritional myelopathy have been attributed to nicotinic acid deficiency (pellagra) but probably are due to several vitamin deficiencies as well as caloric malnutrition.[295,304] There have been rare reports of myelopathy developing in the setting of chronic alcoholism. Whether this is a direct effect of alcohol per se or secondary to associated nutritional deficiencies, liver disease, or other factors is unknown.[305]

Myelopathy Associated with Liver Disease

While encephalopathy is a common manifestation of liver failure, in rare individuals myelopathy secondary to liver disease is encountered. The myelopathy usually occurs in the setting of a surgical portacaval anastomosis or a spontaneously developing shunt.[306–308] Hepatic encephalopathy is usually an associated feature, but chronic progressive myelopathy secondary to hepatic failure may be the sole neurological abnormality.[309,310]

This disorder appears to occur predominantly in men.[307] In one review,[307] myelopathy occurred 1 to 120 months following surgical shunting procedures. The clinical features are those of a chronically progressive symmetric spastic paresis. Difficulty in walking is often, therefore, an early complaint. Sphincter dysfunction is also frequently seen, whereas sensory disturbances are not prominent.[15] On pathological inspection, the spinal cord shows bilateral corticospinal tract degeneration; posterior column degeneration also may be seen.[15,309] The spastic paresis is usually progressive over a course of many years. Pathogenesis of the disorder is unknown.

SPINAL CORD INFARCTION

Although spinal cord infarction is an extremely rare disease, its frequency appears to be increasing. An autopsy study of 3737 cases at the National Hospital, Queen Square in London, between 1909 and 1958 found nine cases (five arterial occlusion and four venous thrombosis) of non-hemorrhagic spinal cord infarction and only two cases of hemorrhage.[311] In this older series based on patients in a neurological hospital, the common causes of vascular disease (that is, hypertension and atherosclerosis) were not found to be the etiology in any of the cases; rather, dislocation of the odontoid (one case), herniated cervical intervertebral disc (three), dissecting aortic aneurysm (one), and subacute necrotic myelitis secondary to thrombosis of spinal veins (four) were found to be the causes.

A more recent study at a general hospital found 52 cases of hypoxic myelopathy among 1200 consecutive autopsies over a five-year period.[312] Furthermore, in a ten-year study from two university hospitals, 44 cases of spinal cord ischemia and infarction were reported by Cheshire et al.[313] The increasing frequency in the two more recent studies may be because they

were done in general hospitals where more patients with systemic diseases that predispose to spinal cord infarction are found and where more invasive procedures that may be complicated by spinal cord infarction take place. For example, in the study of Cheshire et al.[313] 15 of 44 patients had aortic surgery (ten) or traumatic aortic rupture (five) as the cause of spinal cord infarction. The next most common cause in their series was cardiac arrest (four patients). Other causes of spinal cord infarction include aortic dissection, hypotension, atherosclerosis, collagen vascular disease and other inflammatory/infectious diseases, diabetes, caisson disease, spondylosis, and various other invasive procedures[15,78,314–316] (Table 8–6). An interesting but rare cause of spinal cord embolization and infarction is fibrocartilaginous embolization.[317,318]

The prognosis of patients with spinal cord infarction has been summarized by Cheshire et al.[313] Among 158 patients culled from the literature, 22% died, 33% remained essentially unchanged, 25% improved, and 20% markedly improved. Among their own series of 41 patients, 20% died, 46% remained essentially unchanged, 17% improved, and 17% markedly improved.

Arterial Infarction

First described early in this century,[319] anterior spinal artery infarction is far more common than infarction in the territory of the posterior spinal artery. The anatomical distribution of anterior spinal artery infarction is shown in Chapters 1 and 2.

Patients with anterior spinal artery infarction typically develop, below the level of the lesion, acute paralysis, dissociated sensory loss, and loss of sphincter function. Symptoms develop abruptly. Radicular pain in a girdle distribution, or lower extremity pain of a throbbing, burning character is often reported to last for two or three days. Usually the motor paralysis below the level of infarction is initially flaccid and areflexic owing to spinal shock. Tendon reflexes usually return and spas-

Table 8–6. **Causes of Spinal Cord Infarction***

	Ischemic	Emboli
Heart	Hypotension Cardiac arrest	Subacute bacterial endocarditis Atrial myxoma
Aorta	Atherosclerosis Aortic surgery (with clamping) Dissecting aneurysm Coarctation of aorta	Aortic angiography Cholesterol emboli Saddle emboli Aortic trauma Intra-aortic balloon counterpulsation
Vertebra	Vertebral occlusion Vertebral dissection Sickle cell anemia Fracture and spinal dislocations	Vertebral angiography
Intercostal arteries	Thoracoplasty Coarctation operation	
Radicular arteries	Arteriosclerosis Ligation during surgery Cervical spondylosis Cervical sprain Caisson disease Plasmacytoma Reticulum cell sarcoma Lumbar sympathectomy Aneurysm artery of Adamkiewicz	Aortic emboli Spinal angiography
Anterior median spinal artery	Atherosclerosis Diabetes Syphilis Cervical disc	Aorta embolization
Sulcal arteries	Hypertensive lacunae disease Diabetes Polyarteritis nodosa Infection, TB, syphilis	Aorta embolization Renal embolization
Pial microcirculation	In association with AVM Adhesive arachnoiditis Neoplastic spread Subarachnoid hemorrhage Infective and granulomatous meningitis	Emboli from AVM

*From Buchan, AM and Barnett, HJM,[322] p. 712, with permission.

ticity may supervene. Babinski signs are usually absent initially but later develop. A sensory level is typically found at which pain and temperature are perceived, with preservation of posterior column function. Sacral sensation may be spared. Urinary retention usually occurs immediately following infarction.[320]

Anterior spinal artery infarction is most common in the thoracic area because this is the watershed area for blood flow in the rostrocaudal axis.[315] Although the classical view has been that the most vulnerable region is at the T4 level, Cheshire and colleagues[313] reported that the mean deficit in their large series was at the T8 level, and in cases of global ischemia it was at T9. A Brown-Séquard syndrome may occur if only half of the spinal cord has been infarcted.

Posterior spinal artery infarction is rare.[313,321] Damage extends into the posterior horns of the spinal cord, resulting in global anesthesia at the affected level(s).[322] Below the level of infarction, there is loss of vibratory and position sensation.

In addition to anterior and posterior spinal artery infarctions, lacunar infarctions also have been found in the spinal cords of patients with hypertension and atherosclerosis.[323] These lesions are considered the spinal counterpart to lacunae in the basal ganglia.[322] Transient ischemic attacks of the spinal cord also have been reported. These seem to be most commonly due to arteriovenous malformations that steal blood into the low-pressure AVM and away from the normal tissue.[324] The symptoms may also be due to compression of the spinal cord when the AVM distends.[322]

Venous Infarction

Venous infarction of the spinal cord may be either hemorrhagic or nonhemorrhagic. Although venous infarction may occur in the setting of severe systemic disease, such as sepsis or carcinomatosis, many patients have an associated vascular malformations.[322,325,326] In the decompression sickness of scuba divers, nitrogen bubbles may lodge in spinal veins causing venous infarction.[313,327]

The typical clinical presentation of a hemorrhagic venous infarction is sudden onset of back, leg, or abdominal pain, evolving over one to two days to progressive flaccid weakness and loss of sensation below the level of the hemorrhagic infarction, and loss of sphincter function.[325] Because venous hemorrhagic infarction does not respect the distribution of the anterior spinal artery alone, the sensory loss is usually not that of a dissociated sensory disturbance. Nonhemorrhagic venous infarction of the spinal cord may have a subacute evolution consisting of painless progressive lower extremity weakness, sphincter disturbance, and sensory loss below the level of the lesion.[328] Unlike hemorrhagic venous infarction, reported cases of nonhemorrhagic venous infarction have been at T3 or below.[322]

Laboratory Evaluation of Vascular Diseases

As emphasized above, vascular diseases of the spinal cord are sufficiently unusual that other diseases, such as compressive lesions and inflammatory disorders, must be considered first. An MRI excludes extramedullary compressive lesions and can provide anatomical information concerning both the spinal cord and extramedullary tissues.[329] A CT scan has value in detecting hematomas and vertebral fractures. Cheshire et al.[313] found that, acutely, MRI could be normal in spinal cord stroke with profound neurologic deficit. After several days, MRI often shows cord swelling and enhancement and abnormal signal in adjacent vertebral bodies. Months or years later, MRI may reveal cord atrophy. In some cases myelography in the prone and supine positions or spinal arteriography is needed to diagnose arteriovenous malformations.[313]

Evaluation of CSF is useful to exclude inflammatory conditions (both infectious and noninfectious) and demyelinating disease. The CSF in vascular disease of the spinal cord may demonstrate a nonspecific elevation of protein and pleocytosis. A careful systemic workup for associated conditions, such as underlying neoplastic disease, infection, or collagen vascular disease, should be performed when clinically indicated.

AUTOIMMUNE DISEASES

The spinal cord may be the target of a variety of systemic autoimmune diseases, which by their very nature demonstrate a predilection for multiorgan injury. Among others, Sjogren's syndrome, sytemic lupus erythematosus, rheumatoid arthritis, polyarteritis nodosa, Wegener's granulomatosis, lymphomatoid granulomatosis, Takayasu's arteritis, isolated angiitis of the CNS, spinal cord arteritis, giant cell (temporal) arteritis, Behcet's disease, and progressive systemic sclerosis have been reported to involve the CNS.[330–335] Injury of the central and/or the peripheral nervous system may herald the onset of the disease; in such cases, involvement of the brain, the peripheral nervous system, or both may dominate the neurological manifestations. In many cases, there is already evidence of a systemic vasculitis. Rarely, the spinal cord may be the sole manifestation of systemic arteritis. Isolated spinal cord arteritis may rarely be seen in association with heroin addiction.[335] The reader is referred to review articles and textbooks of rheumatology and internal medicine for a more detailed discussion of autoimmune disorders.[334,336]

Sjogren's Syndrome

Sjogren's syndrome is an autoimmune disease that is believed to affect approximately 2% of the population.[337] It characteristically involves the lacrimal and salivary glands, resulting in xerophthalmia and xerostomia. Multiple visceral organs also may be involved, including the central and peripheral nervous system.[330,338]

The prevalence of central nervous system involvement in patients with Sjogren's syndrome is controverial.[339–341] One study[337] reported that approximately 20% of patients with primary Sjogren's syndrome developed CNS involvement. Other studies have reported 2%–12% CNS involvement.[342–344] In such cases, episodic multifocal involvement of the brain and spinal cord may evolve over time. Thus, the presentation of such patients may mimic the clinical course for multiple sclerosis. In addition to cerebral, brain-stem, and cerebellar disturbances, patients may demonstrate an acute or subacute transverse myelopathy, chronic progressive myelopathy, neurogenic bladder, or other spinal cord syndromes.[345] In the study reported by Alexander above,[337] the spinal cord was involved in 85% of cases with CNS involvement; however, in other studies, myelopathy has been rare.[346] In other cases, there is an abrupt onset of pain and myelopathy suggesting a vascular etiology, as described below.

The CSF findings in patients with Sjogren's syndrome and CNS involvement mimic those found in patients with multiple sclerosis.[337] For example, there may be CSF pleocytosis, oligoclonal bands, and elevated IgG indices. In fact, even among patients without clinical neurologic impairment the CSF may show oligoclonal bands.[347] Evoked responses may also be abnormal at multiple sites, as is typically seen with demyelinating diseases.[337] An MRI of the spinal cord and brain also may demonstrate abnormalities similar to those seen in multiple sclerosis.[337,339,348] Although the pathogenesis of CNS involvement is uncertain, an immune vasculopathy has been considered.[330] In two autopsied cases of myelopathy, necrotizing angiitis and necrosis of the spinal cord were reported.[349,350]

The diagnosis of CNS involvement by Sjogren's syndrome may be difficult if the underlying disease has not been recognized. Involvement of multiple organs such as salivary and lacrimal glands, lungs, kidneys, thyroid, muscle, and peripheral nerves may suggest the diagnosis and help distinguish the disease from multiple sclerosis.[330,337] Furthermore, the presence of antibodies to Ro(SS-A) or La(SS-B), and other serologic abnormalities, are often found in these patients.[351] Although there are limited reports of therapy, case reports of responses to plasmapharesis and/or corticosteroids do exist.[345,349]

CASE ILLUSTRATION

A 54-year-old woman with a past medical history significant for discoid lupus and Raynaud's phenomenon developed neck pain and pain radiating into the left arm when her neck was hyperextended during a shampoo. An orthopedic consultation found a left C6 radiculopathy, and she was placed in a cervical collar. Two weeks later, she developed numbness of the left lower face and ascending numbness beginning in the left lower extremity which then extended into the right leg and later ascended up through the trunk to the ulnar aspect of both hands, forearms, and axillae. She was admitted to the hospital for evaluation.

General physical examination was unremarkable. Neurological examination demonstrated slight hyperpathia over the second and third divisions of the left fifth cranial nerve. Hyperpathia and causalgia were present bilaterally from the first thoracic segment caudally, with preservation of temperature and position sensation. On extension of the neck, dysesthesias appeared in the lower back. Motor, cerebellar, and gait examinations were normal. There was a depressed left brachioradialis reflex and plantar responses were flexor.

Laboratory studies revealed a sedimentation rate of 40 and a positive antinuclear antibody (ANA) with a titer of 1:128 consisting of a diffuse and nucleolar pattern. The CSF revealed normal cell count, protein, and glucose, and the IgG index was normal. There were two faint oligoclonal bands in the CSF, which were also present in the serum. Cervical spine film showed narrowing of the disc space at the C5–6 level. An MRI (0.15 teslas) of the brain and cervical spine showed an equivocal small linear periventricular hyperintensity in the left parietal area of unknown significance and compression of the spinal cord at the C5–6 level due to disc protrusion and spondylosis. Triple-evoked responses, including somatosensory latencies from the upper and lower extremities, were normal. Rheumatological consultation revealed no evidence for systemic lupus erythematosus or autoimmune illness involving the CNS. A neurosurgical opinion was obtained and although the presentation was considered atypical, a tentative diagnosis of spinal cord compression and cervical radiculopathy was made, and the patient was discharged with a soft cervical collar.

Five days later, she was readmitted with progressive right leg weakness and a right Babinski sign but no evidence of left leg weakness. She had pain in both hands and forearms and dysesthesias and reduced pin sensation below the C7 level bilaterally. A myelogram demonstrated congenital spinal stenosis with superimposed spinal cord compression at the C5–6 level due to disc protrusion and spondylosis, with bilateral foraminal encroachment at the same level. Repeat MRI of the brain showed no evidence of the previously seen area of hyperintensity in the left parietal area. The clinical presentation was considered atypical for cervical spondylosis but in the absence of a definitive alternative diagnosis and concern that the spinal cord compression could be responsible, the patient underwent an anterior cervical discectomy and fusion of C5–6.

Postoperatively, the patient's myelopathy was significantly improved but she continued to complain of progressive sensory disturbances of the upper extremities and described a progressive, tight, girdle-like sensation in the chest. A repeat MRI of the brain and cervical spine four months postoperatively demonstrated several areas of hyperintensity in both cerebral hemispheres and no evidence of spinal cord compression. Electrodiagnostic studies of the upper extremities demonstrated no evidence of peripheral neuropathy or denervation. Somatosensory-evoked responses of the upper extremities revealed conduction disturbances within the cervical spinal cord.

Over the next several weeks, the patient developed progressive position sense disturbances of the hands with secondary pseudo-athetoid movements. A repeat rheumatological evaluation included serological studies for Sjogren's syndrome, the results of which were positive. A biopsy of minor salivary glands was interpreted as consistent with this diagnosis. The patient was placed on a course of steroids and cyclophosphamide for several months with clinical stabilization of her neurological syndrome. However, MRI continued to show evidence of evolving subclinical cerebral lesions.

Comment. This case illustrates the frequent difficulty of differentiating intramedullary spinal cord disease from spinal cord compression. Although this patient did have spinal cord compression secondary to cervical spondylosis, which may have aggravated the intramedullary spinal cord disease, the latter was primarily responsible for her neurological condition, as ultimately shown by her clinical course. Only with continued close observation and the recognition at the time of surgery that the spondylosis alone might not have been completely responsible for her neurological condition was the diagnosis of neurological involvement by Sjogren's syndrome made. The case also illustrates that a systemic disease such as Sjogren's syndrome may present clinically with spinal cord dysfunction alone.

Systemic Lupus Erythematosus

Systemic lupus erythematosus (SLE) is typically a systemic disease with multiorgan involvement. In occasional patients, however, the CNS is the principal site of clinical involvement, with minimal evidence of skin or articular disease.[352] Furthermore, although much less common than cerebral and brainstem involvement, myelopathy has been well documented as a complication of SLE.[316,353-355]

Among patients with SLE, myelopathy may occur in an acute or subacute fashion.[356] In 26 cases of transverse myelopathy in the setting of SLE,[357] the myelopathy, which could occur at any time during the course of SLE, evolved rapidly in the majority of cases. A sensory level, sphincter disturbance, and paresis or paralysis below the lesion were commonplace. In cases which resemble an anterior artery syndrome, the posterior columns are spared. The antiphospholipid antibody has been found in some such cases, raising the question of whether it is responsible for the pathogenesis of the myelopathy, but this is unproven.[358,359] On pathological examination, extensive destruction of the thoracic and lumbar segments was usually seen, with angiitis and thrombosis of blood vessels secondary to SLE. Prognosis for recovery with this form of myelopathy is considered to be poor.[316]

Other cases of myelopathy in patients with SLE may resemble subacute transverse myelopathy.[316,360,361] As in other cases of transverse myelopathy, the pathogenesis of those cases associated with SLE is unknown.[316]

Occasionally, myelopathy in the setting of SLE may clinically resemble multiple sclerosis.[316,352,362] In such cases, there may be a subacute progressive myelopathy. Furthermore, the patient may show improvement in neurological function, as in some bouts of multiple sclerosis. Patients with SLE also have been reported to develop a necrotic and demyelinative myelopathy and demyelinative optic neuritis.[14,316]

In evaluating patients with systemic lupus erythematosus and myelopathy, spinal cord imaging is important to exclude compressive lesions. In cases of intrinsic cord disease attributed to SLE, MRI may show focal areas of cord edema and T2 signal changes, which have been reported to improve with clinical recovery.[354] The CSF may show oligoclonal bands such as those that occur in multiple sclerosis. In a study of 25 cases of SLE with neurological involvement, 28% had local CNS synthesis of oligoclonal bands.[363] Other studies have shown even higher prevalence of increased intrathecal IgG synthesis rates.[363,364] Reports of successful treatment of lupus myelopathy have been limited, but include treatment with high-dose corticosteroids and other forms of immunosuppression.[365,366]

PARANEOPLASTIC MYELOPATHY

Paraneoplastic myelopathy refers to spinal cord disease in patients with malignancy, where the myelopathy is not due to compression from tumor, effects of treatment, metabolic or electrolyte imbalance, or identifiable disease unrelated to the malignancy (e.g., spondylosis, vitamin B_{12} deficiency)[367] (Table 8–7). Paraneoplastic myelopathies must be considered in the cancer patient with a progressive myelopathy for which no alternative cause is discovered.[286]

Table 8–7. Classification of Spinal Cord Lesions in Cancer Patients

Metastatic Cancer
Epidural
Leptomeningeal
Intramedullary

Toxicity from Therapy
Radiation myelopathy
Myelopathy due to chemotherapy
Infectious disease
Vascular disease
Paraneoplastic syndromes
Diseases unrelated to cancer or its therapy

First described by Mancall and Remedios,[326] the etiology and pathogenesis of paraneoplastic myelopathies is unknown.[368] On pathological examination of the spinal cord, necrotizing myelopathy is characterized by nearly symmetric necrosis involving both gray and white matter.[369] Both myelin sheaths and axons are involved, and there is a predilection for the thoracic spinal cord.[368] Vascular necrotic changes also may be seen, but pathological changes within the spinal cord are not characteristic of ischemic myelopathy.[78]

The clinical picture of paraneoplastic necrotizing myelopathy is that of a rapidly ascending sensorimotor myelopathy. The course is typically short, with death ensuing within a few months.[368] Paraneoplastic myelopathy has most frequently occurred in the setting of a variety of carcinomas and lymphoma.[368] As discussed in Chapter 6, the diagnosis may be difficult to distinguish from intramedullary metastasis, radiation myelopathy, and other diseases because there is no specific laboratory test for paraneoplastic myelopathy. Its rarity compared with the frequent incidence of metastatic disease to the spine or complications of therapy should be recognized by the clinician when this diagnosis is considered.[368]

NEURONAL DEGENERATIONS

There are several neuronal degenerations that may involve the spinal cord, and they thus are considered in the differential diagnosis of spinal cord compression. Some of these disorders are genetic in origin (Table 8–8), and others are of unknown

Table 8–8. **Some Neuronal Degenerations of Genetic Origin**

Spinocerebellar ataxia (Friedreich's ataxia)
Hereditary motor neuron disease
Werdnig-Hoffmann disease
Hereditary spastic paraplegia
Charcot-Marie-Tooth disease
Adrenomyeloneuropathy

etiology and pathogenesis (e.g., motor neuron disease).

The clinical presentations of most of these disorders share several features. Most begin insidiously and are slowly progressive. In those cases of genetic origin, patients may report a history of clumsiness or inability to compete in athletics or perform in the military at an early age. Other signs, such as pes cavus and scoliosis, may precede the clinical presentation. A family history of neurological disease may be obtained. Unlike the case of spinal cord compression, pain is not usually a prominent early feature. Symptoms and signs of involvement of the brain and/or peripheral nerves are frequently encountered, if carefully sought. There may be other signs of systemic involvement, such as heart disease in patients with Friedreich's ataxia or endocrine disturbance in those with adrenomyeloneuropathy. The reader is referred to textbooks of neurology and other sources for a complete discussion.

ACUTE AND SUBACUTE TRANSVERSE MYELOPATHY OF UNKNOWN ETIOLOGY

Despite exhaustive attempts to diagnose the etiology and pathogenesis of acute or subacute noncompressive transverse myelopathy, there are still cases in which no specific diagnosis can be made at the time of clinical presentation. This has led to the concept of noncompressive transverse myelopathy (TM), which is defined as a clinical syndrome of bilateral intramedullary dysfunction which may be ascending or static and often involves several spinal segmental levels; the syndrome occurs without prior history of neurological disease.[3] *Because there is usually no specific laboratory test for transverse myelopathy, the diagnosis of noncompressive TM is often a clinical one after the exclusion of known (and often treatable) causes such as cord compression secondary to neoplasm, abscess, or degenerative joint disease.*

Because, by definition, the etiology of TM is unknown, the neuropathological processes which are discussed earlier in this chapter and elsewhere in this book need to be considered and excluded, such as: postinfectious and postvaccination myelitis, multiple sclerosis, and acute necrotizing myelitis; viral invasion of the spinal cord; spinal cord infarction; radiation myelopathy; vascular malformations; and paraneoplastic syndrome. Even after a clinical diagnosis of TM is made and the specific etiology and pathogenesis remain obscure the clinician should consider TM as a clinical syndrome of diverse etiologies with the expectation that ultimately the etiology may declare itself as the patient is followed.

The clinical challenge in diagnosing TM is seen in a study from the Massachusetts General Hospital.[3] Of 164 patients presenting with acute myelopathy or myelitis, 82 were ultimately found to have an anatomical mass lesion (usually metastatic cancer) responsible for the myelopathy. Because many of the patients reviewed had been initially diagnosed as having TM but were later found to have tumors impinging on the spinal cord, the researchers would only include in their study those patients who had undergone a myelogram to exclude a compressive lesion. This study underscores the necessity to exclude compressive lesions of the cord that are treatable before a diagnosis of TM is made.

The clinical features of 52 patients with TM have been reported in detail.[3] The age at diagnosis ranged from 4 to 83 years and there was no sex preponderance. A recent acute infectious illness was reported to antedate the onset of TM in one-third of patients. (Some of these patients might now be classified as postinfectious demyelinating disease.) The initial symptoms are shown in Table 8–9. In some patients, these symptoms occurred in combination. Paresthesias often began distally and ascended. When pain was the presenting complaint, it usually occurred at the segmental level of neurological dysfunction. The temporal profile of the myelopathy varied in these 52 patients; 21% of the patients developed a myelopathy within 12 hours, 69% progressed smoothly over a period of 1 to 14 days, and 10% had a stuttering progressive

Table 8–9. **Summary of Clinical Data from 52 Patients with Acute and Subacute Noncompressive Transverse Myelopathy***

	Number (%) of Patients	
Preceding Febrile Illness	18	(35%)
Initial Symptoms		
Paresthesias	24	(46%)
Back pain	18	(35%)
Leg weakness	7	(13%)
Sphincter disturbance	3	(6%)
Time to Maximal Deficit		
<1 day	13	(25%)
1 to 10 days	30	(57%)
>10 days	9	(17%)
Multiple Sclerosis	7	(13%)
Outcome		
Good	16	(31%)
Fair	20	(38%)
Poor	12	(23%)
Total	52	

*From Ropper, AH and Poskanzer, DC,[3] p. 58, with permission.

course over a period of 10 days to 4 weeks. Spinal shock was seen in some of the patients with catastrophic onset.

The difficulty in clinically distinguishing intramedullary disease from extramedullary compressive disease has already been reviewed. In a manner similar to patients with TM, patients with epidural abscess or spinal tumor usually present with back pain and a relatively rapid neurological deterioration. Although neoplasms generally run a more chronic course than the inflammatory myelitides, spinal tumors may have a brief course. Although the history of recent infection may be helpful in a diagnosis of postinfectious myelitis, patients with epidural abscess often have a history of recent infection as well. These observations underscore the importance of a high index of suspicion for cord compression and emphasize the role of laboratory and imaging studies in differentiating compressive lesions such as epidural abscess or neoplasm from transverse myelopathy. In arriving at a diagnosis of noncompressive myelitis or myelopathy, the clinician must ask at each juncture, "Can this patient be harboring a compressive lesion?"

The optimal treatment of acute and subacute transverse myelopathy of unknown etiology remains uncertain. In the Massachusetts General Hospital series,[3] half of the patients with adequate follow-up received no specific treatment other than bed rest and analgesia as required. An equal number of patients received adrenocorticotrophic hormone or corticosteroids. If the pathogenesis of the disorder is thought to be demyelinating disease high-dose steroids have been advocated by some authors.[18a,18b] Some of the general principles involving the management of patients with myelopathy are discussed in the section on postinfectious myelitis.

The prognosis for neurological recovery following TM varies from good to poor. Factors that have been found to affect outcome include the tempo of neurological deterioration and the presence of back pain. Patients with a gradual or stuttering progressive myelopathy had a good (41%) or fair (46%) outcome in the series cited above.[3] However, a poor outcome was found in 64% of those with a rapid catastrophic onset and in 53% of those with back pain heralding the onset. Of the 52 patients, 7 (13%) were diagnosed as having multiple sclerosis on follow-up examinations.[3]

SUMMARY

There is a broad spectrum of diseases that afflict the spinal cord and are not due to cord compression. These are called intramedullary diseases. These disorders include (1) inflammatory disorders, such as multiple sclerosis and transverse myelitis; (2) infectious disorders, such as HIV, herpes zoster, or HTLV-1 infection; (3) toxic disorders, such as radiation myelopathy; (4) vitamin deficiencies, such as B_{12} deficiency; and (5) vascular diseases, such as cord infarction. Their clinical manifesta-

tions are protean. The temporal profile may occur over hours, as in the case of infarction, or months as in HTLV-1 myelopathy or B_{12} deficiency. Since biopsy is rarely performed, clinical diagnosis and management rely heavily upon clinical characteristics, associated disease processes, imaging, and CSF analyses.

For example, a patient who develops a transverse myelopathy within a few weeks of a vaccination is more likely to have the inflammatory demyelinating syndrome of transverse myelitis than an individual with a past history of optic neuritis who might be expected to have multiple sclerosis. The long-term management and implications of these two disorders for the patient is quite different. Spirochetal diseases of the spinal cord, due both to syphilis and *B. burgdorferi*, need to be considered. Furthermore, in the immunocompromised patient, opportunistic infectious are more likely to occur. Complications of therapy such as radiation myelopathy and spinal arachnoiditis are to be considered in the appropriate clinical context.

Subacute combined degeneration of the cord due to B_{12} deficiency presents a challenging clinical diagnosis. Patients may not have any hematologic abnormalities, and dominant clinical neurologic signs may suggest peripheral nerve disease or be overshadowed by dementia. Patients with B_{12} deficiency may have neuropsychiatric disturbances and inconsistent neurologic findings, leading the examiner to the erroneous conclusion that their complaints are functional. Furthermore, the diagnosis of B_{12} deficiency is complicated by the fact that some (especially elderly) patients may not be truly deficient and yet have serum levels at or just below the normal range. Other patients may have low normal levels and be, in fact, deficient as documented by measurement of serum methylmalonic acid and, more importantly, response to B_{12} administration. Accordingly, there must be a high level of clinical suspicion in order not to miss cases of this eminently treatable disorder.

Spinal cord infarction was once considered a clinical rarity. However, with the advent of more invasive technologies such as vascular surgery and embolization procedures, spinal cord infarction is more frequently seen. Other causes of spinal cord infarction and demyelination are seen in patients with autoimmune diseases such as Sjogren's syndrome, systemic lupus erythematosus, and the antiphospholipid syndrome. As has been seen in oncology, with the longer survival of these patients, it appears that the neurologic complication rate is also rising. Paraneoplastic myelopathy, a rare disorder, and neuronal degenerations, are also briefly discussed.

Finally, despite exhaustive attempts to diagnose the etiology and pathogenesis of acute and subacute transverse myelopathy, there remain a group of cases in which there is no specific diagnosis. Since the classic paper on transverse myelopathy by Ropper and Poskanzer,[3] the development of MRI, polymerase chain reaction assays, spinal neuroangiography, and other immunological tests has reduced the size of this group but has not eliminated it. As reported by Ropper and Poskanzer, the clinical features of this group are presented, but because, by definition, the etiology and pathogenesis are not known, precise prognostic or therapeutic recommendations are difficult to offer.

REFERENCES

1. Sebire G, Hollenberg H, Meyer L, et al. High dose methylprednisolone in severe acute transverse myelopathy. *Arch Dis Child* 1997;76: 167–8.
2. Harisdangkul V, Doorenbos D, Subramony S. Lupus transverse myelopathy: better outcome with early recognition and aggressive high-dose intravenous corticosteroid pulse treatment. *J Neurol* 1995;242:326–31.
3. Ropper AH, Poskanzer DC. The prognosis of acute and subacute transverse myelopathy based on early signs and symptoms. *Ann Neurol* 1978;4:51–9.
4. Booss J, Esiri MM. *Viral Encephalitis: pathology, Diagnosis and Management.* Oxford: Blackwell Scientific; 1986.
5. Adams RD, Victor M. Diseases of the spinal cord. In Adams RD, Victor M, editors. *Principles of Neurology.* New York: McGraw-Hill; 1985; pp. 665–98.
6. Miller HG, Stanton JB, Gibbons JL. Parainfectious encephalomyelitis and related syndromes: a critical review of the neurological complications of certain specific fevers. *Q J Med* 1956;25:427–505.
7. Spillane JD, Wells EC. The neurology of jennerian vaccination. *Brain* 1964;87:1.
8. Macfarlane PI, Miller V. Transverse myelitis associated with Mycoplasma pneumonia infection. *Arch Dis Child* 1984;59:80–2.
9. Johnson RT, Griffin DE, Hirsch RL, et al. Measles encephalomyelitis—clinical and immunological studies. *N Engl J Med* 1984;310: 137.
10. Miller HG, Stanton JB, Gibbons JL. Acute disseminated encephalomyelitis and related syndromes. *Br Med J* 1957;1:668–72.
11. Reik L. Disorders that mimic CNS infections. *Neurol Clin North Am* 1986;4:223–48.
12. Abramsky O, Teitelbaum D. The autoimmune features of acute transverse myelopathy. *Ann Neurol* 1977;2:36–40.
13. Reik L. Disseminated vasculomyelinopathy: an immune complex disease. *Ann Neurol* 1980;7: 291–6.
14. Croft PB. Para-infectious and post-vaccinal encephalomyelitis. *Postgrad Med* 1969;45:392–400.
15. Hughes JT. *Pathology of the Spinal Cord* Philadelphia: W.B. Saunders; 1978.
16. Choi K, Lee K, Chung S, et al. Idiopathic transverse myelitis: MR characteristics. *AJNR Am J Neuroradiol* 1996;17:1151–60.
17. Tartaglino L, Croul S, Flanders A, et al. Idiopathic transverse myelitis: MR imaging findings. *Radiology* 1996;201:661–9.
18. Provenzale J, Barboriak D, Gaensler E, et al. Lupu-related myelitis: serial MR findings. *AJNR Am J Neuroradiol* 1994;15:1911–7.
18a. Dowling P, Bosch V, Cook S. Possible beneficial effect of high-dose intravenous steroid therapy in acute demyelinating disease and transverse myelitis. *Neurology* 1980;30:33–6.
18b. Kalman B, Lublin FD. Postinfectious encephalomyelitis and transverse myelitis. In Johnson R, Griffin J, editors. *Current Therapy in Neurologic Disease.* St. Louis: B.C. Decker/ Mosby Year Book; 1997; pp. 175–8.
19. Scott T, Weikers N, Hospodar M, Wapenski J. Acute transverse myelitis: a retrospective study using magnetic resonance imaging. *Can J Neurol Sci* 1994;21:133–6.
19a. Scott T, Bhagavatula K, Snyder P, Chieffe C. Transverse myelitis: comparison with spinal cord presentations of multiple sclerosis. *Neurology* 1998;50:429–33.
20. Miller D, Ormerod I, Rudge P, et al. The early risk of multiple sclerosis following isolated acute syndromes of the brainstem and spinal cord. *Ann Neurol* 1989;26:635–9.
21. Altrocchi P. Acute transverse myelopathy. *Arch Neurol* 1963;9:21–9.
22. Peet MM, Echols DH. Herniation of the nucleus pulposus. A cause of compression of the spinal cord. *Arch Neurol Psychiat* 1934;32: 924–32.
22a. Jeffrey D, Mandler R, Davis L. Transverse myelitis: retrospective analysis of 33 cases with differentiation of cases associated with multiple sclerosis and parainfectious events. *Arch Neurol* 1993;50:532–6.

23. Paty D, Noseworthy J, Ebers G. Diagnosis of multiple sclerosis. In Paty D, Ebers G, editors. *Multiple Sclerosis*. Philadelphia: F.A. Davis; 1997; pp. 48–135.

23a. Tippett D, Fishman P, Panitch H. Relapsing transverse myelitis. *Neurology* 1991;41:703–6.

24. Paty D, Ebers G. *Muliple Sclerosis*. Philadelphia: F.A. Davis; 1998.

25. Ebers GC. Multiple sclerosis and other demyelinating diseases. In Asbury AK, McKhann GM, McDonald WI, editors. *Diseases of the Nervous System: Clinical Neurobiology*. Philadelphia: W.B. Saunders; 1986; pp. 1268–81.

26. Lumsden CE. Multiple sclerosis and other demyelinating diseases. In Vinken PJ, Bruyn GW, editors. *Handbook of Clinical Neurology, Volume 9*. Amsterdam: North-Holland; 1970; pp. 217–319.

27. Fog T. Topographic distribution of plaques in the spinal cord in multiple sclerosis. *Arch Neurol Psychiatr* 1950;63:382–414.

28. Oppenheimer DR. The cervical cord in multiple sclerosis. *Neuropathol Appl Neurobiol* 1978;4: 151–62.

29. McDonald W, Miller D, Barnes D. The pathological evolution of multiple sclerosis. *Neuropathol Appl Neurobiol* 1992;18:319–34.

30. Trapp B, Peterson J, Ransohoff R, et al. Axonal transection in the lesions of multiple sclerosis. *N Engl J Med* 1998;338:278–85.

31. Waxman S. Demyelinating diseases—new pathological insights, new therapeutic targets. *N Engl J Med* 1998;338:323–5.

32. Poser S, Hermann-Gremmeis I, Wikstrom J, Poser W. Clinical features of the spinal form of multiple sclerosis. *Acta Neurol Scand* 1978;57: 151–8.

33. Leibowitz U, Halpern L, Alter M. Clinical studies of multiple sclerosis in Israel. V. Progressive spinal syndromes and multiple sclerosis. *Neurology* 1967;17:988–92.

34. Waxman SG. Clinical course and electrophysiology of multiple sclerosis. In Waxman SG, editor. *Functional Recovery in Neurological Disease*. New York: Raven Press; 1988; pp. 151–84.

35. Marshall J. Spastic paraplegia of middle age. *Lancet* 1955;I:643–6.

36. Paty DW, Blume WT, Brown WF, et al. Chronic progressive myelopathy: investigation with CSF electrophoresis, evoked potentials, and CT scan. *Ann Neurol* 1979;6:419–24.

37. Hume AL, Waxman SG. Evoked potentials in suspected multiple sclerosis: diagnostic value and prediction of clinical course. *J Neurol Sci* 1988;83:191–210.

38. Blumhardt LD, Barrett G, Halliday AM. The pattern visual evoked potential in the clinical assessment of undiagnosed spinal cord disease. In Corjon JE, Maugiere F, Revol M, editors. *Clinical Applications of Evoked Potentials in Neurology*. New York: Raven Press; 1982; pp. 463–71.

39. Ropper AH, Miett T, Chiappa KH. Absence of evoked potential abnormalities in acute transverse myelopathy. *Neurology* 1982;32:80–2.

40. Miller DH, McDonald WI, Blumhardt LD, et al. Magnetic resonance imaging in isolated noncompressive spinal cord syndromes. *Ann Neurol* 1987;22:714–23.

41. Paty DW, Asbury AK, Herndon RM, et al. Use of magnetic resonance imaging in the diagnosis of multiple sclerosis: policy statement. *Neurology* 1986;36:1575.

42. Poser C, Paty D, Scheinberg L, et al. New diagnostic criteria for multiple sclerosis. *Ann Neurol* 1983;13:227–31.

43. Miska RM, Pojounas KW, McQuillen MP. Cranial magnetic resonance imaging in the evaluation of myelopathy of undetermined etiology. *Neurology* 1987;37:840–3.

44. McDonald W. Pathophysiology in multiple sclerosis. *Brain* 1974;97:179–96.

45. Clifford D, Trotter J. Pain in multiple sclerosis. *Arch Neurol* 1984;41:1270–2.

46. Stenager E, Knudsen L, Jensen K. Acute and chronic pain syndromes in multiple sclerosis. *Acta Neurol Scand* 1991;84:197–200.

47. Moulin D. Pain in multiple sclerosis. *Neurol Clin* 1989;7:321–31.

48. Vermote R, Ketelaer P, Carton H. Pain in multiple sclerosis: a prospective study using the McGill pain questionnaire. *Clin Neurol Neurosurg* 1986;88:87–93.

49. IFNB. Interferon beta 1-b is effective in relapsing-remitting multiple sclerosis. I. Clinical results of a multi-center, randomized, double-blind, placebo-controlled trial. *Neurology* 1993; 43:655–61.

50. IFNB. Interferon beta-1b in the treatment of multiple sclerosis: final outcome of the randomized controlled trial. *Neurology* 1995;45: 1277–85.

51. Paty D, Li D. Interferon beta-1b is effective in remitting-relapsing multiple sclerosis. II. MRI analysis results of a multicenter, randomized, double blind, placebo-controlled trial. *Neurology* 1993;43:662–7.

52. Jacobs L, Cookfair D, Rudick R, et al. Intramuscular interferon beta-1a for disease progression in relapsing multiple sclerosis (erratum in Ann Neurol 1996;40:480). *Ann Neurol* 1996;39:285–94.

53. Pozzilli C, Bastianello S, Koudriavtseva T, et al. Magnetic reonance imaging changes with recombinant human interferon-beta-1a: a short term study in remitting-relapsing multiple sclerosis. *J Neurol Neurosurg Psychiatry* 1996;61: 251–8.

54. Johnson K, Brooks B, Cohen J, et al. Copolymer 1 reduces relapse rate and improves disability in remitting-relapsing multiple sclerosis: results of a phase III multicenter, double blind placebo-controlled trial. *Neurology* 1995; 45:1268–76.

55. Bornstein M, Mille A, Slagle S, et al. A pilot trial of Cop 1 in exacerbating-remitting multiple sclerosis. *New Engl J Med* 1987;317:408–14.

56. Bornstein M, Miller A, Slagle S, et al. A placebo controlled, double blind, randomized two-center, pilot trial of Cop 1 in chronic pro-

gressive multiple sclerosis. *Neurology* 1991;41: 533–9.

57. Johnson K, et al. Extended use of glatiramer acetate (Copaxone) is well tolerated and maintains its clinical effect on multiple sclerosis relapse rate and degree of disability. *Neurology* 1998;50:701–8.

58. Barnes D, Hughes R, Morris E, et al. Randomized trial of oral and intravenous methylprednisolone in acute relapses of multiple sclerosis. *Lancet* 1997;349:902–6.

59. Fazekas F, Deisenhammer F, Strasser-Fuchs S, et al. Randomized placebo-controlled trial of monthly intravenous immunoglobulin therapy in remitting relapsing multiple sclerosis. Austrian immunoglobulin in multiple sclerosis group. *Lancet* 1997;349:589–93.

60. Sorenson P, Wanscher B, Schreiber K, et al. A double-blind, cross-over trial of intravenous immunoglobulin G in multiple sclerosis: preliminary results. *Multiple Sclerosis* 1997; 3:145–8.

61. Fazekas F, Deissenhammer F, Strasser-Fuchs S, et al. Treatment effects of monthly intravenous immunoglobulin on patients with remitting-relapsing multiple sclerosis: further analyses of the Austrian Immunoglobulin in MS study. *Multiple Sclerosis* 1997;3:137–41.

62. McAlpine D. Familial neuromyelitis optica, occurrence in identical twins. *Brain* 1939;62:227.

63. Waxman SG. The demyelinating diseases. In Rosenberg R, editor. *Clinical Neuroscience.* New York: Churchill Livingstone; 1983; pp. 609–44.

64. Tyler HR. Acute transverse myelitis. In Wyngaarden JB, Smith LH Jr, editors. *Cecil: Textbook of Medicine.* Philadelphia: W.B. Saunders; 1985; pp. 2138–9.

65. Bodian D. Histopathologic basis of clinical findings in poliomyelitis. *Am J Med* 1949;6: 563–78.

66. Johnson RT. Acute anterior poliomyelitis. In Wyngaarden JB, Smith LH Jr, editors. *Cecil: Textbook of Internal Medicine, 17th Edition.* Philadelphia: W.B. Saunders; 1985; pp. 2130–2.

67. Nathanson N, Martin JR. The epidemiology of poliomyelitis: enigmas surrounding its appearance, pathogenicity, and disappearance. *Am J Epidemiol* 1979;110:672–92.

68. Nkowane BM, Wassilak S, Orenstein WA, et al. Paralytic poliomyelitis U.S.: 1973 through 1984. *JAMA* 1987;257:1335–40.

69. Paul JR. *A History of Poliomyelitis.* New Haven: Yale University Press; 1971.

70. Robbins RC, Fox JP, Hopps HE, Horstmann DM, Quinn TC. International symposium on poliomyelitis control. *Rev Infect Dis* 1984; 6(Suppl 6):S301–601.

71. Adams RD, Victor M. Viral infections of the nervous system. In Adams RD, Victor M, editors. *Principles of Neurology.* New York: McGraw-Hill; 1985; pp. 545–68.

72. Curnen EC, Shaw EW, Melnick JL. Diseases resembling nonparalytic poliomyelitis associated with a virus pathogenic for infant mice. *JAMA* 1949;141:894–901.

73. Jarcho LW, Fred HL, Castle CH. Encephalitis and poliomyelitis in the adult due to coxsackie virus group B, type 5. *N Engl J Med* 1963; 268:235–8.

74. Lerner AM, Finland M. Coxsackie viral infections. *Arch Int Med* 1961;108:329.

75. Magoffin RL, Lennette EH, Schmidt NJ. Association of caxsackie viruses with illness resembling mild paralytic poliomyelitis. *Pediatrics* 1961;28:602–13.

76. Steigman AJ. Poliomyelitic properties of certain nonpolio viruses: enteroviruses and Heine-Medin disease. *J Mount Sinai Hosp NY* 1958;25:391–404.

77. Wadia NH, Katrak SM, Misra VP, et al. Polio-like motor paralysis associated with acute hemorrhagic conjunctivitis in an outbreak in 1981 in Bombay, India: clinical and serologic studies. *J Infect Dis* 1983;147:660–8.

78. Plum F, Olson ME. Myelitis and myelopathy. In Baker AB, Baker LH, editors. *Clinical Neurology.* Hagerstown: Harper & Row; 1973; pp. 1–52.

79. Lennette EH, Caplan GE, Magoffin RL. Mumps virus infection simulating paralytic poliomyelitis. *Pediatrics* 1960;25:788–97.

80. Mukherjee SK. Involvement of anterior horn of spinal cord in infectious mononucleosis. *Br Med J* 1965;1:1112.

81. Hurst EW, Pawan JL. Outbreak of rabies in Trinidad, without history of bites, and with symptoms of acute ascending myelitis. *Lancet* 1931;2:622–8.

82. Knutti RE. Acute ascending paralysis and myelitis due to the virus of rabies. *JAMA* 1929; 93:754–8.

83. Dalakas MC, Elder G, Hallet M, et al. A long-term follow-up study of patients with postpoliomyelitis neuromuscular symptoms. *N Engl J Med* 1986;314:959–63.

84. Hensinger RN, Ewen GDM. Congenital anomalies of the spine. In Rothman RH, Simeone FA, editors. *The Spine.* Philadelphia: W.B. Saunders; 1982; pp. 188–315.

85. Dalakas MC, Sever JL, Madden DL, et al. Late postpoliomyelitis muscular atrophy: clinical, virologic, and immunologic studies. *Rev Infect Dis* 1984;6(Suppl 2):562–7.

86. Mulder DW, Dale AJD. Spinal cord tumors and disks. In Baker AB, Baker LH, editors. *Clinical Neurology.* Hagerstown: Harper & Rowe; 1975; pp. 1–28.

87. Cashman NR, Siegel IM, Antel JP. Post-polio syndrome: a review. *Clin Prosthetics Orthotics* 1987;11:74–8.

88. Pezeshkpour GH, Dalakas MC. Long-term changes in the spinal cords of patients with old poliomyelitis. *Arch Neurol* 1988;45:505–8.

89. Cashman NR, Maselli R, Wollman R, et al. Late denervation in patients with antecedent paralytic poliomyelitis. *N Engl J Med* 1987;317: 7–12.

90. Johnson RT. Herpes zoster. In Wyngaarden JB, Smith LH Jr, editors. *Cecil: Textbook of Internal Medicine.* Philadelphia: W.B. Saunders; 1985; pp. 2128–30.

91. Hanakawa T, Hashimoto S, Kawamura J, et al. Magnetic resonance imaging in a patient with segmental zoster paresis. *Neurology* 1997;49: 631–2.

92. Barnes DW, Whitley RJ. CNS diseases associated with varicella zoster virus and herpes simplex virus infection. *Neurol Clin North Am* 1986;4:265–83.

93. Thomas JE, Howard FM. Segmental zoster paresis: a disease profile. *Neurology* 1972;22: 459–66.

94. Hogan EL, Krigman MR. Herpes zoster myelitis. *Arch Neurol* 1973;29:309–13.

95. Rose FC, Brett EM, Burston J. Zoster encephalomyelitis. *Arch Neurol* 1964;11:155–72.

96. Applebaum E, Kreps SI, Sunshine A. Herpes zoster encephalitis. *Am J Med* 1962;32:25–31.

97. deSilva S, Mark A, Gilden D, et al. Zoster myelitis: improvement with antiviral therapy in two cases. *Neurology* 1996;47:929–31.

98. Gilden D, Wright R, Schneck S, et al. Zoster sine herpete, a clinical variant. *Ann Neurol* 1994;35:530–3.

99. Mayo D, Booss J. Varicella-zoster associated neurologic disease without skin lesions. *Arch Neurol* 1989;46:313.

100. Gilden D, Beinlich B, Rubinstein E, et al. Varicella-zoster myelitis: an expanding spectrum. *Neurology* 1994;44:1818–23.

101. Engelter S, Lyrer P, Radu E, Steck A. Acute infectious disorders of the spinal cord and its roots with gadolinium-DTPA enhancement in magnetic resonance imaging. *J Neurol* 1996; 243:191–5.

102. Gilbert RW, Kim JH, Posner JB. Epidural spinal cord compression from metastatic tumor: diagnosis and treatment. *Ann Neurol* 1978;3:40–51.

103. Bleyer WA, Poplack DG. Intraventicular versus intralumbar methotrexate for central nervous system leukemia. *Med Pediatr Oncol* 1979;6:207–13.

104. Osame M, Usuku K, Izumo S. HTLV-1 associated myelopathy, a new clinical entity. *Lancet* 1986;1031–2.

105. Gessain A, Barin F, Vernant JC, et al. Antibodies to human T-lymphotropic virus type-I in patients with spastic tropical paraparesis. *Lancet* 1985;2:407–9.

106. Johnson RT, McArthur JC. Myelopathies and retroviral infections (editorial). *Ann Neurol* 1987;21:113–6.

107. Vernant JC, Maurs L, Gessain A, et al. Endemic tropical spastic paraparesis associated with human T-Lymphotropic virus type 1: a clinical and seroepidemiological study of 25 cases. *Ann Neurol* 1987;21:123–30.

108. Batson OV. The function of the vertebral veins and their role in the spread of metastases. *Ann Surg* 1940;112:138–48.

109. Osame M, Matsumoto M, Usuku K, et al. Chronic progressive myelopathy associated with elevated antibodies to human T-lymphotropic virus type 1 and adult T-cell leukemialike cells. *Ann Neurol* 1987;21:117–22.

110. Jacobson S, Raine C, Mingioli E, McFarlin D. Isolation of an HTLV-1 like retrovirus from patients with tropical spastic paraparesis. *Nature* 1988;331:540.

111. Bhagavati S, Ehrlich G, Kula RW, et al. Detection of human T-cell lymphoma/leukemia virus type I DNA and antigen in spinal fluid and blood of patients with chronic progressive myelopathy. *N Engl J Med* 1988;318:1141–7.

112. Kira J, Itoyama Y, Koyanaga Y, et al. Presence of HTLV 1 proviral DNA in the central nervous system of patients with HTLV-1 associated myelopathy. *Ann Neurol* 1992;31:39–45.

113. Nakamura T, Tsujihata M, Shirabe S, et al. Characterization of HTLV-I in a T-cell line established from a patient with myelopathy. *Arch Neurol* 1989;46:35–7.

114. Wong-Staal F, Gallo RC. Human T-lymphotropic retroviruses. *Nature* 1985;317:395–403.

115. Gessain A, Gout O. Chronic myelopathy associated with human T-lymphotropic virus type I (HTLV-I). *Ann Intern Med* 1992;117:933–46.

116. Lehky T, Fox C, Koenig S, et al. Detection of human T-lymphotropic virus Type 1 (HTLV-1) tax RNA in the central nervous system of HTLV-1-associated myelopathy/tropical spastic paraparesis patients by in situ hybridization. *Ann Neurol* 1995;37:167–75.

117. Power C, Weinshenker B, Dekaban G, et al. Pathological and molecular biological features of a myelopathy associated with HTLV-1 infection. *Can J Neurol Sci* 1991;18:352–5.

118. Tangy F, Vernant J, Coscoy L, et al. A search for human T-cell leukemia virus type 1 in the lesions of patients with tropical spastic paraparesis and polymyositis. *Ann Neurol* 1995;38: 454–60.

119. Ogata A, Nagashima K, Tashiro E, et al. MRI-pathological correlate of brain lesions in a necropsy case of HTLV-1 associated myelopathy. *J Neurol Neurosurg Psychiatry* 1993;56: 194–6.

120. Hollsberg P. Pathogenesis of chronic progressive myelopathy associated with human T-cell lymphotropic virus type 1. *Acta Neurol Scand Suppl* 1997;169:86–93.

121. Murphy E, Fridey J, Smith J, et al. HTLV-associated myelopathy in a cohort of HTLV-I and HTLV-II-infected blood donors. *Neurology* 1997;48:315–20.

122. Gout O, Baulac, Gessain A, et al. Rapid development of myelopathy after HTLV-1 infection acquired by transfusion during cardiac transplantation. *N Engl J Med* 1990;322:383–9.

123. Levin M, Jacobson S. HTLV-1 associated myelopathy/tropical spastic paraparesis (HAM/TSP): a chronic progressive neurologic disease associated with immunologically mediated damage to the central nervous system. *J Neurovirol* 1997;3:126–40.

124. Puccioni-Sohler M, Rieckmann P, Kitze B, et al. A soluble form of tumor necrosis factor receptor in cerebrospinal fluid and serum of human T-lymphotropic virus type 1 associated myelopathy and other neurological diseases. *J Neurol* 1995;242:239–42.

125. Robert-Guroff M, Weiss SH, Giron JA, et al. Prevalence and antibodies to HTLV-I, -II, -III

in intravenous drug abusers from an AIDS epidemic region. *JAMA* 1986;255:3133–7.

126. Rosenblum M, Brew B, Hahn B, et al. Human T-lymphotropic virus type 1-associated myelopathy in patients with acquired immunodeficiency syndrome. *Hum Pathol* 1992;23: 513–9.

127. Lehky T, Flerlage N, Katz D, et al. Human T-cell lymphotropic virus type II-associated myelopathy: clinical and immunologic profiles. *Ann Neurol* 1996;40:714–23.

128. Newton M, Criuckshank K, Miller D, et al. Antibodies to human T-cell lymphotropic virus Type 1 in West Indian-born UK residents with spastic paraparesis. *Lancet* 1987.415–6.

129. Godoy A, Kira J, AHasuo K, Goto I. Characterization of cerebral white matter lesions of HTLV-1-associated myelopathy/tropical spastic paraparesis in comparison with multiple sclerosis and collagen-vasculitis: a semiquantitative MRI study. *J Neurol Sci* 1995;133: 102–11.

130. Kuroda Y, Matsui M, Yukitake M, et al. Assessment of MRI criteria for MS in Japanese MS and HAM/TSP. *Neurology* 1995;45:30–3.

131. Moritoyo H, Arimura K, Arimura Y, et al. Study of lower limb somatosensory evoked potentials in 96 cases of HTLV-1-associated myelopathy/tropical spastic paraparesis. *J Neurol Sci* 1996;138:78–81.

132. Nakagawa M, Nakahara K, Maruyama M, et al. Therapeutic trials in 200 patients with HTLV-1-associated myelopathy/tropical spastic paraparesis. *J Neurovirol* 1996;2:345–55.

133. Goldstick L, Mandybur TI, Bode R. Spinal cord degeneration in AIDS. *Neurology* 1985; 35:103–6.

134. Grafe MR, Wiley CA. Spinal cord and peripheral nerve pathology in AIDS: the roles of cytomegalovirus abd human immunodeficiency virus. *Ann Neurol* 1989;25:561–6.

135. McArthur JC, Johnson RT. Primary infection with human immunodeficiency virus. In Rosenblum ML, Levy RM, Bredesen DE, editors. *AIDS and the Nervous System*. New York: Raven Press; 1988; pp. 183–202.

137. Snider WD, Simpson DM, Nielsen S, et al. Neurological complications of acquired immune deficiency syndrome: analysis of 50 patients. *Ann Neurol* 1983;14:403–18.

138. Tan S, Guiloff R, Scaravilli F. AIDS-associated vacuolar myelopathy. A morphometric study. *Brain* 1995;118:1247–61.

139. Levy JA, Shimabukuro J, Hollander H, et al. Isolation of AIDS associated retroviruses from cerebrospinal fluid and brain of patients with neurological symptoms. *Lancet* 1985;2: 586–8.

140. Levy R, Bredesen DE. Central nervous system dysfunction in acquired immunodeficiency syndrome. In Rosenblum ML, Levy RM, Bredesen DE, editors. *AIDS and the Nervous System*. New York: Raven Press; 1988; pp. 29–63.

141. Rosenblum M, Scheck AC, Cronin K, et al. Dissociation of AIDS-related vacuolar myelopathy and productive human immunodeficiency virus type 1 (HIV-1) infection of the spinal cord. *Neurology* 1989;39:892–6.

142. Kamin S, Petito C. Idiopathic myelopathies with white matter vacuolation in non-acquired immunodeficiency syndrome patients. *Hum Pathol* 1991;22:816–24.

143. Tyor W, Glass J, Baumrind N, et al. Cytokine expression of macrophages in HIV-1-associated vacuolar myelopathy. *Neurology* 1993;43: 1002–9.

144. Tan S, Guiloff R, Henderson D, et al. AIDS-associated vacuolar myelopathy and tumor necrosis factor-alpha (TNFalpha). *J Neurol Sci* 1996;138:134–44.

145. Tyor W, Wesselingh S, Griffin J, et al. Unifying hypothesis for the pathogenesis of HIV-associated dementia complex, vacuolar myelopathy and senssory neuropathy. *J Acquir Immun Defic Syndr Hum Retrovirol* 1995;9:379–88.

146. Petito CK, Navia BA, Cho E-S, et al. Vacuolar myelopathy pathologically resembling subacute combined degeneration in patients with acquired immunodeficiency syndrome. *N Engl J Med* 1985;312:874–9.

147. Silver B, McAvoy K, Mikesell S, Smith T. Fulminating encephalopathy with perivenular demyelination and vacuolar myelopathy as the initial presentation of human immunodeficiency virus infection. *Arch Neurol* 1997;54: 647–50.

148. Berger J, Bender A, Resnick L, Perlmutter D. Spinal myoclonus associated with HTLV 111/LAV infection. *Arch Neurol* 1986;43: 1203–4.

149. Berger J, Tornatore C, Major E, et al. Relapsing and remitting human immunodeficiency virus-associated leukoencephalopathy. *Ann Neurol* 1992;31:34–8.

150. Santosh C, Bell J, Best J. Spinal tract pathology in AIDS: postmortem MRI correlation with neuropathology. *Neuroradiology* 1995;37: 134–8.

151. Rosenblum ML, Levy RM, Bredesen DE. *AIDS and the Nervous System* New York: Raven Press; 1988.

152. Britton DB, Mesa-Tejada R, Fenoglio CM, et al. A new complication of AIDS: thoracic myelitis caused by herpes simplex virus. *Neurology* 1985;35:1071–4.

153. Klastersky J, Cappel R, Snoeck JM. Ascending myelitis in association with herpes simplex virus. *N Engl J Med* 1972;287:182–4.

154. Morgello S, Cho E-S, Nielsen S, et al. Cytomegalovirus encephalitis in patients with acquired immunodeficiency syndrome. *Hum Pathol* 1987;18:289–97.

155. Tucker T, Dix RD, Katzen C, et al. Cytomegalovirus and herpes simplex virus ascending myelitis in a patient with acquired immunodeficiency syndrome. *Ann Neurol* 1985; 18:74–9.

156. Kim Y, Hollander H. Polyradiculopathy due to cytomegalovirus: report of two cases in which improvement occurred after prolonged therapy and review of the literature. *Clin Infect Dis* 1993;17:32–7.

157. Cohen B, McArthur J, Grohman S, et al. Neurologic prognosis of cytomegalovirus polyradicu-

lomyelopathy in AIDS. *Neurology* 1993;43: 493–9.

158. Vinters H, Kwok M, Ho H, et al. Cytomegalovirus in the nervous system of patients with the acquired immunodeficiency syndrome. *Brain* 1989;112:245–68.

159. deGans J, Portegies P, Tiessens G, et al. Therapy for cytomegalovirus polyradiculomyelitis in patients with AIDS. *AIDS* 1990;4:421–5.

160. Fuller G, Gill S, Guiloff R, et al. Ganciclovir for lumbosacral polyradiculopathy in AIDS. *Lancet* 1990;335:48–9.

161. McCutchan J. Clinical impact of cytomegalovirus infections of the nervous system in patients with AIDS. *Clin Infect Dis* 1995; 21(Suppl 2):S196–201.

162. Herskowitz S, Siegel S, Schneider A, et al. Spinal cord toxoplasmosis in AIDS. *Neurology* 1989;39:1552.

163. Woolsey RM, Chambers TJ, Chung HD, McGarry JD. Mycobacterial meningomyelitis associated with human immunodeficiency virus infection. *Arch Neurol* 1988;45:691–3.

164. Melhem E, Wang H. Intramedullary spinal cord tuberculoma in a patient with AIDS. *Am J Neuroradiol* 1992;13:986–8.

165. Poon T, Tchertkoff V, Pares G, et al. Spinal cord toxoplasma lesion in AIDS: MR findings. *J Comput Assist Tomogr* 1992;16:817–9.

166. Mehren M, Burns PJ, Mamani F, et al. Toxoplasmic myelitis mimicking intramedullary spinal cord tumor. *Neurology* 1988;38:1648–50.

167. Berger J. Spinal cord syphilis associated with human immunodeficiency virus infection: a treatable myelopathy. *Am J Med* 1992;92: 101–3.

168. Devinsky O, Cho E, Petito C, Price R. Herpes zoster myelitis. *Brain* 1991;114(Part 3): 1181–96.

169. Chetrien F, Gray F, Lescs M, et al. Acute varicella-zoster virus ventriculitis and meningo-myelo-radiculitis in AIDS. *Acta Neuropathol* 1993;86:659–65.

170. Bermudez MA, Grant KM, Rodvien R, Mendes F. Non-Hodgkin's lymphoma in a population with or at risk for acquired immunodeficiency syndrome: indications for intensive chemotherapy. *Am J Med* 1989;86:71–6.

171. Hochberg FH, Miller DG. Primary central nervous system lymphoma. Review article. *J Neurosurg* 1988;68:835–53.

172. Jordan KG. Modern neurosyphilis—a critical analysis. *West J Med* 1988;149:47–57.

173. Lukehart SA, Hooker EW, Baker-Zander SA, et al. Invasion of the central nervous system by Treponema pallidum: implications for diagnosis and therapy. *Ann Intern Med* 1988;109: 855–62.

174. Merritt HH, Adams RD, Solomon HC. *Neurosyphilis.* New York: Oxford University Press; 1946.

175. Adams RD, Victor M. Nonviral infections of the nervous system. In Adams RD, Victor M, editors. *Principles of Neurology.* New York: McGraw-Hill; 1985; pp. 510–44.

176. Musher DM. How much penicillin cures syphilis? (editorial). *Ann Intern Med* 1988;109: 849–51.

177. Davis LE, Schmitt JW. Clinical significance of cerebrospinal fluid tests for neurosyphilis. *Ann Neurol* 1989;25:50–5.

178. Pachner AR. Spirochetal diseases of the CNS. *Neurol Clin North Am* 1986;4:207–22.

179. Simon RP. Neurosyphilis. *Arch Neurol* 1985;42: 606–13.

180. Bleyer WA, Byrne TN. Leptomeningeal cancer in leukemia and solid tumors. *Curr Probl Cancer* 1988;12:185–238.

181. Hook E. Syphilis. In Scheld W, Whitley R, Durack D, editors. *Infections of the Central Nervous System.* Philadelphia: Lippincott-Raven; 1997; pp. 669–84.

182. CDC. 1989 Sexually transmitted diseases treatment guidelines. *MMWR Morb Mortal Wkly Rep* 1989;38(Suppl 8):9.

183. Steere AC, Broderick TF, Malawista SE. Erythema chronicum migrans and Lyme arthritis: epidemiologic evidence for a tick vector. *Am J Epidemiol* 1978;108:312–21.

184. Steere AC, Grodzicki RL, Kornblatt AN, et al. The spirochetal etiology of Lyme disease. *N Engl J Med* 1983;308:733–40.

185. Steere AC, Malawista SE, Bartenhagen NH, et al. The clinical spectrum and treatment of Lyme disease. *Yale J Biol Med* 1984;57:453–61.

186. Pachner AR, Duray P, Steere AC. Central nervous system manifestations of Lyme disease. *Arch Neurol* 1989;46:790–5.

187. Reik L, Steere AC, Bartenhagen NH, Shope RE, Malawista SE. Neurologic abnormalities of Lyme disease. *Medicine* 1979;58:281–94.

188. Luft BJ, Steinman CR, Neimark HC, et al. Invasion of the central nervous system by Borrelia burgdorferi in acute disseminated infection. *JAMA* 1992;267:1364–7.

189. Reik L. Lyme disease. In Scheld W, Whitley R, Durack D, editors. *Infections of the Central Nervous System.* Philadelphia: Lippincott-Raven; 1997; pp. 685–718.

190. Finkel MF. Lyme disease and its neurological complications. *Arch Neurol* 1988;45:99–104.

191. Coyle PK. Borrelia burgdorferi antibodies in multiple sclerosis patients. *Neurology* 1989;39: 760–1.

192. Halperin JJ, Luft BJ, Anand AK, et al. Lyme neuroborreliosis: central nervous system manifestations. *Neurology* 1989;39:753–9.

193. Logigian EL, Kaplan RE, Steere AC. Chronic neurologic manifestations of Lyme disease. *N Eng J Med* 1990;323:1438–44.

194. Rousseau JJ, Lust C, Zangerle PF, Bigaignon G. Acute transverse myelitis as presenting neurological feature of Lyme disease. *Lancet* 1986; II:1222–3.

195. Christen H, Hanefeld FJ, Eiffert H, Thomssen R. Epidemiology and clinical manifestations of Lyme borreliosis in childhood: a prospective multicentre study with special regard to neuroborreliosis. *Acta Paediatr (Suppl)* 1993;386: 1–76.

196. Hansen K, Lebech A. The clinical and epidemiological profile of Lyme neuroborreliosis in Denmark 1985–1990: a prospective study of 187 patients with Borrelia burgdorferi specific intrathecal antibody production. *Brain* 1992; 115:399–423.
197. Steere A, Berardi V, Weeks K, et al. Evaluation of the intrathecal antibody response to Borrelia burgdorferi as a diagnostic test for Lyme neuroborreliosis. *J Infect Dis* 1990;161:1203–9.
198. Hammers-Berggren S, Hansen K, Lebach A, Karlsson M. Borrelia burgdorferi-specific intrathecal antibody production in neuroborreliosis: a follow-up study. *Neurology* 1993;43:169–75.
199. Nocton J, Bloom B, Rutledge B, et al. Detection of Borrelia burgdorferi DNA by polymerase chain reaction in cerebrospinal fluid in Lyme neuroborreliosis. *J Infect Dis* 1996;174:623–7.
200. Schoen RT. Lyme Disease. In Rakel RE, editor. *Conn's Current Therapy*. Philadelphia: W.B. Saunders; 1989; pp. 866–9.
201. Chaduri RN. Paralytic disease caused by contamination with tricresyl phosphate. *Trans R Soc Trop Med Hyg* 1965;59:98.
202. Smith HV, Spalding JMK. Outbreak of paralysis in Morocco due to ortho-cresyl phosphate poisoning. *Lancet* 1959;2:1019–21.
203. Aring CD. The systemic nervous affinity of tri-orthocresyl phosphate (Jamaica ginger palsy). *Brain* 1942;65:34–47.
204. Killen DA, Foster JH. Spinal cord injury as a complication of aortography. *Ann Surg* 1960;152:211–30.
205. Killen DA, Foster JH. Spinal cord injury as a complication of contrast angiography. *Surgery* 1966;59:969–81.
206. Abeshouse BA, Tiongson AT. Paraplegia, a rare complication of translumbar aortography. *J Urol* 1956;75:348.
207. Roman GC, Spencer PS, Schoenberg BS. Tropical myeloneuropathies: the hidden endemias. *Neurology* 1985;35:1158–70.
208. Adams RD, Victor M. Disorders of the nervous system due to drugs and other chemical agents. In Adams RD, Victor M, editors. *Principles of Neurology*. New York: McGraw-Hill; 1985; pp. 826–58.
209. Dastur DK. Lathyrism. Some aspects of the disease in man and animals. *World Neurol* 1962;3:721–30.
210. Siegal S. Transverse myelopathy following recovery from pneumococcic meningitis treated with penicillin intrathecally: report of a case with note on current methods of therapy. *JAMA* 1945;129:547–50.
211. Sweet KK, Dumont-Stanley E, Dowling HF, Lepper MH. The treatment of pneumococcic meningitis with penicillin. *JAMA* 1945;127:263–7.
212. Walker AE. Toxic effects of intrathecal administration of penicillin. *AMA Arch Neurol Psychiat* 1947;58:39–45.
213. Evans JP, Keegan HR. Danger in the use of intrathecal methylene blue. *JAMA* 1960;174:856–9.
214. Schultz P, Scwarz GA. Radiculomyelopathy following intrathecal instillation of methylene blue. *Arch Neurol* 1970;22:240–4.
215. Davis L, Haven H, Givens JH, Emmett J. Effects of spinal anesthetics on the spinal cord and its membranes: experimental study. *JAMA* 1931;97:1781–5.
216. Dripps RD, Vandam LD. Long-term follow-up of patients who received 10,098 spinal anesthetics: failure to discover major neurological sequelae. *JAMA* 1954;156:1486–91.
217. Paddison RM, Alpers BJ. Role of intrathecal detergents in pathogenesis of adhesive arachnoiditis. *AMA Arch Neurol Psychiat* 1954;71:87–100.
218. Thorsen G. Neurological complications after spinal anesthesia and results from 2,493 follow-up cases. *Acta Chir Scand* 1947;95(Suppl 121).
219. Pendergrass EP, Schaeffer JP, Hodes PJ. *The Head and Neck in Roentgen Diagnosis, 2nd Edition*. Springfield, IL: C.C. Thomas; 1956.
220. Winkelman NW. Neurological symptoms following accidental intraspinal detergent injection. *Neurology* 1952;2:284.
221. Kamman GR, Baker AB. Damage to the spinal cord and meninges following spinal anesthesia: a clinico-pathological study. *Minn Med* 1943;26:786–91.
222. Kennedy F, Effron AS, Perry G. The grave spinal cord paralyses caused by spinal anesthesia. *Surg Gynecol Obstet* 1950;91:385–98.
223. Adams RD, Kubik CS. The morbid anatomy of the demyelinating diseases. *Am J Med* 1952;12:510–46.
224. Luddy RE, Gilman PA. Paraplegia following intrathecal methotrexate. *J Pediatr* 1973;83:988–92.
225. Saiki JH, Thompson S, Smith F, Atkinson R. Paraplegia following intrathecal chemotherapy. *Cancer* 1972;29:370–4.
226. Weiss HD, Walker MD, Wiernik PH. Neurotoxicity of commonly used antineoplastic agents. *N Engl J Med* 1974;291:75–81, 127–33.
227. Wolff L, Zighelbohm J, Gale RP. Paraplegia following intrathecal cytosine arabinoside. *Cancer* 1979;43:83–5.
228. Kaplan RS, Wiernik PH. Neurotoxicity of antineoplastic drugs. *Semin Oncol* 1982;9:103–29.
229. Duttera MJ, Bleyer WA, Pomeroy TC, et al. Irradiation, methotrexate toxicity, and treatment of meningeal leukemia. *Lancet* 1973;2:703–7.
230. Haughton VM, Ho K-C. Arachnoid response to contrast media: a comparison of iophendylate and Metrizamide in experimental animals. *Radiology* 1982;143:699–702.
231. Junck L, Marshall WH. Neurotoxicity of radiological contrast agents. *Ann Neurol* 1983;13:469–84.
232. Williams AG, Seiger RS, Kornfield M. Experimental production of arachnoiditis with glove

powder contamination during myelography. *Am J Neuroradiol* 1982;3:121–5.

233. Lewis VL, Rosenbaum AE. Neurologic complications of radiologic procedures. In Asbury AK, McKhann GM, McDonald WI, editors. *Diseases of the Nervous System*. Philadelphia: W.B. Saunders; 1986; pp. 1592–1603.

233a. Caplan LR, Norohna AB, Amico LL. Syringomyelia and arachnoiditis. *J Neurol Neurosurg Psychiatr* 1990;53:106–13.

234. Calabro JJ. The seronegative spondyloarthropathies: a graduated approach to management. *Postgrad Med* 1986;80:173–88.

235. Grossman CB, Post MJ D. The adult spine. In Gonzalez CF, Grossman CB, Masdeau JC, editors. *Head and Spine Imaging*. New York: John Wiley & Sons; 1985; pp. 781–858.

236. Haughton VM, Williams AL. *Computed Tomography of the Spine*. St. Louis: C.V. Mosby; 1982.

237. Ross JS. Inflammatory disease. In Modic MT, Masaryk TJ, Ross JS, editors. *Magnetic Resonance Imaging of the Spine*. Chicago: Year Book Medical Publishers; 1988; pp. 167–82.

238. Ross JS, Masaryk TJ, Modic MT, et al. MR imaging of lumbar arachnoiditis. *AJNR* 1987; 8:885–92.

239. Sze G. Gadolinium-DTPA in spinal disease. *Radiol Clinics North Am* 1988;26:1009–24.

239a. Dolan R. Spinal adhesive arachnoiditis. *Surg Neurol* 1993;39:479–84.

239b. Wilmink J, Hofman P. MRI of the postoperative lumbar spine: triple-dose gadodiamide and fat suppression (published erratum in Neuroradiology 1997;39:820). *Neuroradiology* 1997;39:589–92.

239c. Laitt R, Jackson A, Isherwood I. Patterns of chronic adhesive arachnoiditis following Myodil myelography: the significance of spinal canal stenosis and previous surgery. *Br J Radiol* 1996;69:693–8.

239d. Fitt G, Stevens J. Postoperative arachnoiditis diagnosed by high resolution fast spin-echo MRI of the lumbar spine. *Neuroradiology* 1995; 37:139–45.

240. Dubuisson D. Nerve root damage and arachnoiditis. In Wall PD, Melzack R, editors. *Textbook of Pain*. Edinburgh: Churchill Livingstone; 1984; pp. 435–50.

241. Shaw MDM, Russell JA, Grossart KW. The changing pattern of spinal arachnoiditis. *J Neurol Neurosurg Psychiaty* 1978;41:97–107.

242. Brown WJ, Kagan AR. Comparison of myelopathy associated with megavoltage irradiation and remote cancer. In Gilbert HJ, Kagan AR, editors. *Radiation Damage to the Nervous System*. New York: Raven Press; 1980; pp. 191–206.

243. Kagan AR, Wollin M, Gilbert HA, et al. Comparison of the tolerance of the brain and spinal cord to injury by radiations. In Gilbert HA, Kagan AR, editors. *Radiation Damage to the Nervous System*. New York: Raven Press; 1980; pp. 183–90.

244. Brenk HASVd, Richter W, Hurley RH. Radiosensitivity of the human oxygenated cervical spinal cord based on analysis of 357 cases

receiving 4 MeV X rays in hyperbaric oxygenation. *Br J Radiol* 1968;41:205–14.

245. Reagan TJ, Thomas JE, Colby MY. Chronic progressive radiation myelopathy: its clinical aspects and differential diagnosis. *JAMA* 1968; 103:106–10.

246. Lhermitte J, Bollak NM. Les douleurs a type de decharge electrique consecutives a la flexion cephalique dans la sclerose en plaque. *Rev Neurol (Paris)* 1924;31:36–52.

247. Word JA, Kalokhe UP, Aron BS, Elson HR. Transient radiation myelopathy (Lhermitte's sign) in patients with Hodgkin's disease treated by mantle radiation. *Int J Radiat Oncol Biol Phys* 1980;6:1731–3.

248. Jones A. Transient radiation myelopathy (with reference to Lhermitte's sign of electrical paresthesia). *Br J Radiol* 1964;37:727–44.

249. Rottenberg DA. Acute and chronic effects of radiation therapy on the nervous system. In Posner JB, editor. *Neuro-Oncology III, Memorial Sloan-Kettering Cancer Center*. New York: MSKCC; 1981; pp. 88–98.

250. Dejong RN. Sensation. In Vinken PJ, Bruyn GW, editors. *Handbook of Clinical Neurology, Volume 1*. Amsterdam: North-Holland; 1969; pp. 80–113.

251. Benninger TR, Patterson VH. Lhermitte's sign as a presenting symptom of B12 deficiency. *Ulster Med J* 1984;53:162–3.

252. Gautier-Smith PC. Lhermitte's sign in subacute degeneration of the cord. *J Neurol Neurosurg Psychiatry* 1973;36:861–3.

253. Sandyk R, Brennan MJW. Lhermitte's sign as a presenting symptom of subacute degeneration of the cord. *Ann Neurol* 1983;13:215–6.

254. Chan RC, Steinboh P. Delayed onset of Lhermitte's sign following head and/or neck injuries. *J Neurosurg* 1984;60:609–12.

255. Khanchandani R, Howe JG. Lhermitte's sign in multiple sclerosis: a clinical survey and review of the literature. *J Neurol Neurosurg Psychiatry* 1982;45:308–12.

256. Walther PJ, Rossitch E, Bullard DE. The development of Lhermitte's sign during cisplatin chemotherapy: possible drug-induced toxicity causing spinal cord demyelination. *Cancer* 1987;60:2170–2.

257. Smith KJ, McDonald WI. Spontaneous and evoked electrical discharges from a central demyelinating lesion. *J Neurol Sci* 1982;55:39–47.

258. Dorfman L, Donaldson S, Gupta P, et al. Electrophysiologic evidence of subclinical injury to the posterior columns of the human spinal cord after therapeutic radiation. *Cancer* 1982;50:2815–9.

259. Chiang C, Mason K, Withers H, et al. Alteration in myelin-associated proteins following spinal cord irradiation in guinea pigs. *Int J Radiat Oncol Biol Phys* 1992;24:929–37.

260. Ruifrok A, Kleiboer B, Kogel AVD. Radiation tolerance and fractionation sensitivity of the developing rat cervical spinal cord. *Int J Radiat Oncol Biol Phys* 1992;24:505–10.

261. Fogelholm R, Haltia M, Andersson LC. Radiation myelopathy of the cervical spinal cord

simulating intramedullary neoplasm. *J Neurol Neurosurg Psychiatry* 1974;37:1177–80.

262. Marty R, Minckler DS. Radiation myelitis simulating tumor. *Arch Neurol* 1973;29:352–4.

263. Pallis CA, Louis S, Morgan RL. Radiation myelopathy. *Brain* 1961;84:460–76.

264. Palmer JJ. Radiation myelopathy. *Brain* 1972; 95:109–22.

265. Sanyal B, Pant GC, Subrahmaniyan K, et al. Radiation myelopathy. *J Neurol Neurosurg Psychiatry* 1979;42:413–8.

266. Byrne TN. Spinal cord compression from epidural metastases. *N Engl J Med* 1992;327: 614–9.

267. Melki P, Halimi P, Wibault P, et al. MRI in chronic progressive radiation myelopathy. *J Comput Assist Tomogr* 1994;18:1–6.

268. Michikawa M, Wada Y, Sano M, et al. Radiation myelopathy: significance of gadolinium-DTPA enhancement in the diagnosis. *Neuroradiology* 1991;33:286–9.

269. Krishnan KR, Smith WT. Intramedullary hemangioblastoma of the spinal cord associated with pial varicosities simulating intradural angioma. *J Neurol Neurosurg Psychiatry* 1961;24: 350–2.

270. Burns RJ, Jones AN, Robertson JS. Pathology of radiation myelopathy. *J Neurol Neurosurg Psychiatry* 1972;35:888–98.

271. Ang K, Price R, Stephens L, et al. The tolerance of primate spinal cord to re-irradiation. *Int J Radiat Oncol Biol Phys* 1993;25:459–64.

272. Powers B, Beck E, Gillette E, et al. Pathology of radiation injury to the canine spinal cord. *Int J Radiat Oncol Biol Phys* 1992;23:539–49.

273. Godwin-Austen RB, Howell DA, Worthington B. Observations on radiation myelopathy. *Brain* 1975;98:557–68.

274. Schultheiss T, Stephens L, Maor M. Analysis of the histopathology of radiation myelopathy. *Int J Radiat Oncol Biol Phys* 1988;14:27–32.

275. Sawaya R, Rayford A, Kona S, et al. Plasminogen activator inhibitor-1 in the pathogenesis of delayed radiation damage in the rat spinal cord in vivo. *J Neurosurg* 1994;81:381–7.

276. Delattre JY, Rosenblum MK, Thaler HT, et al. A model of radiation myelopathy in the rat. Pathology, regional capillary permeability changes and treatment with dexamethasone. *Brain* 1988;111:1319–36.

277. Glantz M, Burger P, Friedman A, et al. Treatment of radiation-induced nervous system injury with heparin and warfarin. *Neurology* 1994;44:2020–7.

278. Greenfield MM, Stark FM. Post-irradiation neuropathy. *Am J Roentgenol Radium Ther Nucl Med* 1948;60:617–22.

279. Kristensen O, Melgard B, Schiodt AV. Radiation myelopathy of the lumbosacral spinal cord. *Acta Neurol Scand* 1977;56:217–22.

280. Sadowsky CH, Sachs E, Ochoa J. Postradiation motor neuron syndrome. *Arch Neurol* 1976;33: 786–7.

281. Lamy C, Mas J, Varet B, et al. Postradiation lower motor neuron syndrome presenting as

monomyelic amyotrophy. *J Neurol Neurosurg Psychiatry* 1991;64:648–9.

282. Malapert D, Brugieres P, Degos J. Motor neuron syndrome in the arms after radiation treatment. *J Neurol Neurosurg Psychiatry* 1991; 54:1123–4.

283. Schold SC, Cho E-S, Somasundaram M, Posner JB. Subacute motor neuronopathy: a remote effect of lymphoma. *Ann Neurol* 1979;5: 271–87.

284. Berlit P, Schwechheimer K. Neuropathological findings in radiation myelopathy of the lumbosacral cord. *Eur Neurol* 1987;27:29–34.

285. Allen J, Miller D, Budzilovich G, et al. Brain and spinal cord hemorrhage in long-term survivors of malignant pediatric brain tumors: a possible late effect of therapy. *Neurology* 1991; 41:148–50.

286. Posner J. *Neurologic Complications of Cancer.* Philadelphia: FA Davis; 1995; Contemporary Neurology Series.

287. Panse F. Electrical lesions of the nervous system. In Vinken PJ, Bruyn GW, editors. *Handbook of Clinical Neurology, Volume 7.* Amsterdam: North-Holland; 1970; pp. 344–87.

288. Farrell DF, Starr A. Delayed neurological sequelae of electrical injuries. *Neurology* 1968;18: 601–6.

289. Jackson FE, Martin R, Davis R. Delayed quadriplegia following electrical burn. *Mil Med* 1965;130:601–5.

290. Russell JSR, Batten FE, Collier J. Subacute combined degeneration of the spinal cord. *Brain* 1900;23:39–110.

291. Healton E, Savage D, Brust J, et al. Neurologic aspects of cobalamin deficiency. *Medicine* 1991; 70:229–45.

292. Kunze K, Leitenmaier K. Vitamin B12 deficiency and subacute combined degeneration of the spinal cord (funicular spinal disease). In Vinken PJ, Bruyn GW, editors. *Handbook of Clinical Neurology, Volume 28.* Amsterdam: North-Holland; 1976; pp. 141–98.

293. Lindenbaum J, Healton EB, Savage DG, et al. Neuropsychiatric disorders caused by cobalamin deficiency in the absence of anemia or macrocytosis. *N Engl J Med* 1988;318:1720–8.

294. Victor M, Lear AA. Subacute combined degeneration of the spinal cord. *Am J Med* 1956; 20:896–911.

295. Farmer TW. Neurologic complications of vitamin and mineral disorders. In Baker AB, Baker LH, editors. *Clinical Neurology.* Hagerstown: Harper & Row; 1979; Chapter 42.

296. Tefferi A, Pruthi R. The biochemical basis of cobalamin deficiency. *Mayo Clin Proc* 1994; 69:181–6.

297. Pennypacker L, Allen RH, Kelly J, et al. High prevalence of cobalamin deficiency in elderly outpatients. *J Am Geriatr Soc* 1992;40:1197–2004.

298. Green R, Kinsella L. Current concepts in the diagnosis of cobalamin deficiency. *Neurology* 1995;45:1435–40.

299. Yao Y, Yao S-L, Yao S-S, et al. Prevalence of vitamin B12 deficiency among geriatric outpatients. *J Fam Pract* 1992;35:524–8.

300. Cruickshank EK. Effects of malnutrition on the central nervous system and the nerves. In Vinken PJ, Bruyn GW, editors. *Handbook of Clinical Neurology, Volume 28*. Amsterdam: North-Holland; 1976; pp. 1–41.

301. Denny-Brown D. Neurological conditions resulting from prolonged and severe dietary restriction. *Medicine* 1947;26:41–113.

302. Grieve S, Jacobson S, Proctor NSF. A nutritional myelopathy occurring in the Bantu on the Witwatersrand. *Neurology* 1967;17:1205–12.

303. Spillane JD. *Nutritional Disorders of the Nervous System*. Edinburgh: Livingstone; 1947.

304. Erbsloh F, Abel M. Deficiency neuropathies. In Vinken PJ, Bruyn GW, editors. *Handbook of Clinical Neurology, Volume 7*. Amsterdam: North-Holland; 1970; pp. 558–663.

305. Dreyfus PM. Amblyopia and other neurological disorders associated with chronic alcoholism. In Vinken PJ, Bruyn GW, editors. *Handbook of Clinical Neurology, Volume 28*. Amsterdam: North-Holland; 1976; pp. 331–47.

306. Bechar M, Freud M, Kott E, et al. Hepatic cirrhosis with post-shunt myelopathy. *J Neurol Sci* 1970;11:101–7.

307. Gauthier G, Wildi E. L'encephalo-myelopathie porto-systemique. *Rev Neurol* 1975;131:319–38.

308. Leigh AD, Card WI. Hepato-lenticular degeneration. A case associated with postero-lateral column degeneration. *J Neuropathol Exp Neurol* 1949;8:338–46.

309. Plum F, Hindfelt B. The neurological complications of liver disease. In Vinken PJ, Bruyn GW, editors. *Handbook of Clinical Neurology, Volume 27*. Amsterdam: North-Holland; 1976; pp. 349–76.

310. Zieve L, Mendelson DF, Goepfert M. Shunt encephalomyelopathy. II. Occurrence of permanent myelopathy. *Ann Intern Med* 1960;53:53–63.

311. Blackwood W. Discussion on the vascular disease of the spinal cord. *Proc R Soc Med* 1958;51:543–7.

312. Vinters HV, Gilbert JJ. Hypoxic myelopathy. *Can J Neurol Sci* 1979;6:380.

313. Cheshire W, Santos C, Massey E, Howard J. Spinal cord infarction; etiology and outcome. *Neurology* 1996;47:321–30.

314. DeJong RN. The neurological manifestations of diabetes mellitus. In Vinken PJ, Bruyn GW, editors. *Handbook of Clinical Neurology, Volume 27*. Amsterdam: North-Holland; 1976; pp. 99–142.

315. Henson RA, Parsons M. Ischaemic lesions of the spinal cord: an illustrated review. *Q J Med* 1967;36:205–22.

316. Richardson EP Jr. Systemic lupus erythematosus. In Vinken PJ, Bruyn GW, editors. *Handbook of Clinical Neurology, Volume 39*. Amsterdam: North-Holland; 1980; pp. 273–92.

317. Bots TAM, Wattendorf AR, Buruma OJS. Acute myelopathy caused by fibrocartilagenous emboli. *Neurology* 1981;31:1250–6.

318. Naiman JL, Donahue WL, Pritchard JS. Fatal nucleus pulposus embolism of spinal cord after trauma. *Neurology* 1961;11:83–7.

319. Preobrajensky PA. Syphilitic paraplegias with dissociated disturbances of sensibility. *J Neuropat Psikhiat* 1904;4:594.

320. Silver JR, Buxton PH. Spinal stroke. *Brain* 1974;97:539–50.

321. Perier O, Demanet JC, Hennaux J, et al. Existe-t-il un syndrome des arteres spinales posterieures? *Rev Neurol* 1960;103:396–409.

322. Buchan AM, Barnett HJM. Infarction of the spinal cord. In Barnett HJM, Mohr JP, Stein BM, Yatsu FM, editors. *Stroke: Pathophysiology, Diagnosis and Management*. New York: Churchill Livingstone; 1986; pp. 707–19.

323. Fieschi C, Gottlieb A, Carolis VD. Ischaemic lacunae in the spinal cord of arteriosclerotic subjects. *J Neurol Neurosurg Psychiatry* 1970;33:138–46.

324. Taylor JR, Allen MWV. Vascular malformation of the cord with transient ischemia attacks. *J Neurosurg* 1969;31:576–8.

325. Hughes JT. Venous infarction of the spinal cord. *Neurology* 1971;21:794–800.

326. Mancall EL, Remedios KR. Necrotizing myelopathy associated with visceral carcinoma. *Brain* 1964;87:639–55.

327. Hallenbeck J, Bove A, Elliott D. Mechanisms underlying spinal cord damage in decompression sickness. *Neurology* 1975;25:308–16.

328. Kim R, Smith HR, Henbest ML, Choi BH. Nonhemorrhagic venous infarction of the spinal cord. *Ann Neurol* 1984;15:379–85.

329. Yuh W, Marsch E, Wang A, et al. MR imaging of spinal cord and vertebral infarction. *AJNR Am J Neuroradiol* 1992;13:145–54.

330. Alexander EL, Provost TT, Stevens MB, Alexander GE. Neurologic complications of primary Sjogren's syndrome. *Medicine* 1982; 61:247–57.

331. Calabrese LH, Mallek JA. Primary angiitis of the central nervous system. *Medicine* 1987;67:20–38.

332. Caselli RJ, Hunder GG, Whisnant JP. Neurologic disease in biopsy-proven giant cell (temporal) arteritis. *Neurology* 1988;38:352–9.

333. Moore PM. Diagnosis and management of isolated angiitis of the central nervous system. *Neurology* 1989;39:167–73.

334. Moore PM, Cupps TR. Neurological complications of vasculitis. *Ann Neurol* 1983;14:155–67.

335. Sigal LH. The neurologic persentation of vasculitis and rheumatologic syndromes. *Medicine* 1987;66:157–80.

336. Moore PM, Fauci AS. Neurologic manifestations of systemic vasculitis. A retrospective and prospective study of the clinicopathologic features and responses to therapy in 25 patients. *Am J Med* 1981;71:517–24.

337. Alexander EL, Malinow K, Lejewski JE, et al. Primary Sjogren's syndrome with central nervous system disease mimicking multiple sclerosis. *Ann Intern Med* 1986;104:323–30.

338. Ferreiro JE, Robalino BD, Saldana MJ. Primary Sjogren's syndrome with diffuse cerebral vasculitis and lymphocytic interstitial pneumonitis. *Am J Med* 1987;82:1227–32.

339. Manthorpe R, Manthorpe T, Sjoberg S. Magnetic resonance imaging of the brain in pa-

tients with primary Sjogren's syndrome. *Scand J Rhematol* 1992;21:148.

340. Moutsopoulos H, Sarmas J, Talal M. Is central nervous system involvement a systemic manifestation of primary Sjogren's syndrome? *Rheum Dis Clin North Am* 1993;19:909.

341. Escudero D, Olive A, Latorre P, et al. Central neurological manifestations of primary Sjogren's syndrome. *Br J Rheumatol* 1992;31:787.

342. Hietaharju A, Yli-Kerttela U, Khakkinen V, et al. Nervous system manifestations in Sjogren's syndrome. *Acta Neurol Scand* 1990;81:144.

343. VBinder A, Snaith M, Isenberg D. Sjogren's syndrome: a study of its neurological manifestations. *Br J Rheumatol* 1988;27:275.

344. Adonopoulos A, Lagos G, Drosos A, et al. The spectrum of neurological involvement in Sjogren's syndrome. *Br J Rheumatol* 1990;29:21.

345. Konttinen YT, Kinnunen E, Bonsdorff MV, et al. Acute transverse myelopathy successfully treated with plasmapharesis and prednisone in a patient with primary Sjogren's syndrome. *Arth Rheum* 1987;30:339–44.

346. Rosenbaum R, Campbell S, Rosenbaum J. *Clinical Neurology of Rheumatic Diseases*. Boston: Butterworth-Heinemann; 1996.

347. Vrethem M, Ernerudh J, Linstrom F, et al. Immunoglobulins within the central nervous system in primary Sjogren's syndrome. *J Neurol Sci* 1990;100:186.

348. Alexander EL, Beall SS, Gordon B, et al. Magnetic resonance imaging of cerebral lesions in patients with the Sjogren syndrome. *Ann Intern Med* 1988;108:815–23.

349. Rutan G, Martinez A, Fieshko J, et al. Primary biliary cirrhosis, Sjogren's syndrome and transverse myelitis. *Gastroenterology* 1986;90: 206.

350. Alexander E, Craft C, Dorsch C, et al. Necrotizing arteritis and spinal subarachnoid hemorrhage in Sjogren's syndrome. *Ann Neurol* 1982;11:632.

351. Lukes SA, Norman D. Computed tomography in acute disseminated encephalomyelitis. *Ann Neurol* 1983;13:567–72.

352. Fulford KWM, Catterall RD, Delhanty JJ, et al. A collagen disorder of the nervous system presenting as multiple sclerosis. *Brain* 1972;95:373–86.

353. Provenzale J, Bouldin T. Lupus-related myelopathy: report of three cases and review of the literature. *J Neurol Neurosurg Psychiatry* 1992;55:830.

354. Boumpas D, Patronas N, Dalakas M, et al. Acute transverse myelitis in systemic lupus erythematosus: magnetic resonance imaging and literature review. *J Rheumatol* 1990;17:89.

355. Propper D, Bucknell R. Acute transverse myelopathy complicating systemic lupus erythematosus. *Ann Rheum Dis* 1989;48:512.

356. Johnson RT, Richardson EP Jr. The neurological manifestations of systemic lupus erythe-

matosus: a clincial-pathological study of 24 cases and review of the literature. *Medicine* 1968;47:337–69.

357. Adrianakos AA, Duffy J, Suzuki M, Sharp JT. Transverse myelopathy in systemic lupus erythematosus: report of 3 cases and review of the literature. *Ann Intern Med* 1975;83:616–24.

358. Dell'Isola B, Vidailhet M, Gatfosse M, et al. Recovery of anterior spinal artery syndrome in a patient with systemic lupus erythematosus and antiphospholipid antibodies. *Br J Rheumatol* 1991;30:314.

359. Lavalle C, Pizzaro S, Drinkard C, et al. Transverse myelitis: a manifestation of systemic lupus erythematosus strongly associated with antiphospholipid antibodies. *J Rheumatol* 1990;17:34.

360. Andrews JM, Cancilla PA, Kimm J. Regressive spinal cord signs in a patient with disseminated lupus erythematosus. *Bull Los Angeles Neurol Soc* 1970;35:78–85.

361. Penn AS, Rowan AJ. Myelopathy in systemic lupus erythematosus. *Arch Neurol* 1968;18: 337–49.

362. Shepherd EI, Downie AW, Best PV. Systemic lupus erythematosis and multiple sclerosis (abstract). *Arch Neurol* 1974;30:423.

363. McLean B, Miller D, Thompson E. Oligoclonal banding of IgG in CSF, blood-brain barrier function, and MRI findings in patients with sarcoidosis, systemic lupus erythematosus, and Behcet's disease involving the nervous system. *J Neurol Neurosurg Psychiatry* 1995;58:548–54.

364. Winfield J, Shaw M, Silverman L, et al. Intrathecal IgG synthesis and blood brain barrier impairment in patients with systemic lupus erythematosus and central nervous system dysfunction. *Am J Med* 1983;74:837–44.

365. Barile L, Lavalle C. Transverse myelitis in systemic lupus erythematosus—the effect of IV pulse methylprednisolone and cyclophosphamide. *J Rheumatol* 1992;19:370.

366. Berlanga B, Rubio F, Moga I, et al. Response to intravenous cyclophosphamide treatment in lupus myelopathy. *J Rheumatol* 1992; 19:829.

367. Norris FH. Remote effects of cancer on the spinal cord. In Vinken PJ, Bruyn GW, editors. *Handbook of Clinical Neurology, Volume 38*. Amsterdam: North-Holland; 1979; pp. 669–77.

368. Ojeda VJ. Necrotising myelopathy associated with malignancy: a clinicopathological study of two cases and literature review. *Cancer* 1984; 53:1115–23.

369. Henson RA, Urich H. *Cancer and the Nervous System*. Oxford: Blackwell; 1982.

370. Matsuo H, Tsujihata M, Satoh A, et al. Plasmapharesis in treatment of HTLV-1 associated myelopathy. *Lancet* 1988;ii:1109–12.

Chapter 9

INFECTIOUS AND NONINFECTIOUS INFLAMMATORY DISEASES AFFECTING THE SPINE

Inflammatory diseases of the spine include both infectious and noninfectious causes. In this chapter, we have chosen to discuss infectious causes that generally cause space-occupying lesions, such as epidural and intramedullary abscesses, tuberculosis, and fungal disease. In addition, we discuss noninfectious inflammatory diseases of the vertebral column, such as ankylosing spondylitis and rheumatoid arthritis. Noninfectious inflammatory diseases of the spinal cord, such as demyelinating disease, and viral infections are reviewed in Chapter 8.

INFECTIOUS DISEASES

Pyogenic Infections Causing Spinal Cord Compression

Bacterial infections of the spinal cord and its coverings (meningitis excluded) may be classified according to location. An abscess may occur in the epidural space or may be subdural or intramedullary.[1,2] Epidural abscesses are responsible for approximately two thirds of surgically significant infections of the spine.[1] Spinal subdural abscesses are rare and often are clinically indistinguishable from epidural abscesses.[3] Pachymeningitis may also occur in the setting of epidural and subdural abscess.[1,4] Rarely, hypertrophic spinal pachymeningitis may occur and cause spinal cord and nerve root compression.[5–7]

The symptoms of spinal cord compression from spinal abscesses are nonspecific, making diagnosis difficult.[8] As discussed below, in some cases of acute epidural abscess, systemic symptoms and signs dominate the clinical picture. Alternatively, in chronic cases, there may be few if any signs of infection, and a neoplasm may be considered when neurological signs appear. Thus, in order to make the diagnosis in the early and most treatable stages, a high index of suspicion must be maintained. Epidural and intramedullary spinal abscesses are discussed separately.

EPIDURAL ABSCESS

Early diagnosis and treatment of spinal epidural abscess is imperative for a successful outcome.[9–12] The diagnostic challenge can be daunting, because this is a rare disorder that may mimic other more commonly encountered diseases (Fig. 9–1).[13]

Spinal epidural abscess is infrequently encountered in both community and referral hospitals, although prevalence appears to be increasing.[11,14] In a series of nontuberculous bacterial infections of the spinal epidural space reported from the New York Hospital, the overall incidence was one case per 12,720 admissions.[15] The disease affects both sexes, and any age may be affected. In the New York Hospital series, the average age was 58 years, with a range of 8 to 81.[15]

Pathogenesis and Pathology

Infection spreads to the epidural space through hematogenous dissemination from an infected remote site or by direct extension from a primary infection in the region of the spine.[15–19] The primary infection may be primary vertebral osteomyelitis[20–22] or may extend from perinephric, retropharyngeal, or other paraspinal locations. Direct extension to the epidural space may also occur due to an infected spinal surgical wound, lumbar puncture, or epidural catheter placement for anesthesia.[15,23–25] Intravenous drug abuse is also a major risk factor for spinal epidural abscess (Fig. 9–1).[10] Rarely, an abscess may form from extension of an infected dermal sinus.

Hematogenous dissemination to the epidural space from an identified distant site occurs in 25% to 50% of cases (Table 9–1). Skin and soft tissue infections are the most common sites of remote primary infection; other primary sources reported include urinary tract infection, upper respiratory infection, periodontal abscess, infected intravenous lines, or intravenous drug abuse.[2,15] No identifiable source is

found in approximately 20%–40% of patients.[15] The route of hematogenous spread to the epidural space and vertebral column is probably via the arterial supply[26] and Batson's plexus.[27,28]

Anatomically, the epidural abscess resides in the dorsal epidural space in approximately 70% of cases, perhaps because it is larger than the ventral epidural space. The lower thoracic and lumbar regions are most frequently involved.[14] Among several series shown in Table 9–2, the thoracic spine was the most common level of involvement, followed by the lumbar and cervical levels, possibly due to the larger epidural space in the caudal half of the spine. In a series from the Massachusetts General Hospital, the average rostrocaudal extent of the abscess was four to five vertebral segments; in three patients, it extended from 11 to 26 vertebrae.[16] In the transverse plane, the majority of abscesses in several series were located dorsally (Table 9–2). Osteomyelitis occurred more frequently in conjunction with ventral abscesses.[15]

Pathological findings of epidural abscess vary widely and include acute purulent material in some patients and chronic granulomatous findings in others. Vertebral osteomyelitis is much more common among patients with chronic epidural abscess than in those with an acute condition.[5,16]

The pathogenesis of neurologic dysfunction involves both neural compression and disturbances of spinal cord circulation without direct neural compression. The latter may be secondary to arterial compression and/or venous thrombosis and thrombophlebitis.[29,30] Direct extension of inflammatory cells into the spinal cord is unusual; the dura mater typically provides an effective barrier to prevent the extension of infection into the central nervous system.[4]

Clinical Features

Spinal epidural abscesses may be classified as either acute or chronic on the basis of the duration of symptoms. Such a distinction is important, because patients with a

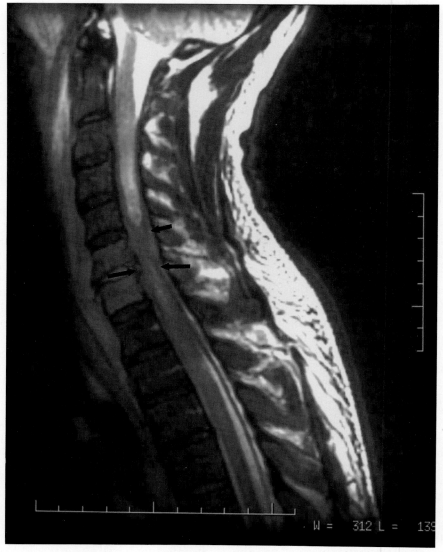

Figure 9–1. A T_1 sagittal MRI of a 47-year-old male intravenous drug abuser with a rapidly progressive quadriparesis. He was initially thought to have Guillain-Barré syndrome. The diagnosis of spinal epidural abscess, however, was made by MRI (arrows). A staphylococcus abscess was drained and treated with antibiotics. Of note is the significant prevertebral soft tissue involvement.

chronic abscess generally present less dramatically. Danner and Hartman[15] identified acute abscesses as those in which symptoms were present for less than 16 days. Using such a distinction, those with

chronic abscesses were less likely to be febrile (average temperature 37.4° ± 0.5° C in chronic cases, compared with 38.4° ± 1.0° C in patients with acute abscesses). Moreover, the mean WBC count was 7.1 ±

Table 9–1. **Primary Sources of Infection in Patients With Epidural Abscess***

Source of Infection	No. of Patients (%) at Indicated Facility During Indicated Period					
	Boston City Hospital 1930–1948	Stoke Mandeville Hospital 1945–1968	Massachusetts General Hospital 1947–1974	Montefiore Hospital 1968–1978	New York Hospital 1971–1982	Total No. of patients (%)
Skin and soft tissue	9 (45)		7 (18)	4 (21)	8 (23)	28 (21)
Bone or joint†	4 (20)		11 (28)		3 (9)	18 (13)
Spinal surgery or procedures	0		9 (23)		5 (14)	14 (10)
Abdomen	1 (5)		1 (3)	2 (11)	1 (3)	5 (4)
Upper respiratory tract	0		4 (10)		4 (11)	8 (6)
Urinary tract	1 (5)		0		2 (6)	3 (2)
IV Drug abuse	0		0§	4 (21)	2 (6)	6 (4)
Specific source not identifiable‡		26 (53)				
No source identified	5 (25)	23 (47)	7 (18)	9 (47)	10 (29)	54 (40)
Total	20 (100)	49 (100)	39 (100)	19 (100)	35 (100)	136 (100)

*From Danner, RL and Hartman, BJ,[15] p. 266, with permission.
†Vertebral osteomyelitis was considered as a primary source by most authors when it was present without any other identifiable focus of infection. In The New York Hospital series, patients with vertebral osteomyelitis without a known antecedent infection were classified as *no source identified*. The three New York Hospital patients with a bone or joint source had a distant osteomyelitis, a hip infection, and an infection of the olecranon bursa, respectively.
‡These patients had an identifiable source that was not specified by the authors. These patients are not included in the calculations for the totals of all the series.
§Two patients were reported to be IV drug abusers.

1.9×10^3 in chronic cases, compared with an average of $12.3 \pm 3.8 \times 10^3$ per cubic millimeter in acute abscesses.

In patients with both chronic and acute spinal epidural abscesses, the most characteristic clinical course progresses through four stages: (1) local pain, (2) radicular pain, (3) motor weakness and sphincter disturbance, and (4) paralysis.[31] A sensory level may also be observed as transverse myelopathy develops. The tempo of progression of these symptoms and signs is quite variable, ranging from hours to several weeks.[15] Cases that commence as vertebral osteomyelitis may evolve slowly in the first two phases, and thus be classified as chronic, only to accelerate rapidly into the final phases.[5] In cases of rapid neurologic deterioration, an erroneous diagnosis of acute transverse myelitis may be considered.[13]

Typically, patients with acute epidural abscess are acutely ill, with signs of toxicity, systemic infection, and fever. The early course is characterized by fever and back pain, often followed by radicular pain. Spasm of paraspinal muscles may occur. Headache is often present, and neck stiffness may be marked. Percussion tenderness over the spine may be pronounced. There may be a history of a recent or remote infection elsewhere.

Despite this characteristic course, the clinical presentation of acute spinal epidural abscess is highly variable, resulting in a delayed diagnosis in many cases. In one series, the diagnosis of spinal epidural abscess was considered initially in only one-fourth of patients.[16] When the abscess arises from a distant focus of infection that disseminates to the spine hematogenously, the clinical presentation

Table 9–2. Location of Abscess in Patients With Spinal Epidural Abscess*

Location of Abscess	No. of Patients at Indicated Facility During Indicated Period							
	Boston City Hospital 1930–1948	Stoke Mandeville Hospital 1945–1968	Massachusetts General Hospital 1947–1974	The Royal Infirmary 1957–1973	Pinderfields General Hospital 1958–1978	Montefiore Hospital 1968–1978	New York Hospital 1971–1982	Total No. of Patients
Anterior	1	13	7	—	—	—	17	28
Posterior	19	36	32	—	—	—	18	105
Cervical	3	—	7	0	1	3	6	20
Thoracic	13	most common site	20	6	10	12	10	71
Lumbar	4	—	12	8	1	4	19	48
Total	20	49	39	14	12	19	35	188
Mean No. of Vertebrae Involved (Range)								
	3.6 (1–7)	—	4.5 (1–26)	4.4 (1–15)	—	1.8 (1–5)	3.8 (2–10)	3.8 (1–26)

*From Danner, RL and Hartman, BJ,[15] p. 269, with permission.

may be dominated by the systemic illness. The patient may not complain of pain, and if lethargic or confused, he or she may fail to complain of weakness. However, once infection of the epidural space occurs, symptoms of local and radicular pain usually ensue rapidly.[2] At that time, the clinical presentation may mimic spinal tumor or disc disease.

In chronic cases (defined as symptoms present for longer than 16 days), the epidural abscess often arises from an adjacent vertebral osteomyelitis.[2] (Spinal epidural abscess is reported to develop in up to 20% of cases of vertebral osteomyelitis.[32]) The progression of symptoms and signs beyond pain, fever, and weakness may evolve over weeks or even months before signs of neural dysfunction occur. Alternatively, the clinical evolution of an indolent chronic abscess may suddenly and unpredictably change, with rapid development of paraplegia. In most (but not all) cases of both chronic and acute epidural abscess, symptoms and signs of spinal cord/cauda equina dysfunction develop following the onset of local and radicular pain.[31]

The clinical setting often provides helpful clues in diagnosis. In addition to remote and local infection, several other factors may be associated with spinal epidural abscess, including diabetes mellitus, nonpenetrating or penetrating back trauma, pregnancy, cancer or spinal tumor, intravenous drug abuse, alcoholism, or degenerative joint disease of the spine.[15,16] A possible association with cancer is especially important to recognize, because the symptoms and signs of epidural abscess may be difficult to distinguish clinically from epidural spinal metastasis. As discussed below, even radiographic studies may not definitively establish a diagnosis of spinal epidural abscess or differentiate it from metastatic cancer.

In summary, although the constellation of fever, back and radicular pain, and percussion tenderness over the spine is characteristic of both chronic and acute epidural abscess, fever and other constitutional symptoms may be entirely absent, particularly in chronic cases.[15,33] Further-more, although local and radicular pain and spinal tenderness occur in over 90% of cases,[2] in occasional patients these findings have been absent.[34,35] Thus, whenever paraparesis develops without a well-defined cause, the clinician must think of epidural abscess. Even prior to the development of weakness, the development of back and/or radicular pain, or spinal tenderness, in the setting of systemic illness should alert the clinician to this possibility. The difficulty encountered in arriving at a correct diagnosis is demonstrated by the reported series of epidural abscess in Table 9–3. In the New York Hospital series, 43% of patients had an initial diagnosis unrelated to the spine (Fig. 9–1); in many instances, patients were incoherent and therefore could not offer an accurate history.

Spinal subdural empyema is a rare cause of spinal cord compression. It is difficult on clinical grounds to differentiate it from spinal epidural abscess; however, vertebral tenderness is usually lacking in patients with subdural empyema.[36,37] An MRI or myelography may distinguish between subdural and epidural collections of pus. Surgical intervention will differentiate between them.

Laboratory Studies

Staphylococcus aureus is the most common bacterium isolated in cases of spinal epidural abscess, although there is an increasing incidence of gram-negative aerobic bacilli, especially *E. coli* and *Pseudomonas*.[38] Although *Mycobacterium tuberculosis* has been excluded from many series, it has been responsible for as many as one-fourth of the cases in some reports.[39] In addition, fungal infections (e.g., *Cryptococcus neoformans* and *Coccidioides immitis*) and several other organisms have been reported.[2,40–42] In cases of tuberculosis and fungal infections, there may be a granulomatous mass or abscess.[43] Infrequently, multiple organisms are found.[5] The microbiology of spinal epidural abscess has been recently reviewed.[14]

Blood cultures are often positive; among those patients with *Staphylococcus aureus*, results were positive in 18 (95%) of 19 pa-

Table 9–3. **Initial Diagnosis for Patients With Spinal Epidural Abscess***

Initial Diagnosis	No. of Patients at Indicated Facility				
	Boston City Hospital	Massachusetts General Hospital	Pinderfields General Hospital	New York Hospital	Total No. of Patients
Spinal epidural abscess	1	10	1	7	19
Vertebral osteomyelitis or infected disk	4	1	0	1	6
Spinal tuberculosis	0	0	0	1	1
Cholecystitis, pyelonephritis, intraabdominal abscess	0	4	0	2	6
Meningitis	3	1	0	0	4
Dental infection	0	1	0	0	1
Bacterial infection, other sites	0	0	1	6	7
Herpes zoster	0	1	0	1	2
Viral syndrome	0	1	0	1	2
Infectious polyneuritis or transverse myelitis	1	1	1	1	4
Spinal tumor or metastatic cancer	4	1	0	6	11
Spinal hematoma	0	0	0	1	1
Extruded disk	0	5	3	3	11
Musculoskeletal pain, arthritis, neuritis	3	6	5	2	16
Fibrositis	0	0	1	0	1
Myocardial infarction	0	1	0	0	1
Cerebrovascular accident or subdural hematoma	0	2	0	1	3
Hysteria	2	2	0	0	4
Anemia	0	1	0	0	1
Benign prostatic hypertrophy	0	0	0	1	1
Drug fever	0	0	0	1	1
None	2	1	0	0	3
Total	20	39	12	35	106

*From Danner, RL and Hartman, BJ,[15] p. 272, with permission.

tients reported from the New York Hospital series.[15] Cerebrospinal fluid cultures appear to yield positive results in far fewer cases; only two were positive out of 31 cases in which the procedure was performed. In the same series, cultures of the abscess were positive in 84% of cases; patients who had been on antibiotics for longer than one week were unlikely to have positive cultures of the abscess.

In routine and CSF studies, the peripheral white blood cell count is usually elevated. Although the erythrocyte sedimentation rate (ESR) is usually high, four patients in the series from the New York Hospital had a normal ESR.[15]

Blood glucose levels may reveal diabetes, and blood chemistries should be scrutinized for signs of renal disease. The cerebrospinal fluid typically shows evidence of a parameningeal infection, with elevated protein, moderate pleocytosis (usually lower than 150 white cells per cubic millimeter) and normal sugar.[2,5] It can be xanthochromic, especially in cases of a subarachnoid block.

If there is suspicion of an epidural abscess, lumbar puncture should be done cautiously to avoid entering the abscess and contaminating the CSF. Lumbar puncture should not be performed at the site of a suspected abscess; if epidural abscess is suspected over the lumbar region, a cisternal tap may be performed. If lumbar puncture is performed in a patient with a possible abscess, gentle suction should be applied to the needle because the abscess may have extended to lumbar areas; aspiration of pus is diagnostic of epidural abscess. It is essential in such cases that the arachnoid not be penetrated by the needle. Furthermore, in the case of spinal block, myelopathy may worsen following lumbar puncture; therefore, routine lumbar puncture should not be performed if epidural abscess is suspected.[5,44]

Plain spinal radiographs may show evidence of osteomyelitis, discitis, compression fracture, or paravertebral mass, but it is common to find no specific abnormalities. Routine radiographs demonstrated osteomyelitis in 37% of patients in the New York Hospital series described above.[15] Radionuclide bone scanning often shows evidence of abnormality, but a substantial number of patients also have normal bone scans.

Until the advent of MRI, myelography was considered the most sensitive technique for identifying epidural abscess.[2,45,46] The myelogram is nearly always abnormal, demonstrating an epidural mass.[2] It may show the longitudinal extent of the abscess and its anteroposterior relationship to the spinal cord.

Although CT has been shown to be sensitive in identifying osteomyelitis, paravertebral infections, and epidural abscesses,[47–49] some authors have found it less accurate than myelography.[15] A CT may be able to detect involvement of the spongy vertebral bone and intervertebral disc before changes are seen on plain radiographs. When combined with myelography, CT may be very sensitive for evaluating bony and epidural tissues.[48,50,51] Paravertebral structures are also seen more readily on CT than with plain films or myelography.

An MRI has been shown to be superior to CT and myelography in evaluating pa-

tients with epidural abscess and vertebral osteomyelitis.[21,52,53] Paramagnetic contrast materials may differentiate active inflammation from chronic granulation tissue.[54–57] Paraspinal abscesses, as well as diskitis, can be visualized.[45] In patients with osteomyelitis, hypointense signal intensity in the vertebral body on T_1-weighted images, abnormal disk signal on both T_1- and T_2-weighted images, and abnormal contrast enhancement were found most commonly (Fig. 9–1).[21]

Therapy

The treatment of spinal epidural abscess includes administration of intravenous antibiotics and urgent surgical drainage of the mass.[2,5,15,58] Some authors[5] recommend initiating antibiotic therapy before surgery, when a presumptive diagnosis can be made. Since *Staphylococcus aureus* is the most common offending organism, initial treatment includes a first-line antistaphylococcal agent.[15] When there are known sources of infection, antibiotic therapy should include coverage for these. For example, epidural abscesses due to gram-negative organisms are more common in the setting of intravenous drug abuse or following spinal operation. *Staphylococcus epidermidis* infection is also more frequent following spinal procedures. Antibiotic therapy can be modified based on the results of Gram and other special stains, and laboratory culture results of operative specimens. The duration of antibiotic therapy is determined in part by the presence or absence of associated osteomyelitis. Recent reviews[2,38,58] suggest six to eight weeks of parenteral antibiotic therapy if osteomyelitis is present. Some suggest subsequent oral antibiotics in selected cases.[15] The prognosis for neurologic recovery is good if treatment is begun before symptoms and signs of myelopathy occur; although patients with paraparesis may be restored to normal neurologic function, the presence of paraplegia for longer than 48 hours carries a poor prognosis for recovery.[2]

As mentioned above, MRI is exceptionally sensitive in detecting small epidural inflammatory lesions or areas (for example, secondary to adjacent infections) that are not true abscesses. These infections may be successfully managed with antibiotics alone, without surgical drainage. In cases in which MRI identifies a small noncompressive inflammatory lesion that is not considered to be a true abscess, some surgeons have been reluctant to attempt urgent open surgical drainage in neurologically intact patients who can be followed with repeated clinical and laboratory examinations and MRI scanning. In some of these patients, treatment with antibiotics alone has been successful,[59] whereas in others, surgical drainage has been required after an unsuccessful trial of antibiotics.[2,15] Because of the risk of rapid neurologic deterioration, it has been suggested that even in neurologically intact patients with cervical or thoracic epidural abscess causing cord compression surgery may benefit those with symp-

toms less than two weeks in duration.[59] With more experience using MRI and carefully performed clinical studies, criteria may be established to identify those patients not requiring urgent surgical drainage. Standard infectious disease references recommend that nonsurgical therapy alone for spinal epidural abscesses be reserved only for patients without neurologic dysfunction.[14,15,58]

Surgery is directed at the site of symptomatic (or potentially symptomatic) compression. In many cases, complete surgical evacuation is not possible. Drainage, decompression, and antibiotic therapy, however, are usually successful in combination. Occasionally, osteomyelitis and/or disc interspace infection accompanies epidural abscess. Spinal stability may, therefore, be compromised, necessitating a spinal stabilization procedure (Fig. 9–2).

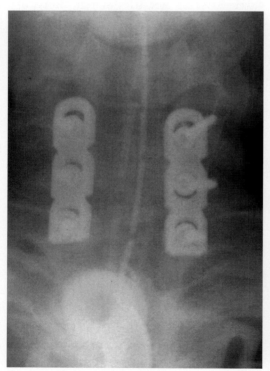
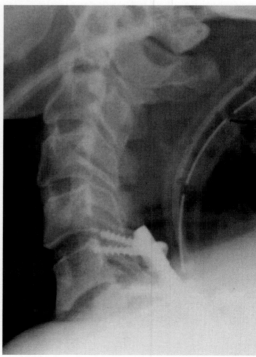

A

B

Figure 9–2. The patient whose preoperative images are depicted in Figure 9–1 underwent a C6 and C7 laminectomy and a dorsal stabilization procedure (lateral mass plates from C6-T1) as depicted by an AP (A) and lateral (B) radiograph.

CASE ILLUSTRATION

A 61-year-old former housepainter with a history of alcoholism was admitted to the medical service after being found in his hotel room. He was in a confused state attributed to a withdrawal syndrome. The patient had a fever of 38° to 38.5°C. No focal neurologic signs were noted. The patient exhibited witzelsucht and did not complain of back pain, but said he was weak and could not get out of bed. A lumbar puncture yielded CSF showing mild xanthochromia, a moderate pleocytosis, protein of about 110 mg per dl, and normal glucose. The patient was treated with antibiotics but, because he remained confined to bed, neurologic consultation was obtained.

The consultant found the patient confused and uncooperative. He denied having any pain. He stated that he was weak and could not walk, but would not attempt to ambulate. The neck was supple and there was no paravertebral spasm, but percussion tenderness was present over the spine at T9–10. Motor examination revealed flaccid paraparesis. Patellar and ankle jerks could not be obtained, but the plantar responses were extensor. The patient was not cooperative for testing of vibratory or position sensation. Although he denied feeling a pin as painful over any part of his body, when the examiner watched for a facial wince on pinprick, a sensory level at the T5–6 level could be appreciated.

Myelography revealed epidural abscess, and the patient was taken to surgery. The abscess was found to extend over five vertebral segments. The confusional state resolved postoperatively, but the patient remained paraparetic.

Comment. This case illustrates some of the difficulties that can be encountered in the diagnosis of epidural abscess. While back pain and neck stiffness are usually encountered, they did not appear to be present in this patient, possibly because they were masked by his confusional state. While this patient complained of weakness, a careful neurologic examination was not carried out initially, and the paraparesis was not appreciated. The initial workup did not include percussion of the vertebral column to determine whether tenderness was present. It is essential for the spinal column to be examined carefully in any patient with back pain,

radicular signs or symptoms, or weakness that includes the legs. In retrospect, the patient's confusional state may have been partially due to the meningitis that accompanied his epidural abscess. This case illustrates that an associated confusional state may make diagnosis difficult.

INTRAMEDULLARY SPINAL CORD ABSCESS

Intramedullary spinal cord abscess is a rare but devastating infection. It usually occurs in the setting of systemic infection with multiple septic foci elsewhere,[4] but occasionally there is no history of prior infection.[60] Chiari's[61] well-studied case of a patient with metastatic spinal cord abscess associated with meningitis and cerebellar abscess secondary to bronchiectasis increased awareness of this clinical syndrome and described its clinical constellation. A further report[62] of a child who recovered following surgical drainage of a staphylococcal abscess of the thoracic spinal cord demonstrates the value of early recognition.

Intramedullary spinal cord abscess is rare. Between Hart's original description in 1830[60] and 1977, only 54 cases had been reported.[63,64] Both DiTullio[63] and Menezes[64] independently reviewed this literature. In 1994, Byrne et al.[65] and in 1995 Bartels et al.,[66/67] reported cases and reviewed the literature. Between 1977 and 1995, Bartels et al. identified an additional 41 cases. Courville[68] found only one case among 40,000 postmortem examinations.

Intramedullary abscess may occur at any age; but there may be a bimodal age distribution with a predominance in patients under 25 and over age 50. In pediatric patients, a dermal sinus tract can be the etiology.[65] The male–female ratio has been reported to be 5:2.[65]

Among other routes, abscess may arise from a remote site by hematogenous spread, an infected dermal sinus, or trauma. In most cases, intramedullary spinal cord abscesses have been metastatic from a pyogenic infection elsewhere. Bronchiectasis and endocarditis are common sources. Less commonly, intramedullary abscesses arise from an adjacent infection;[4,44] for example, they have been reported to follow a stab wound[69] and high lumbar puncture.[70] In those cases in which no source can be identified, the abscesses are called primary. One review [64] found 20% of cases to be primary, with the remainder secondary to known infection.

Abscesses may be classified as single or multiple. Among 55 reported cases,[64] 42 were single and 13 were multiple. The thoracic region was the most common location; 80% were located in this area. Most extend over several segments in the rostrocaudal axis. The entire spinal cord occasionally may be involved.[64]

On pathological examination, intramedullary abscesses may be centrally located, but often the dorsal spinal cord is more involved than the ventral region.[44] The spinal cord is usually swollen, and this may be visualized on radiological studies. The margins of the abscess may be poorly defined, and there may be little glial reaction.[71]

In most cases, the time between onset of symptoms and diagnosis ranges from days to months. One report[72] found the interval between onset and diagnosis to be less than 2 weeks in 43%, 1 to 3 months in 33%, and 4 months to 3 years in 24%. When myelopathy develops over a few days and radiological studies are nondiagnostic, an erroneous diagnosis of acute transverse myelopathy or multiple sclerosis may be made. Subacute and chronic presentations, with radiological studies that usually are nondiagnostic or show enlarged spinal cords, may mimic intramedullary tumors.

The clinical presentation of intramedullary spinal cord abscess varies according to the location of involvement and the chronicity of infection. Fever and signs of infection are usually present in acute cases. Alternatively, in chronic cases clinical evidence of infection is often not as apparent. For example, in the review[65] of cases reported between 1978 and 1994, Byrne et al. found 6 acute cases (symptoms less than 1 week), 4 subacute (symptoms lasting 1 to 6 weeks), and 4 chronic cases. These authors emphasized that pa-

tients with chronic abscesses were typically afebrile. Such patients typically had radicular pain, with radiological studies showing only a widened cord. The only consistent finding in their review of recent cases was that in cases where the CSF was analyzed, there was pleocytosis, protein was elevated, and cultures were negative.

Pain is a common presenting complaint regardless of the site and chronicity.[64] In one review,[72] incontinence was present in 88% of cases, paraplegia in 72%, and anesthetic sensory loss in 61% at the time of diagnosis. In chronic cases, progression of symptoms may be slow and, at times, stuttering in nature.[64]

Laboratory studies are often nondiagnostic. There is usually leukocytosis on the complete blood count and other signs of infection, but in cases of chronic abscess there may be no fever, as noted above. Cerebrospinal fluid may be nonspecifically abnormal or may suggest meningitis.[4,44] In the review by Byrne et al.[65] cited above, the following results of the abscess culture were found: sterile (7); *staphylococci* (4), Gram negative (6), *streptococci* (3), and *Listeria* (1).

Myelography may demonstrate an intramedullary expansion of the spinal cord consistent with an intraspinal mass.[49] A CT following intrathecal injection of contrast material and MRI may be helpful in demonstrating intramedullary expansion of the spinal cord. Experience using MRI for the diagnosis of intramedullary abscess is limited. In the five cases that were reviewed by Byrne et al.,[65] decreased signal intensity was seen on T_{-1} weighted images, and gadolinium enhancement was seen in the three cases in which it was administered. The MRI pattern was thought to be similar to that seen in cerebral abscesses. Bartels et al.[66/67] observed cases in which enhancement did not occur and concluded that the MRI features were not pathognomonic for intramedullary abscess. The differential diagnosis included neoplasm, granulomatous disease, and demyelinating disease. These authors concluded that surgery was the only way to establish a definitive diagnosis premortem.

Treatment of intramedullary spinal cord abscess includes prompt surgical drainage and appropriate parenteral antibiotic therapy.[60,64–66,67] Among the 20 recent cases reviewed,[65] four patients had a complete recovery, nine had a good recovery, and seven had a poor outcome. Prognostic features that correlated with good outcome were an age less than 25 years and duration of severe motor loss less than three days.

Tuberculous Spondylitis

Mycobacterium tuberculosis may injure the spinal cord and cauda equina through involvement of the epidural and intradural locations.[73–76] In the epidural location, involvement of the vertebral body may lead to destruction of the vertebra, epidural abscess, and neural compression (Pott's disease). In the intradural location, tuberculous meningitis and/or space-occupying lesions (tuberculomas) may cause neurologic injury.

Tuberculous spondylitis is the most common condition affecting the spine. Mycobacteria classically destroy the vertebral bodies and intervening disc space and cause a paravertebral abscess, combining to cause spinal cord or cauda equina compression from the abscess's ventral aspect.[4,77,78] Percival Pott[79] called attention to the curvature of the spine and resulting paraplegia that are due to tuberculous involvement. Pott's disease now bears his name. Less commonly, compression may occur secondary to neural arch involvement or extension into the epidural space without radiographic changes of the vertebral bodies and intervening disc space. The frequency of tuberculous epidural abscess was reported to be up to 25% of epidural abscesses during 1968–1978.[80] Permanent kyphosis may result from tuberculous spondylitis after the infection has been cured (Fig. 9–3).

The pathological anatomy and clinical features of tuberculosis involving the nervous system have been reviewed.[74,79] The spine is the most common site of extrapulmonary tuberculous bone involvement.[74,81]

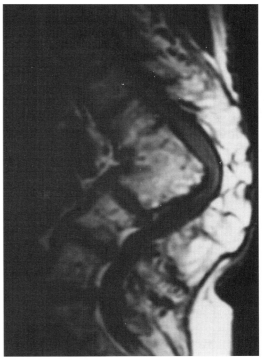

Figure 9–3. An MRI of the thoracolumbar spine showing fused vertebral bodies and gibbus deformity in a 78-year-old woman who had tuberculous spondylitis at age seven. The patient had back pain but no clinical signs of myelopathy.

Most commonly, spinal involvement follows a primary tuberculous infection elsewhere, with either a short or long latency period. The vertebral column usually is seeded hematogenously, immediately from the primary infection, or later from that site or from another extraosseus secondary site.[73] Epidural compression of the spinal cord and nerve root(s) may be due to granuloma formation, abscess, pathological subluxation, or collapse of a vertebral body.[74] Thrombosis of spinal blood vessels may also occur.[74]

Although in developing countries younger patients appear to be at greater risk for spinal involvement than older individuals, in industrialized nations, the age of presentation is usually in the fifth and sixth decade.[73,74,82] Although tuberculous involvement of the spine has not been observed commonly in developed countries, the use of immunosuppressive therapy and the AIDS epidemic may increase the frequency of this disease.[83,84]

CLINICAL FEATURES

The clinical presentation of tuberculous spondylitis may be very similar to that of other infectious or neoplastic processes in the same location.[4,77,85,86] Patients typically complain of pain and tenderness in the region of the infected vertebrae. They often have a low-grade fever, chills, weight loss, and other constitutional symptoms.[74] The average duration of symptoms prior to diagnosis is one year, but it may range from weeks to years.[74,87] Local pain and radicular pain as well as motor, sensory, and sphincter disturbances caudal to the lesion progress if the disease is not recognized and treated.[87,88] According to one review of tuberculous spondylitis, paraplegia occurred with a frequency ranging from 4% to 38%.[74]

Skin testing for tuberculosis has been reported to be negative in up to 20% of patients in some series.[74,87] Furthermore, the chest radiograph has been negative for active or inactive pulmonary tuberculosis in one half of patients with osteoarticular tuberculosis.[74,80] Thus, some patients may not have evidence of tuberculosis elsewhere when they present with tuberculous spondylitis.

The thoracic spine and thoracolumbar region are favored levels for involvement. The cervical spine is much less frequently represented.[17,73,87] Plain radiographs often demonstrate features that resemble pyogenic infections and abscess formation,[18,82,89] or metastatic cancer.[78] The kyphosis that develops from vertebral body and disc involvement may approach 90°. The radionuclide bone scan has been reported negative in 35% of cases, and the gallium scan negative in 70%.[87] When epidural neural compression occurs secondary to extension of a paravertebral mass, the bone scan may be negative. Both CT and MRI may be helpful in demonstrating the vertebral destruction and paravertebral mass associated with tuberculous spondylitis.[90] Lindahl and colleagues[91] described the imaging characteristics of spinal tuberculosis in detail. Of 503 patients with tuberculosis, 63 (13%) had spinal involvement. Among these 63 patients, the spine was the sole location of involvement in 40. The most common MRI findings were destroyed vertebrae with associated paraspinal soft-tissue mass with or without abscess formation, and sometimes epidural extension and gibbus deformity. Single-vertebral-level disease was common, and the imaging characteristics were sometimes indistinguishable from neoplastic disease.

Biopsy of bone, often performed as needle biopsy under fluoroscopy or CT, is important in the confirmation of a diagnosis. Specimens should be sent to test for acid-fast bacilli, fungi, bacteria, and neoplastic disease. Culture of the bone has been reported to yield acid-fast bacilli in only 60% to 80% of cases.[74,80] When cultures are negative, histological studies of the involved bone or other involved tissue may confirm a diagnosis or establish an alternative diagnosis.[75] Superinfection of tuberculous osteomyelitis with pyogenic organisms has been reported.[75] If a diagnosis is not established by needle biopsy or aspirate, extraspinal disease should be sought and, if necessary, an open biopsy and culture should be obtained.

THERAPY

Because the benchmark of microbiologic diagnosis of infection with *M. tuberculosis* is culture of the organism from biopsy or tissue fluids, therapy of tuberculous spondylitis usually must be initiated before culture results are available. Thus, therapy usually is begun on clinical and radiological grounds that are supported by laboratory studies, such as histologic evidence of granulomatous inflammation and lymphocytic reaction, when available. Recently, new techniques, such as serologic tests for *M. tuberculosis*–specific antigens[92,93] and probes to identify *M. tuberculosis* DNA[94] have been developed for diagnosis.[77]

With the advent of effective antituberculous chemotherapy, the need for surgical intervention has become controversial and surgery is less common. One recent review recommends an antituberculous regimen beginning with four drugs.[14] Decompression and spinal fusion are reserved for those with (1) severe loss of neurologic function when first seen, (2) progressive loss of neurologic function while on adequate antituberculous chemotherapy, (3) no improvement of neurologic function after four to six weeks of adequate antituberculous chemotherapy, and (4) an unstable spine.[2,14,81,95,96] Alternatively, despite the apparent success of nonsurgical management, another review[2] generally recommends surgery for all cases of suspected tuberculous epidural abscess with neurologic abnormalities, for both diagnostic and therapeutic reasons. In a recent report by Rezai and colleagues,[97] operative intervention was undertaken in 11 of 20 patients with Pott's disease. Indications for surgery included motor deficits, spinal deformity, nondiagnostic CT-guided needle biopsy, and lack of response to medical therapy. At one-year follow-up, of the nine surviving operated patients, all were neurologically improved or normal without residual infection. The average angulation of the spine was reduced from 31° to 24°.

A short course of corticosteroids may be helpful in cases of progressing myelopathy with concurrent administration of antituberculous chemotherapy. Prolonged antituberculous chemotherapy is required when spondylitis is present. The prognosis for neurologic recovery is good for 75% to 95% of appropriately treated patients with tuberculous spondylitis.[77] However, the emergence of antibiotic-resistant strains of *M. tuberculosis* is expected to complicate the management of this facet of the disease, and the general medical and immunological status of patients with spinal epidural abscess must be considered. Accordingly, management must be individualized.

Tuberculosis Meningitis and Spinal Cord Tuberculoma

Intradural tuberculosis of the spine may be classified as (1) diffuse meningeal inflammation or (2) mass lesions of the spine. In meningitis, or what has been termed radiculomyelitis,[98] there is diffuse inflammation of the leptomeninges, with tuberculous exudate that microscopically reveals caseating granulomas and tubercles. The spinal cord and roots are injured as a result of the diffuse inflammatory process.

The clinical presentation of tuberculous radiculomyelitis has been presented by Wadia and Dastur.[98,99] Patients commonly present with pain, weakness, and sensory disturbances. Radicular findings may obscure the diagnosis of myelopathy. A subacute myelopathy or acute transverse myelitis has been reported.[100,101]

Findings on MRI of the spine include clumping of nerve roots, loss of the subarachnoid space, and edema of the spinal cord.[102,103] The CSF typically shows elevated protein and pleocytosis. The management of this condition is beyond the scope of this text, and the reader is referred to infectious disease references.[95,104]

Space-occupying lesions of the spine may be observed with tuberculosis, but these are rare. For example, intramedullary spinal tuberculomas have been reported,[105–107] and may cause myelopathy in patients with AIDS.[108] Magnetic resonance imaging has identified intramedullary tuberculomas that may show contrast enhancement.[109,110] Because of the increase in drug-resistant tuberculosis and the AIDS epidemic, spinal tuberculosis is expected to continue to be considered in the differential diagnosis of patients at risk for tuberculosis.

Fungal Infections

Several different fungi may invade the spinal cord, either as primary infection or as a manifestation of disseminated disease. As with bacterial infections, fungal infections may involve the intramedullary spinal cord or the leptomeninges or they may cause epidural spinal cord compression. In the spine, many fungal infections behave like masses, compressing the spinal cord or cauda equina.[4] The radiographic appearance of spinal fungal infections may be similar to pyogenic and tuberculous infection.[89]

Cryptococcal involvement of the spine usually occurs as a necrotic granulomatous mass in the intradural location,[4,111] but it may occur secondary to osteomyelitis.[112] *Coccidioides,*[113,114] *Blastomyces,*[4,115] *Aspergillus,*[50,116,117] and *Nocardia*[118,119] have been found to cause myelopathy or cauda equina compression due to granulomas in both intradural and extradural locations. Candidiasis may also rarely involve the spine.[120,121] Spinal involvement from actinomycosis is considered rare, but it may occur due to extension from a paravertebral site or, less commonly, from a vertebra.[89]

Parasitic Disease

Although parasitic disease involving the spine is rare in North America and Europe, it is occasionally observed in patients who have visited endemic areas or who are immunosuppressed.[122] The parasitic diseases most commonly seen are cysticercosis, hydatid disease, and schistosomiasis.[4]

Cysticercosis is a disease that results from ingestion of the pork tapeworm, *Taenia solium.* Involvement of the central nervous system results when embryos disseminate to the brain and, occasionally, to the spinal cord. There they form cysts, or, as occurs in the racemose form in the cerebral ventricles and subarachnoid space, multiple cysts that are grouped together. A case of cysticercosis involving the dorsal spinal cord has been reported.[123]

Hydatid disease is caused by the larval form of the parasite *Taenia echinococcus.* It is rarely encountered in North America. The liver is most often involved;[4] the central nervous system may be involved as a primary site of infection or as a host site for a metastatic cyst. The most common cause of spinal dysfunction is vertebral involvement with secondary spinal canal encroachment. According to a 1955 study by Fischer,[4] there have been a dozen cases of cysts involving the spinal cord but over 200 reports of vertebral column involvement.

Schistosomiasis arises from infection with one of three trematode parasites: *Schistosoma haematobium,* found mainly in Africa; *S. mansoni,* present primarily in Africa and South America; and *S. japonicum,* seen in the Far East.[4] Involvement of the central nervous system is rare with any of the three parasites, yet each reveals a different pattern of CNS invasion. For example, *S. haematobium* primarily affects the spinal cord. *S. japonicum* may involve the brain and almost never invades the spinal cord. *S. mansoni* causes lesions in the brain and spinal cord with similar frequency and is the most common cause of spinal schistosomiasis.[124]

Back pain and leg pain that may be present for a few weeks are often part of the initial clinical presentation of spinal schistosomiasis. These symptoms give way to weakness, sensory loss, and sphincter dysfunction.[125,126] Although the clinical presentation may evolve over several months, the myelopathic signs may develop acutely over several hours or days.[127] Schistosomiasis is to be suspected in the patient who has been in an endemic area. Pathological findings are those of arterial and venous infarction secondary to ova in these blood vessels.[4]

In addition to the above parasitic diseases, myelopathy may rarely be due to toxoplasmosis, paragonimiasis, gnathostomiasis, trichinosis, and malaria.[4,122,128,129]

NONINFECTIOUS INFLAMMATORY DISEASES

Sarcoidosis

Neurologic involvement has been reported in 5% of sarcoidosis cases. Involvement of the spine includes the spectrum of arachnoiditis, cauda equina syndrome and other radiculopathies, intramedullary disease, and extradural disease.[130] The pathogenesis, diagnosis, and management of sarcoidosis have been recently reviewed.[131]

Sarcoidosis may involve the spine or nerve roots secondary to intradural or epidural localization of granulomata. Although rare, there have been isolated reports of sarcoidosis causing a clinical syndrome characterized by an expanding intramedullary mass, and more recently a series of 16 patients with intramedullary sarcoidosis.[130] More commonly, clinical and imaging studies may be consistent with arachnoiditis. The sarcoid granulomata may cause vascular compression with secondary ischemic changes of the spinal cord.[4] Sarcoid may infrequently involve the skeletal system.[89,132] Pulmonary involvement may be seen radiographically in 80% to 90% of patients with osseous sarcoidosis.[89] When the vertebral column is involved, the thoracic and lumbar regions are the most common sites;[133] in such cases, roentgenograms of the spine may show a variable appearance.[73,134–136] The MRI appearance of intramedullary sarcoidosis has been recently reported;[130] among 16 patients, Junger and colleagues found leptomeningeal enhancement, fusiform spinal cord enlargement (either focal or diffuse), and spinal cord atrophy.

Corticosteroids have been used in the treatment of systemic and neurologic manifestations of sarcoidosis.[137,138] Junger and colleagues[130] found that corticosteroids, often in high dose, were the mainstay of therapy; five of 12 patients responded. In cases where corticosteroids are contraindicated or cannot be tolerated, other immunosuppressive agents such as methotrexate, azathioprine, cyclosporine, and antimalarials and radiation therapy have been used.[131,139–142]

Rheumatoid Arthritis

Rheumatoid arthritis (RA), an inflammatory disease affecting synovial joints as well as periarticular tissues, is a well-defined cause of spinal cord compression.[143,144] The most commonly involved level of involvement is the atlanto-axial joint; the damage occurs as a result of ventral subluxation of C1 on C2. This level is vulnerable because the odontoid is bordered ventral and dorsally by synovial joints and dorsally by the transverse atlantal ligament, which may also be involved. Atlanto-axial instability has been reported in 36% of rheumatoid outpatients[145] and in 61% of patients requir-

ing knee or hip arthroplasties (see Fig. 9–4).[146]

Dorsal subluxation is a less frequent cause of compressive myelopathy.[147] Involvement of the occipito-atlanto-axial complex may also permit the skull to settle on the cervical spine, resulting in upward migration of the dens through the foramen magnum. This abnormality has been reported to occur in 5% to 8% of patients with RA and has been variously termed cranial settling,[148–150] atlanto-axial

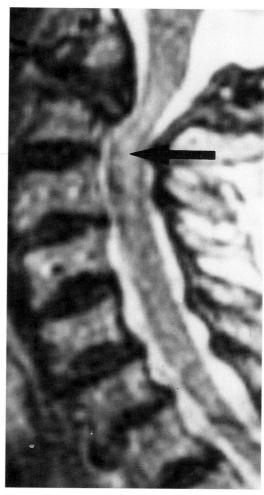

Figure 9–4. An MRI of the craniocervical junction in a patient with rheumatoid arthritis who sustained a fracture of the C2 vertebra (after long-term steroids), causing cord compression. Arrow indicates changes in the spinal cord secondary to compression. (Courtesy of Dr. Richard Becker.)

impaction,[151,152] and pseudobasilar invagination.[153] Brain-stem compression may occur secondary to this vertical migration.

Occasionally, the lower spinal cord and nerve roots are involved as a result of complications of rheumatoid arthritis (Fig. 9–5).[144] For example, there are case reports of rheumatoid pachymeningitis of the spinal dura,[154] and involvement of the epidural space with rheumatoid nodules and granulation tissue[155,156] may cause spinal cord or nerve root compression. Furthermore, the vertebral bodies[157] or intervertebral discs[158] may infrequently be the site of rheumatoid involvement, resulting in subluxation and neural compression. Because of the frequency of atlanto-axial subluxation (AAS), this section will discuss this important aspect of spinal disease in rheumatoid arthritis.

CLINICAL FEATURES AND DIAGNOSTIC IMAGING STUDIES

Symptoms and signs of AAS are protean. Paresthesias, crepitation, and pain are common early symptoms. The pain may radiate to the occiput if the second cervical

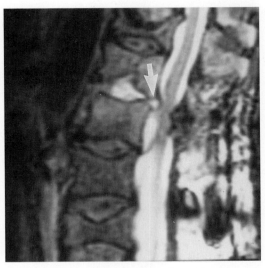

Figure 9–5. An MRI of the lumbar spine showing discitis at L1–2 and secondary epidural abscess causing spinal cord compression (arrow). The patient had severe rheumatoid arthritis and had undergone a laminectomy, following which she developed the discitis. (Courtesy of Dr. Richard Becker.)

root is compressed. Hyperreflexia was the most common early manifestation of myelopathy in a series of 100 patients reported by Stevens et al.[145] Hyperreflexia was observed in 24 of 36 patients with 3 mm or more ventral atlanto-axial subluxation, but it was also observed in 10 patients without subluxation. As myelopathy progresses, Babinski responses and other signs of myelopathy ensue. For example, in a series of 32 rheumatoid patients with cervical spine disease referred for neurologic consultation, Nakano et al.[145a] found (1) that more than half had pain in the C2 dermatome, two had spastic quadriparesis of insidious onset, and progression was seen in nearly all, with rapid progression after minor trauma in occasional patients, and (3) six patients had brain-stem signs that could be precipitated by neck movements.

Radiographs of the spine show a variety of abnormalities in patients with RA.[89,152,159] As noted above, plain radiographs commonly reveal ventral AAS in both unselected rheumatoid outpatients and those with more advanced disease.[145,146] This may not be apparent if flexion and extension views are not obtained, underscoring the importance of obtaining these radiographs.[89,152,160] Since such subluxation may cause spinal cord compression, flexion–extension studies must be performed with caution to avoid neurologic injury. AAS may occur secondary to a variety of other causes, including Down's syndrome,[161–164] trauma, neoplasms,[165] Behcet's syndrome,[166] psoriatic arthritis,[167] achondroplasia,[168] and neurofibromatosis (see Chapter 2).[169]

In addition to plain radiographs, CT has been used to delineate the spinal deformities associated with RA;[170,171] CT myelography has also been used in the radiological evaluation of AAS.[172] Magnetic resonance imaging has become the imaging test of choice for viewing the craniocervical junction, providing excellent resolution of the bone, soft tissues, and brainstem and spinal cord. Magnetic resonance imaging can demonstrate whether spinal cord compression is secondary to subluxation or soft-tissue changes such as pannus formation.[173–175] In addition to the

C1–2 level, subluxation may occur at other levels of the spine, and radiographic abnormalities associated with spinal cord compression at lower levels are occasionally seen (see Fig. 9–5).[89]

NATURAL HISTORY AND THERAPY

Cervical spine involvement and AAS due to RA are commonly observed early in the course of the disease and correlate with its severity elsewhere. Many patients who develop ventral AAS will do so within a few years of onset of RA. In a postmortem study, ventral AAS was found in 11% to 46% of cases.[160] Neurologic signs are noted in up to one third of patients with cervical spine involvement, and neurologic progression may occur in 2% to 36% of cases.[160] However, atlanto-axial instability may persist without clinical change for years. For example, among 41 rheumatoid patients with AAS followed for 10 years or more, 61% showed no significant progression, 27% showed progression of subluxation and 12% showed reduced anterior subluxation, sometimes associated with an increase in vertical subluxation. Among this cohort of 41 patients, three developed progressive neurologic dysfunction.[176] Alternatively, Pellicci et al.[177] reported a higher rate of progression of AAS and neurologic deterioration. In his series, which was followed for six years, 80% showed evidence of progression on imaging studies and 36% revealed neurologic deterioration.

The management of rheumatoid AAS must be individualized; it includes both medical and surgical options. Medical therapy includes treatment of the overall disease process, use of a collar and, antiinflammatory agents, and an exercise program.[178] The indications for surgical intervention are controversial and evolving. Surgical therapy, although not uniformly successful, must be considered in patients with progressive neurologic impairment due to compression or those with incapacitating pain.[179,180] If a patient suffers from progressive neurologic dysfunction due to AAS, and his/her general health permits, surgery is usually considered in an attempt to prevent neurologic deterioration. Because many patients requiring surgery have debilitating intercurrent problems associated with their underlying disease and are thus susceptible to infection and poor wound healing, they are a major surgical challenge and risk.[160] These patients may, in fact, present excessive risks. Ranawat reported a grading system for extent of disability (Table 9–4).[181] In RA patients, the morbidity and mortality in surgically treated patients in class IIIb according to Ranawat's classification is excessive, thus often contraindicating surgery.

There is also controversy in cases of radiologic instability without clinical signs of neurologic involvement. Rosenbaum, et al.[143] state that the only radiographic finding that mandates neck surgery in patients without spinal cord or brain-stem dysfunction is odontoid fracture. They base this recommendation on natural history studies that reveal that only a minority of patients will develop neurologic compromise. They acknowledge that other authors recommend surgery using a measure of subluxation (e.g., 8 mm of ventral atlanto-axial movement or 4 mm of subaxial subluxation, with imaging evidence of spinal cord compression, without clinical signs of neurologic dysfunction).[182–184] These recommendations must be tempered with data that substantiate a significant incidence of sudden death related to AAS in patients with RA.[185]

Due to the risk of injury during intubation among patients with AAS, cervical spine stability prior to endotracheal anesthesia is recommended in rheumatoid patients suspected of having AAS. If instability is found, special precautions need to be taken to protect the neck during intubation and during the anesthesia.

Table 9–4. **Ranawat Classification of Myelopathy**[181]

Class	Neurologic Status
I	Intact
II	Radiculopathy/Mild myelopathy
IIIa	Moderate Myelopathy (but ambulatory)
IIIb	Severe myelopathy (non-ambulatory)

Spondyloarthropathies

The spondyloarthropathies are a group of disorders that include ankylosing spondylitis (AS), Reiter's syndrome and reactive arthritis, psoriatic arthritis, and arthritis associated with inflammatory bowel disease.[143,186] Since they characteristically cause inflammation of the sacroiliac joints, the facet joints, and spinal ligaments, it is not unexpected that patients often complain of back pain and develop spinal complications. The spondyloarthropathies are to be distinguished from diffuse idiopathic skeletal hyperostosis (Forestier's disease), a noninflammatory ossifying disorder affecting the spine which may also cause spinal cord compression. This syndrome predominantly involves ossification of the anterior longitudinal ligament.

A full discussion of the diagnostic criteria for the spondyloarthopathies is beyond the scope of this book. In general, they are inflammatory disorders involving the sacroiliac joints, spine, and larger peripheral joints.[187,188] They usually present between the ages of 20 and 40 years, and men are more commonly affected than women. In cases of ankylosing spondylitis, there is a strong association with the presence of HLA-B27.[189] Extra-articular manifestations often occur and may include anterior uveitis, aortic insufficiency, and pulmonary fibrosis. Back pain, which may be nocturnal, is the most common presenting complaint of AS.[186] Patients often report morning stiffness that improves with activity; a flexed posture is often assumed to alleviate pain.

In addition, major neurologic complications such as vertebral fracture due to minor trauma (Fig. 9–6),[190–192] spinal epidural hematoma,[193,194] spinal cord and nerve root compression, and cauda equina dysfunction[195–197] may occur in patients with ankylosing spondylitis. Several reports have emphasized the extreme vulnerability of the vertebral column to trauma.[191] The cervical spine appears especially prone to fracture and, as is the case with rheumatoid arthritis, patients are vulnerable to spinal deformation during hyperextension of the neck at the time of intubation. Although not as common as in rheumatoid arthritis, subluxation of the atlanto-axial joint is not an infrequent finding in patients with AS.[197,198] Hunter[199] found three cases of odontoid erosions and three cases of atlanto-axial subluxation among 26 unselected patients with ankylosing spondylitis. Epidural hematomas may result from trauma and

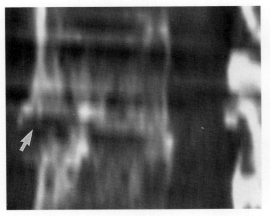 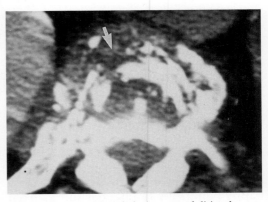

A   B

Figure 9–6. A CT scan of the lower thoracic spine in a 66-year-old man with ankylosing spondylitis who sustained a fracture of the anterior longitudinal ligament. (A, left figure) Reformatted CT scan showing fracture of the anterior longitudinal ligament and anterior vertebral column (arrow). (B, right figure) Axial CT scan showing erosive discovertebral pseudoarthosis (arrow) at the level of the fracture. (Courtesy of Dr. Richard Becker.)

also have been found following spinal anesthesia.[193,194]

CLINICAL FEATURES

Nerve root pain, usually thoracic or lumbar, is the most common neurologic manifestation of the spondyloarthopathies.[197] Such radiculopathies may or may not be associated with abnormal neurologic signs. In a retrospective series of 54 patients, seven described symptoms typical of sciatica.[196] In addition, thoracic radiculopathy may cause girdle pain. Spinal cord compression due to granulomatous tissue and dural thickening may be a potential cause of myelopathy,[196] and multiple sclerosis has been reported at an increased frequency among patients with AS.[187]

A progressive cauda equina syndrome is an infrequent and obscure but well-described complication of the spondyloarthopathies.[200] Its pathogenesis is poorly understood. Pathological studies have typically shown arachnoid diverticula. Although evidence of arachnoiditis is not routinely observed, arachnoid cysts and cauda equina syndrome may be late sequelae of arachnoiditis.[196] Furthermore, Charlesworth and colleagues[201] have recently shown evidence for arachnoiditis on MRI, which they conclude provides evidence for arachnoiditis in the pathogenesis of the cauda equina syndrome in AS.

Cauda equina syndrome appears to be a late complication of spondyloarthopathies. It is often observed years after the disease has become quiescent. The shortest interval reported between diagnosis of AS and the development of cauda equina syndrome was four years; one-third of patients suffer from the disease for over 30 years before the syndrome evolves.[197] Fourteen patients with cauda equina syndrome secondary to AS were reported from the Mayo Clinic;[195] the interval ranged from 17 to 53 years and averaged 35 years. Furthermore, AS had gone into remission in 10 of the 14 patients prior to the onset of neurologic symptoms. Once diagnosed, cauda equina syndrome is usually slowly progressive.[195] The clinical manifestations of the syndrome are typical of cauda equina syndrome due to other causes: sphincter disturbances, impotence, a lax anal sphincter, pain, loss of sensation over the sacral and lower lumbar dermatomes, and weakness and wasting of muscles innervated by the cauda equina. In the Mayo Clinic series,[195] the most common finding on neurologic examination was sensory loss, usually symmetrical, in the distribution of multiple nerve roots at and below the L5, S1, S2, and S3 level. In the same series, weakness (often asymmetric) was found in the distribution of the L5 and sacral roots. Deep tendon reflexes are depressed routinely at the ankles, and occasionally at the knees.

LABORATORY STUDIES AND DIAGNOSTIC IMAGING STUDIES IN THE CAUDA EQUINA SYNDROME

The electromyogram commonly shows evidence of denervation of muscles innervated by multiple lumbar and sacral nerve roots. Cerebrospinal fluid findings usually do not show typical signs of arachnoiditis; rather, normal or modestly elevated protein is commonly found.[195] Conventional radiography usually shows involvement of the sacroiliac joints, which are almost always affected.[202–204] Spinal inflammation accompanies this involvement, and it eventually may result in a "bamboo" appearance on x-ray, which has earned it the name "bamboo spine."[204]

Myelography may be normal, especially if the procedure is done with the patient in a prone position. However, if the patient is in a supine position, myelography often reveals multiple arachnoid diverticula,[196] which usually erode the adjacent vertebrae. The thecal sac may be widened in the lumbosacral region.

Lumbar puncture is difficult to perform in patients with AS, and there is a risk of transient neurologic worsening after myelography.[195,205] In some patients, CT may eliminate the need for myelography. Among other abnormalities, CT may show scalloping of the laminae, multiple dorsal diverticula, and calcification of ligaments and discs associated with dural ectasia and posterior diverticula.[195,206,207] Magnetic resonance imaging has been reported to reveal characteristic expansion of the lumbar spinal canal, with scalloping of the pedicles, laminae, and spinous processes along with dural diverticula. As mentioned above, arachnoiditis has been reported to be seen on MRI.[201] Magnetic resonance imaging and CT are the preferred modalities for imaging these patients.[208,209]

THERAPY

The treatment of AS includes the use of antiinflammatory agents and strengthening exercises.[210] Extension exercises, hydrotherapy, and swimming appear very effective. Bartleson and colleagues[195] report no effective therapy for cauda equina syndrome secondary to longstanding AS and advise that surgical intervention be avoided. More recently, there have been case reports of apparent benefit derived from shunting between the lumbar subarachnoid space and the peritoneum.[211,212]

SUMMARY

Both infectious and noninfectious inflammatory diseases may cause spinal cord and root compression, thereby causing neurologic manifestations. These disorders are presented in this chapter and are to be distinguished from primary inflammatory diseases of the spinal cord such as demyelinating diseases. This distinction is made because the imaging findings usually separate these two groups of disorders. Furthermore, the clinical manifestations are often distinguishable.

Initially pyogenic diseases which may cause epidural abscess have been discussed at length. Epidural abscess is a rare disorder, but its frequency appears to be increasing. The infection may spread from a known infection elsewhere or may appear initially in the vertebral column with secondary extension into the spinal canal. The dura mater is effective in limiting its spread, but the spinal cord and roots are compressed as the abscess extends into the spinal canal. *Staphylococcus aureus* is the most common organism isolated from

epidural abscesses, although there is an increasing incidence of other bacteria, especially Gram-negative bacilli. Magnetic resonance imaging is the diagnostic imaging test of choice because paravertebral abscesses, discitis, osteomyelitis and epidural extension of the abscess can be identified. Therapy includes antibiotics and surgery. Principles used in the decision for surgical intervention are discussed in the text. Intramedullary pyogenic abscesses are rare and are also reviewed.

Neural compression from tuberculosis may occur secondary to tuberculous spondylitis or tuberculous meningitis. In addition, examples of spinal cord compression from vertebral column deformities (e.g., kyphosis) found years after tuberculous spondylitis are also seen. Magnetic resonance imaging is helpful in diagnosis; however, the findings are not pathognomonic. The principles of therapy for tuberculosis are mentioned but current infectious disease references should be consulted for management of this and the other infectious diseases reviewed in this book. Fungal infections and parasitic diseases are also briefly reviewed.

Noninfectious inflammatory diseases are discussed in this chapter. Among them, sarcoidosis, rhematoid arthritis and ankylosing spondylitis are discussed in some detail. Rheumatoid arthritis presents unique problems for the spine since the atlanto-axial joint is frequently involved, which may lead to atlanto-axial subluxation. Spinal cord or root compression may occur at other levels due to pannus formation or complications of the disease or immunosuppressive therapy. The principles involved in management of the neurologic complications of rheumatoid arthritis are reviewed.

The spondyloarthropathies include ankylosing spondylitis, Reiter's syndrome, psoriatic arthritis, and arthritis associated with inflammatory bowel disease. The spinal complications of ankylosing spondylitis, as the prototype for this group of diseases, are presented in this chapter. Axial and root pain are the most common neurologic manifestations of the disease. Furthermore, vertebral fracture due to minor trauma is a feared complication which may occur in these patients. An infrequent complication of the spondyloarthropathies is a progressive cauda equina syndrome. The pathogenesis is not understood but the clinical manifestations and diagnostic imaging features are presented. The management of inflammatory diseases of the spine requires integration of an understanding of (1) the biology of the underlying disease process, (2) clinical manifestations, (3) diagnostic imaging findings, and (4) biomechanics of the spine.

REFERENCES

1. D'Angelo CM, Whisler WW. Bacterial infections of the spinal cord and its coverings. In Vinken PJ, Bruyn GW, editors. *Handbook of Clinical Neurology, Volume 33.* Amsterdam: North-Holland; 1978; pp. 187–94.
2. Verner EF, Musher DM. Spinal epidural abscess. *Med Clin North Am* 1985;69:375–84.
3. Heindell CC, Ferguson JP, Kumarasamy T. Spinal subdural empyema complicating pregnancy. Case report. *J Neurosurg* 1974;40:654–6.
4. Hughes JT. *Pathology of the Spinal Cord.* Philadelphia: W.B. Saunders; 1978.
5. Greenlee JE. Epidural abscess. In Mandell GL, Douglas RG, Bennett JE, editors. *Principles and Practice of Infectious Diseases, 2nd Edition.* New York: John Wiley; 1985; pp. 594–6.
6. Guidetti B, LaTorre E. Hypertrophic spinal pachymeningitis. *J Neurosurg* 1967;26:496.
7. Oonishi T, Ishiko T, Arai M, et al. Pachymeningitis cervicalis hypertrophica. *Acta Pathol Jpn* 1982;32:163.
8. Boharas S, Koskoff YD. The early diagnosis of acute spinal epidural abscess. *JAMA* 1941;117:1085–8.
9. Khanna R, Malik G, Rock J, Rosenblum M. Spinal epidural abscess: evaluation of factors influencing outcome. *Neurosurgery* 1996;39:958–64.
10. Broner F, Garland D, Zigler J. Spinal infections in the immunocompromised host. *Orthop Clin North Am* 1996;27:37–46.
11. Hlavin M, Kaminski H, Ross J, et al. Spinal epidural abscess: a ten year perspective. *Neurosurgery* 1990;27:177–84.
12. Redekop G, Maestro RD. Diagnosis and management of spinal epidural abscess. *Can J Neurol Sci* 1992;19:180–7.
13. Altrocchi PH. Acute spinal epidural abscess vs acute transverse myelopathy. *Arch Neurol* 1963; 9:17–25.
14. Gellin B, Weingarten K, FW Gamache J, Hartman B. Epidural abscess. In Scheld W, Whitley R, Durack D, editors. *Infections of the Central Nervous System, 2nd Edition.* Philadelphia: Lippicott-Raven; 1997; pp. 507–22.
15. Danner RL, Hartman BJ. Update of spinal epidural abscess: 35 cases and review of the literature. *Rev Infect Dis.* 1987;9:265–74.
16. Baker AS, Ojemann RJ, Swartz NM, et al. Spinal epidural abscess. *N Engl J Med* 1975;293:463–8.
17. Goldman AB, Freiberger RH. Localized infectious and neuropathic diseases. *Skeletal Radiol* 1979;14:19–32.
18. Griffiths HED, Jones DM. Pyogenic infection of the spine: a review of 28 cases. *J Bone Joint Surg* 1971;53B:383–91.
19. Hensner AP. Nontuberculous spinal epidural infections. *N Engl J Med* 1948;239:845–54.
20. Torda A, Gottlieb T, Bradbury R. Pyogenic vertebral osteomyelitis. Analysis of 20 cases and review. *Clin Infect Dis* 1995;20:320–8.
21. Dagirmanjian A, Schils J, McHenry M, Modic M. MR imaging of vertebral osteomyelitis. *AJR Am J Roentgenol* 1996;167:1539–43.
22. Ozuna R, Delamarter R. Pyogenic vertebral osteomyelitis and postsurgical disc space infections. *Orthop Clin North Am* 1996;27:87–94.
23. Knight J, Cordingley J, Palazzo M. Epidural abscess following epidural steroid and local anesthesic injection. *Anaesthesia* 1997;52:576–8.
24. Horlocker T, McGregor D, Matsushige D, et al. A retrospective review of 4767 consecutive spinal anesthetics: central nervous system complications. Perioperative Outcomes Group. *Aneath Analg* 1997;84:578–84.
25. Fine P, Hare B, Zahniser J. Epidural abscess following epidural catheterization in a chronic pain patient. *Anesthesiology* 1988;69:422–4.
26. Ratcliffe JF. Anatomic basis for the pathogenesis and radiologic features of vertebral osteomyelitis and its differentiation from discitis: a microarteriographic investigation. *Acta Radiol (Diagn)* 1985;26:137–43.
27. Batson OV. The function of the vertebral veins and their role in the spread of metastases. *Ann Surg* 1940;112:138–48.
28. Sapico FL, Montgomerie J. Pyogenic vertebral osteomyelitis: report of nine cases and review of the literature. *Rev Infect Dis* 1976;1:754–76.
29. Allen SS, Kahn EA. Acute pyogenic infection of the spinal epidural space. *JAMA* 1932;98:875–8.
30. McLaurin RL. Spinal suppuration. *Clin Neurosurg* 1967;14:314.
31. Rankin RM, Flothow PG. Pyogenic infection of the spinal epidural space. *West J Surg Obstet Gyn* 1946;54:320–3.
32. Ross PM, Fleming JL. Vertebral body osteomyelitis. *Clin Orthop* 1976;118:190–8.
33. Heusner AP. Nontuberculous spinal epidural infections. *N Engl J Med* 1948;239:845–54.
34. Hakin RN, Burt AA, Cook JB. Acute spinal epidural abscess. *Paraplegia* 1979;17:330–6.
35. Hancock DO. A study of 49 patients with acute spinal extradural abscess. *Paraplegia* 1973;10:285–8.

36. Fraser RAR, Ratzan K, Wolpert SM, et al. Spinal subdural empyema. *Arch Neurol* 1973; 28:235–8.

37. Patronas NJ, Marx WJ, Duda EE. Radiographic presentation of spinal abscesses in the subdural space. *Am J Radiol* 1979;132:138–9.

38. Darouiche R, Hamill R, Greenberg S, et al. Bacterial spinal epidural abscess. Review of 43 cases and literature survey. *Medicine* 1992;71: 369–85.

39. Kaufman DM, Kaplan JG, Litman N. Infectious agents in spinal epidural abscesses. *Neurology* 1980;30:844–50.

40. Goodhart SP, Davison C. Torula infection of the nervous system. *AMA Arch Neurol Psychiat* 1937;37:435–9.

41. Lifeso RM, Harder E, McCorkell SJ. Spinal brucellosis. *J Bone Joint Surg* 1985;67B: 345–51.

42. Smith FB, Crawford JS. Fatal granulomatosis of the central nervous system due to a yeast (Torula). *J Path Bact* 1930;33:291–6.

43. Rahman NU. Atypical forms of spinal tuberculosis. *J Bone Joint Surg* 1980;62:162–5.

44. Plum F, Olson ME. Myelitis and myelopathy. In Baker AB, Baker LH, editors. *Clin Neurol.* Hagerstown: Harper & Row; 1973; pp. 1–52.

45. Post MJD, Quencer RM, Montalvo BM, et al. Spinal infection: evaluation with MR imaging and intraoperative ultrasound. *Radiology* 1988;169:765–71.

46. Erntell M, Holtas S, Norlin K, et al. Magnetic resonance imaging in the diagnosis of spinal epidural abscess. *Scand J Infect Dis* 1988;20: 323–7.

47. Brant-Zawadzki M, Burke VD, Jeffrey RB. CT in the evaluation of spine infection. *Spine* 1983;8:358–64.

48. Golimbu C, Firoonzia H, Rafil M. CT of osteomyelitis of the spine. *AJR Am J Roentgenol* 1984;142:159–63.

49. McGeachie RE, Ford WJ, Nelson MJ, et al. Neuroradiology case of the day. *AJR Am J Roentgenol* 1987;148:1053–8.

50. Ferris B, Jones C. Paraplegia due to aspergillosis: successful conservative treatment of two cases. *J Bone Joint Surg* 1985;67B: 800–3.

51. Price AC, Allen JH, Eggers FM, et al. Intervertebral disc-space infection: CT changes. *Radiology* 1983;149:725–9.

52. Modic MT, Feiglin DH, Piraino DW, et al. Vertebral osteomyelitis: assessment using MR. *Radiology* 1985;151:157–66.

53. Modic MT, Pflanze W, Feiglin DH, Belhobek G. Magnetic resonance imaging of musculoskeletal infections. *Radiol Clin North Am* 1986;24:247–58.

54. Sandhu F, Dillon W. Spinal epidural abscess: evaluation with contrast-enhanced MR imaging. *AJNR Am J Neuroradiol* 1991;12:1087–93.

55. Teman A. Spinal epidural abscess: early detection with gadolinium magnetic resonance imaging. *Arch Neurol* 1992;49:743–6.

56. Numaguchi Y, Rigamonti D, Rothman M, et al. Spinal epidural abscess: evaluation with gadolinium-enhanced MR imaging. *Radiographics* 1993;13:545–59.

57. Sadato N, Numaguche Y, Rigamonte D, et al. Spinal epidural abscess with gadolinium-enhanced MRI: serial follow-up studies and clinical correlations. *Neuroradiology* 1994;36: 44–8.

58. Baker AS. Spinal epidural abscess. In Braude AI, Davis CE, Fierer J, editors. *Infectious Disease and Medical Microbiology, 2nd Edition.* Philadelphia: W.B. Saunders; 1986; pp. 1101–3.

59. Mampalam T, Rosegay H, Andrews B, et al. Nonoperative treatment of spinal epidural infections. *J Neurosurg* 1989;71:208–10.

60. Blacklock JB, Hood TW, Mazwell RE. Intramedullary cervical spinal cord abscess: case report. *J Neurosurg* 1982;57:270–3.

61. Chiari H. Uber myelitis suppurativa bei bronchiektasie. *Z Heilk* 1900;1:351–72.

62. Woltman HW, Adson AW. Abscess of the spinal cord: functional recovery after operation. *Brain* 1926;49:193–206.

63. Di Tullio M. Intramedullary spinal abscess. Case report with a review of 53 previously reported cases. *Surg Neurol* 1977;7:351–3.

64. Menezes AH, Graf CJ, Perret GE. Spinal cord abscess: a review. *Surg Neurol* 1977;8:461–7.

65. Byrne R, Roenn KV, Whisler W. Intramedullary abscess: a report of two cases and a review of the literature. *Neurosurgery* 1994;35: 321–6.

66/67. Bartels R, Gonera E, Spek Jvd, et al. Intramedullary spinal cord abscess: a case report. *Spine* 1995;20:1199–204.

67. Ibid.

68. Courville CB. *Pathology of the Central Nervous System.* Mountain View, CA.; 1950.

69. Wright RL. Intramedullary spinal cord abscess: report of a case secondary to stab wound with good recovery following operation. *J Neurosurg* 1965;23:208–10.

70. Rifaat M, El Shafei I, Samra K, Sorour O. Intramedullary spinal abscess following spinal puncture. *J Neurosurg* 1973;38:366–7.

71. Keener EB. Abscess formation in the spinal cord. *Brain* 1955;78:394–400.

72. Ditulio MV. Intramedullary spinal abscess: a case report with a review of 53 previously described cases. *Surg Neurol* 1977;7:351–4.

73. CPC. A 34 year-old man with a destructive sacral lesion and a left gluteal mass. *N Engl J Med* 1988;318:306–12.

74. Gorse GJ, Pais MJ, Kusske JA, Cesario TC. Tuberculous spondylitis: a report of six cases and review of the literature. *Medicine (Baltimore)* 1983;62:178–93.

75. Martini M, Adjrad A, Boudjemaa A. Tuberculous osteomyelitis: a review of 125 cases. *Int Orthop* 1986;10:201–7.

76. Walton JN. Subarachnoid hemorrhage of unusual etiology. *Neurology* 1953;3:517–43.

77. Gandy SE. Tuberculosis of the central nervous system: recent experience and reappraisal. In Plum F, editor. *Advances in Contemporary Neurology.* Philadelphia: F.A. Davis; 1988; pp. 153–84.

78. Mann JS, Cole RB. Tuberculous spondylitis in the elderly: a potential diagnostic pitfall. *Br Med J* 1987;294:1149–50.
79. Griffiths D, Seddon HJ, Roaf R. *Pott's Paraplegia*. London: Oxford University Press; 1956.
80. Kaufman D, Kaplan J, Litman N. Infectious agents in spinal epidural abscess. *Neurology* 1980;30:844–50.
81. Waldvogel F, Medoff G, Swartz M. Osteomyelitis: a review of clinical features, therapeutic considerations and unusual aspects. *N Engl J Med* 1970;282:198–206, 260–6, 316–22.
82. Weaver P, Lifeso RM. The radiological diagnosis of tuberculosis of the adult spine. *Skeletal Radiol* 1984;12:178–86.
83. Mallolas J, Gatell JM, Rovira M, et al. Vertebral arch tuberculosis in two human immunodeficiency virus-seropositive heroin addicts. *Arch Intern Med* 1988;148:1125–7.
84. Nemir RL, Krasinki K. Tuberculosis in children and adolescents in the 1980's. *Pediatr Infect Dis J* 1988;7:375–9.
85. Mackay AD, Cole RB. The problems of tuberculosis in the elderly. *Q J Med* 1984;212:497–510.
86. Pattison PRM. Pott's paraplegia: an account of the treatment of 89 consecutive patients. *Paraplegia* 1986;24:77–91.
87. Lifeso RM, Weaver P, Harder EH. Tuberculous spondylitis in adults. *J Bone Joint Surg* 1985;67A:1405–13.
88. Bailey HL, Gabriel M, Hodgson AR, et al. Tuberculosis of the spine in children: operative findings and results in one hundred consecutive patients treated by removal of the lesion and anterior grafting. *J Bone Joint Surg* 1972;54A:1633–57.
89. Kricun ME. Conventional radiography. In Kricun ME, editor. *Imaging Modalities of Spinal Disorders*. Philadelphia: W.B. Saunders; 1988; pp. 59–288.
90. Roos A, Meerten EP, Bloem JL, Bluemm RG. MRI of tuberculous spondylitis. *AJR Am J Roentgenol* 1986;147:79–82.
91. Lindahl S, Nyman R, Brismar J, et al. Imaging of tuberculosis. IV. Spinal manifestations in 63 patients. *Acta Radiol* 1996;37:506–11.
92. Ma Y, Wang Y-M, Daniel TM. Enzyme-linked immunosorbent assay using Mycobacterium tuberculosis Antigen 5 for the diagnosis of pulmonary tuberculosis in China. *Am Rev Respir Dis* 1986;134:1273.
93. Raymond CA. Ushering in a new generation of diagnostics. *JAMA* 1986;256:3330.
94. Eisenach KD, Crawford JT, Bates JH. Genetic relatedness among strains of Mycobacterium tuberculosis complex. *Am Rev Respir Dis* 1986;133:1065.
95. Haas D, Prez RD. Mycobacterium tuberculosis. In Mandell G, Bennett J, Dolan R, editors. *Principles and Practices of Infectious Diseases, 4th Edition*. New York: Churchill Livingstone; 1995; pp. 2213–43.
96. Fancourt G, Ebden P, Garner P, et al. Bone tuberculosis: results and experience in Leicestershire. *Br J Dis Chest* 1986;80:265–72.
97. Rezai A, Lee M, Cooper P, et al. Modern management of spinal tuberculosis. *Neurosurgery* 1995;36:87–97.
98. Wadia N, Dastur D. Spinal meningitides with radiculomyelopathy. *J Neurol Sci* 1969;8(Part 1):239–60.
99. Dastur D, Wadia N. Spinal meningitides with radiculomyelopathy. Pathology and pathogenesis. *J Neurol Sci* 1969;8(Part 2):261–93.
100. Vleck B, Burchiel KJ, Gordon T. Tuberculous meningitis presenting as an obstructive myelopathy. *J Neurosurg* 1984;60:196–9.
101. Brooks W, Fletcher A, Wilson R. Spinal cord complications of tuberculous meningitis. *Q J Med* 1954;23:275–90.
102. Gupta R, Gupta S, Kumar S, et al. MRI in intraspinal tuberculosis. *Neuroradiology* 1994;36:39–43.
103. Kumar A, Montanera W, Willinsky R, et al. MR features of tuberculous arachnoiditis. *J CAT* 1993;17:127–30.
104. Zuger A, Lowy F. Tuberculosis. In Scheld W, Whitley R, Durack D, editors. *Infections of the Central Nervous System, 2nd Edition*. Philadelphia: Lippincott-Raven; 1997; pp. 417–43.
105. Dastur DK, Lalitha VS. The many facets of neurotuberculosis: an epitome of neuropathology. In Zimmerman HM, editor. *Progress in Neuropathology*. New York: Grune & Stratton; 1973; pp. 351–408.
106. Davison C, Keschner M. Myelitic and myelopathic lesions (a clinico-pathologic study): I. Myelitis. *Arch Neurol Psychiat* 1933;29:332–43.
107. Lin TH. Intramedullary tuberculoma of the spinal cord. *J Neurosurg* 1960;17:497–9.
108. Woolsey RM, Chambers TJ, Chung HD, McGarry JD. Mycobacterial meningomyelitis associated with human immunodeficiency virus infection. *Arch Neurol* 1988;45:691–3.
109. Lin S, Wu T, Wai Y. Intramedullary spinal tuberculomas during treatment of tuberculous meningitis. *Clin Neurol Neurosurg* 1994;96:71–8.
110. Rhoton E, Ballinger W, Quisling R, et al. Intramedullary spinal tuberculoma. *Neurosurgery* 1988;22:733–6.
111. Skulety FM. Cryptococci granuloma of the dorsal spinal cord. *Neurology* 1961;11:1066–70.
112. Matsushita T, Suzuki K. Spastic paraparesis due to cryptococcal osteomyelitis. *Clin Orthop* 1985;196:279–84.
113. Delaney P, Niemann B. Spinal cord compression by Coccidioides immitis abscess. *Arch Neurol* 1982;39:255–6.
114. McGahan JP, Graves DS, Palmer PES. Coccidioidal spondylitis. usual and unusual radiographic manifestations. *Radiology* 1980;136:5–9.
115. Osmond JD, Schweitzer G, Dunbar JM, Villet W. Blastomycosis of the spine with paraplegia. *S Afr Med J* 1971;45:431–4.
116. Mawk JR, Erickson DL, Chou SN, Seljeskog EL. Aspergillus infections of the lumbar disc spaces: report of three cases. *J Neurosurg* 1983;58:270–1.

117. McKee DF, Barr WM, Bryan CS, et al. Primary aspergillosis of the spine mimicking Pott's paraplegia. *J Bone Joint Surg* 1984;66A:1481–3.

118. Epstein S, Holden M, Feldshuh J, Singer JM. Unusual cause of spinal cord compression: nocardiosis. *New York J Med* 1963;63:3422–7.

119. Welsh JD, Rhoades ER, Jaques W. Disseminated nocardiosis involving spinal cord. *Arch Int Med* 1961;73:108.

120. Hayes WS, Berg RA, Dorfman HD. Candida discitis and vertebral osteomyelitis at L1–L2 from hematogenous spread. Case report 291. *Skeletal Radiol* 1984;12:184–287.

121. Hirschmann JV, Everett ED. Candida vertebral osteomyelitis: case report and review of the literature. *J Bone Joint Surg* 1976;58A:573–5.

122. Mehren M, Burns PJ, Mamani F, et al. Toxoplasmic myelitis mimicking intramedullary spinal cord tumor. *Neurology* 1988;38:1648–50.

123. Hesketh KT. Cysticercosis of the dorsal cord. *J Neurol Neurosurg Psychiatry* 1965;28:445–8.

124. Herskowitz A. Spinal cord involvement with Schistosoma mansoni. *J Neurosurg* 1972;36:494–8.

125. Marcial-Rojas RA, Fiol RE. Neurological complications of schistosomiasis. *Ann Intern Med* 1963;59:215.

126. Queiroz LD, Nucci A, Facure NO, Facure JJ. Massive spinal cord necrosis in schistosomiasis. *Arch Neurol* 1979;36:517–9.

127. Bird AV. Acute spinal schistosomiasis. *Neurology* 1964;14:647–56.

128. Meltzer LE, Bockman AA. Trichinosis involving the nervous system: treatment with corticotrophin (ACTH) and cortisone. *JAMA* 1957;164:1566–9.

129. Merritt HH, Rosenbaum M. Involvement of the nervous system in trichinosis. *JAMA* 1936;106:1646–9.

130. Junger S, Stern B, Levine S, et al. Intramedullary spinal sarcoidosis: clinical and magnetic resonance imaging characteristics. *Neurology* 1993;43:333–7.

131. Newman L, Rose C, Maier L. Sarcoidosis. *NEJM* 1997;336:1224–34.

132. Saroris DJ, Resnick D, Resnick C, et al. Musculoskeletal manifestations of sarcoidosis. *Semin Roentgenol* 1985;20:376–86.

133. Brodey PA, Pripstein S, Strange G, et al. Vertebral sarcoidosis: a case report and review of the literature. *AJR Am J Roentgenol* 1976;126:900–2.

134. Beck RN, Brower TD. Vertebral sarcoidosis. *Radiology* 1964;82:660–3.

135. Delaney P. Neurologic manifestations in sarcoidosis: review of the literature, with a report of 23 cases. *Ann Intern Med* 1977;87:336–45.

136. Zener JC, Alpert M, Klainer LM. Vertberal sarcoidosis. *Arch Int Med* 1963;111:696–702.

137. Martin CA, Murall R, Trasi SS. Spinal cord sarcoidosis: case report. *J Neurosurg* 1984;61:981–2.

138. Stern BJ, Krumholz A. Neurosarcoidosis. In Johnson RT, editor. *Current Therapy in Neurologic Disease—2* Toronto: B.C. Decker; 1987; pp. 135–7.

139. Sharma O. Effectiveness of chloroquine and hydroxychloroquine in treating selected patients with sarcoidodid with neurological involvement. *Arch Neurol* 1998;55:1248–54.

140. Lower E, Boederick J, Brott T, et al. Diagnosis and management of neurological sarcoidosis. *Arch Int Med* 1997;157:1864–8.

141. Stren B, Schonfeld A, Sewell C, et al. The treatment of neurosarcoidosis with cyclosporin. *Arch Neurol* 1992;49:1065–72.

142. Agbogu B, Stern B, Sewell C, Yang G. Therapeutic considerations in patients with refractory neurosarcoidosis. *Arch Neurol* 1995;52:875–9.

143. Rosenbaum R, Campbell S, Rosenbaum J. *Clinical Neurology of Rheumatic Diseases*. Boston: Butterworth-Heinemann; 1996.

144. Krane SM, Simon LS. Rheumatoid arthritis: clinical features and pathogenetic mechanisms. *Adv Rheumatol* 1986;70:263–84.

145. Stevens J, Cartlidge N, Saunders M, et al. Atlanto-axial subluxation and cervical myelopathy in rheumatoid arthritis. *Q J Med* 1971;40:391.

145a. Nakano KK, Schoene WS, Baker A, et al. The cervical myelopathy associated with rheumatoid arthritis: analysis of 32 patients with postmortem cases. *Ann Neurol* 1978;3:144.

146. Collins D, Barnes C, Fitzrandolph R. Cervical spine instability in rheumatoid patients having total hip or knee arthroplasty. *Clin Orthop* 1991;272:135.

147. Lipson S. Cervical myelopathy and posterior atlanto-axial subluxation in patients with rheumatoid arthritis. *J Bone Joint Surg* 1985;67-A:593–7.

148. El-Khoury GY, Wener MH, Menezes AH, et al. Cranial settling in rheumatoid arthritis. *Radiology* 1980;137:637–42.

149. Coggeshall RE, Applebaum ML, Fazen M, et al. Unmyelinated axons in human ventral roots, a possible explanation for the failure of dorsal root rhizotomy to relieve pain. *Brain* 1975;98:157–66.

150. Weissman BNW, Aliabadi P, Weinfeld MS, et al. Prognostic features of atlantoaxial subluxation in rheumatoid arthritis patients. *Radiology* 1982;144:745–51.

151. Redlund-Johnell I, Pettersson H. Radiographic measurements of the cranio-vertebral region; designed for evaluation of abnormalities in rheumatoid arthritis. *Acta Radiol (Diagn)* 1984;25:23–8.

152. Reynolds H, Carter SW, Murtaugh FR, Rechtine GR. Cervical rheumatoid arthritis: value of flexion and extension views in imaging. *AJR Am J Roentgenol* 1987;164:215–8.

153. Martel W. The occipito-atlanto-axial joints in rheumatoid arthritis and ankylosing spondylitis. *AJR Am J Roentgenol* 1961;86:223–40.

154. Guttmann L, Hable K. Rheumatoid pachymeningitis. *Neurology* 1963;13:901–5.

155. Friedman H. Intraspinal rheumatoid nodule causing nerve root compression. Case report. *J Neurosurg* 1970;32:689–91.

156. Kudo H, Iwano K, Yoshizawa H. Cervical cord compression due to extradural granulation tissue in rheumatoid arthritis. A review of five cases. *J Bone Joint Surg* 1984;66B:426–30.

157. Lorber A, Pearson CM, Rens RM. Osteolytic vertebral lesions as a manifestation of rheumatoid arthritis and related disorders. *Arthritis Rheum* 1961;4:514–32.

158. Bywaters EGL. Thoracic intervertebral discitis in rheumatoid arthritis due to costovertebral joint involvement. *Rheumatol Int* 1981;1: 83–97.

159. Breedveld FC, Algra PR, Vielvoye CJ, Cats A. Magnetic resonance imaging in the evaluation of patients with rheumatoid arthritis and subluxation of the cervical spine. *Arthritis Rheum* 1987;30:624–30.

160. Lipson SJ. Rheumatoid arthritis in the cervical spine. *Clin Orthop* 1989;239:121–7.

161. Burke SW, French HG, Roberts JM, et al. Chronic atlanto-axial instability in Down's syndrome. *J Bone Joint Surg* 1985;67A:1356–60.

162. Dawson EG, Smith L. Atlanto-axial subluxation in children due to vertebral anomalies. *J Bone Joint Surg* 1979;61A:582–7.

163. Hungerford GD, Akkaraju V, Rawe SE, et al. Atlanto-axial dislocations with spinal cord compression in Down's syndrome: a case report and review of the literature. *Br J Radiol* 1981;54:758–61.

164. Moore RA, McNicholas KW, Warran SP. Atlantoaxial subluxation with symptomatic spinal cord compression in a child with Down's syndrome. *Anesth Analg* 1987;66:89–90.

165. Hastings DE, Macnab I, Lawson V. Neoplasms of the atlas and axis. *Can J Surg* 1968;11:290–6.

166. Koss JC, Dalinka MA. Atlantoaxial subluxation in Behcet's syndrome. *AJR Am J Roentgenol* 1980;134:392–3.

167. Killebrew K, Gold RH, Sholkoff SD. Psoriatic spondylitis. *Radiology* 1973;108:9–16.

168. Gulati DR, Rout D. Atlantoaxial dislocation with quadriparesis in achondroplasia: case report. *J Neurosurg* 1974;40:394–6.

169. D'Aprile P, Krajewska G, Perniola T, et al. Congenital dislocation of dens of the axis in a case of neurofibromatosis. *Neuroradiology* 1984;26:405–40.

170. Braunstein EM, Weissman BN, Seltzer SE, et al. Computed tomography and conventional radiographs of the craniocervical region in rheumatoid arthritis. *Arthritis Rheum* 1984;27:26–31.

171. Toolanen G, Garsson S-E, Fagerlund M. Medullary compression in rheumatoid atlanto-axial subluxation evaluated by computerized tomography. *Spine* 1986;11:191–4.

172. Laasonen EM, Kankaanpaa U, Paukku P, et al. Computed tomographic myelography (CTM)

173. in atlanto-axial rheumatoid arthritis. *Neuroradiology* 1985;27:119–22.

173. Dickman C, Mamourian A, Sonntag V, et al. Magnetic resonance imaging of the transverse atlantal ligament for the evaluation of atlantoaxial instability. *J Neurosurg* 1991;75:221.

174. Aisen A, Martel W, Ellis J, et al. Cervical spine involvement in rheumatoid arthritis. *Radiology* 1987;165:159.

175. Dvorak J, Grob D, Baumgartner H, et al. Functional evaluation of the spinal cord by magnetic resonance imaging in patients with rheumatoid arthritis and instability of the upper cervical spine. *Spine* 1989;14:1057.

176. Rana N. Natural history of atlanto-axial subluxation in rheumatoid arthritis. *Spine* 1989; 14:1054.

177. Pellicci P, Ranawat C, Tsairis P, et al. A prospective study of the progression of rheumatoid arthritis of the cervical spine. *J Bone Joint Surg (Am)* 1981;63:342.

178. Bland JH. *Disorders of the Cervical Spine: diagnosis and Medical Management*. Philadelphia: W.B. Saunders; 1987.

179. Larsson S-E, Toolanen G. Posterior fusion for atlanto-axial subluxation in rheumatoid arthritis. *Spine* 1986;11:525–30.

180. Rothman RH, Simeone FA. *The Spine*. Philadelphia: W.B. Saunders; 1982.

181. Ranawat C, O'Leary P, Pellicci P. Cervical fusion in rheumatoid arthritis. *J Bone Joint Surg* 1979;51A:1003.

182. Clark C, Goetz D, Menezes A. Arthrodesis of cervical spine in rheumatoid arthritis. *J Bone Joint Surg (Am)* 1989;71:381.

183. Papadopoulos S, Dickman C, Sonntag V. Atlantoaxial stabilization in rheumatoid arthritis. *J Neurosurg* 1991;74:1.

184. Boden S, Dodge L, Bohlman H, et al. Rheumatoid arthritis of the cervical spine: a long term analysis with predictors of paralysis and recovery. *J Bone Joint Surg (Am)* 1993;75:1282.

185. Smith PH, Benn RT, Sharp J. Natural history of rheumatoid cervical subluxations. *Ann Rheum Dis* 1972;31:431–9.

186. Calabro JJ. The seronegative spondyloarthropathies: a graduated approach to management. *Postgrad Med* 1986;80:173–88.

187. Thomas D, Kendall MJ, Whitfield AGW. Nervous system involvement in ankylosing spondylitis. *Br Med J* 1974;1:148–50.

188. Wu PC, Fang D, Ho EKW, Leong JCY. The pathogenesis of extensive discovertebral destruction in ankylosing spondylitis. *Clin Orthop* 1988;230:154–61.

189. Jajic I, Kerhin V, Kastelen A. Ankylosing spondylitis in patients without HLA-B27. *Brit J Rheum* 1983;22(Suppl 2):136.

190. Harding JR, McCall IW, Park WM, Jones BF. Fracture of the cervical spine in ankylosing spondylitis. *Br J Radiol* 1985;58:3–7.

191. Murray GC, Persellin RH. Cervical fracture complicating ankylosing spondylitis: report of eight cases and review of the literature. *Am J Med* 1981;70:1033–41.

192. Weinstein PR, Karpman RR, Gall EP, Pitt M. Spinal cord injury, spinal fracture and spinal stenosis in ankylosing spondylitis. *J Neurosurg* 1982;57:609–16.

193. Gustafson H, Rutberg H, Bengtsson M. Spinal haematoma following epidural analgesia. Report of a patient with ankylosing spondylitis and a bleeding diathesis. *Anesthesia* 1988;43: 220–22.

194. Hissa E, Boumphrey F, Bay J. Spinal epidural hematoma and ankylosing spondylitis. *Clin Orthop* 1986;208:225–27.

195. Bartleson JO, Cohen MD, Harrington TM. Cauda equina syndrome secondary to long-standing ankylosing spondylitis. *Ann Neurol* 1983;14:662–9.

196. Matthews WB. The neurological complications of ankylosing spondylitis. *J Neurol Sci* 1968;6:561–73.

197. Whitfield AGW. Neurological complications of ankylosing spondylitis. In Vinken PJ, Bruyn GW, editors. *Handbook of Clinical Neurlogy, Volume 38*. Amsterdam: North-Holland; 1979; pp. 505–20.

198. Sharp J, Purser DW. Spontaneous atlanto-axial dislocation in ankylosing spondylitis and rheumatoid arthritis. *Ann Rheum Dis* 1961;20: 47–77.

199. Hunter T. The spinal complications of ankylosing spondylitis. *Semin Arthritis Rheum* 1989; 19:172.

200. Bowie EA, Glasgow GL. Cauda equina lesions associated with ankylosing spondylitis. *Br Med J* 1961;2:24–7.

201. Charlesworth C, Savy L, Stevens J, et al. MRI demonstration of arachnoiditis in cauda equina syndrome of ankylosing spondylitis. *Neuroradiology* 1996;38:462–5.

202. Dihlmann W. Current radiodiagnostic concept of ankylosing spondylitis. *Skeletal Radiol* 1979;4:179–88.

203. Lehtinen K, Kaarela K, Antilla P, et al. Sacroilitis in inflammatory joint diseases. *Rheumatology* 1984;52:19–22.

204. Resnick D. Radiology of seronegative spondyloarthropathies. *Clin Orthop* 1979;143:38–45.

205. Young A, Dixon A, Getty J, et al. Cauda equina syndrome complicating ankylosing spondylitis: use of electromyography and computerised tomography in daignosis (case report). *Ann Rheum Dis* 1981;40:317–22.

206. Grosman H, Gray R, Louis ELS. CT of long-standing ankylosing spondylitis with cauda equina syndrome. *AJNR Am J Neuroradiol* 1983;4:1077–80.

207. Kricun R, Kricun ME. Computed tomography. In Kricun ME, editor. *Imaging Modalities in Spinal Disorders*. Philadelphia: W.B. Saunders; 1988; pp. 376–467.

208. Sparling M, Bartleson J, McLeod R, et al. Magnetic resonance imaging of arachnoid diverticula associated with cauda equina syndrome in ankylosing spondylitis. *J Rheumatol* 1989;16:1335.

209. Avrahami E, Wigler L, Stern D, et al. Computed tomographic demonstration of calcification of the ligamentum flava of the lumbosacral spine in ankylosing spondylitis. *Ann Rheum Dis* 1988;47:62.

210. Roberts WN, Larson MG, Liang MH, et al. Sensitivity of anthropometric techniques for clinical trials in ankylosing spondylitis. *Br J Rheumatol* 1989;28:40–5.

211. Confavreux C, Larbre J-P, Lejeune E, et al. Cerebrospinal fluid dynamics in the tardive cauda equina syndrome of ankylosing spondylitis. *Ann Neurol* 1991;29:221.

212. Okada S, Hase H, Hirasawa Y, et al. A case report of lumboperitoneal shunt for cauda equina syndrome in ankylosing spondylitis. *Spine* 1992;17:S59.

Chapter 10

SYRINGOMYELIA AND SPINAL HEMORRHAGE

SYRINGOMYELIA

Syringomyelia is characterized by cavitation of the spinal cord, resulting in myelomalacia and cystic cavitation. Although it has protean manifestations, traditionally it has been considered to be a chronically progressive disorder that is clinically manifested by brachial amyotrophy, dissociated anesthesia, neurogenic arthropathies, and long tract signs.[1] Its pathogenesis is controversial. Barnett et al.[1] have suggested that syringomyelia be classified into communicating and noncommunicating forms (Table 10–1). The communicating types are usually associated with obstructive lesions of the foramen magnum, leading some authors[2] to propose a hydrody-namic theory for its development. The noncommunicating type is usually associated with other diseases of the spinal cord, discussed below.

Pathology

Syringomyelia most commonly affects the cervicothoracic region of the spine. The cavity often extends at least one-half of the rostrocaudal extent of the spinal cord; the largest portion of the cavity is often in the cervical region, although it is usually absent at the first cervical segment.[3,4] A syrinx commonly extends into the lower end of the thoracic spinal cord. The lumbosacral spinal cord is rarely involved, although occasionally the cavity may extend the entire length of the cord and even into the brain stem or cerebrum.[5]

At the level of the syrinx, the spinal cord may be of normal transverse size, wider than usual, or occasionally thinner than normal.[6] The cavity is usually located within the gray matter of the spinal cord, dorsal to the central canal[3] (Fig. 10–1), and is usually filled with clear fluid that has the composition of cerebrospinal fluid.[4] Occasionally, the fluid may be xanthochromic or may reveal signs of hemorrhage.[7] As the cavity enlarges, it may involve the lateral and posterior funiculi and may extend to the pial surface. Although a communication with the central

Table 10–1. **Classification of Syringomyelia***

1. Communicating (syringo-hydromyelia)
   a. Associated with developmental abnormalities of the cranial–cervical junction and posterior fossa (e.g., Chiari malformation)
   b. Associated with acquired obstructive lesions of the foramen magnum (e.g., basilar meningitis)
2. Secondary to traumatic myelopathy
3. Secondary to spinal arachnoiditis
4. Secondary to spinal cord tumors
5. Idiopathic (unrelated to the above causes)

*Adapted from Barnett, HJM, et al.,[1] p. 312.

canal may be present, this is not found in all cases.

The wall of the cavity varies in histological appearance. It may be irregular and may contain degenerated neuroglial elements, strands of collagen, and blood vessels. When it communicates with the central canal, the cavity frequently is lined by ependymal cells.[3] This process is often termed hydromyelia, reflecting its communicating nature. In noncommunicating cases associated with neoplasms, trauma, and arachnoiditis, these pathological conditions are present, usually making the etiology obvious. In both communicating and noncommunicating syringomyelia, other associated pathological processes such as scoliosis and developmental disturbances may be present and should be considered.

Pathogenesis

Syringomyelia is associated with a diverse group of disorders. This thwarts attempts to develop a unified understanding of its pathogenesis and leads to intense debate.[1,2,8,9]

COMMUNICATING SYRINGOMYELIA

Communicating syringomyelia may be part of a dysraphic state (for example, myelomeningocele, basilar invagination, Chiari malformation [I or II], or Klippel-Feil anomaly) (Fig. 10–2). Gardner[2] proposed that communicating syringomyelia arises secondary to the obstruction of normal CSF flow through the outlets of the fourth ventricle. He suggested a water-hammer effect in which CSF pulsations

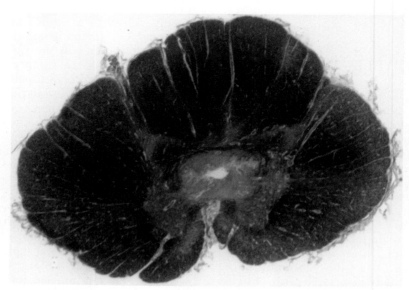

Figure 10–1. Transverse section of cord showing syrinx in the central gray matter surrounded by gliosis. (Courtesy of Lysia Forno.)

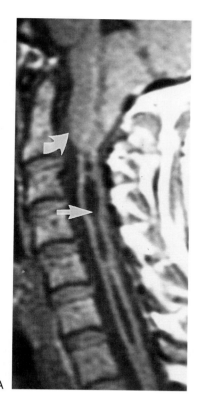

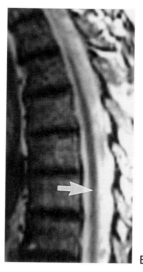

A

B

Figure 10–2. An MRI of the craniocervical junction (A) and thoracic spine (B) of a patient with Chiari malformation and syringomyelia. The patient presented at age 15 with acute myelopathy and sensory level in the midthoracic region. No imaging or CSF analysis was done, but she was told she had multiple sclerosis, and gradually improved. She presented again at age 36 with nystagmus, gait ataxia, and lower extremity spasticity. (A) An MRI revealed descended cerebellar tonsils (curved arrow) and syrinx (arrow) in the cervical spine. (B) The syrinx (arrow) extends into the thoracic spine.

are transmitted to the central canal due to this obstruction (Fig. 10–3A and B). He postulated that the central canal thus dilates and, with rupture of the ependymal lining, a cystic cavity is formed within the spinal cord. This theory may apply in cases of syringomyelia associated with craniocervical anomalies.

Williams[10] suggested that differences in the intracranial, intraspinal, and venous and CSF pressures are important in the pathogenesis of syringomyelia. Coughing and other Valsalva maneuvers result in engorgement of the epidural venous plexus (Fig. 10–3C), causing displacement of spinal CSF intracranially. If there is any obstruction of CSF outflow from the fourth ventricle, then, CSF is postulated to enter the central canal. When the epidural venous plexus fills, the fluid within the central canal and syrinx is displaced to the area of least resistance and lowest pressure. According to this view, these fluid shifts result in extension of the cavity to other areas of the spinal cord. Ball and Dayan[11] propose that CSF under in-

creased pressure tracks along Virchow-Robin spaces to form cystic cavitations within the spinal cord (Fig. 10–3D). This theory explains the passage of intrathecal contrast material into noncommunicating syrinxes.

Obstruction of the subarachnoid pathways via a coning effect seems to be a common factor with communicating syringomyelia. The theories of both Williams and Gardner are based on the assumption that the pathology is related to passage of CSF through the central canal from the obex to the syrinx. However, a more plausible and clinically consistent theory, posed by Oldfield et al.[12] is that the Chiari I malformation partially occludes the subarachnoid space and completely occludes it during systole. The cerebellar tonsils descend (during systole) and act as a piston that causes a descending wave of subarachnoid CSF. This, in turn, compresses the spinal cord in a wave-like fashion. This wave of external spinal cord pressure is thought to propel syrinx fluid caudally, gradually dissecting the spinal cord and

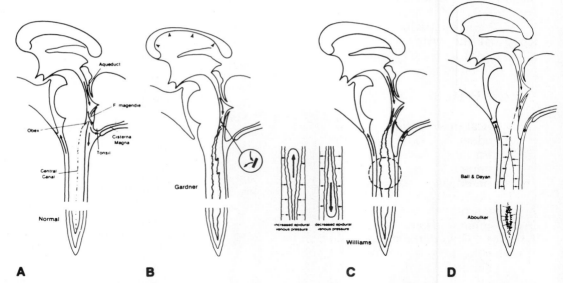

Figure 10–3. Diagrammatic representations of pathophysiological theories of syringomyelia. (A) Normal CSF flow. Note incomplete central canal of spinal cord. (B) Gardner's theory emphasizing imperforate foramen of Magendie (blocked arrow, insert). (C) William's theory emphasizing the "ball-valve" effect of foramen magnum obstruction. Movement of intracranial CSF into the spinal canal is impeded and redirected into the central canal. The CSF movements in the syrinx are depicted (inset). (D) Theory of Ball and Dayan and Albouker. Movement of CSF from the spinal canal into the cranial space is impeded (blocked arrow). The CSF passes into the cord. (From Sherman et al.,[24] with permission.)

increasing syrinx size.[12,13] Decompression and the elimination of the coning phenomenon appear to be curative in a majority of cases (see below).[13–17] In fact, in cases where it was not effective, persistent compression was observed.[18]

NONCOMMUNICATING SYRINGOMYELIA

Cases of noncommunicating syringomyelia may be associated with intramedullary tumors, posttraumatic states, spinal arachnoiditis, infarction, acute transverse myelopathy, and, rarely, extramedullary cord compression.[19,20] Extensions of the cavities observed after spinal cord trauma may be due to transmission of venous back pressure, to the spinal cord precipitated by Valsalva maneuvers.[1] Experimental studies have suggested that ischemia of the spinal cord caused by spinal arachnoiditis and tethering may be important in cases of syringomyelia associated with posttraumatic states and spinal arachnoiditis.[1]

The cystic cavitations associated with intramedullary spinal cord tumors are similar to the cysts formed in association with cerebral neoplasms. Poser[21] found that of 245 cases of syringomyelia, 40 patients (16%) had intramedullary spinal cord tumors, while among 209 patients with a diagnosis of spinal tumor, 65 cases (31%) had syringomyelia. The most common spinal tumors associated with syringomyelia are those in von Hippel–Lindau disease and von Recklinghausen's disease.[1] Approximately 20% of patients with von Recklinghausen's neurofibromatosis harboring multiple intraspinal and intracranial nerve sheath tumors or meningiomas also had spinal cord cavitation.[22] A high incidence of syringomyelia is found when spinal hemangioblastoma is a manifestation of von Hippel–Lindau disease.[23]

In addition to being a sensitive modality for the diagnosis of syringomyelia, MRI may be valuable in elucidating its pathogenesis.[20] Using MRI, 58 cases of syringomyelia were classified as communicating (those associated with Chiari malformation), 40%; traumatic, 29%; neoplastic, 15%; and idiopathic, 15%. The average length of the syrinx was approximately seven spinal segments.[24]

Clinical Features

The clinical presentation of syringomyelia is dependent upon the location of the syrinx and the associated pathological changes noted above. Thus in some cases, an associated pathological condition such as Arnold-Chiari malformation (present in more than 60% of cases in some series) or hydrocephalus may overshadow the spinal findings.[10,25] As noted above, although syringomyelia may occur at any level, its most common location is in the cervicothoracic region, and the most typical syndrome includes brachial amyotrophy, dissociated segmental sensory loss, trophic disturbances, and long tract findings.

Syringomyelia may present at any age but most commonly occurs between the ages of 25 and 40. Men are somewhat more frequently affected than are women.[26] Although familial occurrence has been reported infrequently, syringomyelia is considered a sporadic disease in most instances.[27]

The symptoms and signs of syringomyelia are shown in Table 10–2. Sensory abnormalities are the most common presenting complaint, with 52% of patients reporting sensory loss, pain, or paresthesias. The sensory loss is typically in a cape distribution, a pattern that is secondary to involvement of the decussating pain and temperature pathways, with preservation of posterior column function. Occasionally, such sensory involvement will result in painless burns of one or both upper extremities as a presenting manifestation. When advanced, sensory disturbances may result in painless ulcers and dystrophic changes (Morvan's syndrome). Infrequently, the posterior columns may also be involved and complete anesthesia may be seen.

Pain may be a presenting manifestation of syringomyelia.[28] In one study it was reported in one third to one-half of patients

Table 10–2. First Signs and Symptoms of Syringomyelia Noted By Patients*

SYMPTOM/SIGN	NO. OF PATIENTS (N = 172)	
Muscular weakness	52	(30%)
Sensory disturbances	32	(19%)
Paresthesias	32	(19%)
Pain	25	(14%)
Neurogenic arthropathy and scoliosis	11	(6%)
Muscular wasting	9	(5%)
Spastic gait	5	(3%)
Brain-stem signs	3	(2%)
Trophic skin disorders	3	(2%)

*From Schliep, G,[27] p. 260, with permission.

with idiopathic syringomyelia or with obstruction of the foramen magnum.[29] The pain is usually of a burning or aching nature and is often seen at the borders of sensory impairment. Exacerbation by a Valsalva maneuver suggests an associated compressive lesion such as an Arnold-Chiari malformation.

Muscle weakness, the second most common presenting complaint (see Table 10–2), is present in 30% of cases. It often is associated with wasting and diminution of the deep tendon reflexes. Kyphoscoliosis and neurogenic arthropathies account for approximately 6% of the presenting manifestations.[27] Kyphoscoliosis may reflect involvement of the tracts projecting to axial musculature. Neurogenic arthropathies in the areas of anesthesia are observed in approximately 25% of cases throughout the course of the disease.[30]

Autonomic involvement, in the form of trophic disturbances of the skin, Horner's syndrome, or sphincter disturbance, is frequently encountered. Horner's syndrome may occur secondary to involvement of the descending sympathetic pathways or involvement of the intermediolateral cells at C8, T1, and T2. Trophic changes in the upper extremities are also reported. Involvement of descending autonomic fibers may cause a neurogenic bladder, but this is usually a late phenomenon.

When syringomyelia is of the communicating variety, brain-stem and cerebellar signs (for example, ataxia, nystagmus, hoarseness, dysphagia, and hydrocephalus) may be present and dominate the clinical presentation. When a spinal cord tumor is the cause, the motor and sensory disturbances often extend over several segments.

Somatosensory-evoked potentials have been used to evaluate intramedullary spinal cord tumors and syringomyelia.[31] According to Restuccia and colleagues, the somatosensory-evoked potential was frequently more sensitive than the clinical neurologic examination in defining the extent of involvement. This modality may provide an adjunct to the clinical examination and MRI scan in evaluating response to therapy, especially in patients with subtle neurologic signs.

Although the clinical onset is usually insidious and the temporal course is most commonly progressive, the course may vary. Among[32] patients followed for up to 20 years, Schliep[27] defined four different temporal profiles of syringomyelia: (*1*) chronic progression, 50%; (*2*) no progression during period of follow-up, 22%; (*3*) stationary and progressive stages, 25%; and (*4*) partial remission, 3%. The observation[33–35] that no progression of signs or symptoms may be found in a substantial number of patients over several years has led to difficulty in the differential diagnosis and in evaluating therapies.

Diagnostic Imaging Studies

Plain radiographs or MRI of the cervical spine may show a dilated cervical canal (Fig. 10–4), and the craniocervical junction may show developmental abnormalities such as basilar impression, atlantoaxial dislocation, and occipitalization of the atlas.[36] For example, McRae[37] was able to demonstrate bony abnormalities in the region of the foramen magnum in 38% of patients with a clinical diagnosis of syringomyelia. Occasionally, fused vertebrae, bifid spinous processes, Klippel-Feil deformity, and other vertebral anomalies may be observed, as well as anomalies in the thoracic and lumbosacral spines.[27]

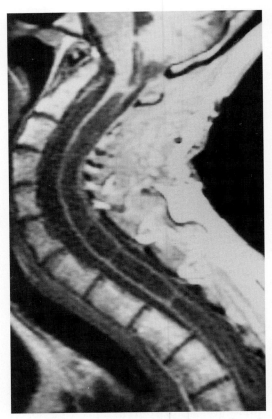

Figure 10–4. An MRI of the cervical–upper thoracic cord showing a massively dilated spinal cord due to syrinx. The spinal canal is enlarged due to the chronic cord dilatation. (Courtesy of Dr. Richard Becker.)

The cystic cavitation of syringomyelia may change in shape and size, and thus has been difficult in many cases to demonstrate myelographically.[38] Its appearance may vary depending upon whether air or positive contrast is used and whether the patient is in a sitting or reclining position. This phenomenon has given rise to the so-called collapsing cord sign that can present difficulties in the diagnosis of syringomyelia.[32,39]

In 1975, Di Chiro and colleagues[40] described the value of CT in the diagnosis of syringomyelia. Administering of intrathecal contrast material revealed the cystic cavity filled with contrast. Since that time, the criteria for CT diagnosis of syringomyelia have evolved.[41–43] On CT, the transverse diameter of the spinal cord may be small, normal, or expanded.[41]

Magnetic resonance imaging (see Figs. 10–2 and 10–4) has been found to be exceedingly sensitive in the diagnosis of intramedullary spinal cord disease.[44] Magnetic resonance imaging is equivalent or superior to CT myelography in the diagnosis of many cases of syringomyelia,[8,45] and it may be able to differentiate intramedullary neoplasms from intramedullary cysts.[46] In addition, arachnoid cysts associated with syringomyelia have been reported using MRI.[47]

Therapy

Complications of syringomyelia, such as burns and decubiti, may be prevented if patients are aware of these risks. Neuropathic pain is a common problem, which may respond to routine analgesics, amitriptiline, or carbamazepine. Because this is a chronic disorder, the use of narcotic analgesics should be limited or avoided. Baclofen or diazepam may be effective for spasticity.[48]

Because management decisions in patients with syringomyelia are usually difficult, patients should be treated by physicians with a wide experience with this disorder. Syringomelia is commonly managed via surgical intervention. Neurosurgical consultation, therefore, should usually be obtained. Nevertheless, the neurosurgeon, the referring physician, and the patient should be cognizant of the three predominant treatment strategies: (1) observation without surgery, (2) spinal decompression operations, and (3) syrinx drainage operations.

Syringomyelia, as mentioned, is multifactorial. This essentially necessitates multiple, potential therapies, and thus controversy. Therefore, the clinical decision-making process is extremely complex and difficult. Nonsurgical management has been recommended in patients with (1) advanced, longstanding neurologic deficits, (2) progressive arachnoiditis, (3) no significant motor deficit or mild nonprogressive neurologic deficit, (4) no response to cyst puncture, or (5) high surgical risk.[48] Since the temporal course of neurologic function is frequently variable,

with long periods of clinical stabilization, the efficacy of surgical therapy has been difficult to establish. Nonetheless, surgical intervention has been advocated in selected patients: (1) with early and/or rapid neurologic defect or deterioration, (2) with Chiari malformation associated with hydrocephalus and/or neurologic deficit or neurologic deterioration, and (3) who previously benefited from surgery and have since deteriorated. There are a variety of surgical procedures (e.g., foramen magnum decompression, ventriculoperitoneal shunt, syringoperitoneal shunt[49,50]) that have been used in patients with syringomyelia and associated problems.[14,15,17,18,51,52] When syringomyelia is associated with neoplasm, the underlying neoplasm is treated.

OBSERVATION WITHOUT SURGERY

Not all syrinxes are the same. Their etiologies differ, as do the characteristics of the patients in which they lie. For example, an asymptomatic small syrinx in an elderly or a high-medical-risk patient should usually be observed with serial imaging studies (MRI). The emergence of symptoms, however, significantly alters the decision-making process, particularly if the symptoms are progressive.

Moderate-sized or large syrinxes in asymptomatic patients present significant clinical challenges, as these patients may neurologically deteriorate abruptly and occasionally catastrophically. This probably occurs more commonly in patients with larger syrinxes. Therefore, patients must be counseled regarding the risks and benefits of both operative and nonoperative management.

The etiology of the syrinx also plays a significant role in the decision-making process. Syrinxes caused by compressive lesions, such as Chiari I or II malformation, respond well to decompression surgery. Furthermore, this surgery is relatively noninvasive, with respect to spinal cord manipulation and operative spinal cord manipulation and injury. Additionally, these operations are often successful, with excellent long-term prognoses. Syrinxes that are caused by trauma or tumor are often managed by syrinx drainage procedures. These operations, which require spinal cord manipulation, often fail due to shunt tube obstruction. Hence they are often not associated with a good long-term prognosis. These factors must be taken into consideration in each patient with syringomyelia.

SPINAL DECOMPRESSION OPERATIONS

Spinal canal compressive lesions in cases of communicating syringomyelia, particularly at the craniocervical junction, can cause a syrinx caudal to the site of spinal cord en-croachment.[12,13] This communicating syringomyelia phenomenon most commonly occurs in association with the Chiari I and II malformations. Spinal cord decompression via laminectomy with duraplasty, with or without suboccipital decompression, routinely results in syrinx resolution or in a diminution of its size. If such does not occur following the decompression operation, the diagnosis of inadequate decompression must be *strongly* entertained.[18]

SYRINX DRAINAGE OPERATIONS

Syrinxes that are caused by trauma or tumor are often managed by syrinx drainage procedures. These usually entail placing a

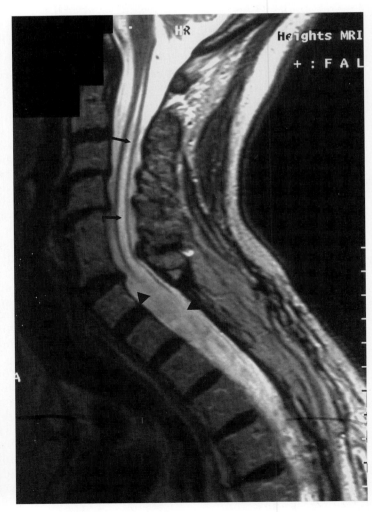

Figure 10–5. A T_2-weighted image of the cervical spine in a patient who incurred a traumatic incomplete spine injury 30 years previously, Note the syrinx (arrows) and a region of cystic myelomalacia (arrowheads). A shunting procedure only temporarily halted neurologic deterioration.

shunt tube into the syrinx cavity with drainage to an external site such as the subarachnoid space, the pleural cavity, or the peritoneal cavity. Simple syrinx drainage by incision of the spinal cord or terminal ventriculostomy (incising of the conus medullaris to drain the syrinx) used to drain the syrinx into the subarachnoid space may also be employed.

Obviously, these strategies are more invasive than a simple decompression operation. They require transgression of the spinal cord, and are associated with a high incidence of failure, usually because of shunt tube obstruction. This correlates with the natural history of the treated posttraumatic syrinx patient. Their clinical course is one of a ratcheting downhill nature, interspersed with multiple drainage operations that are first successful and then fail (Fig. 10–5).[52] Obviously syringomyelia caused by tumor is best managed by tumor resection.

ARACHNOID CYSTS

Arachnoid cysts are leptomeningeal diverticula that may occur in the extradural, intradural, or perineural location. They are often assymptomatic and are observed incidentally on radiological studies or at postmortem. They are rare causes of spinal cord or nerve root compression.[53] Most arachnoid cysts communicate with the subarachnoid space and represent diverticula rather than closed cavities.[54,55] Arachnoid cysts share a common pathogenesis; their location depends on local abnormalities of tissue and hydrodynamic factors.[56] Their histopathology, which consists of arachnoidal tissue, is also similar in these different locations.[56]

Extradural Arachnoid Cysts

Arachnoid cysts extend into the extradural space through a defect in the dura mater. They may be congenital or secondary to a rent from trauma or previous surgical intervention (Fig. 10–6).[55] Communication may be found between the cyst and the subarachnoid space. In a surgical series of extradural arachnoid cysts,[57] a communication was observed in 58% of cases and was demonstrated on myelography in 46%. Congenital extradural arachnoid cysts preferentially occur at the junction of the radicular dural sheath and the spinal dura mater or more laterally along the radicular dural sheath.[55]

Extradural arachnoid cysts are usually single. Although the age of clinical presentation may vary enormously, symptoms frequently begin in adolescence. Arachnoid cysts are much more common in men than in women. The most commonly involved region is the thoracic spine dorsal to the spinal cord.[58] In one review,[57] 65% of cases were found in the thoracic region.

Clinical symptoms and signs are similar to those of other space-occupying lesions of the spine and include pain, radicular dysfunction, and myelopathic manifestations. Symptoms may change dramatically in relation to postural changes. For example, one patient developed transient paraplegia during the exertion of defecation.[59] Transient paraplegia was also described in a pilot after a dive.[60] At times, the history of remissions and exacerbations may mimic multiple sclerosis. In some cases, periods of transient neurologic disturbance last weeks or months.

Lumbar puncture may reveal normal results or show nonspecific elevation of protein. At times, a block may be encountered. Some patients seem to show improvement following lumbar puncture, which may be due to reduction in CSF pressure with secondary emptying of a communicating cyst.

Extradural arachnoid cysts may cause erosion of the pedicles or other spinal elements at the level of the cyst and enlargement of the adjacent intervertebral foramen if the cyst extends into the paravertebral area. These findings may be observed on plain radiographs of the spine. If the cyst extends into the paravertebral region, it may be seen radiologically. These abnormalities may also be revealed by CT and MRI. Kyphoscoliosis has been reported to occur with greater frequency in patients with extradural arachnoid cysts.[55] Myelography usually reveals evidence of an extradural mass. The treat-

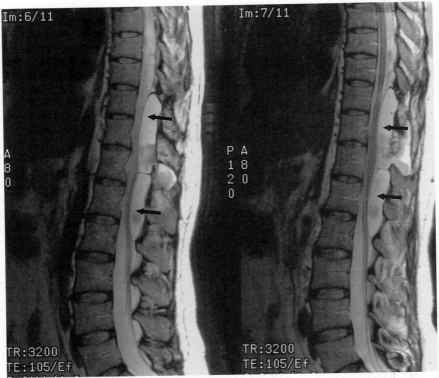

Figure 10–6. A postoperative thoracic epidural arachnoid cyst. A sagittal T_2-weighted image of a patient who previously underwent surgery for an intradural arachnoid cyst. Note the epidural extension of the cyst (arrow) through a dural vent.

ment of spinal cord compression from an extradural arachnoid cyst is surgery, if feasible. However, it is only appropriate if clinical symptoms, neurological deficit, or impending spinal deformity is present in a patient with an acceptable medical risk.

Intradural Arachnoid Cysts

Intradural arachnoid cysts are frequently encountered as asymptomatic findings on spinal imaging studies. One study[61] reported a 10% frequency of these diverticula incidentally found in patients undergoing myelography. However, because these lesions are usually dorsally located, myelography may not identify them unless the dorsal region of the intradural space is imaged and the patient is in a supine position.[55,62]

Intradural arachnoid cysts may be congenital, posttraumatic, familial, or associated with intramedullary cysts.[47,53,54,63] They may occur at any level of the spinal axis, but they are most commonly observed in the thoracic region. Unlike extradural arachnoid cysts, they are often multiple in number. They often become symptomatic in middle age.[55,56]

The clinical manifestations of intradural arachnoid cysts are similar to those of their extradural counterparts. Although not always present, the most characteristic feature is the fluctuation of symptoms in relation to changes in posture. Clinical symptoms and signs often worsen with muscular exertion and increased thoracic and abdominal pressure.[55] The fluctuating symptoms may suggest multiple sclerosis. The clinical course may be acute or extend over several years.

Plain radiographs of the spine are usually unrevealing. Due to mixing of the dye with CSF, myelography with water-soluble agents may fail to demonstrate the cyst if it freely communicates with the subarachnoid space.[54] A CT may be very helpful, especially when performed following the administration of intrathecal contrast material. Magnetic resonance imaging also is a sensitive imaging modality for these lesions (Fig. 10–7).[47]

The treatment of intradural arachnoid cysts depends upon their clinical manifestations, since many are asymptomatic. Some authors advocate rest in a recumbent position several times daily to alleviate minor symptoms.[55] The most definitive treatment of spinal cord compression from intradural arachnoid cysts is surgery. If the location and circumstances permit, resection of the cyst may be performed.

Alternatively, if resection is considered too hazardous, some advocate marsupialization or shunting of the cyst.[54] Recurrence following surgery is common. This should be taken into consideration during the decision-making and patient counseling process.

SPINAL HEMORRHAGE

Spinal hemorrhage may occur in the spinal cord itself, the subarachnoid space, the subdural space, or the epidural space. In each setting, the clinical presentation is typically sudden pain followed by neurologic symptoms and signs determined by

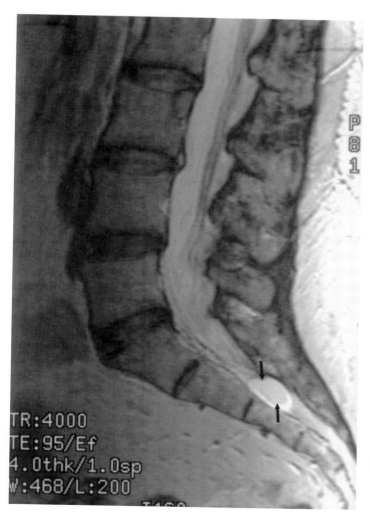

Figure 10–7. A T_2-weighted MRI of a patient with an intradural sacral arachnoid cyst (arrow) and an S2 radiculopathy.

the level of the hematoma. Some cases are due to trauma, but in many the etiology is a coagulopathy, anticoagulant therapy, or a vascular malformation.[64–66]

Intramedullary Hemorrhage

Although commonly secondary to trauma, nontraumatic hematomyelia is encountered rarely. It may occur secondary to bleeding from a spinal arteriovenous malformation (AVM), venous infarction, AVM with aneurysm, neoplasm, syrinx, or bleeding diathesis such as hemophilia, anticoagulant therapy, or coagulopathy.[65–67] According to Buchan and Barnett,[67] neither congophilic hemorrhage nor hypertensive hemorrhage, both of which are occasionally observed in patients with intracerebral hemorrhages, has been reported.

The clinical presentation most commonly observed is that of sudden severe back pain with or without a radicular component. The neurologic symptoms and signs largely depend on the level and extent of the hemorrhage. The hemorrhage may cause a central cord syndrome; a complete cord transection may develop in massive hemorrhage. The CSF usually demonstrates evidence of hemorrhage. The myelogram may show an enlarged spinal cord. Magnetic resonance imaging may be significant in evaluating these patients.

Treatment of nontraumatic hematomyelia depends upon the underlying cause. Drainage of the hematoma may be beneficial in appropriately selected patients.[67] Those with no myelopathy or with a complete myelopathy may be managed nonoperatively. Those with an incomplete myelopathy, particularly if progressive, are often managed surgically.

Spinal Subarachnoid Hemorrhage

Spontaneous spinal subarachnoid hemorrhage, as distinguished from hemorrhage related to major trauma, is a rare disorder; it accounts for less than 1% of all cases of subarachnoid hemorrhage.[67,68] While aneurysm is a frequent cause of intracra-nial subarachnoid hemorrhage, spontaneous spinal subarachnoid hemorrhage is commonly associated with arteriovenous malformations, coagulopathy, neoplastic and infectious meningitis, extreme physical exertion, collagen vascular disease, and lumbar puncture.[67,69–71]

Among these diverse etiologies, the most common cause appears to be an arteriovenous malformation (AVM) of the spinal cord.[69,71] Nearly 10% of patients with spinal AVMs present with a spinal subarachnoid hemorrhage; these AVMs may be associated with spinal artery aneurysms.[71] Spinal tumor appears to be a less common cause.

A 1984 review[70] found that only 55 cases of spinal subarachnoid hemorrhage were attributable to spinal neoplasm; 89% of these were in the region of the conus medullaris and cauda equina. Although several different histological types have been reported, ependymomas are the most frequent tumor responsible.[70,71]

The clinical presentation of spinal subarachnoid hemorrhage is usually that of sudden severe back or neck pain.[70,72] Michon[73] termed the presenting complaint *le coup de poignard* (the strike of the dagger). The pain may be localized to the spine, or may radiate into the legs or trunk and thereby suggest a visceral catastrophe.[71] There may be a history of prior, repeated, less severe pain suggesting earlier hemorrhage. When the nerve roots or spinal cord is involved, there is associated radiculopathy or myelopathy. Auscultation of the spine may reveal a bruit in patients with an AVM.[74] Intracranial symptoms and signs may develop as the blood circulates over the cerebral hemispheres.[75]

The CSF typically demonstrates evidence of hemorrhage. The bleeding may be diluted by CSF, but occasionally a hematoma may form due to massive hemorrhage resulting in mass effect that may be observed on imaging studies. Subarachnoid hemorrhage may be associated with a subdural hematoma.[71] When a spinal AVM is the cause, it may be seen in imaging studies.

The treatment of spinal subarachnoid hemorrhage depends upon the cause. Patients with a bleeding diathesis are treated with appropriate measures. Those with a spinal AVM are evaluated for definitive treatment of this lesion.[67,76] If a subarachnoid hematoma is found to cause spinal cord compression, evacuation of the clot may be necessary.[67]

Spinal Epidural Hemorrhage

Since first described in 1869 by Jackson, there have been approximately 250 cases of nontraumatic spinal epidural hematoma reported up to 1987.[64] Most traumatic cases share predisposing factors similar to those with spinal subdural hemorrhage. For example, many patients were receiving anticoagulant therapy[77] or had a bleeding diathesis due to thrombocytopenia or liver disease. Many cases occur in such patients following lumbar puncture or epidural anesthesia.[78] The Food and Drug Administration has published an advisory alerting physicians that several patients have developed epidural or spinal hematomas with the concurrent use of low molecular weight heparin and spinal/epidural anesthesia or spinal puncture.[79] Patients with ankylosing spondylitis are reported to be at increased risk,[80] and vascular malformations also may be responsible. Occasionally, no explanation can be found other than exertion or Valsalva maneuver.

Spinal epidural hemorrhage has a clinical presentation similar to the less common spinal subdural hemorrhage.[67] Although an epidural hematoma rarely may develop without pain,[81] patients nearly always complain of axial pain, which may radiate in a radicular distribution.[64] The motor, sensory, and sphincter functions are disrupted dependant upon the level of the spinal axis involved. Symptoms and signs of spinal cord and/or cauda equina dysfunction generally follow within minutes, hours, or (less commonly) days.[64] The thoracic and thoracolumbar areas are the most commonly involved regions; the hematoma may extend over several segments and is usually in the posterior epidural space.[64,82]

The CSF may be clear, have an elevated protein, or be bloody. The most useful laboratory studies are imaging techniques. In the past, myelography[64] and CT have been widely used,[83–85] but MRI has now become the imaging test of choice (Fig. 10–8).[86]

Spinal Subdural Hemorrhage

Spinal subdural hematoma unrelated to major trauma is a rarely described clinical entity, with only about 60 reported cases noted in a 1987 review.[64] It usually occurs in conjunction with vascular malformation, coagulopathies such as hemophilia or

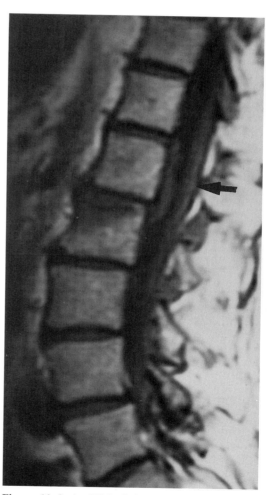

Figure 10–8. An MRI of the lumbar spine demonstrating a spontaneous epidural hematoma in a patient on coumadin for prosthetic heart valve. The hematoma is present both posterior (arrow) and anterior to the thecal sac. (Courtesy of Dr. Richard Becker.)

thrombocytopenia, the administration of anticoagulant therapy, following lumbar puncture, or following spinal surgery.[77,87,88] Lumbar puncture in the setting of a co-agulation disturbance is an important etiology.[64,87,89]

Because the subdural space harbors few blood vessels, the source of bleeding in spinal subdural hematomas has been a source of conjecture and debate.[89] The greater frequency of spinal epidural hemorrhage than subdural hemorrhage may reflect the greater density of blood vessels in the epidural space.[87] Spinal subdural hematomas occur most commonly in the thoracic and thoracolumbar regions.[90]

The clinical presentation of spinal subdural hematoma is usually acute in onset and evolution. Patients usually present with severe back or neck pain with or without a radicular component. Paraplegia, sensory loss, and bowel/bladder dysfunction may rapidly ensue over several minutes, hours, or (less commonly) days.[64] Although less frequent, chronic subdural hematomas have been described.[67,89] These patients may show fluctuating neurologic signs.[89]

The cerebrospinal fluid may show blood if there is an associated subarachnoid hemorrhage. A complete block due to a hematoma may result in a dry tap. Myelography may demonstrate a filling defect from a hematoma in the subdural space. A CT may show a clot if the level of the hematoma is imaged. An MRI avoids the risks of lumbar or cisternal puncture (Fig. 10–9). Hence, it is usually the imaging modality of choice.

Differential Diagnosis of Spinal Hematoma

At the time that patients have only local and/or radicular pain, the differential diagnosis of spinal hematoma is exceedingly broad, including diseases of the spine as well as visceral diseases such as myocardial infarction and dissecting aortic aneurysm. When neurologic symptoms and signs of spinal cord or cauda equina dysfunction develop, the differential diagnosis in-cludes those diseases that may cause rapidly evolving paraparesis or tetraparesis, such as herniated discs, neoplasm (extradural, intradural–extramedullary, and intramedullary), abscess, as well as sequelae of trauma. Intramedullary diseases such as acute and subacute transverse myelitis, demyelinating disease, spinal cord infarction, and infectious diseases also need to be considered.[64]

Therapy

Spinal cord compression secondary to non-traumatic spinal subdural and epidural hematoma is a neurologic and neurosurgical emergency. Patients with impaired hemostasis due to thrombocytopenia should receive platelet transfusions. In patients receiving anticoagulation, fresh frozen plasma, and, when indicated, phytonadione should be administered urgently to correct the bleeding diathesis.[64] Prompt surgical decompression of the compressed spinal cord and/or cauda equina is recommended, because the prognosis for neurologic recovery depends upon the preoperative neurologic status and the duration of neurologic dysfunction.[64,67] In patients with noncorrectable bleeding disorders, however, the risks of surgical intervention may outweigh the benefits.[87]

The prognosis for neurologic recovery depends on several factors. Many patients with incomplete motor and sensory paralysis preoperatively can be expected to enjoy a good recovery, whereas those with complete sensorimotor paralysis have an exceedingly small chance of successful recovery.[64] Other prognostic factors include the time course of sensorimotor paralysis and the rostrocaudal location of the hematoma. Those with hematomas at the cervical and thoracic levels fare more poorly than those with lumbar hematomas.[64]

SUMMARY

Syringomyelia is a chronic progressive disorder of the spinal cord characterized pathologically by cavitation of the central

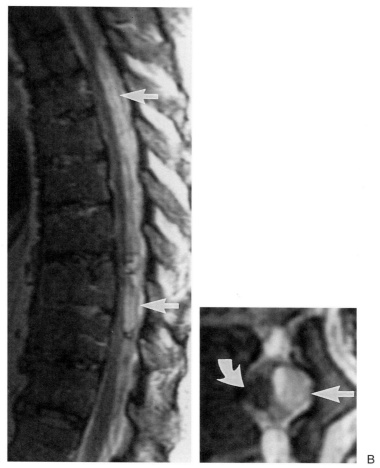

Figure 10–9. An MRI of the thoracic spine demonstrating spinal subdural hemorrhage. A 76-year-old man on coumadin for atrial fibrillation (INR of 2.1) and who had a history of prostate cancer presented with acute onset of back pain and rapidly progressive paraplegia over 24 hours. Clinically it was thought that he had metastatic spinal cord compression, but the MRI demonstrated a hematoma. (A) Extensive clot along the posterior aspect of the thoracic cord (arrows). The axial scan demonstrates a clot (arrow) posterior to the cord (curved arrow). The patient was given fresh frozen plasma and vitamin K, and underwent drainage of the subdural clot. He regained bowel and bladder function and could walk with assistance postoperatively. No tumor was found at the time of surgery.

portion of the cord and clinically by brachial amyotrophy and dissociated sensory loss. Although any level of the cord may be involved, most commonly the cervical region is affected and, secondarily, the adjacent medulla oblongata or thoracic cord may be affected.

Syringomyelia may be classified into communicating or noncommunicating types. The communicating forms are often associated with obstructions of the foramen magnum such as hindbrain developmental abnormalities (e.g., Chiari malformation). Noncommunicating forms are usually associated with intramedullary diseases of the cord such as spinal cord tumors, traumatic myelopathy, and arachnoiditis. The pathogenesis of syringomyelia is controversial and a number of putative mechanisms are discussed. Magnetic resonance imaging is the diagnostic imaging test of choice and can be used to follow the size of the cystic cavitation. Since syringomyelia is multifactorial in origin the potential therapies are multiple and, as might be expected, controversial. The principles surrounding both nonsurgical and surgical treatments are presented.

Spinal arachnoid cysts may be in either an intradural or epidural location. They may be incidental findings on MRI. Alternatively, they may cause neural compression and require surgical decompression. Their clinical presentation and management are discussed.

Spinal hemorrhage may be intramedullary, subarachnoid, subdural, and epidural. Clinical presentation is usually the acute onset of pain and myelopathy. The etiologies include coagulopathy, trauma, vascular malformations, lumbar puncture, spinal anesthesia, and surgery. Diagnostic imaging studies, using MRI and CT, have been reviewed, as have as the principles of management.

REFERENCES

1. Barnett HJM, Foster JB, Hudgson P. *Syringomyelia*. Philadelphia: Saunders; 1973.
2. Gardner WJ. *The Dysraphic States From Syringomyelia to Anencephaly*. Amsterdam: Excerpta Medica; 1973.
3. Hughes JT. Diseases of the Spinal Cord. In Blackwood W, Corsellis JAN, editors. *Greenfield's Neuropathology*. Chicago: Year Book Medical; 1976; pp. 652–87.
4. Hughes JT. *Pathology of the Spinal Cord*. Philadelphia: W.B. Saunders; 1978.
5. Spiller WG. Syringomyelia, extending from the sacral region of the spinal cord through the medulla oblongata, right side of the pons and right cerebral peduncle to the upper part of the right internal capsule (syringobulbia). *Br Med J* 1906; 2:1017.
6. Finlayson AI. Syringomyelia and related conditions. In Baker AB, Baker LH, editors. *Clinical Neurology, Volume 3*. Hagerstown: Harper & Row; 1980.
7. Perot P, Feindel W, Lloyd-Smith D. Hematomyelia as a complication of syringomyelia. Gowers syringal haemorrhage. *J Neurosurg* 1966;25: 447–51.
8. Brunberg JA, Latchaw RE, Kanal E, et al. Magnetic resonance imaging of spinal dysraphism. *Radiol Clin North Am* 1988;26:181–205.
9. Peerless SJ, Durward QJ. Management of syringomyelia: a pathophysiological approach. *Clin Neurosurg* 1983;30:531–76.
10. Williams B. On the pathogenesis of syringomyelia: a review. *R Soc Med* 1980;73:798– 806.
11. Ball MJ, Dayan AD. Pathogenesis of syringomyelia. *Lancet* 1972;2:799.
12. Oldfield E, Muraszko K, Showker T, Patronas N. Pathophysiology of syringomyelia associated with Chiari I malformation of the cerebellar tonsils: implications for diagnosis and treatment. *J Neurosurg* 1994;80:3–15.
13. Armond R, Heiss J, Oldfield E. Craniocervical decompression reduces subarachnoid and syrinx fluid velocity with syringomyelia resolution. *J Neurosurg* 1994;80:399A.
14. Levy W, Mason L, Hahn J. Chiari malformation presenting in adults: a surgical experience in 127 cases. *Neurosurgery* 1983;12:377–89.
15. Logue V, Edwards MR. Syringomyelia and its surgical treatment—an analysis of 75 cases. *J Neurol Neurosurg Psychiatry* 1981;44:273.
16. Dahlin DC. Giant cell tumor of the vertebrae above the sacrum: a review of 31 cases. *Cancer* 1977;39:1350–6.
17. Pillay P, Awad I, Little J, Hahn J. Surgical management of syringomyelia: a five year experience in the era of magnetic resonance imaging. *Neurol Res* 1991;13:3–9.
18. Pare L, Batzford U. Syringomyelia persistence after Chiari decompression as a result of pseudomeningocele formation: implications for syrinx pathogenesis: report of three cases. *Neurosurgery* 1998;43:945–8.
19. Anton HA, Schweigel JF. Posttraumatic syringomyelia: the British Columbia experience. *Spine* 1986;11:865–8.
20. Castillo M, Quencer RM, Green BA, Montalvo BM. Syringomyelia as a consequence of compressive extramedullary lesions: postoperative clinical and radiological manifestations. *AJR Am J Roentgenol* 1988;150:391–6.
21. Poser CM. *The Relationship Between Syringomyelia and Neoplasm*. Springfield, IL: C.C. Thomas; 1956.
22. Rodriguez HA, Berthrong M. Multiple intracranial tumors in von Recklinghausen's neurofibromatosis. *Arch Neurol* 1966;14:467–75.
23. Melmon KG, Rosen SW. Lindau's disease. *Am J Med* 1964;36:695–703.
24. Sherman JL, Barkovich AJ, Citrin CM. The MR appearance of syringomyelia: new observations. *AJR Am J Roentgenol* 1987;148:381–91.
25. Cahan LD, Bentson JR. Considerations in the diagnosis and treatment of syringomyelia and the Chiari malformation. *J Neurosurg* 1982;57:24–31.
26. McIlroy WJ, Richardson JC. Syringomyelia: a clinical review of 75 cases. *Can Med Assoc J* 1965; 93:731–4.
27. Schliep G. Syringomyelia and syringobulbia. In Vinken PJ, Bruyn GW, editors. *Handbook of Clinical Neurology, Volume 32*. Amsterdam: North-Holland; 1978; pp. 255–326.
28. Spiller WG. Central pain in syringomyelia and dysesthesia and overreaction to sensory stimuli in lesions below the optic thalamus. *AMA Arch Neurol Psychiat* 1923;10:491.
29. Adams RD, Victor M. Diseases of the spinal cord. In Adams RD, Victor M, editors. *Principles of Neurology*. New York: McGraw-Hill; 1985; pp. 665–98.
30. McCrae DL. Asymptomatic intervertebral disc protrusions. *Acta Radiol* 1956;46:9–27.
31. Restuccia D, Di Lazzaro V, Valeriano M, et al. Spinal responses to median and tibial nerve stim-

ulation and magnetic resonance imaging in intramedullary cord lesions. *Neurology* 1996;46: 1706–14.

32. Conway LW. Radiographic studies of syringomyelia. *Trans Am Neurol Assoc* 1961;86: 205–6.

33. Adelstein LJ. The surgical treatment of syringomyelia. *Am J Surg* 1938;40:384–95.

34. Brain R, Wilkinson M. Cervical arthropathy in syringomyelia, tabes dorsalis and diabetes. *Brain* 1958;81:275–89.

35. Netsky MG. Syringomyelia. *Arch Neurol Psychiat* 1953;70:741–77.

36. Spillane JD, Pallis C, Jones AM. Developmental abnormalities in the region of the foramen magnum. *Brain* 1957;80:11–48.

37. McRae DL. Bony abnormalities in the region of the foramen magnum: correlation of the anatomic and neurologic findings. *Acta Radiol* 1953; 40:335–54.

38. Pendergrass EP, Schaeffer JP, Hodes PJ. *The Head and Neck in Roentgen Diagnosis, 2nd Edition.* Springfield, IL: C.C. Thomas; 1956.

39. Conway LW. Hydrodynamic studies in syringmyelia. *J Neurosurg* 1967;27:501–14.

40. DiChiro G, Axelbaum SP, Schellinger D, et al. Computerized tomography in syringomyelia. *N Engl J Med* 1975;292:13–6.

41. Fitz CR. The pediatric spine. In Gonzalez CF, Grossman CB, Masdeu JC, editors. *Head and Spine Imaging.* New York: John Wiley; 1985; pp. 759–80.

42. Grossman CB, Post MJD. The adult spine. In Gonzalez CF, Grossman CB, Masdeau JC, editors. *Head and Spine Imaging.* New York: John Wiley; 1985; pp. 781–858.

43. Haughton VM, Williams AL. *Computed Tomography of the Spine.* St. Louis: C.V. Mosby; 1982.

44. Council ScientificAffair. Magnetic resonance imaging of the central nervous system. *JAMA* 1988;259:1211–22.

45. Kanaze MG, Gado MH, Sartor KJ, Hodges FJ. Comparison of MR and CT myelography in imaging the cervical and thoracic spine. *AJR Am J Roentgenol* 1988;150:397–403.

46. Williams AL, Haughton VM, Pojunas KW, et al. Differentiation of intramedullary neoplasms and cysts by MR. *AJR Am J Roentgenol* 1987;149: 159–64.

47. Andrews BT, Weinstein PR, Rosenblum ML, Barbaro NM. Intradural arachnoid cysts of the spinal canal associated with intramedullary cysts. *J Neurosurg* 1988;68:544–9.

48. McIlroy WJ, Stowe RM. Syringomyelia. In Johnson RT, editor. *Current Therapy in Neurologic Disease—2.* Toronto: B.C. Decker; 1987; pp. 94–7.

49. Shannon N, Simon L, Logue V. Clinical features, investigation, and treatment of post-traumatic syringomyelia. *J Neurol Neurosurg Psychiatry* 1981; 44:35.

50. Tator CH, Meguro K, Rowed DW. Favorable results with syringosubarachnoid shunts for treatment of syringomyelia. *J Neurosurg* 1982;56: 517–23.

51. Hida K, Iwasaki Y, Koyanagi I, et al. Surgical indication and results of foramen magnum decom-

pression versus syringo-subarachnoid shunting for syringmyelia associated with Chiari I malformation. *Neurosurgery* 1995;37:673–8.

52. Umbach H. Post-spinal cord injury syringomyelia. *Paraplegia* 1991;29:219–21.

53. Aarabi B, Pasternak G, Hurko O, Long DM. Familial intradural arachnoid cysts: report of two cases. *J Neurosurg* 1979;50:826–9.

54. Galzio RJ, Zenobil M, Lucantoni D, Cristuib-Grizzi L. Spinal intradural arachnoid cyst. *Surg Neurol* 1981;17:388–91.

55. Gimeno A. Arachnoid, neurenteric and other cysts. In Vinken PJ, Bruyn GW, editors. *Handbook of Clinical Neurology, Volume 32.* Amsterdam: North Holland; 1978; pp. 393–447.

56. Fortuna A, Torre EL, Ciapetta P. Arachnoid diverticula: a unitary approach to spinal cysts communicating with the subarachnoid space. *Acta Neurochir* 1977;39:259–68.

57. Cloward RB. Congenital extradural cysts: case report with a review of the literature. *Ann Surg* 1968;168:851–64.

58. Rexed B. The cytoarchitectonic atlas of the spinal cord in the cat. *J Comp Neurol* 1954;100: 297–379.

59. Dandy W. A sign and symptom of spinal cord tumors. *Arch Neurol Psychiatry* 1920;16:435–41.

60. Hamlin H, Garrity RW, Golden JB. Extradural spinal cyst. A case report. *J Neurosurg* 1949;6: 260–3.

61. Teng P, Rudner N. Multiple arachnoid diverticula. *Arch Neurol* 1960;2:348–56.

62. Chan RC, Thompson GB, Bratty PJA. Symptomatic anterior spinal arachnoid diverticulum. *Neurosurgery* 1985;16:663–5.

63. Zuccarello M, Scanarini M, D'Avella D, et al. Spontaneous spinal extradural hematoma during anticoagulant therapy. *Surg Neurol* 1980;14: 411.

64. Mattle H, Sieb JP, Rohner M, Mumenthaler M. Nontraumatic spinal epidural and subdural hematomas. *Neurology* 1987;37:1351–8.

65. Papo I, Luongo A. Massive intramedullary hemorrhage in a patient on anticoagulants. *J Neurosurg Sci* 1974;18:268.

66. Schenk VWD. Hemorrhages in spinal cord with syringomyelia in a patient with hemophelia. *Acta Neuropathol (Berlin)* 1963;2:306.

67. Buchan AM, Barnett JM. Vascular malformations and hemorrhage of the spinal cord. In Barnett HJM, Mohr JP, Stein BM, Yatsu FM, editors. *Stroke: pathophysiology, Diagnosis and Management.* New York: Churchill Livingstone; 1986; pp. 721–30.

68. Walton JN. Subarachnoid hemorrhage of unusual etiology. *Neurology* 1953;3:517–43.

69. Henson RA, Croft PB. Spontaneous spinal subarachnoid hemorrhage. *Q J Med* 1956;25: 53.

70. Roscoe MWA, Barrington TW. Acute spinal subdural hematoma. A case report and review of literature. *Spine* 1984;9:672–5.

71. Swann KW, Ropper AH, New PJF, Poletti CE. Spontaneous spinal subarachnoid hemorrhage and subdural hematoma. *J Neurosurg* 1984;61: 975–80.

72. Plotkin R, Ronthal M, Froman C. Spontaneous spinal subarachnoid hemorrhage. Report of 3 cases. *J Neurosurg* 1966;25:443–6.
73. Michon P. Le coup de poignard rachidien symptome initial de certaines hemorragies sous-arachnoidennes. Essai sur les hemorragies meningees spinales. *Presse Med* 1928;36:964–6.
74. Hook O, Lidvall H. Arteriovenous aneurysms of the spinal cord. A report of two cases investigated by vertebral angiography. *J Neurosurg* 1958;15:84–91.
75. Caroscio JT, Brannan T, Budabin M, et al. Subarachnoid hemorrhage secondary to spinal arteriovenous malformation and aneurysm. Report of a case and review of the literature. *Arch Neurol* 1980;37:101–3.
76. Michelsen WJ. Arteriovenous malformation of the brain and spinal cord. In Johnson RT, editor. *Current Therapy in Neurologic Disease—2*. Toronto: B.C. Decker; 1987:170–3.
77. Silverstein A. Neurological complications of anticoagulation therapy. A neurologist's review. *Arch Intern Med* 1979;139:217–20.
78. Gustafson H, Rutberg H, Bengtsson M. Spinal haematoma following epidural analgesia. Report of a patient with ankylosing spondylitis and a bleeding diathesis. *Anesthesia* 1988;43:220–2.
79. Lumpkin M. FDA Public Health Advisory: reports of epidural or spinal hematomas with the concurrent use of low molecular weight heparin and spinal/epidural anesthesia or spinal puncture. *FDA Public Health Advisory* December 15, 1997.
80. Hissa E, Boumphrey F, Bay J. Spinal epidural hematoma and ankylosing spondylitis. *Clin Orthop* 1986;208:225–7.
81. Senelick RC, Norwood CW, Cohen CH. Painless spinal epidural hematoma during anticoagulant therapy. *Neurology* 1976;26:213–5.
82. Beatty RM, Winston KR. Spontaneous cervical epidural hematoma. Consideration of etiology. *J Neurosurg* 1984;61:143–8.
83. Haykal HA, Wang A-M, Zamani AA, Rumbaugh CL. Computed tomography of spontaneous acute cervical epidural hematoma. *J Comput Assist Tomogr* 1984;8:229.
84. Lanzieri CF, Sacher M, Solodnik P, Moser F. CT myelography of spontaneous spinal epidural hematoma. *J Comput Assist Tomogr* 1985;9:393–4.
85. Levitan LH, Wiens CW. Chronic lumbar extradural hematoma: CT findings. *Radiology* 1983;148:707–8.
86. Holtas S, Heiling M, Lonntoft M. Spontaneous spinal epidural hematoma: findings at MR imaging and clinical correlation. *Radiology* 1996;199:409–13.
87. Edelson RN, Chernik NL, Posner JB. Spinal subdural hematomas complicating lumbar puncture. Occurrence in thrombocytopenic patients. *Arch Neurol* 1974;31:134–7.
88. Yomarken JL. Spinal subdural hematoma. *Ann Emerg Med* 1985;14:261–3.
89. Khosla VK, Kak VK, Mathuriya SN. Chronic spinal subdural hematomas. Report of two cases. *J Neurosurg* 1985;63:636–9.
90. Russell NA, Vaughnan R, Morley TP. Spinal epidural infection. *Can J Neurol Sci* 1979;6: 325–8.

Chapter 11

SPINE TRAUMA, SPINAL CORD INJURY, AND SPINAL STABILITY

Most spinal cord injuries (SCI) are caused by closed trauma (nonpenetrating injuries, usually via spinal column failure); some arise from missile, or less commonly, impalement (penetrating injuries). The presence and extent of spinal cord injuries depend on how much kinetic energy is imparted to the spine, the extent of spinal column failure, the extent of neural compression, the presence of persistent neural compression or neural element transection, and the resilience of the spinal cord and nerve roots in the face of injury. Each of these factors must be considered separately. Many have a variable effect that is dependent upon the region of the spine injured. Therefore, region-specific anatomical and biomechanical factors must be understood and repetitively assessed.[1,2]

UPPER CERVICAL SPINE INJURY MECHANISMS AND PATTERNS

The upper cervical spine is prone to injury due to (1) its unique anatomical arrangement, (2) the substantial spinal movements allowed in this region, and (3) exposure to significant pathological stresses.[1] Most upper cervical spine injuries result from blows to the head.[1,3–9] However, a deceleration of the torso combined with a restriction of movement of the cervical spine creates a flexion–distraction force complex that can result in an applied bending moment (see below).[1]

Factors Affecting Pattern of Injury

Orientation of an applied force vector predominantly dictates a given pattern or type of injury. The relative intrinsic strengths of C1 and C2, as well as the surrounding spinal elements (including the adjacent vertebrae, calvarium, and sup-

359

porting ligaments), also affect the pattern of injury by "setting the stage" for dissipating the energy of the applied force vector.[10] The kinetic energy of the applied force predominantly dictates the magnitude of the injury.[1]

Injury Mechanisms and Patterns of Injury

Figure 11–1 shows force vectors that cause a variety of upper cervical fractures and dislocations. Several of the injury types

that result from these force vectors have been underemphasized previously.[1] These injury types are discussed in the order of force vector application, starting with the judicial hangman's fracture and proceeding in a clockwise manner; then lateral (coronal plane) and finally rotatory injuries are discussed (Fig. 11–1).

JUDICIAL HANGMAN'S FRACTURE

Judicial hanging causes a combination of distraction (the abrupt and violent application of tension via the noose and rope)

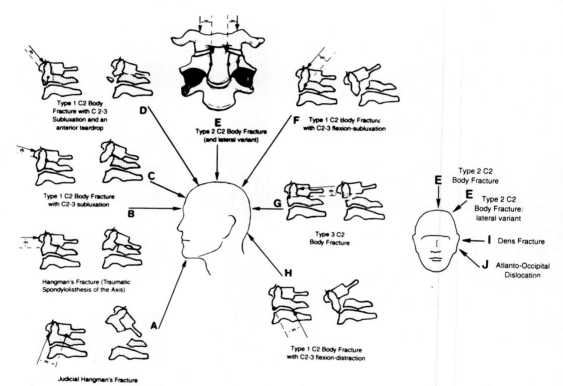

Figure 11–1. Schematic diagrams of the most probable mechanisms involved in upper cervical spine injuries; sagittal plane (left) and coronal plane (right). The moment arm (m) applied by the force vector (arrows) is depicted for each mechanism of injury (A–J). (A) Judicial hangman's fracture; (B) traumatic spondylolisthesis of the axis (hangman's fracture); (C) coronally oriented vertical fracture of the posterior C-2 vertebral body (Type 1 C-2 body fracture) with C2–3 hyperextension-subluxation; (D) coronally oriented vertical fracture of the dorsal C-2 vertebral body (Type 1 C-2 body fracture) with C2–3 hyperextension-subluxation and an anterior teardrop; (E) sagittally oriented vertical C-2 pedicle burst fracture (Type 2 C-2 body fracture), its lateral variant, or a C-1 burst fracture (Jefferson fracture); (F) coronally oriented vertical fracture of the posterior C-2 vertebral body (Type 1 C-2 body fracture) with C2–3 flexion-subluxation; (G) Type 3 C-2 body fracture (formerly the Type III odontoid process fracture of Anderson and D'Alonzo[1]) or rupture of transverse ligament of the atlas; (H) coronally oriented vertical fracture of the posterior C-2 vertebral body (Type 1 C-2 body fracture) with C2–3 flexion-distraction; (I) dens fracture (formerly Anderson and D'Alonzo Type II odontoid process fracture); and (J) atlanto-occipital dislocation. Taken from references 1,10.

and capital hyperextension if the noose is placed in the submental position (injury mechanism A; Fig. 11–1). This results in a fracture through the pars interarticularis with or without ventral subluxation of the C2 on the C3 vertebral body. Falls with a rostrally oriented force vector applied to the submental position can cause a similar injury, although this is not common.[1,11,12]

DORSAL DISLOCATION OF C1 ON C2

Dorsal C1–2 dislocations are rare.[13] They are purported to be caused by injury mechanism A (Fig. 11–1). The ventral arch of C1 rides dorsally over the dens, becoming "locked" behind it.[1]

TRAUMATIC SPONDYLOLISTHESIS OF THE AXIS (HANGMAN'S FRACTURE)

Capital hyperextension of the head, without an associated distraction component, causes the commonly observed hangman's fracture (traumatic spondylolisthesis of the axis)(injury mechanism B; Fig. 1).[1,5,6] The mechanism of injury is similar to the judicial hangman fracture, except it is without a distraction component vector (no abrupt or violent application of tension via the noose). Spinal cord compression is uncommon because the spinal canal is widened via the separation of the dorsal from the ventral elements (via a fracture of the pars interarticularis), rather than narrowed.

VERTICAL CORONALLY ORIENTED DORSAL C2 BODY FRACTURE, WITH C2–3 EXTENSION–SUBLUXATION

With slightly less capital extension than the hangman's fracture, and a small axial load component (injury mechanism C; Fig. 11–1), this injury may result in the bony fault passing through the dorsal C2 vertebral body instead of the pars interarticularis of C2, as occurs with a hangman's fracture.[1,4,5,10] The fracture line passes slightly ventral to the pars interarticularis

in comparison to the hangman's fracture. This fracture is also termed a type I C2 body fracture with C2–3 extension-subluxation.

VERTICAL CORONALLY ORIENTED DORSAL C2 BODY FRACTURE WITH C2–3 EXTENSION–SUBLUXATION AND A VENTRAL TEARDROP

A force vector applied to the high forehead region may result in the application of an axial load and capital hyperextension forces to the upper cervical spine (injury mechanism D; Fig. 11–1).[1] This is similar to the immediately aforementioned injury, with the addition of a "teardrop" component (avulsed chip of vertebral body that is akin to a teardrop). The axial load component is of relatively greater magnitude in this case. This fracture is also termed a type I C2 body fracture with C2–3 extension–subluxation and a ventral teardrop.[10]

C1 BURST FRACTURE

Axial loads applied to the vertex of the calvarium (injury mechanism E; Fig. 11–1) can cause several types of injuries. The most common of these is the C1 burst fracture (Jefferson fracture). Bursting of the C1 ring occurs because of the radially oriented resultant forces applied by the condyles of the occiput and the facet joints of C2. The oblique orientation of the condyles causes a laterally directed resultant force, resulting in several fractures (two or more; usually four) about the ring of C1.[1] This type of fracture is uncommonly associated with spinal cord injury. Since the spinal canal is widened, rather the compressed. As with most of the aforementioned fractures, it usually heals well with bracing alone, without the need for surgery.

OCCIPITAL CONDYLE FRACTURE

Although several occipital condyle fracture types exist,[14,15] type I and II fractures usually result from an axially applied load (injury mechanism E; Fig. 11–1). Type I fracture is a medial disruption of the condyle (impacted occipital condyle) as a result of a medially applied resultant force caused by the oblique orientation of the occipital condyle–C1 facet complex. Type II fracture (an extension of a basilar skull fracture) most likely also occurs as a result of an axially applied load (Fig. 11–1).[1,14,15] These fractures are often obscure. They usually heal without the need for surgery.

VERTICAL SAGITTALLY ORIENTED C2 BURST/PEDICLE FRACTURE

Axial loads applied to the skull vertex (injury mechanism E; Figure 1) may cause a C2 body (type II) fracture, though this is rare. If other spinal elements do not fail first (resulting in an occipital condyle fracture, a Jefferson fracture or a subaxial cervical spine burst fracture), the load applied to the articular pillars of C2 may result in a comminuted sagittal fracture of the C2 body.[1,10] A lateral component of the axial load may shift the location of the fracture further (Fig. 11–1), causing a more laterally situated sagittal C2 fracture.[1,7,10] This fracture may pass through the foramina transversarium and along the pars interarticularis of C2.[1] It is often associated with severe head injury. Fortunately, it is relatively uncommon.

C1 ARCH FRACTURE

Axial loads, with or without a hyperextension component (injury mechanism type C, D, or E; Fig. 11–1), may result in a fracture through the weakest point of the ring of C1 (dorsal arch in region of the groove for the vertebral artery), causing a C1 arch fracture.[1] This is a stable fracture that must not be confused with a Jefferson's fracture. The former is benign, where the latter may be unstable. With the former, the ring of C1 is disrupted in two dorsal locations. With the Jefferson fracture, the ring of C1 is usually disrupted in four locations, although fracture in only two locations may be observed if one is ventral and the other is dorsal.

VERTICAL CORONALLY ORIENTED DORSAL C2 BODY TEARDROP FRACTURE WITH C2–3 FLEXION–SUBLUXATION

The application of a dorsally applied force vector with an axial load component (injury mechanism F; Fig. 11–1) may result in the opening of the dorsal aspect of the C2–3 disc interspace (capital neck flexion), thus causing an accompanying avulsion teardrop fracture of the dorsal aspect of the caudal C2 vertebral body. Since the C2–3 disc interspace is slanted in a downward direction, the orientation of this disc interspace is nearly in line with the applied force vector. This then results in a subluxation between C2 and C3.[1] This injury is uncommon. However, it is frequently "missed" due to inadequate imaging or misdiagnosis and confusion with similar injuries. Fortunately, the injury is relatively benign in nature. This fracture is also termed a type I C2 body fracture with flexion–subluxation.

HORIZONTAL ROSTRAL C2 BODY FRACTURE

A dorsal blow to the head (injury mechanism G; Fig. 11–1) may result in true neck flexion. By virtue of previously reported data,[8] if the C2 region "fails," a horizontal fracture through the rostral portion of the body of C2 occurs. This fracture was defined by Anderson and D'Alonzo.[16] This injury is through the region of the C2 body, not the odontoid process.[1,10,15] It therefore should not be considered an "odontoid process fracture," as others have argued.[16] It is also termed a type III C2 body fracture. It is usually treated efficiently with bracing alone.

TRANSVERSE LIGAMENT OF THE ATLAS RUPTURE

If the odontoid process does not yield to a failure-producing force applied by injury mechanism G (Fig. 11–1), the transverse ligament of the atlas may rupture.[1,8,17] This injury may be difficult to diagnose, and instability could result in dorsal "migration" of the dens into the spinal canal, with catastrophic results. A high index of suspicion for the diagnosis of this injury is thus warranted.

VERTICAL CORONALLY ORIENTED DORSAL C2 BODY FRACTURE WITH FLEXION–DISTRACTION

If a capital (upper cervical) flexion injury is combined with a distraction component, usually caused by a deceleration over the fulcrum (e.g., shoulder harness), a flexion–distraction force complex is applied (injury mechanism H, Fig. 11–1).[1] This is an uncommon mechanism of injury (flexion–distraction), since most cervical spine injuries result from a blow to the head. It is also termed a type I C2 body fracture with flexion–distraction.

DENS FRACTURE

The type II odontoid process fracture of Anderson and D'Alonzo[16] is perhaps more appropriately termed a dens fracture.[15] It most probably results from a lateral blow to the head (injury mechanism I; Fig. 11–1),[8] perhaps combined with vertical compression.[1,10,18] This fracture heals poorly. In patients with advanced age, significant displacement, or multiple comminuted fracture fragments, surgery may be indicated.

OCCIPITAL CONDYLE FRACTURE (TYPE III)

A lateral blow to the head (injury mechanism I, Fig. 11–1) may result in a medial avulsion of the occipital condyle, a type III occipital condyle fracture.[1,14,15] This is often a severe injury with lower cranial nerve involvement and associated head injury.

ATLANTO-OCCIPITAL DISLOCATION

A lateral (with or without a hyperextension component) deceleration injury causes a lateral bending–rotation–distraction injury force application (injury mechanism J, Fig. 11–1), resulting in atlanto-occipital dislocation. Others have postulated hyperextension–distraction mechanisms.[1,3,19] Cranio-

cervical integrity disruption is catastrophic. It is commonly caused by motor vehicle accidents, death frequently occurs at the scene. Survival is uncommon.

DENS AVULSION FRACTURES

A distraction of the spine, not unlike that which might be incurred in a judicial hanging (injury mechanism A, Fig. 11–1) or as a result of a lateral force vector component (injury mechanism J, Fig. 11–1), may result in an avulsion of the tip of the dens.[1] This is uncommon. Stability may be compromised by this injury.

ROTATORY SUBLUXATION INJURIES

If a torque (bending moment) is created about the long axis of the spine (about the dens), a rotational injury may occur,[20] resulting in rotatory subluxation of C1 on C2.[1] This is an uncommon injury sometimes associated with pharyngeal infections in children (Grissel's syndrome).

Clinical Strategies

Most upper cervical spinal injuries are not associated with neurological injury. This, combined with the fact that bony healing often ensues if unimpeded, allows nonsurgical management (bracing) in most cases. Notable exceptions are transverse ligament ruptures and dens (type II odontoid) fractures.

SUBAXIAL CERVICAL, THORACIC, AND LUMBAR INJURY MECHANISMS AND PATTERNS

Factors Affecting Pattern of Injury

Denis described fracture types and accompanying modes of failure for the subaxial spine (Table 11–1).[21] This scheme is widely utilized.

The manner in which a load is applied affects the bending moment applied (the

Table 11–1. **Fracture Types by Mode of Failure**

	COLUMN		
TYPE OF FRACTURE	ANTERIOR	MIDDLE	POSTERIOR
Compression	Compression	None	None or severe distraction
Burst	Compression	Compression	None
"Seatbelt" (flexion–distraction)	None or compression	Distraction	Distraction
Fracture-dislocation	Compression rotation shear	Distraction rotation shear	Distraction rotation shear

product of the applied force and the moment arm [level arm] through which it acts) (Fig. 11–2). This, in turn, alters the stresses placed on a spinal segment. Bending moments cause a concentration of stresses to be applied to the spine, thus increasing the chance that spinal column failure will occur.

Injury Mechanisms and Patterns of Injury

VENTRAL WEDGE COMPRESSION FRACTURES

Ventral wedge compression fractures are the product of an axial load, and a ven-trally oriented bending moment (to failure), where the axial load is eccentrically placed (Fig. 11–3).[1,2] This results in a flexion deformity of the fractured bone.

BURST FRACTURES

If a pure axial load (to failure) is applied to a vertebral body, a wedge fracture is unlikely. A symmetrical compression of the vertebral body results. This is termed a burst fracture.[1,22–30] This "pancaking" of the vertebral body often causes retropulsion of bony fragments into the spinal canal and dural sac compression (Fig. 11–4).[1,21,31]

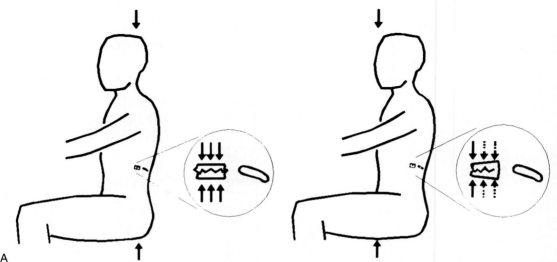

Figure 11–2. (A) If an axial load is sufficient to result in vertebral body failure, the failure is of a burst-fracture nature. (B) If, however, a load is applied in a plane ventral to the instantaneous axis of rotation (IAR), a pair of asymmetrical bending moment forces will be applied to the IAR, resulting in a wedge compression fracture.[1]

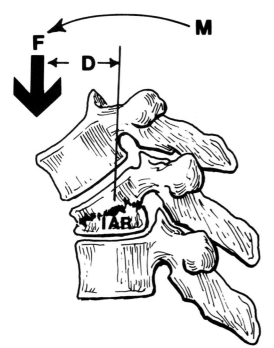

Figure 11–3. A depiction of the injury force vector causing a ventral wedge compression fracture. F = applied force vector; D = length of moment arm (from IAR to plane of F); M = bending moment.

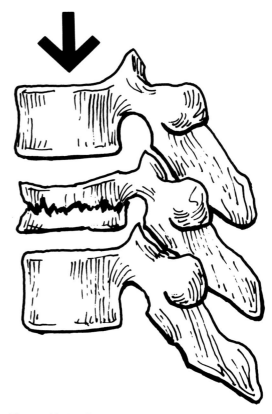

Figure 11–4. The mechanism of injury of a burst fracture: true axial loading without a moment arm and bending moment.

FLEXION–DISTRACTION (CHANCE) FRACTURES

If a lap belt is worn without a shoulder harness by a person involved in a deceleration motor vehicle accident, distraction and flexion of the lumbar spine result (Fig. 11–5).[1,22,32–35]

DORSAL ELEMENT FRACTURES

Dorsal element fractures are not uncommon particularly when the spine assumes a lordotic posture and the vertebral segments are small; e.g. the subaxial cervical spine. In the cervical region, spinal extension thrusts the opposing facet surfaces together, thus subjecting them to significant stress (Fig. 11–6).

Rotation may also cause dorsal element injury by forcing opposing inferior and superior articulating facets against each other. These are not often isolated injuries, because the applied forces are of such magnitude that vertebral body fracture or disc interspace disruption simultaneously occurs.[1,36]

The lumbar spine, which also assumes a lordotic posture, has a lesser incidence of isolated dorsal element fractures because of the more massive nature of the vertebrae and the somewhat sagittal orientation of the facet joints. These fractures are nearly always associated with other injuries to the spinal column complex; i.e. compression fractures, rotational injuries, or translational injuries. A violent rotational component of the injury may disrupt the dorsal elements as well as the integrity of the ventral axial load-resisting substructure (vertebral bodies) (Fig. 11–6).

Spinous process and laminar fractures may result from extreme flexion or extension. Similarly, extreme lateral bending may result in transverse process fracture(s) on the convex side of the bend.

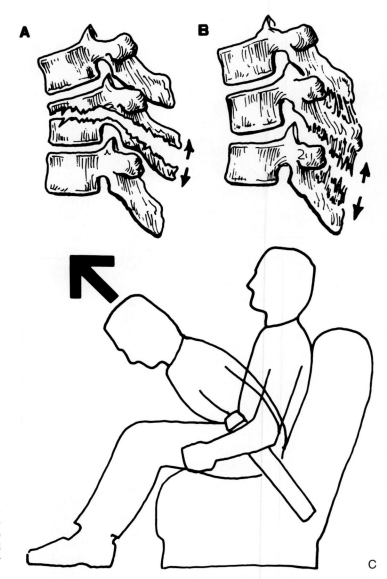

Figure 11–5. There are two fundamental types of Chance (flexion-distraction) fracture. (A) Diastasis fracture through the pedicles and vertebral body; (B) fracture through the vertebral end plate or disk; (C) the mechanism of injury is depicted.

LIGAMENTOUS INJURIES

Isolated ligamentous injuries predominantly occur in the cervical region. This is due in part to cervical flexibility, which allows for a greater strain to be placed on the ligaments. The more massive and less flexible lumbar spine does not rely as much on ligamentous support. In fact, the dorsal ligaments, particularly the interspinous and supraspinous ligaments in the low lumbar region, are weak or essentially nonexistent. Therefore, isolated ligamentous injuries occur at a lesser frequency in this region.[1]

FACET DISLOCATION

Facet dislocation frequently occurs in the cervical and, to a lesser degree, in the thoracic region. It is rare in the lumbar re-

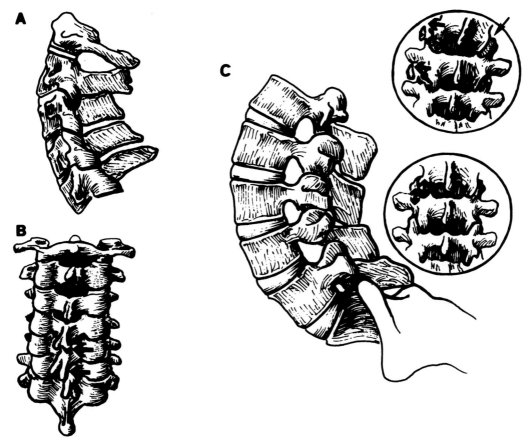

Figure 11–6. The mechanism of injury of dorsal element fractures. Cervical spine extension forcibly approximates the facet joints and/or the laminae, potentialy resulting in facet fracture (A); cervical rotation causes the coronally oriented facet joints to slide past each other, producing isolated ligamentous disruption or dislocation (B), in the lumbar region, the facet joints are able to slide past each other during extension, thus minimizing the chance for facet fracture by this mechanism (C). Lumbar rotation, however, results in one facet's abutting against another, resulting in facet fracture if the force is substantial (C, upper inset). Conversely, extension or flexion causes the sagittally oriented facet joints to slide past each other (C, lower inset).

gion. This is due to the relative coronal orientation of the facet joints in these regions. Exaggerated flexion causes normal facet joint mobility limits to be exceeded. This, in turn, causes the joints themselves to fracture, perch, or lock (Fig. 11–7).

PEDIATRIC SPINE INJURY

Pediatric spinal cord injury (SCI) comprises 5%–10% of all spinal injuries.[37–39] Injury patterns, however, differ from those of adults because the child's spine differs geometrically and biomechanically. Facet joints are more horizontal, ossification centers are still present, vertebral bodies are wedge shaped, and the uncinate processes are incompletely developed. Rotation and flexion are thus poorly resisted. Superimposed upon this is an increased laxity of supporting ligaments and joint capsules (Fig. 11–8).[40]

Pediatric spine injuries may be classified as follows: (1) fracture alone, (2) fracture with subluxation, (3) subluxation alone, and (4) spinal cord injury without radio-

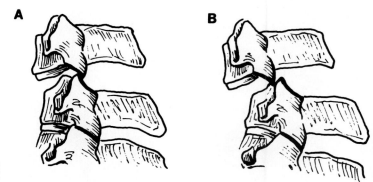

Figure 11–7. Cervical spine facet dislocation: perched (A) and locked (B).

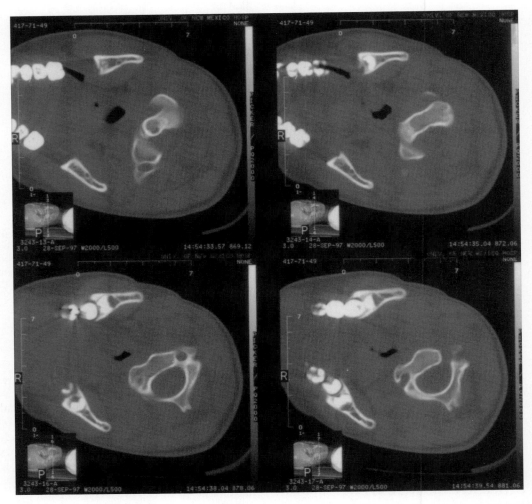

Figure 11–8. Rotatory C1–C2 subluxation in a 5 year-old. This was caused, in part, by a pharyngeal infection (Grissel's syndrome) that exaggerated the normal laxity present in the pediatric population. Note the rotation of C1 (upper right) with respect to the body of C2 (remaining images).

graphic abnormality (SCIWORA). With SCIWORA, neurological deficit associated with an anatomically intact spinal column is present. The mobility of the immature spine is most certainly a causative factor.

Pediatric fractures are the most common injuries. Fractures with subluxation follow closely. Both occur in older children, whose anatomical and biomechanical characteristics more closely approximate those of adults. Younger children are prone to subluxation alone or SCI-WORA.[37–40] Atlanto-occipital dislocation, atlanto-axial rotatory luxation, hangman's fracture, odontoid fracture, and SCI-WORA are relatively common in the pediatric population.

RECOVERY FROM CLOSED SPINAL CORD INJURY

The extent of closed SCI varies considerably. Recovery is related to the extent of injury, as patients with incomplete injuries recover to a much greater extent than those with complete injuries. Therefore, it is important to differentiate them clearly. The patient with a complete myelopathy retains no voluntary motor or sensory function below the level of injury, while an incomplete injury preserves some. Therefore, spine surgeons are likely to take a more aggressive surgical decompression posture with incomplete than with complete injuries (due to the increased chance for recovery of neurological function in the former). Surgery, however, may be required for instability reasons alone.

PENETRATING SPINE INJURIES

Penetrating spine injuries differ from closed injuries in the nature of associated complications, the prognosis for recovery, the incidence of spinal instability, the potential for CSF fistula formation, and the incidence and type of infection.[41] A variety of penetrating SCI types exist, which may be broken down into two basic groups:

missile and nonmissile. Missile injuries may be broken down into high-velocity (predominantly wartime) and low-velocity (predominantly civilian) injuries. The nonmissile injuries are usually caused by acts of violence from stab wounds.[41]

Missile Injuries

Spinal gunshot wounds are unfortunately becoming increasingly common in civilian life in the United States. Therefore, they are an increasingly common cause of spinal injuries.[41]

Military gunshot wound injuries are usually caused by high-velocity projectiles; civilian injuries are more often caused by low-velocity projectiles. Tissue damage inflicted by a missile is determined in part by its kinetic energy. Velocity is more significant than the mass of the bullet (energy = mass × velocity^2) because velocity is exponentially involved.[42] Military injuries, due to their high kinetic energy, are capable of producing SCI by the concussive effect of the bullet penetrating close to the spinal cord, but not through the spinal canal.[41] Civilian injuries, on the other hand, usually require direct spinal canal penetration.[41] In fact, a large percentage of civilian gunshot SCIs are complete injuries (no motor or sensory function below the level of injury).[43–46] Their prognosis for neurologic improvement is worse than with any other SCI type.[41]

Stab Wounds

Spinal cord injuries from stab wounds comprise less than 5% of SCIs worldwide. In South Africa, however, stab wounds account for a quarter of all SCIs.[47] Most stab wounds are due to knives; however, a variety of agents, including axes, screwdrivers, ice picks, scissors, and glass fragments, have been reported.[47,48] The thoracic region is the most common site of injury; there is a lesser incidence in the cervical and lumbar regions. Most have a dorsal or lateral entry point.

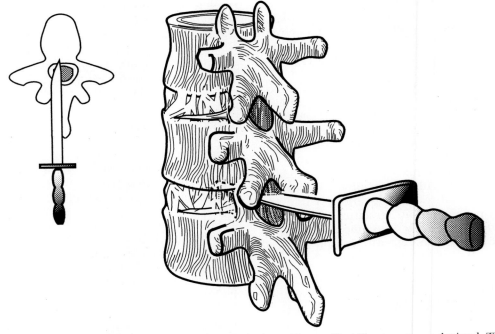

Figure 11–9. A knife is more likely to pass into the spinal canal in an off-midline manner as depicted. This is due to the propensity created by bony confines.

In contrast to gunshot wounds, stab wounds tend to produce incomplete SCIs (two-thirds of the patients).[47] Most patients exhibit a variant of the Brown-Séquard syndrome.[48–51] It has been hypothesized that the anatomy of the dorsal elements in the thoracic region contributes to this pattern of injury (Fig. 11–9).[49] Overall, neurological improvement is common.[47–51]

STABILITY DETERMINATION AND MANAGEMENT

Objective Assessment

The determination of spinal stability is often difficult.[52–74] Point systems have been devised to assist with this process (Table 11–2).[1] A stretch test and flexion–extension radiographs have been recommended. Both, however, may be associated with a high risk of false-negatives.[1]

Column Concepts

The aforementioned point systems are usually based on a "column" concept of spinal structural integrity such as those described by (1) Louis, (2) Bailey et al., and (3) Denis (Fig. 11–10).[21,63,75,76] The use of "columns" in defining the extent of instability is of some value since it assists the physician in conceptualizing and categorizing case-specific phenomena.[1]

Categorization of Instability

Instability is divided into two categories: acute and chronic.[1] Four subcategories of instability exist: (1) overt instability, (2) limited instability, (3) glacial instability, and (4) instability associated with dysfunctional segmental motion. The first two are acute and the second two are chronic.[1] Although addressed in Chapter 1, a brief review of spinal instability is appropriate here.

Table 11–2. Quantitation of acute instability for subaxial cervical, thoracic, and lumbar injuries* (point system†)[1]

CONDITION	POINTS ASSIGNED
Loss of integrity of anterior (and middle) column‡	2
Loss of integrity of posterior column(s)‡	2
Acute resting translational deformity§	2
Acute resting angulation deformity§	2
Acute dynamic translation deformity exaggeration¶	2
Acute dynamic angulation deformity exaggeration¶	2
Neural element injury#	3
Acute disc narrowing at level of suspected pathology	1
Dangerous loading anticipated	1

*Modified from White and Panjabi[15] with care taken to avoid duplication or over-lapping of point criteria.

†A score of five points or more implies the presence of overt instability (see text). A score of two to four points implies the presence of limited instability (see text).

‡By clinical examination, MRI, CT, or radiography. A single point may be allotted if incomplete evidence exists; for example, only MRI evidence of dorsal ligamentous injury (i.e., evidence of only interspinous ligament injury on T_2-weighted images). Columns are as defined by Denis.[21]

§From static resting anteroposterior and lateral spine radiographs. Must be the result of an acute clinical process. Tolerance for this criteria is variable with respect to surgeon and clinical circumstances. Guidelines as per White and Panjabi.[15]

¶From dynamic (flexion and extension) spine radiographs. Recommended only after other mechanisms of instability assessment have been exhausted and then only by an experienced clinician. Usually indicated only in cervical region. Must be the result of an acute clinical process. Tolerance for this criterion is variable with respect to surgeon's opinion and clinical circumstances. Guidelines as per White and Panjabi.[15]

#Three points for cauda equina, two points for spinal cord, or one point for isolated nerve root neurologic deficit. *The presence of neural element injury indicates that a significant spinal deformation occurred at the time of impact; implying that structural integrity may well have been disturbed.*

ACUTE INSTABILITY

Overt instability is the inability of the spine to support the torso during normal activity.[1] The integrity of the spine is insufficient to prevent the development of spinal deformity or the exaggeration of such. A circumferential loss of spinal integrity is present (Fig. 11–11).[1,2]

Limited instability is defined as the loss of ventral *or* dorsal spinal integrity with the preservation of the other. This is sufficient to support some normal activities (Fig. 11–12).

CHRONIC INSTABILITY

Glacial instability is a type of instability that is not overt and that does not demonstrate a significant chance for the rapid development or progression of kyphotic, scoliotic, or translational deformities. However, like a glacier, the deformity progresses gradually over time if substantial external forces causing movement or progression of deformity are avoided.[1,2]

Other etiologies of glacial instability include spondylosis, tumor, congenital abnormalities, and infection.

Dysfunctional segmental motion is defined as *a type of instability that is related to disc interspace or vertebral body degenerative changes, tumor, or infection that results in the potential for pain of spinal origin.*[1] It involves neither overt disruption of spinal integrity nor deformity progression. Most patients with glacial instability can also be considered to have a dysfunctional motion seg-

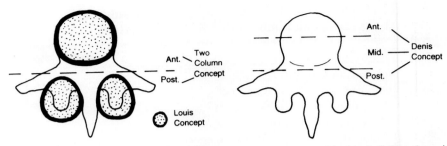

Figure 11–10. "Column" concepts of spinal instability. The concept described by Louis (left) assigns significance to the vertebral body and the facet joint complexes (lateral masses) on either side of the dorsal spine. This two-column construct (left) relies on anatomically defined structures, the vertebral body (anterior column) and the posterior elements (posterior column). Denis's three-column concept (right) assigns significance to the region of the neutral axis and the integrity of the dorsal vertebral body wall (the middle column). (From White and Panjabi,[15]).

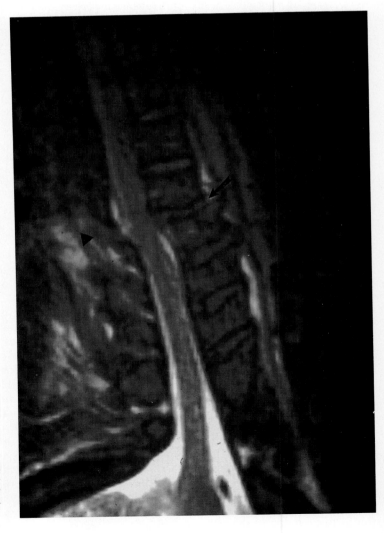

Figure 11–11. Circumferential instability. Note both ventral (arrow) and dorsal element (arrow head) disruption in this T_2-weighted image.

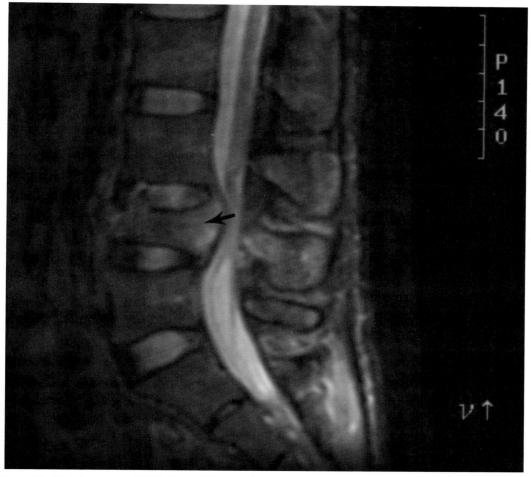

Figure 11–12. A T_2-weighted MRI of an L4 "burst" fracture (arrow). Note only loss of ventral element integrity.

ment. However, all types of glacial insta-bility have, as a component of their insta-bility, deformity progression, with or with-out excessive motion.

The disc interspace depicted in Figure 11–13 shows a dysfunctional motion seg-ment.

SUMMARY

The spine is often subjected to excessive loads. These can result in a loss of struc-tural integrity and neural element injury. Craniocervical and upper cervical spine injuries can be categorized, in part, by the force vectors causing the injury (loads). Most are secondary to a blow to the head.

Subaxial spine injuries can also be cate-gorized by considering the applied loads. Injury mechanisms are, in general, more complex than with craniocervical and up-per cervical injuries.

Pediatric SCI and penetrating spine in-juries present unique problems to the clin-ician. An awareness of their unique nature is imperative.

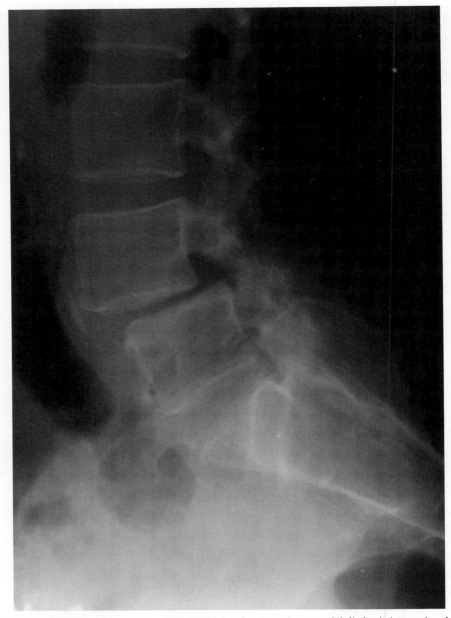

Figure 11–13. Dysfunctional segmental motion. An L4/5 degenerative spondylolisthesis is associated with dysfunctional segmental motion. Note the listhesis, as well as the degenerative changes at the disc interspace.

REFERENCES

1. Benzel EC. Biomechanics of Spine Stabilization: Principles and Clinical Practice. McGraw-Hill; New York 1995.
2. Benzel EC. Biomechanics of lumbar and lumbosacral spine fracture. In Rea GL, editor. *Spinal Trauma: current evaluation and management*. Park Ridge, Illinois: AANS Publications.
3. Bucholz RW, Burkhead WZ. The pathological anatomy of fatal atlanto-occipital dislocations. *JBJS* 1979;61A:248–50.
4. Burke JT, Harris JH. Acute injuries of the axis vertebra. *Skeletal Radiol* 1989;18:335–46.
5. Brashear HR, Venters GC, Preston ET. Fractures of the neural arch of the axis: a report of twenty-nine cases. *JBJS* 1975;57A:879–87.
6. Francis WR, Fielding JW. Traumatic spondylolisthesis of the axis. *Orthop Clin North Am* 1978;9: 1011–27.
7. Francis WR, Fielding JW, Hawkins RJ, Pepin J, Hensinger R. Traumatic spondylolisthesis of the axis. *JBJS* 1981;63B:313–8.
8. Mouradian WH, Fietti VG, Cochran GVB. Fractures of the odontoid: a laboratory and clinical study of mechanisms. *Orthop Clin North Am* 1978; 9:985–1001.
9. Williams TG. Hangman's fracture. *JBJS* 1975;57B:82–8.
10. Benzel EC, Hart BL, Ball PA, Baldwin NG, Orrison WW, Espinosa M. Vertical C2 body fractures. *J Neurosurg* 1994;81:206–12.
11. Levine AM, Edwards CC. Treatment of injuries in the C1–C2 complex. *Orthop Clin North Am* 1986;17:31–44.
12. Wood-Jones F. The ideal lesion produced by judicial hanging. *Lancet* 1913;1:53.
13. Patzakis MJ, Knopf A, Elfering M, Hoffer M, Harvey JP Jr. Posterior dislocation of the atlas on the axis: a case report. *J Bone Joint Surg* 1974; 56A:1260–2.
14. Anderson PA, Montesano PX. Morphology and treatment of occipital condyle fractures. *Spine* 1988;13:731–6.
15. White AA, Panjabi MM. *Clinical Biomechanics of the Spine, 2nd Edition*. Philadelphia, PA: JB Lippincott; 1990; pp. 30–342.
16. Anderson LD, D'Alonzo RT. Fractures of the odontoid process of the axis. *JBJS* 1974;56A: 1663–74.
17. Fielding JW, Cochran GVB, Lawsing JF, Hohl M. Tears of the transverse ligament of the atlas. A clinical and biomechanical study. *J Bone Joint Surg* 1974;56A:1683–91.
18. Altoff B. Fracture of the odontoid process. An experimental study. *Acta Orhop Scand Suppl* 1979; 177(suppl)61–95.
19. Montane I, Eismont FJ, Green GA. Traumatic occipitoatlantal dislocation. *Spine* 1991;16:112–6.
20. Garber JN. Abnormalities of the atlas and the axis: vertebral, congenital and traumatic. *J Bone Joint Surg* 1964;46A:1782.
21. Denis F. The three-column spine and its significance in the classification of acute thoracolumbar spine injuries. *Spine* 1983;8:817–31.
22. Bucholz RW, Gill K. Classification of injuries to the thoracolumbar spine. *Orthop Clin North Am* 1986;17:67–83.
23. Cope R, Kilcoyne RR, Gaines RW. The thoracolumbar burst fracture with inner posterior elements. Implications for neurologic deficit and stability. *Neuro-orthopedics* 1989;7:83–7.
24. Court-Brown CM, Gertzbein SD. The management of burst fractures of the fifth lumbar vertebrae. *Spine* 1987;12:308–12.
25. Holdsworth FW. Fractures, dislocations and fracture dislocations of the spine. *J Bone Joint Surg* 1970;52A:1534–51.
26. Jelsma RK, Kirsch PT, Rice JF, Jelsma LF. the Radiographic description of thoracolumbar fractures. *Surg Neurol* 1982;18:230–6.
27. Keene JS. Radiographic evaluation of thoracolumbar fractures. *Clin Orthop* 1984;189:58–64.
28. Kelly RP, Whitesides TE Jr. Treatment of lumbodorsal fracture-dislocations. *Ann Surg* 1968; 167:705–17.
29. McAfee PC, Yuan HA, Frederickson BE, Lubicky JP. The value of computed tomography in thoracolumbar fractures. *J Bone Joint Surg* 1983;65A: 461–73.
30. McEnvoy RD, Bradford DS. The management of burst fractures of the thoracic and lumbar spine. Experience in 53 patients. *Spine* 1985;10:631–7.
31. Hashimoto T, Kaneda K, Abumi K. Relationship between traumatic spinal canal and neurologic deficits in thoracolumbar burst fractures. *Spine* 1988;13:1268–72.
32. Chance GQ. Note on a type of flexion fracture of the spine. *Br J Radiol* 1948;21:452–3.
33. Gertzbein SD, Court-Brown CM. Flexion-distraction injuries of the lumbar spine. *Clin Orthop* 1988;227:52–60.
34. Rennie W, Mitchell N. Flexion distraction fractures of the thoracolumbar spine. *J Bone Joint Surg* 1973;55A:386–90.
35. Smith WS, Kaufer H. Patterns and mechanisms of lumbar injuries associated with lap seat belts. *J Bone Joint Surg* 1969;51A:239–54.
36. Whitesides TE, Jr. Traumatic kyphosis of the thoracolumbar spine. *Clin Orthop* 1977;128:78–92.
37. Hadley MN, Zabramski JM, Browner CM, Rekate H, Sonntag VR. Pediatric spinal trauma. Review of 122 cases of spinal cord and vertebral column injuries. *J Neurosurg* 1988;68:18–24.
38. Kewalramani LS, Tori JA. Spinal cord trauma in children: neurologic patterns, radiologic features, and pathomechanics of injury. *Spine* 1980; 5:11–8.
39. Osenbach RK, Menezes AH. Pediatric spinal cord and vertebral column injury. *Neurosurgery* 1992;30:385–90.
40. Osenback RK, Menezes AH. Pediatric spinal cord injury. In Benzel EC, Tator CH, editors. Contemporary Management of Spinal Cord Injury (AANS Neurosurgical Topics Series). Park Ridge, Illinois: American Association of Neurological Surgeons, pp. 187–94.
41. Benzel EC, Ball PA. Controversies: penetrating injuries. In Garfin SR and Northrup B, editors. Principles and Techniques in Surgery for Spinal Cord Injuries. New York: Raven Press, 1993; pp. 269–79.

42. DeMuth WE, Jr. Bullet velocity and design as determinants of wounding capability: an experimental study. *J Trauma* 1996;6:222–32.
43. Benzel EC, Hadden TA, Coleman JE. Civilian gunshot wounds to the spinal cord and cauda equina. *Neurosurgery* 1987;20:281–5.
44. Coleman JE, Benzel EC, Hadden T. Gunshot wounds to the spinal cord and cauda equina in civilians. *Surg Forum* 1986;37:496–8.
45. Heiden JS, Weiss MH, Rosenberg AW, Kurze T, Apuzzo MLJ. Penetrating gunshot wounds of the cervical spine in civilians: review of 38 cases. *J Neurosurg* 1975;42:575–9.
46. Six E, Alexander E, Kelly DL, Davis CH, McWhorter JM. Gunshot wounds to the spinal cord. *South Med J* 1979;72:699–702.
47. Peacock WJ, Shrosbree RD, Key AG. A review of 450 stab wounds of the spinal cord. *S Afr Med J* 1977;51:961–4.
48. Lipschitz R, Block J. Stab wounds of the spinal cord. *Lancet* 1962;2:169–72.
49. Rand CW, Patterson GH. Stab wounds of the spinal cord: report of seven cases. *Surg Gynecol Obstet* 1929;48:652–61.
50. Rosenberg AW. Stab wounds of the spinal cord: report of 3 cases. *Bull LA Neurol Soc* 1957;22:79–84.
51. St. John JR, Rand CW. Stab wounds of the spinal cord. *Bull LA Neurol Soc* 1953;18:1–24.
52. Bucholz RW, Gill K. Classification of injuries to the thoracolumbar spine. *Orthop Clin North Am* 1986;17:67–83.
53. Clark WM, Gehweiler JA, Laib R. Twelve significant signs of cervical spine trauma. *Skeletal Radiol* 1979;3:201.
54. Cope R, Kilcoyne RF, Gaines RW. The thoracolumbar burst fracture with intact posterior elements. Implications for neurologic deficit and stability. *Neuroorthopedics* 1989;7:83–7.
55. Cyron BM, Hutrton WL. Variation in the amount and distribution of cortical bone across the pars interarticularis of L5: a predisposing factor in spondylolysis? Spine 1979;4:163.
56. DuPuis PR, Yong-Hing K, Cassidy JD, Kirkaldy-Willis WH. Radiologic diagnosis of degenerative lumbar spinal instability. Spine 1985;10:262–76.
57. Dvorak J, Fohlich D, Penning L, Baumgaertner H, Panjabi MM. Functional radiographic diagnosis of the cervical spine: flexion/extension. Spine 1988;13:748–55.
58. Dvorak J, Panjabi MM, Chang DG, Theiler R, Grob D. Functional radiographic diagnosis of the lumbar spine: flexion-extension and lateral bending. *Spine* 1991;16:562–71.
59. Dvorak J, Panjabi MM, Novotny JE, Chang DG, Grob D. Clinical validation of functional flexion-extension roentgenograms of the lumbar spine. *Spine* 1991;16:943–50.
60. Friberg O. Lumbar instability: a dynamic approach by traction-compression radiography. *Spine* 1987;12:119–29.
61. Froning EC, Frohman B. Motion of the lumbosacral spine after laminectomy and spine fusion. *J Bone Joint Surg* 1968;50A:897–918.
62. Henley EN, Matteri RE, Frymoyer JW. Accurate roentgenographic determination of lumbar flexion-extension. *Clin Orthop* 1976;115:145–8.
63. Holdsworth FW. Fractures, dislocations and fracture dislocations of the spine. *J Bone Joint Surg* 1963;45B:6.
64. Holdsworth FW. Fractures, dislocations and fracture dislocations of the spine. *J Bone Joint Surg* 1970;52A:1534–51.
65. Jelsma RK, Kirsch PT, Rice JF, Jelsma LF. The radiographic description of thoracolumbar fractures. *Surg Neurol* 1982;18:230–6.
66. Kaneda K, Kuniyoshi A, Fujiya M. Burst fractures with neurologic deficits of the thoracolumbar-lumbar spine. *Spine* 1984;788–95.
67. Keene JS. Radiographic evaluation of thoracolumbar fractures. *Clin Orthop* 1984;189:58–64.
68. McAfee PC, Yuan HA, Frederickson BE, Lubicky JP. The value of computed tomography in thoracolumbar fractures. *J Bone Joint Surg* 1983;65A:461–73.
69. Pearcy M, Shepherd J. Is there instability in spondylolisthesis? *Spine* 1985;10:175–7.
70. Penning L, Blickman JR. Instability in lumbar spondylolisthesis: a radiologic study of several concepts. *AJR Am J Roentgenol* 1980;134:293–301.
71. Penning L, Wilmink JT, van Woerden HH. Inability to prove instability. A critical appraisal of clinical-radiological flexion-extension studies in lumbar disc degeneration. *Diagn Imaging Clin Med* 1984;53:186–92.
72. Riggins RS, Kraus JF. The risk of neurological damage with fractures of the vertebrae. *J Trauma* 1977;17:126.
73. Smith WS, Kaufer H. Patterns and mechanisms of lumbar injuries associated with lap seat belts. *J Bone Joint Surg* 1969;51A:239–54.
74. Whitesides TE, Jr. Traumatic kyphosis of the thoracolumbar spine. *Clin Orthop* 1977;128:78–92.
75. Kelly RP, Whitesides TE. Treatment of lumbodorsal fracture-dislocations. *Ann Surg* 1968;167:705–17.
76. Louis R. Spinal stability as defined by the three-column spine concept. *Anat Clin* 1985;7:33–42.

Chapter 12

MANAGEMENT OF THE SPINALLY IMPAIRED PATIENT

The incidence of spinal cord injury (SCI) ranges from 11.5 to 53.4 hospitalized patients, per million, per year. The definition of SCI used, however, affects these statistics.[1] For example, an aggressive definition of SCI, that included an isolated nerve root deficit or a vertebral body fracture without nerve element injury, would result in a higher incidence of SCI computed to a less aggressive definition.

Life expectation tables have been used to determine the relationship between survival, and age, extent, and level of injury.[2] It has been shown that an improved outcome is achieved when specialized SCI centers are utilized.[3] Early aggressive care of the SCI patient is imperative.

In the pages that follow, the treatment strategies for spine injury and SCI are reviewed. Medical, structural spine and neural element issues are addressed.

PREVENTION

The first line of spinal cord injury (SCI) management is prevention. In North America, SCI prevention strategies have been, perhaps, indirectly spearheaded by the automotive industry and directly spearheaded by the Think First Foundation. Perhaps in no other field or aspect of medicine is the phrase "an ounce of prevention is worth a pound of cure" more applicable than it is with SCI. The emotional, physical, and financial costs of SCI are profound, yet its prevention is, more often than not, simple. Automotive safety devices, for example, most certainly can make the difference regarding the outcome of an accident. It is obvious, however, that de novo accident prevention is the most appropriate method of SCI prevention.

377

The Think First Foundation, sponsored predominantly by neurosurgeons, has made tremendous strides in diminishing the incidence of SCI via careless and/or impulsive behavior through an aggressive education and behavior modification program. These issues have been studied and addressed by the Think First Foundation. Further work in this area is clearly indicated.

NONOPERATIVE MANAGEMENT

Treatment Strategies

Surgical decompression, fusion, and aggressive resuscitation of the SCI patient typically improve survival and the quality of the patient's outcome.[4] These techniques can include aggressive and improved surgical procedures, volume status management, thermoregulatory management, cardiovascular management, and pharmacological management.[5] The importance of the secondary injury phenomenon and the neural regeneration process has been addressed, at least in part, by both laboratory and clinical investigations.[4,6–8] However, nonneurological medical treatment strategies are also of extreme importance. Therefore, they are addressed first.

TURNING TECHNIQUE

Turning techniques for the minimization of pressure-related skin injury were introduced during World War II. An understanding and awareness of the points of potential excessive pressure and the methods designed to avoid skin breakdown over these points is critical. Turning beds and frames, and specialty care beds, have been reported to be useful for integument care, pulmonary care, etc.[9–13] However, controlled prospectively acquired data regarding the superiority of these expensive modes of therapy compared to good nursing and respiratory care do not exist. Early mobilization of the patient, therefore, most likely provides the greatest advantage.[8]

DEEP VEIN THROMBOPHLEBITIS PROPHYLAXIS

Deep vein thrombophlebitis prophylaxis minimizes but does not eliminate the potentially catastrophic complications of immobilization (i.e., pulmonary embolism).[14–16] Minimal risks usually outweigh advantages, and both low-dose subcutaneous heparin and mechanical intermittent extremity compression techniques appear to offer some protection. Therefore, one or both should usually be employed.[17]

BLOOD PRESSURE AND ORTHOSTASIS

Blood pressure and vascular volume status management are complex in the SCI patient. This is particularly so in patients without central control of their sympathetic nervous system.[18–20]

Quadriplegic and high paraplegic patients commonly experience orthostasis (excessive position-dependent blood pressure changes). The lack of a functional sympathetic nervous system results in blood pooling in the peripheral venous system and the absence of autoregulatory control of vascular volume. Abdominal binders, gradual adaptation to erect positioning, and pressors are useful therapeutic adjuncts for the patients.[21]

SPINAL SHOCK

The physiology of spinal shock (a manifestation of acute SCI that is characterized by hypotension, bradycardia, areflexia, and flaccid bladder) is poorly defined.[22–24] Its manifestations, however, are consistent with the presence of an "apparent" lower motor neuron injury (areflexia, hypotension, flaccid bladder, etc.) in the presence of an upper motor neuron injury. As the phase of spinal shock passes, the gradual onset of the manifestations of an upper motor neuron injury (hyperreflexia, upper motor neuron neurogenic bladder, etc.) emerge.[17]

PULMONARY COMPLICATIONS

Both the acute and long-term management of SCI require prophylaxis for pulmonary complications. Many techniques are used for this purpose,[9,25–27] and an aggressive approach to pulmonary care is the most important factor. Suctioning, postural drainage, incentive spirometry, and ventilator management all may be appropriate.

NUTRITION

Nutritional deficits become manifest soon after SCI. Their aggressive management is essential in this nutritionally compromised patient population.[28,29] It is impossible to achieve a positive nitrogen balance in patients the first few weeks following SCI. Aggressive attempts at such will result in overfeeding.[30,31] One must, therefore, apply known nutritional guidelines to this patient population.[30,31]

COST CONSIDERATIONS

The cost to rehabilitate SCI patients is high. Paraplegic rehabilitation costs have approached $100,000 per patient, whereas those for quadriplegic rehabilitation have far exceeded this. The cost of total and complete rehabilitation of the ventilator-dependent quadriplegic has exceeded $200,000.[32] These costs have risen dramatically. Only recently have they plateaued.[17]

SURGERY FOR SPINE TRAUMA

Surgery for spine trauma has one or both of two indications: (1) decompression of neural elements and (2) the acquisition and maintenance of a structurally stable spine. The ultimate goal is to achieve and maintain a nonpathological relationship between the neural elements and their bony and soft-tissue confines. Decompression of the spinal cord, cauda equina, and nerve roots is performed at the surgeon's (and patient's) discretion. Both usually go hand in hand.

The surgeon must make several major decisions regarding surgical options. These depend on the age of the patient, medical candidacy for surgery, surgeon philosophy, available facilities and equipment, the region of the spine injured, and the extent of the injury. Nevertheless, the decision-making process centers around several important factors: (1) the decision to perform or to not perform surgery (indication for surgery), (2) the timing of surgery, and (3) the surgical approach and technique (surgical strategy).

Indications for Surgery

Excessive deformity and/or instability is an indication in and of itself for spine surgery. There is obviously a large "gray zone," however, regarding this decision-making component in the overall process.

Surgical decompression of compressed neural elements has been controversial, although the controversy has waned in recent years. Neural element decompression is indicated when the recovery of neurological function could be enhanced or neurologic function deterioration could be prevented. Patients who harbor an incomplete neurologic deficit and persistent neural compression are usually considered to be candidates for surgery. Similarly, those without neurologic deficit and in whom neurologic function is seriously threatened are also potential operative candidates. This latter group includes patients with significant neural compression and no neurological deficit or those without neurological deficit but with an unstable spine. The surgical decision-making process regarding patients with a complete myelopathy (no long tract function, sensory or motor, below the segmental level of injury) is controversial.[34,35] Some authorities feel that these patients have no meaningful chance for significant recovery; others disagree. Obviously, a clear delineation of the presence or absence of preserved long tract function is critical. A meticulous neurological examination and a cooperative patient are mandatory before an accurate determination can be made in this regard.

Finally, even in patients harboring complete myelopathies, decompression may be warranted. This is particularly relevant with regard to cervical SCI.[34]

Timing of Surgery

The timing of surgery for trauma has been debated. The controversies focus on two separate issues: (1) optimal timing from a medical and, thus, nonneurologic perspective, and (2) optimal timing from the perspective of recovery of neurological function.

"Medical stability" is usually suboptimal following trauma. Pulmonary, neurologic, extremity, and visceral injury can adversely compromise the outcome of a planned operative procedure. Furthermore, an optimal surgical environment may not always be available to the surgeon.

Some surgeons feel that early or emergent surgical intervention increases the chances for neurological recovery. Clinical information regarding the benefits of early or emergent surgery, however, is not compelling. Therefore, the topic remains controversial.[34,35] The potential medical and neurological benefits of early or emergent surgery must be weighed against the potential risks associated with such intervention.

Surgical Strategies

Once the decision to operate has been made, the spine surgeon must prioritize many components of the decision-making process. The region of injury significantly affects the decision-making process. Other relevant factors include the presence or absence of neural element injury, the ability to adequately decompress from a ventral versus dorsal approach, and the need for deformity correction or spinal stabilization.

The surgeon usually decides first the approach and technique to take for neural element decompression. Neural element decompression most often further destabilizes the spine, complicating the stabilization component of an operation, if indicated.

Ventral compressive "lesions" usually are decompressed via a ventral surgical approach and dorsal "lesions" via a dorsal approach. Ventral fusion and stabilization techniques are often performed following a ventral decompression procedure. Long dorsal stabilization techniques (seven on more spinal segments) may be indicated when extensive circumferential instability exists, particularly in the thoracic and lumbar spine. Obviously, many variations and combinations are possible and appropriate.

Cervical traction is used to maintain stability acutely, reduce dislocations, and decompress neural elements. There are attendant risks (including neurologic deterioration, the complication of obligatory bedrest [pneumonia venous thrombosis, decubiti, etc.], and delayed decompression) associated with spinal traction. They must be carefully weighed against their benefits.

The specific surgical strategy chosen for any given clinical situation is surgeon dependent. Although this chapter focuses on trauma, the surgical strategies are discussed in general. They are often applicable not only to trauma but also to degenerative disease and tumor surgery.

NEURAL ELEMENT DECOMPRESSION

The goal of neural element decompression is to provide an optimal environment for neurologic recovery.

DORSAL APPROACHES

Laminectomy and its variants are commonly used to decompress neural elements (Fig 12–1), providing dorsal decompression for trauma, tumor, degenerative and other pathologies. A laminotomy (small opening in the lamina) approach is often used for disc disease. Dorsolateral and lateral approaches are frequently used. "Pure" dorsal approaches are not optimal, usually due to a suboptimal trajectory.

VENTRAL APPROACHES

Ventral approaches to the spine are usually more surgically challenging, predominantly related to the anatomical structures

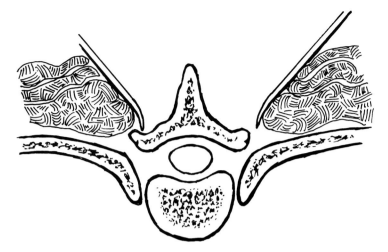

Figure 12–1. A dorsal approach to the subaxial spine, seen in an axial view.

traversed during the surgical exposure. This increases both the degree of difficulty and the risks associated with the ventral approach.

For ventral cervical spine exposures, the esophagus and trachea are retracted medially and the carotid artery, jugular vein, and vagus nerve are retracted laterally. This provides access to the ventral cervical spine for discectomy or vertebrectomy (single or multiple level) for trauma, tumor, or degenerative disease (Fig. 12–2).

The sternum is often an obstacle in selected low cervical or cervicothoracic cases.

The ventral thoracic spine may be exposed from a transthoracic or a lateral extracavitary approach (Fig. 12–3). Each has advantages and disadvantages; however, both are relatively invasive. Each technique places visceral structures at risk and is associated with significant soft-tissue and bony dissection. The thoracolumbar junction presents specific and additional

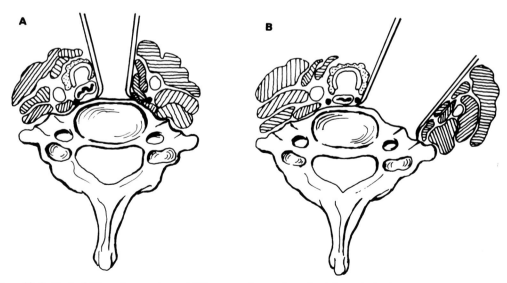

Figure 12–2. Ventral (A) and ventrolateral (B) approaches to the subaxial cervical spine, as seen in an axial view.

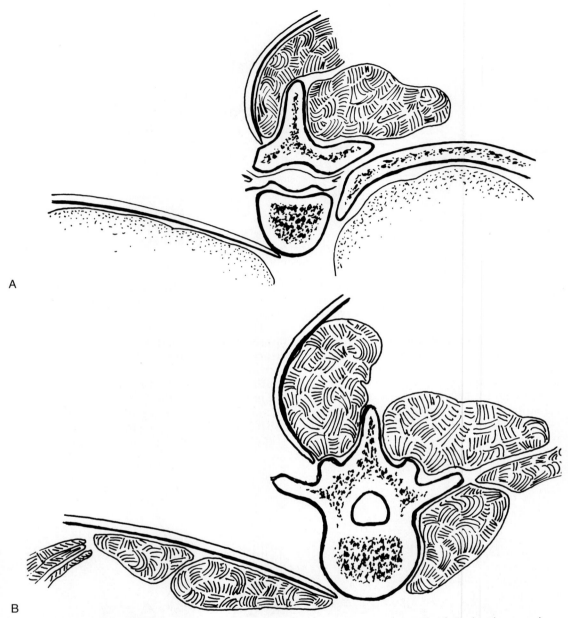

Figure 12–3. Ventral transthoracic (A) and lateral extracavitary (B) approaches to the thoracic spine, seen in an axial view.

challenges. These are predominantly related to the juxtaposition of the diaphragm and other vital structures to the region of pathology.

Ventral exposures of the lumbar spine usually involve a retroperitoneal approach (Fig. 12–4). Occasionally, a transperitoneal approach is employed. In addition to the thoracolumbar junction, the lumbosacral junction poses substantial anatomical constraints due to the juxtaposition of the aorta and vena cava bifurcation sites (into the iliac vessels) and the ventral lumbosacral junction.

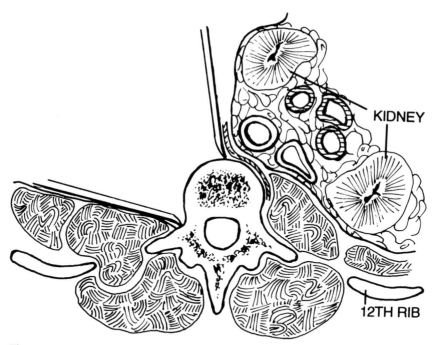

Figure 12–4. The retroperitoneal approach to the lumbar spine, seen in an axial view.

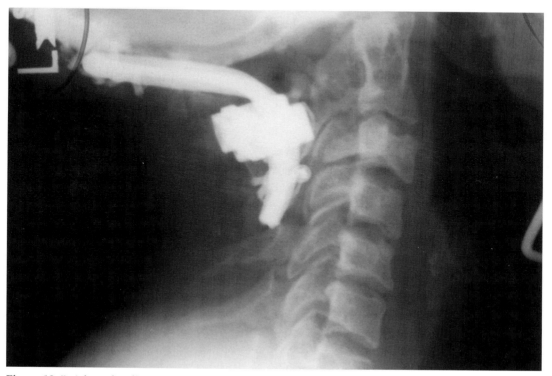

Figure 12–5. A lateral radiograph of a patient following a dorsal occipitocervical fusion and instrumentation that was performed for a tumor causing both neural compression and instability.

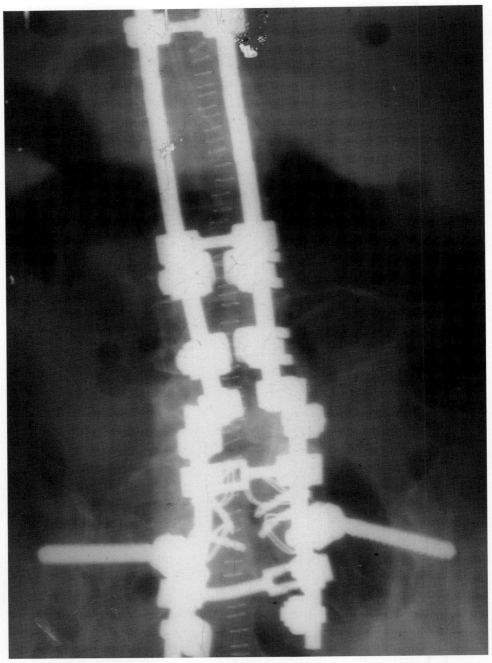

Figure 12–6. An AP radiograph of a patient following a lumbo-sacral-pelvic fusion and instrumentation that was performed for postoperative spinal instability. Note that the fusion is a dorsal onlay type. Immediately following bone grafting, the onlay fusion does not bear a load (see Figure 12–8).

384

SPINAL FUSION AND INSTRUMENTATION

Spinal fusion and instrumentation techniques are often complex, creating significant surgical challenges. The choice of strategies and techniques is also complex. A brief discussion with illustrative techniques follows.

DORSAL FUSION AND INSTRUMENTATION TECHNIQUES

Dorsal fusion and instrumentation techniques vary from region to region. In the upper cervical spine, the occiput is often employed as a site for fusion as well as fixation (Fig. 12–5).

In the lower lumbar spine, the sacrum and ilium may be similarly used (Fig.12–6). Between these extremes, fixation strategies are somewhat simpler. Screws, hooks, and wires attached to plates or rods are usually used to provide spinal stability.

Spinal implants are used to acquire immediate stability. However, since bone is a biological tissue, it remodels in response to the stresses placed upon it; e.g., via spinal implants. Thus, implants usually loosen their "grip" on the spine as time passes following surgery. Therefore, it is ultimately incumbent upon the surgeon to attempt aggressively to achieve bony fusion. This bony fusion must be "realized" prior to implant failure. Dorsal implants must provide adequate spinal support and

weight-bearing ability while the dorsal fusion "matures" (Fig. 12–6).

BONE GRAFTING

Ventral (interbody) bone grafts are often immediately structural in nature; i.e., they contribute to the spine's ability to support loads immediately following surgery (Fig. 12–7). They also generally heal more rapidly than dorsal bone grafts.

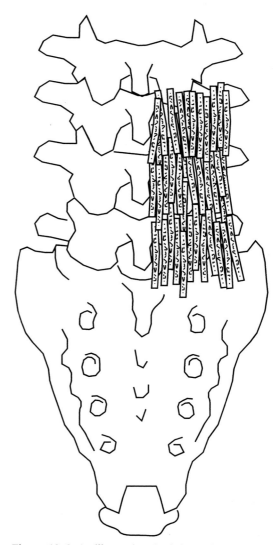

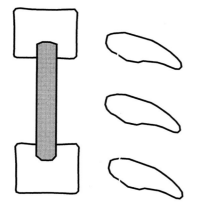

Figure 12–7. An illustration depicting a ventral interbody fusion. This fusion can bear axial loads immediately because of its interbody position.

Figure 12–8. An illustration depicting a dorsal onlay fusion. It cannot bear loads until a solid fusion is achieved.

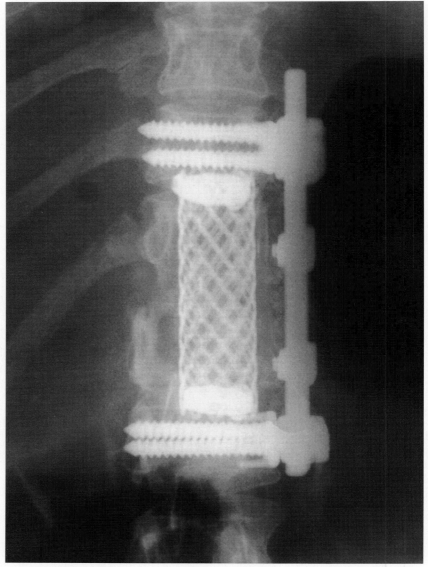

Figure 12–9. AP (A) and lateral (B) radiographs of a patient with an L1 fracture treated with a ventral screw-rod implant and interbody fusion.

Dorsal bone grafts do not bear loads until fusion is achieved (usually 4 months to 2 years) and they heal more slowly. They are usually onlay (non–weight bearing) as opposed to interbody grafts (Fig. 12–8). This latter point explains their lack of ability to provide immediate structural support, particularly for axial load bearing. Since bone heals most rapidly when compressed, ventral interbody grafts, which are usually compressed during the assumption of the upright posture,

heal more rapidly than dorsal grafts (Fig. 12–8).

VENTRAL INSTRUMENTATION AND FUSION TECHNIQUES

Ventral instrumentation and fusion techniques are fraught with many of the same problems that accompany ventral surgical approaches for decompression. Most ventral techniques are short i.e., encompass relatively few segmental levels.

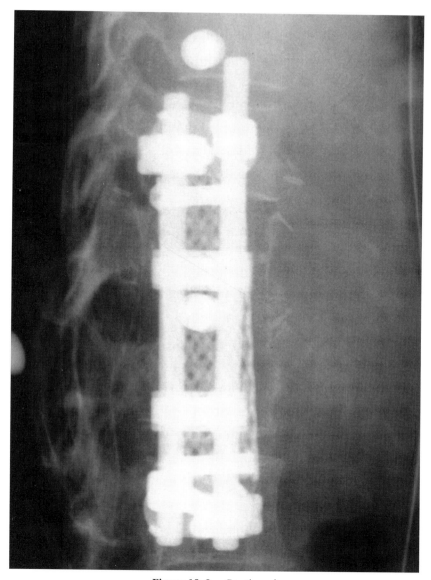

B

Figure 12–9.—Continued

Screws attached to rods or plates usually are used for the acquisition of immediate stability (Fig. 12–9). Short implants cannot apply as much leverage as longer ones, thus rendering them less efficacious.

The greater loads placed on the thoracic and lumbar spine, compared to the cervical spine, create increasingly greater "structural challenges" as one descends the spine. The upper cervical and low lumbar spinal regions present particular challenges regarding ventral instrumenta-

tion application. In fact, the lumbosacral junction is rarely instrumentated from a ventral exposure.

PHARMACOLOGICAL MANAGEMENT

Until the past decade, there were no documented, clinically efficacious, pharmacological treatment alternatives for the management of SCI. In 1990, the Second

National Acute Spinal Cord Injury Study (NASCIS 2)[7,8] concluded that in patients with acute SCI, treatment with high-dose methylprednisolone improves neurological recovery when the medication is given in the first 8 hours. Subsequently, NASCIS 3 compared the efficacy of methylprednisolone administered for 24 hours with methylprednisolone administered for 48 hours.[8a,8b] All patients received an intravenous bolus of methylprednisolone (30 mg/kg) before randomization. Patients in the 24-hour regimen group received a methylprednisolone infusion of 5.4 mg/kg per hour for 24 hours and those in the 48-hour regimen group received a methylprednisolone infusion of 5.4 mg/kg per hour for 48 hours (See articles [8a,8b] for treatment regimen and results). The NASCIS 3 investigators concluded that: *(1)* For patients in whom methylprednisolone therapy is initiated within 3 hours of injury, the 24-hour treatment regimen is appropriate. *(2)* Patients starting therapy 3 to 8 hours after injury should be maintained on the regimen for 48 hours unless there are complicating medical factors.[8a,8b] Similarly, GM-1 ganglioside has also been shown to enhance recovery.[6] Additional trials are needed and are pending.

SPINAL BRACING

Spinal braces and orthotics are effective methods of spinal stabilization for the ambulatory patient. They are, however, also inhibitors of the rehabilitation process by virtue of their bulk and inconvenience. One must deal with this "double-edged sword." The balance, however, is usually in favor of safety, and aggressive bracing is the norm.

FUNCTION AUGMENTATION

Post-SCI, the augmentation of function can be achieved in a number of ways. These include reconstructive surgery, orthoses, and functional electrical stimulation.

Reconstructive Surgery

Reconstructive upper extremity surgery can often enable the quadriplegic patient to achieve a higher functional status.[37–39] These gains may be small; however, to the severely impaired patient they may be significant. The techniques appear to provide a significant cost-effective benefit in appropriately selected cases.

Orthosis-Assisted Ambulation

The ambulation of the complete paraplegic patient with knee–ankle–foot orthoses requires excessive energy expenditure, such that most individuals do not use this form of ambulation. The advantages of weight-bearing (predominantly osteoporosis prevention) and the functional advantages realized by some patients imply that their use in a highly selected patient population is warranted.[40]

Functional Electrical Stimulation

Functional electrical stimulation (FES) has received attention regarding ambulation assistance of the spinally injured.[41–49] This area of research, however, is still in its infancy. Currently, the expense and lack of proven efficacy and efficiency have limited its use.

PROGNOSTICATION AND OUTCOME PREDICTION

The chance for neurological recovery following SCI has been clearly outlined.[50–55] Admission neurological grade is the most significant predictor of neurological outcome.[50,51] For example, a patient with a complete motor myelopathy has a low potential for recovery.

Mobility Gains

We can reliably predict mobility gains by utilizing a mobility index.[53] In patients with cervical spine injuries, important predictive variables regarding mobility gains have been shown to include gender, rectal tone, reflexes, combination medical and surgical management, motor and sensory neurological history since injury, neurological status, and initial mobility score.[53]

Delayed Neurological Changes

Delayed neurological changes are common following incomplete SCI. Piepmeier and Jenkins observed that the majority of neurological improvement occurs within the first year following injury.[56] They also observed, however, that changes in neurological status continued for many years. For example, at 3 years postinjury, 23.3% of the patients continued to improve, whereas 7.1% deteriorated. At 5+ years 12.5% improved, while 5% deteriorated.[56] Conversely, others have shown that the chance for recovery exists only for about 6 months.[57]

Approximately 5% of SCI patients were observed to deteriorate in the early postinjury period.[58] Most had cervical injuries and were associated with specific management events that included timing (e.g., early surgery) and method of immobilization (e.g., traction).

"Complete" Myelopathy

Some authors have never observed neurological recovery following identification of a complete myelopathy.[59,60] Others have observed recovery. The crux of these differing observations is that the definition of complete myelopathy may vary from surgeon to surgeon. Furthermore, this definition is often unclear in the literature. Because the term "complete myelopathy" implies the absence of long tract neural transmission across the segmented level of injury and because this determination may be difficult in the early postinjury period, the clinician must be careful in making this diagnosis.[61]

In patients in which complete motor and sensory myelopathies have been observed, about 20% have had distal sensory function return. This has been associated with a normal or near normal admission blood pressure and pulse (personal communication; Michael Rosner). Perhaps this phenomenon reflects some preservation of autonomic function or of long tract axons that initially fail to conduct as a result of demyelination. This preservation of function, however minimal, indicates that at least some long tract function persists. Therefore, some additional return of function may ensue in the future. Aggressive examination techniques may be useful to help better determine prognosis.[57]

Survival

Survival after SCI has varied from a less than one-year survival rate 50 years ago to a recently reported life expectancy approaching normal overall.[62–68] Life–time table techniques may be effectively employed in this regard.[63,68]

VENTILATOR-DEPENDENT QUADRIPLEGIA

The incidence of long-term ventilator dependency decreases with descending injury level.[17,22] This is because the long-term outlook for ventilator-dependent quadriplegic patients is poor.[26,27,32] Pulmonary failure and related complications are the most common causes of death in SCI patients. At five years after injury, only 33% of the ventilator-dependent patients remain alive, whereas 84% of the ventilator-independent patients are alive.[32]

REHABILITATION

Goals and Expectations of the Rehabilitation Process

SCI rehabilitation has three fundamental goals: (1) to optimize physical restoration and achieve the patient's ultimate physical potential; (2) to optimize occupational (functional) restoration, achieve the patient's ultimate occupational potential, and assist in community re-entrance; and (3) to optimize the patient's psychological adaptation and education.[17]

A fundamental principle of SCI rehabilitation is that the process of rehabilitation does not augment neurological recovery.

It merely "takes advantage" of "existing function" or "recovered function." The caregivers, patients, and families must, therefore, "guide" their expectations, goals, and plans for the future by continuously reiterating this principle.[17]

Predicted life expectancy and mobility gains vary so much that each case must be individualized regarding outcome prediction. SCI radically affects sexual function (erection, pregnancy, orgasm), lifestyle, mobility, vocational gains (independent, employed, employed and independent, employed and independent and financially independent), and psychological function.[59,68] Nevertheless, some predictions may (and should) be made, and treatment plans may be guided by these predictions. Knowledge of the permanency of an injury and its associated neurological deficit can assist in developing and employing an appropriate rehabilitation program and long-term living arrangement.[8]

Today, SCI patients can reasonably expect to achieve a higher-quality lifestyle than that achieved by similarly injured patients several decades ago. Consider, if you will, a typical SCI victim of the World War II era. Commonly, this patient died of renal sepsis or pulmonary complication within several months of injury. Many of those few who survived the initial period succumbed to the ravages of decubiti-related complications (see below). Today, a near-normal life expectancy and a high grade quality of life can often be achieved. One can reasonably expect motivated individuals to regain self-esteem and to become productive, reasonably independent, and self-fulfilled.[17]

Rehabilitation Techniques

Management schemes for SCI should focus on the three aforementioned goals of rehabilitation and medical follow-up (discussed below).

PHYSICAL RESTORATION TECHNIQUES

The strengthening of functioning motor groups is the primary physical restoration goal of the rehabilitation process.[17,69–73]

Strength improvement lays the foundation for skill development. For example, wheelchair operation is facilitated by improved upper extremity strength. There is no good evidence to indicate that the rehabilitation process augments neurological recovery. It can, however, prepare the patient's body (and mind) for neurological recovery, should it occur, and optimize the patient's use of existing capabilities (via education and training). Secondary physical restoration goals include contracture prevention, stimulation of potentially functional muscle groups to prevent atrophy, and patient education.[17] Biofeedback may even play a role.[69]

FUNCTIONAL RESTORATION

Techniques that enhance quality of life (e.g., ambulation skills, transfer skills) naturally consume a large portion of the rehabilitation "effort."[70–73] Many of these techniques and skills are required for community re-entrance.[17]

PSYCHOLOGICAL ADAPTATION AND EDUCATION

A primary overall goal of both the acute and long-term rehabilitation process is patient education.[17] The patients' understanding of his/her pathological and physiological status plays a major role in the early detection of infection, skin care, appropriate medical follow-up, etc. This, in turn, directly affects the rapidity with which community re-entrance is achieved, the incidence of long-term institutionalization, and ultimately longevity and mortality. *The greater the level of independence achieved, the more cost-effective the rehabilitation process.*[17]

MEDICAL FOLLOW-UP

Physiatrists, neurologists, orthopedic surgeons, plastic surgeons, neurosurgeons, urologists, and internists may play roles in the medical follow-up of the SCI patient. A single physician, however, should direct this process. This physician should maintain a high index of suspicion for the multitude of potential complications that may ensue and also play an active role in their prophylaxis.[17] Prevention and management of these complications are best achieved by following a predetermined schedule.[74,75] The most common problems and complications include pain, decubiti, urologic complications, bowel-related complications, and other miscellaneous complications.

PAIN MANAGEMENT

Pain is common after SCI. Its etiologies include pain of nerve root origin, hyperalgesic border reactions, central pain syndromes, phantom sensations, visceral pain, and pain of mechanical origin (pseudoarthrosis). Thus, pain of recent onset should be viewed as a warning of a new medical complication. Prevention and early management are prudent.[76]

DECUBITI PREVENTION

Prevention of decubitus ulcers (pressure sores) is directly related to patient motivation and education.[17] However, the employment of appropriate wheelchair cushions, appropriately utilized and frequent pressure release activities, and appropriate transfer techniques, etc., are also integral to successful prevention.[77]

UROLOGICAL AND BOWEL MANAGEMENT

Urological and bowel management schemes and patient education should be aggressively addressed by the treating team.[78–88] A medically appropriate, yet convenient, bowel and bladder management regimen is critical. An inordinately difficult program may lead to noncompliance, yet an overly simplistic scheme may be ineffective regarding complication prevention. Patient education is mandatory in this process.

MISCELLANEOUS COMPLICATIONS

Physicians assist with patient well-being by paying particular attention to orthostasis prophylaxis;[21] long-term respiratory management;[25] and the management and prevention of spasms,[22] autonomic dysreflexia,[89] heterotopic ossification,[29,90] sexual dysfunction,[52,91–93] spinal neuroarthropathy,[94] occult gallstone formation,[95] burns,[96] alcoholism,[97] and limb fractures.[98,99] Complication avoidance is globally enhanced by overall conditioning (i.e., the increasing of exercise tolerance).[100] All of these complications should be regularly considered by the treating physician, with a high index of suspicion for diagnosis and a low threshold for prophylaxis.[17]

REHABILITATION PROGRAM SELECTION

Questions regarding the quality of the rehabilitation process, the provision of ongoing medical management and follow-up, psychological management, postrehabilitation follow-up, and the quality of patient and family education and counseling must be answered satisfactorily by a rehabilitation institution prior to patient transfer from the acute care setting.[3,17]

SUMMARY

The management of the spinally impaired patient truly begins with implementation of injury-prevention strategies. Once injury has occurred, a multitude of medical, structural, and neurologically oriented strategies come into play.

Finally, functional restoration strategies are employed to optimize the community re-entrance process and to optimize the individual's functional level and quality of life.

The aforementioned strategies, used in combination, can be used to create an optimal milieu for recovery and subsequent community re-entrance and function. Therefore, a multimodality and multidisciplinary approach is needed.

REFERENCES

1. Kraus JF. Injury to the head and spinal cord: the epidemiological relevance of the medical literature published from 1960 to 1978. *J Neurosurg* 1980;53:S3–10.
2. DeVivo MJ, Fine PR, Maetz HM, Stover SL. Prevalence of spinal cord injury. A reestimation employing life table techniques. *Arch Neurol* 1980;37:707–8.
3. Heinemann AW, Yarkony GM, Roth EJ, Lovell L, Hamilton B, Ginsburg K, Brown JT, Meyer PR. Functional outcome following spinal cord injury. A comparison of specialized spinal cord

center vs general hospital short-term care. *Arch Neurol* 1989;46:1098–102.

4. Albin MS. Resuscitation of the spinal cord. *Crit Care Med* 1978;6:270–6.

5. Giffin JP, Grush K. Spinal cord injury treatment and the anesthesiologist. In Lee B, Ostrander L, Cochran G, Shaw W, editors. *The Spinal Cord Injured Patient: comprehensive Management.* Philadelphia: WB Saunders 1991;183–201.

6. Geisler FH, Dorsey FC, Coleman WP. Recovery of motor function after spinal cord injury. A randomized placebo-controlled trial with GM-1 ganglioside. *N Engl J Med* 1992;324:1829–38.

7. Bracken MB, Shepard MJ, Collins WF, Holford TR, Young W, Baskin DS, Eisenberg HM, Flamm E, Leo-Summers L, Maroon J, et al. National acute spinal cord injury study group: a randomized, controlled trial of methylprednisolone and naloxone in the treatment of acute spinal cord injury. *N Engl J Med* 1990; 332:1405–11.

8. Bracken MB, Shepard MJ, Collins, WF, et al. Methylprednisolone or naloxone treatment after acute spinal cord injury: 1-year follow-up data. Results of the second National Acute Spinal Cord Injury Study. *J Neurosurg* 1992;76:23–31.

8a. Bracken MB, Shepard MJ, Holford TR, et al. Administration of methylprednisolone for 24 or 48 hours or tirilazad mesylate for 48 hours in the treatment of acute spinal cord injury. Results of the Third National Acute Spinal Cord Injury randomized controlled trial. *JAMA* 1997;277:1597–1604.

8b. Bracken MB, Shepard MJ, Holford TR, et al. Methylprednisolone or tirilazad mesylate administration after acute spinal cord injury: 1-year follow up. Results of the Third National Acute Spinal Cord Injury randomized controlled trial. *J Neurosurg* 1998;89:699–706.

9. Brackett TO, Condon N. Comparison of the wedge turning frame and kinetic treatment table in the acute care of spinal cord injury patients. *Surg Neurol* 1984;22:53–6.

10. Gonzales-Arias SM, Goldberg ML, Baumgartner R, Hoopes D, Ruben B. Analysis of the effect of kinetic therapy on intracranial pressure in comatose neurosurgical patients. *Neurosurgery* 1983;13:654–6.

11. Krouskop TA. The role of mattresses and beds in preventing pressure sores. In Lee B, Ostrander L, Cochran G, Shaw W, editors. *The Spinal Cord Injured Patient: comprehensive Management.* Philadelphia: WB Saunders; 1991; pp. 231–42.

12. McGuire RA, Green BA, Eismont FJ, Watts C. Comparison of stability provided to the unstable spine by the kinetic therapy table and the Stryker frame. *Neurosurgery* 1988;22:842–5.

13. Smith TK, Whitaker J, Stauffer ES. Complications associated with the use of the circular electrical turning frame. *J Bone Joint Surg Am* 1975;57A:711–3.

14. Lee BY. Deep venous thrombosis in spinal cord injured patients. In Lee B, Ostrander L, Cochran G, Shaw W, editors. *The Spinal Cord Injured Patient: comprehensive Management.* Philadelphia: WB Saunders; 1991; pp. 13–7.

15. Sachs BL, Bargar WL, Rechtine GR, Marsolais EB. An improvised passive motion apparatus. *V Orthop* 1985;194:205–6.

16. Turpie AGG. Thrombosis prevention and treatment in spinal cord injured patients. In Bloch RF, Basbaum M, editors. *Management of Spinal Cord Injuries.* Baltimore: Williams and Wilkins; 1986; pp. 212–40.

17. Benzel EC. Fundamentals, techniques, and expectations of the rehabilitation process. In Benzel EC, Tator CH, editors. Contemporary Management of Spinal Cord Injury. Park Ridge, Illinois: *AANS*, 1994; pp. 239–46.

18. Dolan EJ, Tator CH. The effect of blood transfusion, dopamine, and gamma hydroxybutyrate on posttraumatic ischemia of the spinal cord. *J Neurosurg* 1982;56:350–8.

19. Dolan EJ, Tator CH. The treatment of hypotension due to acute experimental spinal cord compression injury. *Surg Neurol* 1980;13:380–4.

20. Haghighi SS, Chehrazi BB, Wagner FC. Effect of Nimodipine-associated hypotension on recovery from acute spinal cord injury in cats. *Surg Neurol* 1988;29:293–7.

21. Hoeldtke RD, Cavanaugh ST, Huges JD. Treatment of orthostatic hypotension: interaction of pressor drugs and tilt table conditioning. *Arch Phys Med Rehabil* 1988;69:895–8.

22. Bedbrook GM. Physiologic studies. In Bedbrook G, editor. *The Care and Management of Spinal Cord Injuries.* New York: Springer-Verlag; 1981; pp. 255–69.

23. Hughes JT. The new neuroanatomy of the spinal cord (invited lecture). *Paraplegia* 1989; 27:90–8.

24. Schwartzman RJ, Eidelberg E, Alexander GM, Yu J. Regional metabolic changes in the spinal cord related to spinal shock and later hyperreflexia in monkeys. *Ann Neurol* 1983;14:33–7.

25. Mansel JK, Norman JR. Respiratory complications and management of spinal cord injuries. *Chest* 1990;97:1446–52.

26. Morgan MDL, Silver JR, Williams SJ. The respiratory system of the spinal cord patient. In Bloch RF, Basbaum M, editors. *Management of Spinal Cord Injuries.* Philadelphia: WB Saunders, 1991; pp. 78–115.

27. Rinehart ME, Nawoczenski DA. Respiratory care. In Buchanan LE, Nawoczwnaki, editors. *Spinal Cord Injury: concepts and Management Approaches.* Baltimore: Williams and Wilkins, 1987, pp. 63–79.

28. Agarwal N, Lee BY. Nutrition in spinal cord injured patients. In Lee B, Ostrander L, Cochran G, Shaw W, editors. *The Spinal Cord Injured Patient: comprehensive Management.* Philadelphia: WB Saunders, 1991, pp. 330–5.

29. Rossier AB, Favre H, Valloton MB. Body composition and endocrine profile in spinal cord injured patients. In Lee B, Ostrander L, Cochran G, Shaw W, editors. *The Spinal Cord Injured Patient: comprehensive Management.* Philadelphia: WB Saunders; 1991; pp. 163–170.

30. Rodriguez DJ, Clevenger FW, Osler TM, Demarest GB, Fry DE. Obligatory negative nitrogen balance following spinal cord injury. *JPEN* 1991;15:319–22.

31. Rodriguez DJ, Benzel EC, Clevenger FW. The metabolic response to spinal cord injury. *Spinal Cord* 1997;35:599–604.

32. Wicks AB, Menter RR. Long-term outlook in quadriplegic patients with initial ventilator dependency. *Chest* 1986;90:406–10.

34. Benzel EC, Larson SJ. Recovery of nerve root function after complete quadriplegia from cervical spine fractures. *Neurosurgery* 1986;19: 809–12.

35. McAfee PC, Bohlman HH, Yuan HA. Anterior decompression of traumatic thoracolumbar fractures with incomplete neurological deficit using a retroperitoneal approach. *J Bone Joint Surg Am* 1985;67:89–104.

37. Johnstone BR, Jordan CJ, App B, Buntine JA. A review of surgical rehabilitation of the upper limb in quadriplegia. *Paraplegia* 1988;26:317–39.

38. Lamb DW. Reconstructive surgery for the upper limb and hand in traumatic tetraplegia. In Lee B, Ostrander L, Cochran G, Shaw W, editors. *The Spinal Cord Injured Patient: comprehensive Management*. Philadelphia: WB Saunders; 1991; pp. 231–42.

39. Moberg E. The present state of surgical rehabilitation of the upper limb in tetraplegia. *Paraplegia* 1987;25:351–6.

40. Dan BB. One small step for paraplegics, a giant leap for bioengineering. *JAMA* 1983;249: 1113–4.

41. Graupe D, Kohn KH. Patient-responsive EMB-controlled electrical stimulation to facilitate unbraced walking of paraplegics. In Lee B, Ostrander L, Cochran G, Shaw W, editors. *The Spinal Cord Injured Patient: comprehensive Management*. Philadelphia: WB Saunders; 1991; pp. 251–7.

42. Marsolais EB, Kobetic R. Functional walking in paralyzed patients by means of electrical stimulation. *V Orthop* 1983;175:30–6.

43. Nene AV, Jennings SJ. Hybrid paraplegia locomotion with the ParaWalker using intramuscular stimulation: a single subject study. *Paraplegia* 1989;27:125–32.

44. Peckham PH, Marsolais EB, Mortimer JT. Restoration of key grip and release in the C6 tetraplegic patient through functional electrical stimulation. *J Hand Surg* 1980;5:462–70.

45. Peckham PH, Mortimer JT, Marsolais EB. Alternation in the force and fatigability of skeletal muscle in quadriplegic humans following exercise induced by chronic electrical stimulation. *V Orthop* 1976;114:326–33.

46. Peckham PH, Mortimer JT, Marsolais EB. Controlled prehension and release in the C5 quadriplegic elicited by functional electrical stimulation of the paralyzed forearm musculature. *Ann Biomed Eng* 1980;8:369–88.

47. Peckham PH, Mortimer JT, Marsolais EB. Upper and lower motor neuron lesions in the upper extremity muscles of tetraplegics. *Paraplegia* 1976;14:115–21.

48. Peckham PH, Poon CW, Ko WH, Marsolais EB, Rosen JJ. Multichannel implantable stimulator for control of paralyzed muscle. *IEEE Trans Biomed Eng BME* 1981;28:530–6.

49. Woltring HJ, Marsolais EB. Optoelectric (Selspot) gait measurement in two-and three-dimensional space—a preliminary report: technical Note. *Bull Prosthet Res* 1980;17:46–52.

50. Benzel EC, Larson SJ. Functional recovery after decompressive operation for thoracic and lumbar spine fractures. *Neurosurgery* 1986;19: 772–8.

51. Benzel EC, Larson SJ. Functional recovery after decompressive operation for cervical spine fractures. *Neurosurgery* 1987;20:742–46.

52. Berard EJJ. The sexuality of spinal cord injured women: physiology and pathophysiology. A review. *Paraplegia* 1989;27:99–112.

53. Mason RL, Gunst RF. Prediction of mobility gains in patients with cervical spinal cord injuries. *J Neurosurg* 1976;45:677–82.

54. Schmidek HH, Gomes FB, Seligson D, Mc Sherry JW. Management of acute unstable thoracolumbar (T11–L1) fractures with and without neurological deficit. *Neurosurgery* 1980;7:30–5.

55. Suwanwela C, Alexander E Jr, Davis CH. Prognosis in spinal cord injury, with special reference to patients with motor paralysis and sensory preservation. *J Neurosurg* 1962;19:220–7.

56. Piepmeier JM, Jenkins NR. Late neurological changes following traumatic spinal cord injury. J Neurosurg 1988;69:399–402.

57. Tator CH, Rowed DW, Schwartz ML. Sunnybrook cord injury scales for assessing neurological injury and neurological recovery. In Tator CH, editor. *Early Management of Acute Spinal Cord Injury*. New York: Raven Press; 1982; pp. 7–24.

58. Marshall LF, Knowlton S, Gardin SR, Klauber MR, Eisenberg HM, Kopaniky D, Miner ME, Tabbador K, Clifton GL. Deterioration following spinal cord injury. *J Neurosurg* 1987;66:400–4.

59. Bohlman HH, Freehafer A, Dejak J. The results of treatment of acute injuries of the upper thoracic spine with paralysis. *J Bone Joint Surg Am* 1985;67A:360–9.

60. Stauffer ES. Diagnosis and prognosis of acute cervical spinal cord injury. *V Orthop* 1975;112: 9–15.

61. Schrader SC, Sloan TB, Toleikis JR. Detection of sacral sparing in acute spinal cord injury. *Spine* 1987;12:533–5.

62. Dick TBS. Traumatic paraplegia pre-Guttmann. *Paraplegia* 1969;7:173–8.

63. Mesard L, Carmody A, Mannarino E, Ruge D. Survival after spinal cord trauma. *Arch Neuro* 1978;35:78–83.

64. Nakajima A, Honda S, Yoshimura S, Ono Y, Kawamura J, Moriai N. The disease pattern and causes of death of spinal cord injured patients in Japan. *Paraplegia* 1989;27:163–71.

65. Ohry A, Ohry-Kossoy K. *Spinal Cord Injuries in the 19th Century*. Edinburgh, UK: Churchill Livingston, Robert Stevenson House; 1989.

66. Ravichandran G, Silver JR. Survival following traumatic tetraplegia. *Paraplegia* 1982;20: 264–9.

67. Sneddon DG, Bedbrook G. Survival following traumatic tetraplegia. *Paraplegia* 1982;20: 201–7.

68. Bosch A, Stauffer ES, Nickel VL. Incomplete traumatic quadriplegia. A ten year review. *JAMA* 1971;216:473–202.

69. Goldsmith M. Computerized biofeedback training aids in spinal injury rehabilitation. *JAMA* 1985;253:1097–9.

70. Hussey RW, Stauffer ES. Spinal cord injury: requirement for ambulation. *Arch Phys Med Rehabil* 1973;54:544–7.

71. Kostuik JP, Stauffer ES. The rehabilitation of the patient with neurologic dysfunction as a result of injuries to the thoracolumbar spine. In Frymoyer JW, editor. *The Adult Spine: principles and Practice*. New York: Raven Press; 1991; pp. 1353–66.

72. Stauffer ES. The rehabilitation of the patient with neurologic dysfunction as a result of cervical trauma. In Frymoyer JW, editor. *The Adult Spine: principles and Practice*. New York: Raven Press; 1991; pp. 1131–41.

73. Yarkony GM. Spinal cord injury rehabilitation. In Lee Ostrander L, Cochran G, Shaw W, editors. *The Spinal Cord Patient: comprehensive Management*. Philadelphia: WB Saunders; 1991; pp. 265–82.

74. Cioschi H, Staas WE. Follow-up care. In Buchanan LE, Nawoczwnaki DA, editors. *Spinal Cord Injury: Concepts and Management Approaches*. Baltimore: Williams and Wilkins; 1987; pp. 221–34.

75. Meyers AR, Branch LG, Cupples A, Lederman RI, Feltin M, Master RJ. Predictors of medical care utilization by independently living adults with spinal cord injuries. *Arch Phys Med Rehabil* 1989;70:471–6.

76. Tunks E. Pain in spinal cord injured patients. In Bloch RF, Basbaum M, editors. *Management of Spinal Cord Injuries*. Baltimore: Williams and Wilkins; 1986; pp. 180–211.

77. Nawoczenski DA. Pressure sores: prevention and management. In Buchanan LE, Nawoczwnaki, editors. *Spinal Cord Injury: concepts and Management Approaches*. Baltimore: Williams and Wilkins; 1987; pp. 101–21.

78. Achong MR. Urinary tract infections in the patient with a neurogenic bladder. In Bloch RF, Basbaum M, editors. *Management of Spinal Cord Injuries*. Baltimore: Williams and Wilkins; 1986; pp. 164–79.

79. Binnie NR, Creasey GH, Edmond P, Smith AN. The action of cisapride on the chronic constipation of paraplegia. *Paraplegia* 1988;26:151–8.

80. de Groot GH, de Pagter GF. Effects of cisapride on constipation due to a neurological lesion. *Paraplegia* 1988;26:159–61.

81. Etienne M, Verlinden M, Brassinne A. Treatment with cisapride of the gastrointestinal and urological sequelae of spinal cord transection: case report. *Paraplegia* 1988;26:162–4.

82. Herschorn S, Gerridzen RG. The management of the neurogenic bladder. In Bloch RF, Basbaum M, editors. *Management of Spinal Cord Injuries*. Baltimore: William and Wilkins; 1986; pp. 117–33.

83. Kraft C. Bladder and bowel management. In Buchanan LE, Nawoczwnaki DA, editors. *Spinal Cord Injury: concepts and Management Approaches*. Baltimore: Williams and Wilkins; 1987; pp. 83–98.

84. Lloyd LK, Kuhlemeier KV, Fine PR, Stover SL. Initial bladder management in spinal cord injury: does it make a difference? *J Urol* 1986;135:523–7.

85. Seaton T, Hollingworth R. Gastrointestinal complications in spinal cord injuries. In Bloch RF, Basbaum M, editors. *Management of Spinal Cord Injuries*. Baltimore: Williams and Wilkins; 1986; pp. 134–48.

86. Sugarman B, Brown D, Musher D. Fever and infection in spinal cord injury patients. *JAMA* 1982;248:66–70.

87. Vaziri ND. Renal insufficiency in patients with spinal cord endocrine profile in spinal cord injured patients. In Lee Ostrander L, Cochran G, Shaw W, editors. *The Spinal Cord Patient: comprehensive Management*. Philadelphia: WB Saunders; 1991; pp. 135–55.

88. Zejdlik CM. Establishing bowel control. In Zejdlik C, editor. *Management of Spinal Cord Injury*. Monterey, CA: Wadsworth Health Sciences Division; 1983; pp. 331–55.

89. Bloch RF. Autonomic dysfunction. In Bloch RF, Basbaum M, editors. *Management of Spinal Cord Injuries*. Baltimore: Williams and Wilkins; 1986; pp. 149–63.

90. Stover SL. Heterotopic ossification after spinal cord injury. In Bloch RF, Basbaum M, editors. *Management of Spinal Cord Injuries*. Baltimore: Williams and Wilkins; 1986; pp. 284–301.

91. Beretta G, Chelo E, Zanollo A. Reproductive aspects in spinal cord injured males. *Paraplegia* 1989;27:113–18.

92. Chapelle PA, Roby-Brami A, Yakovleff A, Bussel B. Neurological correlations of ejaculation and testicular size in men with a complete spinal cord section. *J Neurol Neurosurg Psychiatry* 1988;51:197–202.

93. Szasz G. Sexual health care. In Zejdlik CM, editor. *Management of Spinal Cord Injury*. Monterey, CA: Wadsworth Health Sciences Division; 1983; pp. 125–51.

94. Crim JR, Bassett LW, Gold RH, Mirra JM, Mikulics M, Dawson EG, Eckhardt JJ. Spinal Neuroarthropathy after traumatic paraplegia. *JNR* 1988;9:359–63.

95. Apstein MD, George B, Tchakarova B. The incidence of gallstones following spinal cord injury: a prospective study. Abstract at American Paraplegia Society 39th annual conference, Las Vegas, September 1993.

96. Formal C, Goodman C, Jacobs B, McMonigle D. Burns after spinal cord injury. *Arch Phys Med Rehabil* 1989;70:380–1.

97. Heinemann AW, Donohue R, Schnoll S. Alcohol use by persons with recent spinal cord injury. *Arch Phys Med Rehabil* 1988;69:619–24.

98. Ingram RR, Suman RK, Freeman PA. Lower limb fractures in the chronic spinal cord injured patient. *Paraplegia* 1989;27:133–9.

99. McMaster WC, Stauffer ES. The management of long bone fracture in the spinal cord injured patient. *Clin Orothop* 1975;112:44–52.

100. McAdam R, Natvig H. Stairclimbing and ability to work for paraplegics with complete lesions— A sixteen-year follow-up. *Paraplegia* 1980;18:197–203.

APPENDIX

Segmental and Peripheral Innervation of the Muscles and Their Function*†

Nerve/Muscle	Function	Spinal Segments
Spinal accessory	Elevates shoulder/arm	C3, C4
Trapezius	Fixes scapula	
Phrenic		C3, C4, C5
Diaphragm	Inspiration	
Dorsal scapular		
Rhomboids	Draw scapula up and in	C4, **C5**, C6
Levator scapulae	Elevates scapula	C3, C4, C5
Long thoracic		
Serratus anterior	Fixes scapula on arm raise	C5, C6, C7
Anterior thoracic		
Pectoralis major (clavicular)	Pulls shoulder forward	**C5**, C6
Pectoralis major (sternal)	Adducts and medially rotates arm	C6, **C7**, C8, T1
Pectoralis minor	Depresses scapula, pulls shoulder forward	C6, C7, C8
Suprascapular		
Supraspinatus	Abducts humerus	**C5**, C6
Infraspinatus	Rotates humerus laterally	**C5**, C6
Subscapular		
Subscapularis	Rotates humerus medially	C5, C6
Teres major	Adducts, medially rotates humerus	C5, C6, C7
Thoracodorsal		
Latissimus dorsi	Adducts, medially rotates humerus	C6, **C7**, C8
Axillary		
Teres minor	Adducts, laterally rotates humerus	C5, C6
Deltoid	Abducts arm	**C5**, C6
Musculocutaneous		
Coracobrachialis	Flexes and adducts arm	C6, **C7**
Biceps brachii	Flexes and supinates arm	C5, C6
Brachialis	Flexes forearm	C5, C6
Radial		
Triceps	Extends forearm	C6, **C7**, C8
Brachioradialis	Flexes forearm	C5, **C6**
Extensor carpi radialis	Extend wrist, abduct hand	C5, **C6**
(longus and brevis)		
Posterior interosseus		
Supinator	Supinates forearm	C6, C7
Extensor carpi ulnaris	Extends wrist, adducts hand	**C7**, C8
Extensor digitorum	Extends fingers at proximal phalanx	**C7**, C8
Extensor digiti quinti	Extends little finger at proximal phalanx	**C7**, C8
Abductor pollicis lungus	Abducts thumb in the plane of palm	**C7**, C8
Extensor pollicis	Extend thumb	**C7**, C8
(longus and brevis)		
Extensor indicis	Extends index finger, proximal phalanx	**C7**, C8

Nerve/Muscle	Function	Spinal Segments
Median		
Pronator teres	Pronates and flexes forearm	C6, C7
Flexor carpi radialis	Flexes wrist, abducts hand	C6, C7
Palmaris longus	Flexes wrist	C7, **C8**, T1
Flexor digitorum superficialis	Flexes middle phalanges	C7, **C8**, T1
Flexor digitorum profundus (digits 2, 3)	Flexes distal phalanges	C7, **C8**
Abductor pollicis brevis	Abducts thumb at right angles to palm	C8, **T1**
Flexor pollicis brevis (superficial)	Flexes first phalange of thumb	C8, **T1**
Opponens pollicis	Flexes, opposes thumb	C8, **T1**
Lumbricals (I, II)	Flex proximal interphalangeal joint, extend other phalanges	C8, **T1**
Anterior interosseus		
Flexor digitorum profundus (digits 2, 3)	Flexes distal phalanges	C7, **C8**
Flexor pollicis longus	Flexes distal phalanx of thumb	C7, **C8**
Pronator quadratus	Pronates forearm	C7, **C8, T1**
Ulnar		
Flexor carpi ulnaris	Flexes wrist, adducts hand	C7, **C8**, T
Flexor digitorum profundus (digits 4, 5)	Flexes distal phalanges	C7, **C8**
Hypothenar muscles	Abduct, adduct, flex, rotate digit 5	C8, **T1**
Lumbricals (III, IV)	Flex proximal interphalangeal joint, extend other phalanges	C8, **T1**
Palmar interossei	Abduct fingers, flex proximal phalanges	C8, **T1**
Dorsal interossei	Adduct fingers	C8, **T1**
Flexor pollicis brevis (deep)	Flexes and adducts thumb	C8, **T1**
Adductor pollicis	Adducts thumb	C8, **T1**
Obturator		
Obturator externus	Adducts and outwardly rotates leg	**L2, L3,** L4
Adductor longus		
Adductor magnus		
Adductor brevis	Adduct thigh	**L2, L3,** L4
Gracilis		
Femoral		
Iliacus	Flexes leg at hip	**L1, L2,** L3
Rectus femoris		
Vastus lateralis		
Vastus intermedius	Extend leg	L2, **L3, L4**
Vastus medialis		
Pectineus	Adducts leg	**L2, L3,** L4
Sartorius	Inwardly rotates leg, flexes thigh and leg	**L2, L3,** L4
Sciatic		
Adductor magnus	Adducts thigh	L4, L5, S1
Semitendinosus	Flexes and medially rotates knee, extends hip	L5, **S1,** S2
Biceps femoris	Flexes leg, extends thigh	L5, **S1,** S2
Semimembranosus	Flexes and medially rotates knee, extends hip	L5, **S1,** S2
Tibial		
Gastrocnemius	Plantar flexes foot	S1, S2
Plantaris	Spreads, brings together, and flexes proximal phalanges	L4, L5, S1
Soleus	Plantar flexes foot	S1, S2
Popliteus	Plantar flexes foot	L4, L5, S1

Nerve/Muscle	Function	Spinal Segments
Tibialis posterior	Plantar flexes and inverts foot	L4, L5
Flexor digitorum longus	Flexes distal phalanges, aids plantar flexion	L5, **S1, S2**
Flexor hallucis longus	Flexes great toe, aids plantar flexion	L5, **S1, S2**
Small foot muscles	Cup sole	S1, S2
Common peroneal		
Superficial peroneal		
Peroneus longus	Plantar flexes and everts foot	L5, S1
Peroneus brevis	Plantar flexes and everts foot	L5, S1
Deep peroneal		
Tibialis anterior	Dorsiflexes and inverts foot	**L4**, L5
Extensor digitorum longus	Extends phalanges, dorsiflexes foot	**L5**, S1
Extensor hallucis longus	extends great toe, aids dorsiflexion	**L5**, S1
Peroneus tertius	Plantar flexes foot in pronation	L4, **L5**, S1
Extensor digitorum brevis	Extends toes	L5, S1
Superior gluteal		
Gluteus medius/minimus	Abduct and medially rotate thigh	**L4, L5**, S1
Tensor fasciae latae	Flexes thigh	**L4, L5**, S1
Inferior gluteal		
Gluteus maximums	Extends, abducts, laterally rotates thigh and extends lower trunk	**L5, S1**, S2

*From Devinsky, O and Feldmann, E: Examination of the Cranial and Peripheral Nerves. Churchill Livingstone, New York, 1988, pp. 22–25, with permission.

†Muscles are listed in the order of innervation, except when presented in groups as for the quadriceps. Boldface type signifies predominant innervation.

INDEX

Page numbers followed by f and t indicate figures and tables, respectively.

399